SUFFOLK UNIVERSITY
MILDRED F. SAWYER LIBRARY
8 ASHBURTON PLACE
BOSTON, MA 02108

American Association of Physicists in Medicine.
Summer School (1985: University of Portland)

MEDICAL PHYSICS MONOGRAPH NO. 14

NMR IN MEDICINE: THE INSTRUMENTATION AND CLINICAL APPLICATIONS

Edited by

Stephen R. Thomas, Ph.D.
University of Cincinnati
Department of Radiology
Cincinnati, Ohio

and

Robert L. Dixon, Ph.D.
Bowman Gray School of Medicine
Department of Radiology
Winston-Salem, North Carolina

Manuscripts were originally prepared for the 1985 AAPM Summer School held at the University of Portland, Portland, Oregon, August 4–9, 1985.

Published for the
American Association of Physicists in Medicine
by the American Institute of Physics

Further copies of this report may be obtained from:

American Institute of Physics
Publications Sales Dept.
335 East 45 Street
New York, New York 10017

Library of Congress Catalog Card Number: 86-71085
International Standard Book Number: 0-88318-497-4
International Standard Serial Number: 0163–1802

Copyright © 1986 by the American Association
of Physicists in Medicine

All rights reserved. No part of this publication may be
reproduced, stored in a retrieval system, or transmitted
in any form or by any means (electronic, mechanical,
photocopying, recording, or otherwise) without the
prior written permission of the publisher.

Published by the American Institute of Physics, Inc.
335 East 45 Street, New York, NY 10017

Printed in the United States of America

FOREWORD

The subject of nuclear magnetic resonance (NMR) goes back just 50 years to 1936, when Gorter recognized the possibility of radiofrequency resonances between nuclear Zeeman levels in bulk matter, though he failed to realize them experimentally. In 1939 Rabi and his co-workers had success in finding NMR in molecular beams, but NMR in bulk matter had to wait until the war was over. Then, just 40 years ago in 1946, Bloch and Purcell and their colleagues, with good attention to relaxation problems, did have success. At first NMR was the province of physicists. Each decade brought its advances and a widening of applications. The fifties saw the development of high-resolution NMR spectroscopy and the arousal of the strong and continuing interest of chemists in NMR. The onward march of NMR across the scientific disciplines had begun. In the sixties Fourier transform procedures, coupled with the remarkable development of computers, enormously extended the sensitivity of NMR and its application to nuclei of low receptivity, a process greatly aided by the concurrent strides in superconducting magnet technology.

The interests of NMR spectroscopists moved from small to large molecules, to perfused organs, to intact small animals and finally to man, spreading the excitement of NMR to biologists and physicians. This progression of NMR spectroscopy from molecules to man was continuous. By contrast, the use of NMR to give medical images burst suddenly upon the scene in the seventies, leading to a tremendous eruption of medical applications accompanied by new developments in technology, new NMR professions, new conferences and summer schools, and new journals.

This volume records the proceedings of an AAPM summer school held in Portland, Oregon in 1985. It covers theory and techniques, all major parts of the system—magnets, gradient coils, radiofrequency coils, data acquisition and manipulation—contrast agents, flow measurement, and clinical applications to all parts of the body. There are chapters on *in vivo* NMR spectroscopy and chemical shift imaging, together with sections on site planning, specifications and quality control, economics and safety. There is something here for everyone in a comprehensive treatment at a not too elementary level. There is even a recapitulation of electromagnetic theory and an American College of Radiology approved glossary of NMR terminology.

NMR imaging has already proved its worth to the clinician and has been accepted as a regular modality of diagnostic radiology. At present there are some 300 whole-body NMR imaging systems installed in hospitals worldwide. Before long we may expect to find an NMR scanner in every major hospital. As the market continues to shake down, it will be of great interest to see whether cheaper, lower-field systems will find a significant place in everyday hospital treatment.

NMR spectroscopy has already shown its value as a medical and biochemical research tool, and it will be interesting to see whether this branch of NMR in medicine will also prove to be of general value in regular patient care as whole-body, high-resolution magnets come on-line in greater numbers.

Overall, NMR appears to have found a secure place in medicine and its future seems indeed to be bright.

E. Raymond Andrew, Ph.D., Sc.D., F.R.S.
J. Hillis Miller Health Center
University of Florida

PREFACE

Over the past decade, we have witnessed a dramatic acceleration in the application of magnetic resonance techniques within the medical sciences. Following the original experimental demonstration of the NMR phenomenon by Bloch and Purcell in 1946, emphasis was directed toward the study of physical materials; however, in the 1950's and 1960's, research was reported on the use of NMR to investigate the properties of biological materials including cell systems, excised muscle tissue and certain *in vivo* models.

The publications of Damadian (Science **171**, 1151 [1971]), which demonstrated the differentiation of normal and malignant tissue based on proton NMR properties, and of Lauterbur (Bull. Am. Phys. Soc. **18**, 86 [1972]; Nature **242**, 190 [1973]), which described methods for the utilization of NMR techniques to provide spatially encoded data allowing image formation, ushered in this new age. We are now impressively aware of the intense academic, industrial, and commercial research and development efforts which have emerged over the past ten years. Some examples of the areas generating considerable interest include: *in vivo* spectroscopic studies of metabolism involving various nuclei; magnetization transfer techniques to explore reaction kinetics; chemical shift imaging allowing quantitative determination of certain tissue components; blood flow imaging; and, of course, high resolution clinical imaging to provide exquisite anatomical and pathological detail under contrast presentation which may be varied by the mode of operation.

Thus, the demonstrated potential of NMR in medicine has produced enthusiasm and raised expectations as new, increasingly sophisticated applications continue to appear. This 1985 AAPM Summer School was structured to provide an intermediate level survey of the concepts and techniques employed in this emerging modality.

The program was divided into two major categories: (1) instrumentation, engineering and scientific principles; and (2) clinical applications. The instrumentation and science oriented lectures provided comprehensive, state-of-the-art details of various components and techniques. The clinical presentations were designed to give the basic, non-clinical scientist an appreciation of how the physical aspects and operational protocols for NMR systems contribute to the diagnostic information contained in a patient imaging study. The faculty included many nationally and internationally known experts in the field of NMR who have been actively engaged in various branches of research and/or teaching within academic, clinical, or industrial environments.

ACKNOWLEDGMENT: The Editors would like to thank the following persons for their assistance in reviewing manuscripts prior to final publication:
    Kenneth E. Ekstrand, Bowman Gray School of Medicine
    Larry Rothenberg, Memorial Sloan Kettering Cancer Center
    Perry Sprawls, Emory University

CONTENTS

Foreword iii

Preface v

AAPM 1985 Summer School ix

Faculty xi

PHYSICAL FOUNDATIONS OF PROTON NMR: PART I 1
    Robert L. Dixon and Kenneth E. Ekstrand

PHYSICAL FOUNDATIONS OF PROTON NMR: PART II—THE MICROSCOPIC DESCRIPTION 32
    Robert L. Dixon, Kenneth E. Ekstrand, and P. R. Moran

METHODS OF RELAXATION TIME MEASUREMENTS 59
    R. Mark Henkelman

PULSE SEQUENCES FOR MAGNETIC RESONANCE IMAGING 71
    Peter M. Joseph

MAGNET DESIGN AND TECHNOLOGY FOR NMR IMAGING 85
    Keith G. Dobson

GRADIENT COIL TECHNOLOGY 111
    Stephen R. Thomas, Lawrence J. Busse, and John F. Schenck

RADIO FREQUENCY COILS 142
    Cecil E. Hayes, William A. Edelstein, and John F. Schenck

DESIGN CONCEPTS OF PULSED FOURIER TRANSFORM NMR SPECTROMETERS 166
    G. Neil Holland and George J. Misic

DATA ACQUISITION AND COMPUTER REQUIREMENTS FOR MAGNETIC RESONANCE IMAGING 180
    Lawrence E. Crooks, J. C. Hoenninger, J. C. Watts, and M. Arakawa

NMR RELAXATION IN TISSUE 201
    M. S. Brown and John C. Gore

SIGNAL–TO–NOISE AND CONTRAST IN MR IMAGING 216
    Felix W. Wehrli

MAGNETIC RESONANCE IMAGING OF THE BRAIN AND SPINE: CLINICAL CONSIDERATIONS 229
    Michael T. Modic

NMR SPECTROSCOPY FOR *IN VIVO* DETERMINATION OF METABOLISM: AN OVERVIEW 249
    Ray L. Nunnally

APPLICATIONS OF FLUORINE IMAGING 269
    Stephen R. Thomas

CHEMICAL SHIFT IMAGING 281
    Ian L. Pykett

PARAMAGNETIC PHARMACEUTICALS IN BIOMEDICAL MAGNETIC RESONANCE ...289
George E. Wesbey

FLOW EFFECTS IN MAGNETIC RESONANCE IMAGING ...326
Leon Axel and Daniel Morton

CLINICAL APPLICATIONS: CARDIAC ...339
Ronald M. Peshock

MAGNETIC RESONANCE IMAGING OF THE ABDOMEN AND PELVIS ...350
Nolan Karstaedt

MAGNETIC RESONANCE IMAGING: CLINICAL RESULTS IN THE CHEST AND BREAST ...364
C. Leon Partain, Madan V. Kulkarni, Martin P. Sandler, James A. Patton, and Ronald R. Price

CLINICAL APPLICATIONS OF CORRELATIVE IMAGING: MRI/NM/US/CT ...372
C. Leon Partain, Madan V. Kulkarni, and Martin P. Sandler

SITE PLANNING FOR MAGNETIC RESONANCE IMAGING ...387
Paul L. Carson, Stephen R. Thomas, M. Koskinen, Margit Lassen, William Pavlicek, Ronald R. Price, Michael J. Bronskill

CONCEPTS OF QUALITY ASSURANCE AND PHANTOM DESIGN FOR NMR SYSTEMS ...414
Ronald R. Price, James A. Patton, J. J. Erickson, D. R. Pickens, C. Leon Partain, and A. Everette James, Jr.

SYSTEMS SPECIFICATIONS AND ACCEPTANCE TESTING ...445
Charles W. Coffey, II, Ronald T. Droege, and Kenneth E. Ekstrand

ECONOMIC CONSIDERATIONS IN MAGNETIC RESONANCE ...476
William Pavlicek, Meredith A. Weinstein, Thomas F. Meaney, and Paul Intihar

BIOLOGICAL EFFECTS AND PHYSICAL SAFETY ASPECTS OF NMR IMAGING AND *IN VIVO* SPECTROSCOPY ...493
Thomas S. Teneforde and Thomas F. Budinger

APPENDIX A: ELECTRICITY AND MAGNETISM FOR NMR—A REVIEW OF BASIC CONCEPTS ...549
Kenneth E. Ekstrand and Robert L. Dixon

APPENDIX B: GLOSSARY OF NMR TERMS ...564
American College of Radiology (1983)

INDEX ...591

1985 AAPM SUMMER SCHOOL

NMR IN MEDICINE:
The Instrumentation and Clinical Applications

University of Portland
Portland, Oregon

August 4–9, 1985

Program Directors:

    Stephen R. Thomas, Director
    Department of Radiology
    University of Cincinnati
      Medical Center
    Cincinnati, OH 45224

    Robert L. Dixon, Co-Director
    Department of Radiology
    Bowman Gray School of Medicine
    Winston-Salem, NC 27103

Local Arrangements Committee:

    D. Bryan Hughes, Chairman
    Department of Radiation Oncology
    St. Vincent Hospital and
      Medical Center
    Portland, OR 97225

    Raymond Fry, Co-Chairman
    Department of Radiation Therapy
    Oregon Health Sciences
      University
    Portland, OR 97201

Organizational Contributors:
    NMR Committee, AAPM
    Continuing Education Committee, AAPM
    Education Council, AAPM
    Publications Committee, AAPM

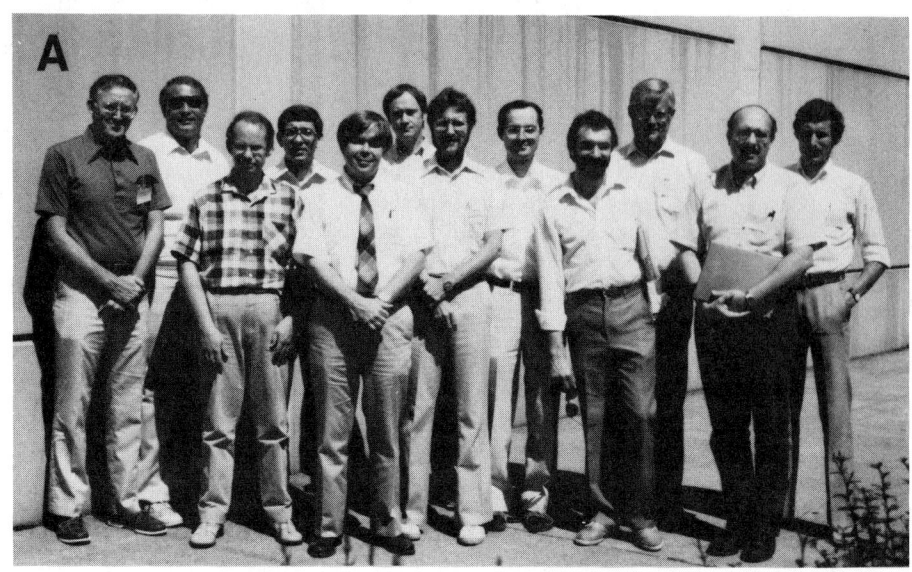

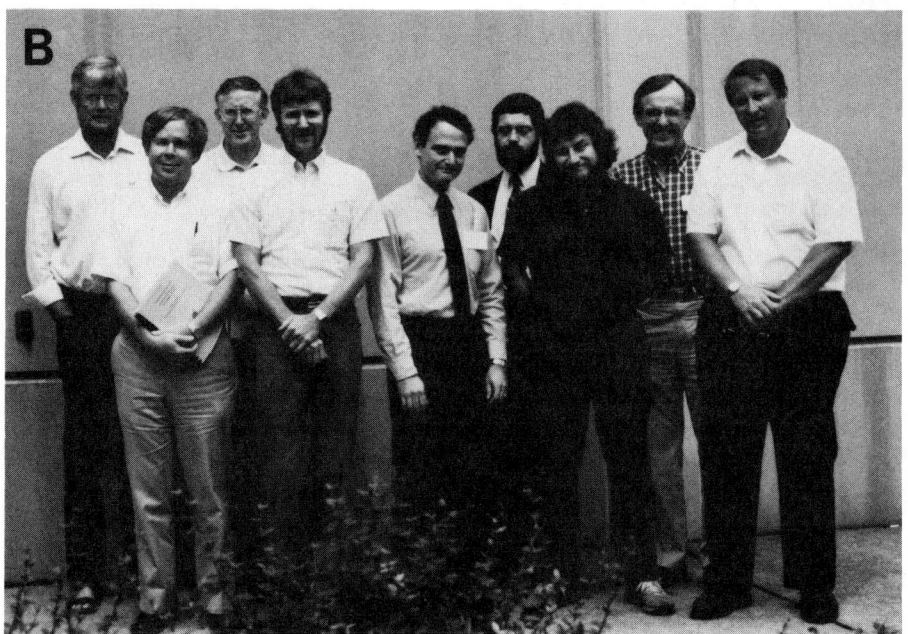

Some of the faculty members of the 1985 AAPM Summer School on "NMR in Medicine: The Instrumentation and Clinical Applications."

(A) (L to R): R.R. Price, W. Pavlicek, K. Dobson, C.W. Coffey, II, R.L. Dixon, J.C. Gore, S.R. Thomas, L.E. Crooks, G.N. Holland, R.M. Henkelman, R.L. Nunnally, F.W. Wehrli.

(B) (L to R): R.M. Henkelman, R.L. Dixon, R.R. Price, S.R. Thomas, L. Axel, I.L. Pykett, M.T. Modic, C.L. Partain, W. Pavlicek.

FACULTY

The presenter of each paper is listed.

LEON AXEL, Ph.D., M.D., Department of Radiology, University of Pennsylvania Hospital, Philadelphia, PA 19104

PAUL L. CARSON, Ph.D., Department of Radiology, University of Michigan Medical Center, Ann Arbor, MI 48109

CHARLES W. COFFEY, II, Ph.D., Department of Radiation Medicine, University of Kentucky, Lexington, KY 40536

LAWRENCE E. CROOKS, Ph.D., Radiologic Imaging Laboratory, University of California, San Francisco, CA 94080

ROBERT L. DIXON, Ph.D., Department of Radiology, Bowman Gray School of Medicine, Winston-Salem, NC 27103

KEITH DOBSON, Ph.D., Oxford Instruments Limited, Oxford OX2 ODX, England

JOHN C. GORE, Ph.D., Department of Diagnostic Radiology, Yale University School of Medicine, New Haven, CT 06510

CECIL E. HAYES, Ph.D., Applied Science Laboratory, General Electric Medical Systems, Milwaukee, WI 53201

R. MARK HENKELMAN, Ph.D., Division of Physics, The Ontario Cancer Institute, Toronto, ON M4X 1K9, Canada

G. NEIL HOLLAND, M. Phil., Director, NMR Engineering and Advanced Development, Picker International, Highland Heights, OH 44143

PETER M. JOSEPH, Ph.D., Department of Radiology, University of Pennsylvania, Philadelphia, PA 19104

NOLAN KARSTAEDT, M.D., Department of Radiology, Bowman Gray School of Medicine, Winston-Salem, NC 27103

MICHAEL T. MODIC, M.D., Department of Radiology, The Cleveland Clinic Foundation, Cleveland, OH 44106

RAY L. NUNNALLY, Ph.D., Department of Radiology, University of Texas Health Science Center at Dallas, Dallas, TX 75235

C. LEON PARTAIN, M.D., Ph.D., Division of Nuclear Medicine and Magnetic Resonance Imaging, Vanderbilt University, Nashville, TN 37232

WILLIAM PAVLICEK, M.S., Department of Radiology, The Cleveland Clinic Foundation, Cleveland, OH 44106

RONALD M. PESHOCK, M.D., Departments of Internal Medicine and Radiology, University of Texas Health Science Center at Dallas, Dallas, TX 75235

RONALD R. PRICE, Ph.D., Department of Radiology, Vanderbilt University School of Medicine, Nashville, TN 37232

IAN L. PYKETT, Ph.D., President, Advanced NMR Systems, Inc., Woburn, MA 01801

THOMAS S. TENFORDE, Ph.D., Biology and Medicine Division, Lawrence Berkeley Laboratory, Berkeley, CA 94720

STEPHEN R. THOMAS, Ph.D., Department of Radiology, University of Cincinnati, Medical Center, Cincinnati, OH 45267

FELIX W. WEHRLI, Ph.D., Manager, MR Applications, General Electric Company, Milwaukee, WI 53201

GEORGE E. WESBEY, M.D., University of Washington, Division of NMR Research, Seattle, WA 98195

PHYSICAL FOUNDATIONS OF PROTON NMR - I

Robert L. Dixon and Kenneth E. Ekstrand
Department of Radiology, The Bowman Gray School of Medicine of
Wake Forest University, Winston-Salem, NC 27103

ABSTRACT

The physics of pulse NMR which is pertinent to an understanding of proton NMR imaging has been condensed and directed toward the medical physicist. The basic physical principles of spin manipulations using RF pulses are presented, and the relation between the quantum mechanical and the classical descriptions is covered in a rigorous fashion. The physics of relaxation is described and the relaxation times T_1 and T_2 are explained in some detail. Application of these spin manipulation techniques is illustrated by showing how they may be used in creating an image.

I. INTRODUCTION

Unlike the advent of CT, for which the fundamental physics of x-ray attenuation was well-understood by the medical physics community, pulse NMR techniques are relatively unfamiliar to most medical physicists and have a greater subtlety in terms of the numerous system properties which can be measured. In order for the physicist to understand the many different imaging methods used by the various NMR imaging groups, it is necessary to have a firm grounding in the basic principles of pulse NMR (which is quite different from continuous wave NMR) and to understand the various spin manipulations which are possible.

We have taken material from a wide variety of sources (1-6); condensed it; and directed it toward the medical physicist who will be expected by the radiology community, in the immediate future, to understand and teach NMR. We have stressed proton NMR for simplicity and have concentrated on getting the physics across to the reader. There have been some "popularizations" of NMR published in which quantum mechanics and physical rigor have been suppressed. This is not the case in the present work, since this approach leads to a superficial understanding.

This work consists of two parts. Part I contains some quantum physics, but is basically a classical (macroscopic) description and contains only an overview of relaxation processes. Part II expands the quantum (microscopic) description and covers relaxation in greater detail, including derivation of formulae for T_1 and T_2 in liquids.

A. Basic Considerations

Before proceeding into the formalism, it is useful to consider a few simple analogies.

A proton by virtue of its spin angular momentum $\vec{S}$ possesses a proportional magnetic dipole moment $\vec{\mu} = \gamma\vec{S}$ where γ is the gyromagnetic ratio. If one thinks of a proton as a charged sphere, then a spinning proton represents a current flowing in a loop around the axis of rotation, thereby generating a dipolar magnetic field. We can therefore think of the proton as a "tiny magnet," having a magnetic moment $\vec{\mu}$.

The neutron also possesses a magnetic moment which is opposite to its spin direction. Although the neutron has no net charge, if the charge distribution were non-uniform (negative charge near the periphery and positive charge near the axis), then a spinning neutron would possess just such a magnetic moment. One should not carry this "spinning top" analogy too far, however, since the intrinsic spin angular momentum of the proton and neutron is no doubt due to some internal structure (quarks). Nuclei with either an odd number of protons or an odd number of neutrons also posses magnetic moments and are thus potential candidates for NMR, whereas even-even nuclei have zero magnetic moments. The unpaired nucleon is primarily responsible for the magnetic moment. If the unpaired nucleon is a proton, there can be an orbital as well as a spin contribution to the magnetic moment of the nucleus since the proton is charged, although the shell model cannot accurately predict the magnitude of the nuclear moment [23]. Nuclei other than hydrogen which have been used for NMR imaging are ^{31}P, ^{23}Na, ^{19}F, ^{13}C [24]. We will restrict our discussion to proton NMR since the sensitivity is several orders of magnitude greater than for other nuclei in tissue.

It is useful to first consider the behaviour of a tiny magnet, such as a compass needle, in an external magnetic field (Figure 1).

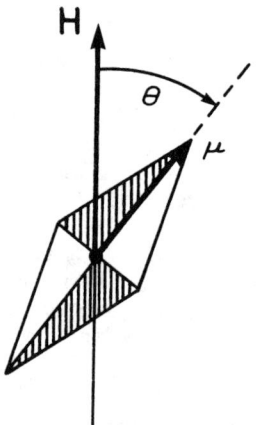

Fig. 1. Compass needle with magnetic moment $\vec{\mu}$ in a magnetic field $\vec{H}$.

The torque on the needle is given by $\vec{\mu} \times \vec{H}$ and the potential energy is $-\vec{\mu} \cdot \vec{H} = -\mu H \cos\theta$ where θ is the angle between $\vec{\mu}$ and $\vec{H}$.

The potential energy is a minimum when $\vec{\mu}$ is aligned with the field ($\theta = 0$, $\cos\theta = 1$). A compass needle on a frictionless bearing would, however, never line up with the external field. If it were initially displaced by an angle θ_o, it would merely oscillate about the field direction with a constant amplitude θ_o. If a coupling between the magnet and its surroundings is added, such as bearings with friction (this is somewhat analogous to the spin-lattice interaction); and, if the nature of this coupling is such that the surroundings can absorb energy from the oscillating magnet, then the magnet will gradually relax until it is in its lowest energy state, i.e., aligned with the external field. In the case of a frictional damping force, the alignment would proceed exponentially with a time constant T_1 called the relaxation time.

The spins of the protons in a sample placed in a magnetic field will eventually arrange themselves such that the net magnetization (magnetic moment) of the sample $\vec{M}$ (where $\vec{M} = \Sigma\vec{\mu_i}$ is the vector sum of the individual proton magnetic moments) lies along the field direction. This, however, requires coupling of the spins to an external system so that thermal equilibrium can be established.

II. CLASSICAL DESCRIPTION OF A SPIN IN A MAGNETIC FIELD

The classical motion of a magnetic moment $\vec{\mu}$ associated with an angular momentum $\vec{S}$ is a bit different from that of a compass needle due to the angular momentum. The kinetic energy of such a system is contained primarily in its spinning motion. When a force is exerted on a spinning object, it tends to move at right angles to the force. A spinning gyroscope in a gravitational field does not fall over, but rather precesses around the gravitational field direction. The classical motion of a spin in a magnetic field can be derived by setting the torque equal to the rate of change of angular momentum.

$$\frac{d\vec{S}}{dt} = \vec{\mu} \times \vec{H} \quad (1)$$

Since $\vec{\mu}$ is proportional to $\vec{S}$ ($\vec{\mu} = \gamma\vec{S}$) we have

$$\frac{d\vec{\mu}}{dt} = \vec{\mu} \times \gamma\vec{H} \quad (2)$$

Since $d\vec{\mu}$ is perpendicular to both $\vec{\mu}$ and $\vec{H}$ (because of the cross product), the magnitude of $\vec{\mu}$ remains constant, and the classical motion is a precession of $\vec{\mu}$ about the magnetic field $\vec{H}$ (Figure 2). It is easy to show from eqn (2) and (Figure 2) that the angular frequency of precession is

$$\omega = \gamma H \quad (3)$$

which is called the Larmor frequency.

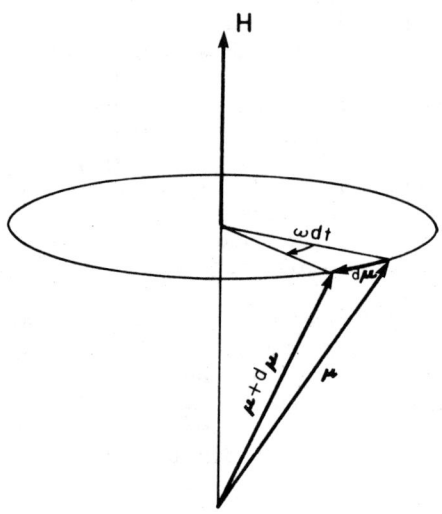

Fig. 2. Precession of a classical angular momentum $\vec{S}$, having a proportional magnetic moment $\vec{\mu} = \gamma\vec{S}$, about a magnetic field $\vec{H}$.

There is still no tendency for a group of <u>isolated</u>, classical spins to align with the magnetic field--rather they would precess about it ad-infinitum.

III. QUANTUM MECHANICAL DESCRIPTION OF A SPIN IN A MAGNETIC FIELD

A quantum mechanical treatment of a spin (i.e., a particle having a magnetic moment) in a magnetic field is easily made by setting the Hamiltonian equal to the potential energy $\mathcal{H} = -\vec{\mu} \cdot \vec{H}$ (unlike a classical spinning top, the magnitude of the angular momentum of a quantum mechanical spin cannot change, hence the "kinetic energy" associated with the spinning motion is constant and thus does not need to be considered in the Hamiltonian). In a time-independent magnetic field H_o along the z-axis, $\mathcal{H} = -\gamma H_o S_z$, hence the stationary states of the system are the eigenstates of the angular momentum operator S_z and the energy levels are given by

$$E_{m_s} = -\gamma \hbar H_o m_s, \quad -s \leq m_s \leq s \quad (4)$$

For a particle with spin 1/2 such as a proton, only two energy states are allowed, corresponding to spins parallel/antiparallel to the field ($m_s = \pm\frac{1}{2}$) as shown in Figure 3, and having an energy separation of $\Delta E = \gamma \hbar H_o$. In the upper energy state, the spin direction is opposite the field direction ("spin down"). A transition from the lower to the upper state can be made by absorption of energy (for example RF energy) of angular frequency ω_o where $\hbar \omega_o = \Delta E$, hence

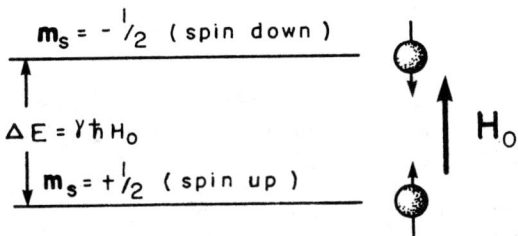

Fig. 3. Stationary energy states for a proton spin in a constant magnetic field $\vec{H}_0$.

$$\omega_o = \gamma H_o \qquad (5)$$

ω_o can be recognized as the classical Larmor precession frequency, $\omega_o = \gamma H_o$. For a proton, this resonant frequency for energy absorption, $\nu_o = \omega_o/2\pi$, is

$$\nu_o (\text{MHz}) = 4.258 H_o (\text{kgauss}) \qquad (6)$$

The magnetic field strength can also be expressed in Tesla (0.1 Tesla = 1 kgauss). RF irradiation of a spin system at this frequency can cause spin-flip transitions. The transitions are magnetic dipole transitions which are influenced only by the magnetic component $\vec{H}'$ of the RF field, and then only by the x or y component of $\vec{H}'$ since the transition matrix element $<m_s'|\vec{\mu}\cdot\vec{H}'|m_s>$ is non-zero only for μ_x and μ_y. RF irradiation at the resonant frequency can also cause de-excitation of a proton spin in the upper energy state by stimulated emission of a photon. Although the angular frequency ω_o obtained from the Hamiltonian is the same as the classical Larmor frequency, the motion of a quantum mechanical spin in one of the aforementioned stationary states should not be interpreted as a precession, since the wave function is independent of time, and the expectation value of the magnetic moment is time independent, i.e., $<\mu_x> = <\mu_y> = 0$, $<\mu_z> = \pm \frac{1}{2}\gamma\hbar$. Recall that the expectation value represents the average result of a series of measurements on a group (or ensemble) of identical spins.

The preceding description of stationary states (time independent wave functions in constant magnetic fields) is insufficient for understanding pulse NMR, since we need to follow the motion of the spins undergoing time dependent perturbations by varying magnetic fields, where the wave functions are time dependent and consist of a mixture of the spin-up and spin-down states. For a proton spin having a wave function which is an equal mixture of both spin-up and spin-down states such that $S_x = \frac{1}{2}$ at t = 0, it can be shown (8) that $<\vec{\mu}>$ evolves with time as

$$\langle\mu_x\rangle = \tfrac{1}{2}\gamma\hbar\cos\omega_o t$$
$$\langle\mu_y\rangle = -\tfrac{1}{2}\gamma\hbar\sin\omega_o t \qquad (7)$$
$$\langle\mu_z\rangle = 0$$

which describes a precession of $\langle\vec{\mu}\rangle$ in the xy plane.

We are fortunate in this regard to be able to make the following simplification. We cannot observe the behavior of a single spin, but rather we observe the collective motion of a group of spins (an ensemble) via the net magnetization $\vec{M}$. The expectation value of the magnetic moment of an ensemble of spins (i.e. the average magnetic moment for the ensemble) follows the quantum mechanical rule for the equation of motion of an operator[7]

$$\frac{d}{dt}\langle\vec{\mu}\rangle = \frac{i}{\hbar}\langle[\mathcal{H},\vec{\mu}]\rangle \qquad (8)$$

where $[\mathcal{H},\vec{\mu}]$ is the commutator of the Hamiltonian $\mathcal{H}$ and $\vec{\mu}$. It may be shown in a straight forward manner[9] using the commutation properties of angular momentum operators, $[S_x,S_y] = i\hbar S_z$, $[S_y,S_z] = i\hbar S_x$, $[S_z,S_x] = i\hbar S_y$, that

$$\frac{d}{dt}\langle\vec{\mu}\rangle = \langle\vec{\mu}\rangle \times \gamma\vec{H} \qquad (9)$$

This is a general result that is valid for a time dependent magnetic field $\vec{H}$, and is the same as the equation of motion for a classical spin with an associated magnetic moment.

For an ensemble of N non-interacting spins, the net magnetization, which is the observable quantity, is given by

$$\vec{M} = N\langle\vec{\mu}\rangle \qquad (10)$$

hence $\vec{M}$ satisfies the classical equation of motion

$$\frac{d\vec{M}}{dt} = \vec{M} \times \gamma\vec{H} \qquad (11)$$

Thus, even though individual spins may undergo complicated behavior, the net magnetization $\vec{M}$ which is the observable quantity, follows the familiar classical equation, i.e., in a constant magnetic field $\vec{M}$ will precess around the field at the Larmor frequency.

IV. MOTION OF $\vec{M}$ IN AN RF FIELD

We have shown for a system of non-interacting spins that the magnetization $\vec{M}$ follows equation (11).

For a static magnetic field $\vec{H}_o$ along the z-axis, $\vec{M}$ will precess around the field (in a clockwise direction when viewed along the z-axis) at the Larmor frequency $\omega_o = \gamma H_o$.

If an RF coil is wound around the sample along the x-axis and driven with an RF oscillator at frequency ω, an oscillating magnetic field $\vec{H}_x(t)$ is generated along the x-axis which can be written as

$$\vec{H}_x(t) = \vec{i}\, 2H_1 \cos\omega t \qquad (12)$$

Since the magnitude of this oscillating field is small compared to the static field H_o, it might be expected to have little effect on the motion of $\vec{M}$. (For pulse NMR $H_x \sim 50$ gauss whereas $H_o \sim 10^3$ gauss).

It is useful to decompose $\vec{H}_x(t)$ into two rotating components $\vec{H}_x = \vec{H}_1 + \vec{H}_1{}'$, where

$$\begin{aligned} \vec{H}_1{}' &= H_1[\vec{i}\cos\omega t + \vec{j}\sin\omega t] \\ \vec{H}_1 &= H_1[\vec{i}\cos\omega t - \vec{j}\sin\omega t] \end{aligned} \qquad (13)$$

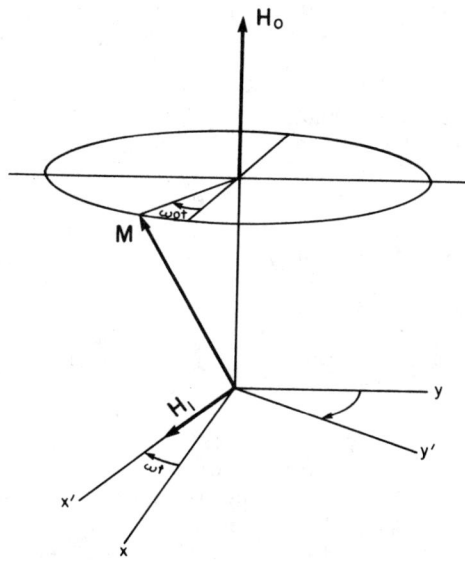

Fig. 4. Rotating frame axes x', y' rotate about the z axis with the frequency ω of the applied rf field $\vec{H}_1$. $\vec{H}_1$ is fixed in the rotating frame along the x' axis. The magnetization $\vec{M}$ precesses about the field $\vec{H}_o$ in the same sense as $\vec{H}_1$ but with frequency ω_o.

so that $\vec{H}_1$ rotates clockwise in the xy plane viewed from above (the same direction as $\vec{M}$) as shown in Figure 4, and $\vec{H}_1'$ rotates counterclockwise. (It is easy to verify this rotation by evaluating $\vec{H}_1$ at ωt values of 0, 90°, 180°, and 270°). Since the torque exerted on $\vec{M}$ by the RF field is $\vec{M} \times \gamma \vec{H}_x$, and since $H_1 \ll H_0$, it can be seen that this torque is small compared to the precessional driving torque due to $\vec{H}_0$, $\vec{M} \times \gamma \vec{H}_0$, and it can therefore have no great effect unless it remains constant for a long period of time. Since $\vec{H}_1'$ rotates in the opposite sense to $\vec{M}$, it is clear that the torque exerted will average to zero, hence we can ignore $\vec{H}_1'$ and write equation (11) as

$$\frac{d\vec{M}}{dt} = \vec{M} \times \gamma [\vec{H}_0 + \vec{H}_1(t)] \qquad (14)$$

It is also clear that $\vec{H}_1$ can have no great effect unless it rotates at the same angular frequency at which $\vec{M}$ precesses, so that it remains in constant phase with $\vec{M}$. That is, there is no significant effect unless the RF frequency ω is equal to the Larmor precession frequency $\omega_0 = \gamma H_0$. If $\omega \neq \omega_0$, $\vec{H}_1$ would either outrun or fall behind $\vec{M}$ and the effect would average to zero, i.e., $\vec{H}_1$ would only cause $\vec{M}$ to wobble a bit. If, however, $\omega = \omega_0$, then $\vec{H}_1$ stays in a constant position relative to $\vec{M}$. Thus, even though $\vec{H}_1$ exerts a small torque on $\vec{M}$, the torque is constant; and, if the torque lasts over many precessions of $\vec{M}$, it can have a significant effect. That is, if the RF signal is applied at the resonant frequency ω_0 for a time large compared to the Larmor precessional period $2\pi/\omega_0$, it will cause a significant effect on $\vec{M}$. This description is the classical explanation of magnetic resonance. By way of analogy, a series of small pushes on a child's swing will have no net effect unless the pushes are timed to coincide with the natural (resonant) frequency of the swing, in which case they can produce a significant increase in the motion.

Equation (14) can be solved by looking at the motion in a frame of reference rotating with the applied RF field $\vec{H}_1$ at angular frequency ω as shown in Figure 4. The rotating frame axes are denoted by (x', y', z'), however, the z' axis is coincident with the z axis of the laboratory system (x,y,z). One can think of the x' and y' axes as being fixed to a turntable rotating with angular frequency ω about the vertical (z', z) axis, whereas the xyz axes are stationary in the laboratory. The field $\vec{H}_1$ lies along the x' axis and rotates with it (Figure 4).

It can be shown[10] that the time derivative of a vector in the laboratory system $d\vec{M}/dt$ can be related to its time derivative in a coordinate system rotating about the z-axis with an angular velocity $\vec{\Omega} = -\omega \hat{k}$ as

$$\frac{d\vec{M}}{dt} = \frac{\delta \vec{M}}{\delta t} + \vec{\Omega} \times \vec{M} \qquad (15)$$

where $\delta\vec{M}/\delta t$ is the derivative in the rotating system. That is, a vector $\vec{M}$ fixed in the rotating system ($\delta\vec{M}/\delta t = 0$) would exhibit a time derivative in the lab system of $\vec{\Omega} \times \vec{M}$ which we recognize as a precession about the z-axis. Applying this transformation to equation (14), the motion of $\vec{M}$ in the rotating system can be determined as

$$\frac{\delta\vec{M}}{\delta t} = \vec{M} \times \gamma\vec{H}_{eff} \qquad (16)$$

where

$$\vec{H}_{eff} = (H_o - \omega/\gamma)\vec{k} + H_1\vec{i}' \qquad (17)$$

Thus the motion of $\vec{M}$ in the rotating frame is the same as the familiar equation of motion (e.g., equation 11) with the field replaced by an effective field $\vec{H}_{eff}$. Note that $\vec{H}_{eff}$ is independent of time, i.e., it is fixed in the rotating frame. The motion in the rotating frame is therefore simply a precession of $\vec{M}$ about $\vec{H}_{eff}$. At resonance ($\omega = \gamma H_o$) note that $\vec{H}_{eff} = H_1\vec{i}'$ lies entirely in the xy plane along the rotating x´ axis thus, by stepping into a reference

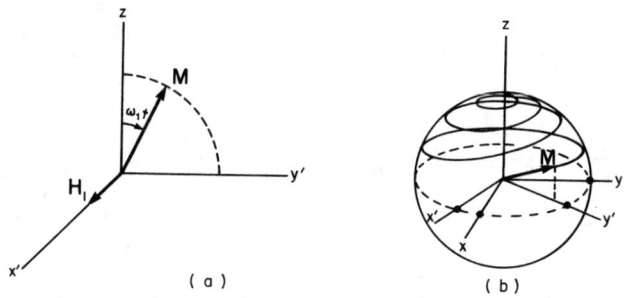

(a) (b)

Fig. 5. Nutation of $\vec{M}$ away from its equilibrium position along the z axis under the influence of rf irradiation $\vec{H}_1$ at the resonant frequency ω_0 as seen in (a) the rotating frame and (b) the laboratory frame.

frame rotating at the Larmor frequency, we have caused the static field H_o to dissappear and we see only the RF field $\vec{H}_1$ which appears as a static field in this rotating frame. Thus if $\vec{M}$ initially lay along the z-axis, the motion in the rotating frame would be a nutation (slow precession) of $\vec{M}$ about the x´ axis with frequency $\omega_1 = \gamma H_1$ as shown in Figure 5a. The vector $\vec{M}$ remains in the y´z plane, rotating about the x´ axis at a frequency ω_1, where $\omega_1 \ll \omega_o$, for as long as the RF irradiation persists. Figure 5b shows the corresponding motion in the laboratory frame. In the lab system, $\vec{M}$ simply spirals down from the z-axis over many precessional periods since $\omega_1 \ll \omega_o$.

If ω is not near resonance, $\vec{H}_{eff}$ lies just a bit off the z-axis in the x´z plane. Since $\vec{M}$ must precess about $\vec{H}_{eff}$, $\vec{M}$ would merely nutate a little. That is, if $\vec{M}$ initially lay along the z-axis, it would periodically dip away from the z-axis by a small angle and return to the z-axis again, with $\vec{H}_{eff}$ defining the center of the cone of nutation.

To observe this resonance phenomenon, an RF pulse at frequency ω_o of duration Δt can be applied such that $\omega_1 \Delta t = \gamma H_1 \Delta t = \pi/2$ (this is called a 90° pulse since such a pulse will rotate the magnetization by 90°). If $\vec{M}$ initially lies along the z-axis, as it will at equilibrium, it will be rotated by 90° such that, at the end of the pulse, it will lie along the y´ axis in the rotating frame (Figure 6a); which means that it will precess in the xy plane in the

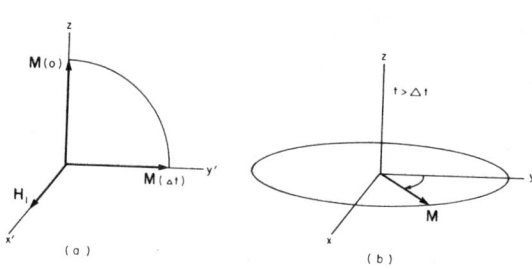

Fig. 6. (a) Nutation of $\vec{M}$ away from its equilibrium position onto the rotating frame y´ axis produced by a 90° rf pulse at resonance. (b) Continued free precession of the magnetization $\vec{M}$ in the laboratory equatorial plane after termination of the rf pulse.

lab system as shown in Figure 6b. $\vec{M}$ will continue to precess in the xy plane at frequency ω_o, as shown, after termination of the RF pulse. This motion can be observed as follows. Such a motion is analogous to spinning a magnet having a dipole moment $\vec{M}$ around inside the RF coil (which you recall is wrapped around the lab x-axis). Such a changing magnetic flux will induce an alternating emf in the coil at frequency ω_o which may be detected by connecting the coil to a receiver after termination of the RF pulse from the transmitter. This signal is the so-called free-precession (or free induction) signal. The magnetic induction $\vec{B}$ produced in a magnetized sample having magnetization $\vec{M}$ is $\vec{B} = 4\pi\vec{M}$ (11). The magnetic flux through a coil having n turns and a cross-sectional area A is approximately $\phi = B_x nA = 4\pi M_x nA$. If a 90° pulse is applied to a sample initially at equilibrium having a magnetization M_o; then, following the pulse, M_x will have the form $M_x = M_o \sin\omega_o t$. The emf induced in the coil is therefore

$$V = -\frac{1}{c}\frac{d\phi}{dt} = (4\pi/c)nA\,M_o\omega_o\cos\omega_o t \qquad (18)$$

The maximum signal strength will be produced by a 90° RF pulse since it is only the component of $\vec{M}$ in the transverse xy plane which induces any signal in the coil. A pulse of duration longer or shorter than $\Delta t = \pi/2\gamma H_1$ will produce a smaller signal, and a 180° pulse ($\Delta t = \pi/\gamma H_1$) will produce no signal at all since $\vec{M}$ will be rotated over to the minus z-axis, thereby having no transverse component. The length of these RF pulses are generally of the order of microseconds and are much shorter than the relaxation times encountered in liquids or tissues. For $H_1 = $ 50 gauss, a 90° pulse would have a length of about 1.2 μsec.

Recall, it has been assumed that the system of protons we have been considering neither interact with each other nor their surroundings, save for the externally applied magnetic field $\vec{H}_o$, which has been presumed to be uniform over the sample (i.e., the same for all protons). In this case, following, say, a 90° pulse, the protons will freely precess in the xy plane, "singing" together in unison into the pickup coil. They would sing forever under the aforementioned idealized conditions, however, relaxation will eventually take place as we will discuss in the next section.

It is worthy of note at this point that the applied oscillating field $H_x = 2H_1\cos\omega t$ resulted in $\vec{H}_1$ lying along the x' axis in the rotating frame. It can be shown that if the RF signal is phase shifted by 90° such that $H_x = 2H_1\sin\omega t$, then an $\vec{H}_1$ is generated along the y' axis in the rotating frame. Thus $\vec{H}_1$ can be put along any axis in the rotating frame simply by electrically phase shifting the RF signal without moving the coil.

The strength of the free precession signal at resonance will increase as the square of the external magnetic field strength since: 1) the initial (equilibrium) magnetization is larger in a larger field, and 2) the emf induced by the rotating magnetization depends on its time derivative and hence is proportional to the precession frequency. Since the thermal equilibrium population ratio of the spin-up and spin-down states depicted in Figure 3 is given by $\exp(-\Delta E/kT)$, it can be shown that the equilibrium magnetization M_o for N proton spins having $\mu = \frac{1}{2}\hbar\gamma$ is given by

$$M_o \simeq (\frac{N\mu^2}{kT})H_o \tag{19}$$

This relation will be derived in section V.

Using equation (18) for the induced emf, and replacing ω_o by γH_o and M_o with equation (19), the free-precession signal following a 90° pulse is

$$V = (4\pi/c)nA\gamma H_o^2(\frac{N\mu^2}{kT})\sin\omega_o t \tag{20}$$

Since the strength of the free-induction signal is proportional to the square of the static magnetic field, the importance of a strong magnetic field in improving the signal-to-noise ratio is evident. It is for this reason that NMR spectroscopy is generally done at frequencies of 24 MHz and above. The signal-to-noise ratio is, however, more complex than the above expression for the induced emf. The noise generated in the coil depends on the coil resistance which in turn depends on frequency, due to the fact that at the frequencies of interest in NMR the current in the coil flows near the surface of the wires, and the skin depth is frequency dependent. For spectroscopy (small samples) the frequency dependence of the signal-to-noise ratio[22] is approximately $\omega^{7/4}$. For NMR imaging noise is also generated by the patient (e.g., induced magnetic eddy currents), as described by Hoult[20]. In addition, at very high frequencies, the RF may be significantly attenuated by the patient.

We can at this point pause to get a brief glimpse of the powerful imaging capabilities available with NMR. If a 90° pulse is applied to an entire sample (e.g., a human head) in a uniform field $\vec{H}_o$, the spins will all precess in the xy plane at the resonant frequency $\omega_o = \gamma H_o$. If, after termination of the 90° RF pulse, it could be arranged (by applying magnetic field gradients) to have the z-component of the magnetic field slightly different (and unique) at each spatial point $\vec{r}$ in the sample in a known fashion, then the precession frequency will be a function of position $\omega_o(\vec{r})$. After application of such gradients, protons at each spatial point will begin to "sing" (precess) at different frequencies. By listening to one frequency at a time one could tell, by the signal strength, the proton density at each spatial point. Or, more efficiently yet, one could perform a spectral analysis of the pickup coil signal $V(t)$ and derive the spatial information using a Fourier transformation,

$$F(\omega) = \int_{-\infty}^{\infty} V(t) e^{-i\omega t} dt \qquad (21)$$

The magnitude of $F(\omega)$ at each ω gives the relative proton density at the corresponding spatial point $\vec{r}$ if $\omega(\vec{r})$ is known. Thus, in principle, with a single RF pulse one could obtain three-dimensional information from which to construct an image without resorting to any CT reconstruction techniques whatsoever. (In reality, it is not quite this simple).

V. RELAXATION

A. T_1 Relaxation

In order to understand relaxation it is necessary to look again at the quantum mechanical model for the energy states of a proton in a magnetic field (Figure 3).

From atomic physics we recall that an atom in an excited state will de-excite in $\sim 10^{-8}$ sec by spontaneous emission. In addition, electromagnetic radiation having a frequency such that hν is equal to the spacing between energy levels can cause either excitation of the atom if it is in the lower energy state; or, with equal probability, the de-excitation of an atom in the upper state by stimulated emission of a photon. Theoretically, the situation is the same in NMR except that a proton in the upper energy state (spin opposite the applied field) has a characteristic time for spontaneous emission of $\sim 10^{13}$ years (12) due to the fact that the spontaneous emission probability is proportional to the cube of the frequency. A 90° RF pulse causes equal population of the two spin states ($M_z = 0$); however, after termination of the RF pulse, we know from experience that the net magnetization will return to the z-axis in a time of the order of 1 second which means that at equilibrium there are more protons in the lower (spin-up) energy state than in the upper (spin-down) state. The reason for the excess population in the lower state is because our system of proton spins, through interaction with the surroundings (the lattice), has come into thermal equilibrium with the surroundings. If the number of protons in the spin-up and spin-down states is denoted by n_+ and n_-, respectively, then at equilibrium the relative populations are given by the Boltzman distribution

$$\frac{n_-}{n_+} = e^{-\Delta E/kT} \qquad (22)$$

where ΔE is the spacing of the energy levels ($\Delta E = \hbar\omega_o$) and T is the temperature. The net z component of the magnetization is proportional to the excess population in the spin-up state

$$M_z = (n_+ - n_-)\mu \qquad (23)$$

where $\mu = \tfrac{1}{2}\hbar\gamma$ is the proton magnetic moment ($<\mu_z> = \pm \tfrac{1}{2}\hbar\gamma$). Since $\Delta E \ll kT$ for NMR, the excess population is very small. For a total of $N = (n_+ + n_-)$ proton spins, it is easy to show, using (22) and (23) that the equilibrium value of M is

$$M_o = N\mu \tanh\left(\frac{\Delta E}{2kT}\right) \qquad (24)$$

Since $\Delta E \ll kT$ and $\Delta E = \gamma\hbar H_o = 2\mu H_o$, eqn (24) may be approximated by

$$M_o \simeq \left(\frac{N\mu^2}{kT}\right) H_o \qquad (25)$$

hence it can be seen that M_o is proportional to the external field strength H_o and the square of the magnetic moment μ.

The characteristic time for return to thermal equilibrium is called the spin-lattice relaxation time T_1, such that in a static field along the z-axis the z component of the magnetization obeys

$$\frac{dM_z}{dt} = -\frac{(M_z - M_o)}{T_1} \qquad (26)$$

which is called the Bloch equation [21]. This form of the more general Bloch equations applies only in the absence of externally applied RF fields; however, it is all we shall require, since the duration of the RF pulses used is short compared to the relaxation times encountered in tissues. That is, we can assume equation (16) describes the motion of $\vec{M}$ during the RF pulse, and equation (26) applies after (or between) RF pulses. Solving (26) by integrating over (0,t) we have

$$M_z(t) = M_o + [M_z(0) - M_o] e^{-t/T_1} \qquad (27)$$

hence equation (26) predicts an exponential return to equilibrium with time constant T_1. That is, any difference in the initial magnetization $M_z(0)$ from the equilibrium value M_o (the term in brackets) disappears exponentially with time constant T_1. Following a 90° pulse, $M_z(0) = 0$, hence

$$M_z(t) = M_o(1 - e^{-t/T_1}) \qquad (27a)$$

Following a 180° pulse, $M_z(0) = -M_o$, and we have

$$M_z(t) = M_o[1 - 2e^{-t/T_1}] \qquad (27b)$$

In order for a spin system initially perturbed from equilibrium by an RF pulse to return to equilibrium (say a 180° pulse which gives an excess population in the upper state), energy must be transferred to the surroundings (the lattice). This is evident from the fact that the total energy of the spin system in a field $\vec{H}_o$ is given by $E = -\vec{M} \cdot \vec{H}_o = -M_z H_o$, hence any change in the net z component of the magnetization after termination of an RF pulse requires an energy transfer to or from the lattice. The transitions from the upper to the lower energy states are not spontaneous but are stimulated by fluctuating magnetic fields produced by molecular motions. If these internal fluctuating fields have frequency components at the resonant (Larmor) frequency, they can stimulate the de-excitation of proton spins in the upper state, this energy being transferred from the spin system into thermal kinetic energy of the lattice (or heat reservoir). T_1 is therefore a measure of the time required to establish thermal equilibrium between the spins and their surroundings. If a static field $\vec{H}_o$ is applied to an initially unmagnetized sample, T_1 is also the characteristic time for the equilibrium magnetization $\vec{M}_o$ to be established.

These fluctuating internal fields can be produced by a wide variety of sources. One source is the dipole-dipole interaction between nuclear spins. That is, a spin by virtue of its magnetic moment $\vec{\mu}$ can exert a magnetic field on a neighboring spin of the order μ/r^3, where r is the separation distance[13]. The separation distance of the two protons in a water molecule is 1.5 Å, hence the magnitude of this local field is about 4 gauss. Let us take the point of view of a proton on a water molecule, and suppose that both protons in the H_2O molecule are in a spin-up state. They will both remain aligned with the external field $\vec{H}_o$ as the molecule tumbles in its random thermal motion, and hence one proton feels a fluctuating magnetic field due to the magnetic moment of its neighbor changing its relative position. In addition, other molecules which collide with the H_2O molecule will present it with a variety of neighboring spins in random orientations which will also produce a fluctuating magnetic field at the position of the proton.

Paramagnetic ions can provide a powerful relaxation mechanism. These ions have an unpaired electron and hence have a magnetic moment equal to that of an electron spin. The magnetic moment of an electron spin is 700 times that of a proton, hence a very large fluctuating field can be provided by the random thermal motion of water molecules near paramagnetic ions. Examples of paramagnetic ions are transition group elements (Fe, Mn, Cu, Cr, Co, Ni, Ti) and rare earth elements. Adding only 20 ppm of Fe^{3+} to pure water will reduce T_1 from 3.6 sec to 20 msec. The O_2 molecule is also paramagnetic, hence dissolved oxygen can also shorten the T_1 of water. Paramagnetic ions can therefore serve as contrast media for NMR imaging by altering relaxation times.

It is only the component of these fluctuating magnetic fields at the Larmor frequency which is efficient in inducing T_1 relaxation. Although the time behavior of the thermal motion is random, it can be Fourier analyzed to determine its component at the Larmor frequency. A method of analysis of this random motion is the following. The molecular environment is considered to be constant for a time, and then changes abruptly but randomly to another configuration. The probability of the environment not changing in a time t is proportional to $\exp(-t/\tau_c)$, where τ_c is the correlation time, or a measure of the average time required for the environment to change significantly. For water at room temperature, $\tau_c \sim 10^{-12}$ sec. The magnitude of τ_c depends on the temperature, i.e., at high temperatures where molecular motion is rapid, τ_c will be short. A Fourier analysis of this type of function gives a spectral power density

$$J(\omega) = k \frac{\tau_c}{1 + \omega^2 \tau_c^2} \qquad (28)$$

where k is a function of the spin separation distance. The form of $J(\omega)$ is shown in Figure 7.

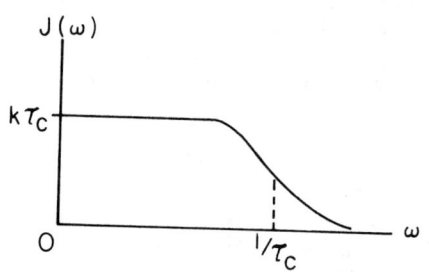

Fig. 7. Spectral power density $J(\omega)$ of random molecular motion for correlation time τ_c.

It is the magnitude of $J(\omega)$ at the Larmor frequency ω_o which is important in stimulating T_1 relaxation. If τ_c is very long such that $\omega_o \gg 1/\tau_c$, there are no components of molecular motion at the Larmor frequency, hence T_1 would be very long. If τ_c is very short, such that $\omega_o \ll 1/\tau_c$, we have a wide frequency range of a molecular motion, however, the magnitude of $J(\omega)$ at any frequency is reduced since the total power available for molecular motion is constant and it is spread over a wide frequency range. From Figure 7 we see that the intercept of $J(\omega)$ at zero frequency is proportional to τ_c such that $\int_0^\infty J(\omega)d\omega =$ constant. Relaxation is most efficient (T_1 is shortest) when $\omega_o \sim 1/\tau_c$.

It can be seen from the above that relaxation times will depend on both resonant frequency and temperature.

B. T_2 relaxation

T_1 (spin-lattice) relaxation is concerned with the z-component of the magnetization. There is, however, another characteristic relaxation time called T_2 (or spin-spin) relaxation which is a measure of the time of disappearance of the transverse component of the magnetization; that is

$$\frac{dM_{xy}}{dt} = -\frac{M_{xy}}{T_2} \qquad (29)$$

$$M_{xy}(t) = M_{xy}(0)e^{-t/T_2}$$

When we tip the magnetization into the transverse plane with a 90° pulse, we have a coherent mixture of spin states such that the precessing spins maintain a constant phase relationship to each other during precession. Processes which affect this phase coherence cause the disappearance of M_x and M_y and hence loss of the free induction signal. Of course, T_1 relaxation processes can also cause loss of the transverse component since random spin-flip transitions are occurring. That is, regrowth of the z-component will occur at some expense to the transverse component. The maximum transverse component is produced by an in-phase _equal_ mixture of spin-up and spin-down states. The T_1 relaxation processes will increase the spin-up component at the expense of the spin-down component and thereby reduce the transverse component. This is the so-called "T_1 contribution to T_2." The transverse component can also disappear due to de-phasing, as mentioned, without any energy transfer to the lattice, and this is called the secular contribution to T_2. It will be shown in PART II that for isotropic fluctuating fields

$$\frac{1}{T_2} = \frac{1}{T_2'} + \frac{1}{2T_1} \qquad (30)$$

where $1/T_2'$ is the secular contribution and $1/2T_1$ is the "T_1 contribution to T_2" or the "lifetime component". In general $T_2 \leq T_1$, with $T_2 = T_1$ in the case of rapid molecular motion in non-viscous liquids. One should not get the idea that the magnetization vector $\vec{M}$, following a 90° pulse, maintains a constant magnitude and just rotates back on to the z-axis as has been depicted in some video tapes on the subject. This is not the case even if $T_1 = T_2$. If $T_2 \ll T_1$, the transverse component will disappear long before a significant regrowth of $\vec{M}$ appears along the z-axis; that is, the magnetization $\vec{M}$ simply disappears and then gradually reappears along the z-axis. This is approximately the case in tissue where $T_2 \sim 1/5\ T_1$.

T_2 relaxation can be understood as follows. If the magnetization is tipped into the xy plane with a 90° pulse, the individual protons would remain in phase with each other if each one felt exactly the same magnetic field H_o. If, however, different protons in the system were to feel slightly different magnetic fields, they would undergo free precession at slightly different frequencies. This would cause the transverse component of the magnetization $\vec{M}$ to disappear as the protons got out of phase with each other, and the free induction signal would therefore disappear. The free-induction signal is often called the FID (free induction decay).

1. Static Field Inhomogeneity

Let us assume a field inhomogeneity which is constant in time such that various groups of protons in the sample experience slightly different fields. If $\vec{m}_i$ denotes the magnetization due to the i th proton group, then the net magnetization, which is the observable quantity, is given by the vector sum

$$\vec{M} = \sum_i \vec{m}_i \qquad (31)$$

Following a 90° pulse all the $\vec{m}_i$ will lie along the y' axis in the rotating frame; however, due to the slightly different free precession frequencies, they will dephase in the rotating frame as depicted in Figure 8 and the vector sum $\vec{M}$ will gradually disappear.

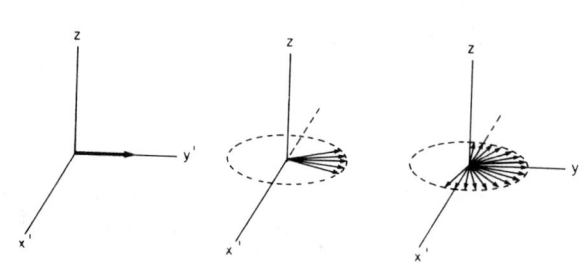

Fig. 8. Dephasing of spins in the rotating frame due to differences in the local magnetic field felt by the various spins.

That is, if the field over the sample varies over the range $H_o \pm \Delta H$, the set of spins which feel the field H_o will remain fixed in the rotating frame (which rotates in the lab with a frequency $\omega_o = \gamma H_o$); however, those spins that feel a field $H_o + \Delta H$ will precess faster by $\Delta\omega = \gamma\Delta H$, and those experiencing a field $H_o - \Delta H$ will precess slower. The net magnetization $\vec{M}$ will completely disappear when the fastest and slowest group of spins dephase in the rotating frame by 180°. This will occur in a time $\pi/\gamma\Delta H$. The time required for the free induction signal to decay by 1/e, assuming an exponential decay, is $\sim 1/\gamma\Delta H$. A 90° pulse has been chosen merely for ease of illustration. The transverse component of the magnetization would disappear in the same amount of time following an RF pulse of less than 90° or greater than 90°.

This type of field inhomogeneity could result from either a non-uniform external field or from an internal field due to neighboring spins. That is, a spin, by virtue of its magnetic moment μ, can exert a magnetic field on a neighboring spin of the order of μ/r^3, where r is the separation distance. The magnitude of the field generated by a proton at a distance of 2Å is 1.8 gauss. This would result in a dephasing time $1/\gamma\Delta H$ of only 20 μsec. In a solid, where neighboring spins maintain a fixed relationship to each other, transverse relaxation times are relatively short. Decay of the transverse magnetization caused by internal fields (static or otherwise) is regarded as true T_2 relaxation, whereas decay produced by external field inhomogeneity is not a T_2 process.

2. $\underline{T_2 \text{ relaxation due to fluctuating internal fields}}$

In a liquid, the protons in our system are the nuclei of hydrogen atoms on molecules which are tumbling and translating about with thermal kinetic energies, such that the internal magnetic field does not contain a large static component. This will increase T_2 significantly over that of a solid, e.g., T_2 of water is ~ 3 sec whereas T_2 for ice is ~ 10 μsec. Even if the time average of this randomly fluctuating field were zero, it could still cause transverse dephasing by causing the spins to execute a random walk in the rotating frame away from the y' axis (figure 8); producing the secular contribution to T_2.

In addition, if the fluctuating field has frequency components at the Larmor frequency, it will provide a lifetime (or T_1) contribution to T_2 since such fluctuations can cause spin flip transitions. Recall that a small oscillating $\vec{H}_1$ field could produce a significant effect if its frequency were near the resonant frequency, since at that frequency it would remain fixed in the rotating frame of the magnetization and could exert a constant torque over a period of time. The same holds true for a fluctuating internal field.

Decay of the transverse magnetization due to these <u>internal</u> fields (static or fluctuating) proceeds exponentially with a time constant denoted by T_2. Since it is the transverse magnetization component in the rotating frame which produces the signal, the free induction signal would decay with a time constant T_2 (if the external field were perfectly homogeneous). T_2 is called the spin-spin relaxation time. For pure water, T_2 is approximately 3 sec.

In a liquid, the major factor influencing the decay of the transverse magnetization and the FID is the inhomogeneity of the external field. For example, if we have an external magnetic field of 1500 gauss which is uniform over the sample to $\pm$ 10 ppm ($\Delta H/H_o = 10^{-5}$), the transverse decay time would be $1/\gamma\Delta H = 2.5$ msec, whereas T_2 in tissue is about 80 msec. The FID signal will decay with an effective time constant T_2^* where

$$\frac{1}{T_2^*} = \gamma\Delta H + \frac{1}{T_2} \qquad (32)$$

If the true intermolecular relaxation time T_2 is long compared to $1/\gamma\Delta H$ (as it generally will be in a liquid), then the free induction decay (FID) will be governed by $1/\gamma\Delta H$. We therefore cannot measure T_2 directly by looking at the FID signal, but must resort to the clever spin echo technique, originally devised by Hahn[14], which will be discussed shortly.

3. Relaxation summary

In summary, it has been seen that fluctuating internal fields having frequency components at the Larmor frequency can cause both T_1 and T_2 relaxation. T_2 relaxation can be produced by all three spatial components of the fluctuating field (x,y,z) whereas T_1 relaxation can only be caused by the transverse (x,y) components. This is due to the fact that the only non-zero matrix elements between energy states are due to the operators μ_x and μ_y. In addition, T_2 relaxation can be produced by a static component of the internal field [i.e., the zero frequency component of $J(\omega)$].

In a pure liquid or gas where molecular motion is random and rapid, $T_1 = T_2$. In a solid or viscous liquid where the internal field can have a large static component $T_2 \ll T_1$. A liquid might have $T_1 = T_2$ above the freezing point, and when the liquid freezes we get a sudden drop in T_2 (and an increase in T_1 due to reduced molecular motion) such that $T_2 \ll T_1$. In an NMR experiment on tissue, our signal is obtained from protons on unbound water molecules or protons in fat; however, due to exchange between water bound to macromolecules and free water, $T_2 < T_1$. In pure water, $T_1 \sim T_2 \sim 3$ sec, however, in brain tissue, at a resonant frequency of 2.7 MHz (corresponding to a field of 634 gauss), $T_1 = 285$ msec and $T_2 = 75$ msec. At 15 MHz, the relaxation times for brain tissue are $T_1 = 488$ msec, $T_2 = 78$ msec. Tissues which have a high water content (e.g., tumor or edematous tissue) have a greater proportion of unbound water and hence a longer T_1.

In addition it has been noted that T_1 and T_2 are dependent on the Larmor frequency (hence the magnetic field strength) and the sample temperature. Note also that in a practical experiment, the free induction signal will decay in a time much shorter than T_2 due to inhomogeneities in the external field.

C. Measurement of T_1

A technique commonly used for T_1 measurements is inversion recovery. The pulse sequence is $180° - \tau - 90°$ as described below. If a 180° pulse is applied to a sample (initially at equilibrium with a magnetization M_o along the z-axis) the magnetization will be rotated onto the -z axis. The z-component of the magnetization would then relax from $-M_o$, through 0, to $+M_o$. If the Bloch equation (26) is solved with the initial conditions $M_z(0) = -M_o$, we obtain

$$M_z(t) = M_o(1 - 2e^{-t/T_1}) \qquad (33)$$

The transverse component would remain equal to zero and a FID signal would never be obtained. We can, however, sample M_z at any time by applying a 90° pulse at a time τ after the 180° pulse. This will rotate whatever component of M_z is present at time τ into the xy plane to give a FID signal. If, as usual, the RF signal $\vec{H}_1$ is applied along the x' axis, such that $\vec{M}$ nutates clockwise around the x' axis in the rotating frame onto the y' axis, the FID signal will be proportional to $M_{y'}$. If the 90° pulse were applied immediately after the 180° pulse, then $M_{y'} = -M_o$ ($\vec{M}$ would lie along the $-y'$ axis). Figure 9 shows the effect of the 90° pulse in the rotating frame at various times τ. If

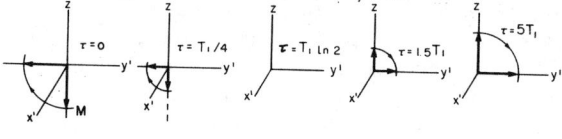
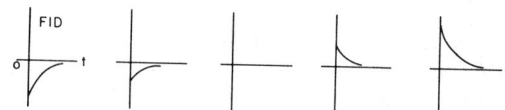

Fig. 9. Inversion-recovery sequence (180° - τ - 90°) used for measuring T_1. The result of the 90° pulse is depicted for various time intervals τ.

the interval τ is varied until the signal passes through zero and then grows positive, T_1 could be found by noting the null point $τ_{null} = T_1 \ln 2$. A better method would be to vary τ over a wide range, and fit the data with equation (33).

D. Measurement of T_2 (spin echoes)

As previously mentioned, true T_2 relaxation often is masked by external field inhomogeneities which cause a rapid decay of the FID signal. If we consider a sample which is divided into incremental segments, each one small enough to feel a uniform external field, and each one having an incremental magnetization $\vec{m}_i$, then the individual $\vec{m}_i$ will dephase in the rotating frame as previously illustrated in Figure 8, such that the net magnetization $\vec{M} = \Sigma \vec{m}_i$ disappears due to the external field inhomogeneity. For illustrative purposes, consider a three region sample as shown in Figure 10. If a 90° pulse is applied with $\vec{H}_1$ along the x′ axis in the rotating frame in order to rotate all the $\vec{m}_i$ onto the y′ axis (Figure 11a); after termination of the pulse, $\vec{m}_o$ will remain at rest in the rotating system, $\vec{m}_+$ will precess faster than $\vec{m}_o$, and $\vec{m}_-$ slower than $\vec{m}_o$ in the lab, hence we get dephasing in the rotating system as shown in Figure 11b.

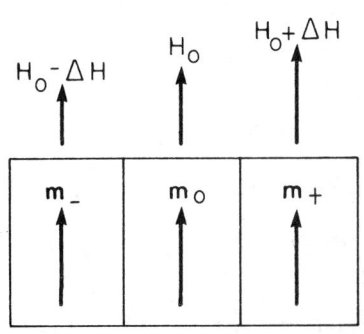

Fig. 10. A sample in a nonuniform external field, divided into segments small enough such that the magnetization in each incremental segment experiences a uniform, external magnetic field.

Suppose that a 180° pulse having $\vec{H}_1$ along the y′ axis is then applied at a time τ after the 90° pulse (recall that the pulse can be shifted from the x′ to the y′ axis simply by phase shifting the RF signal by 90°). This will cause the $\vec{m}_i$ vectors to precess clockwise about $\vec{H}_1$ in the rotating frame (i.e., about the y′ axis). Since $\vec{m}_o$ already lies along the y′ axis, it will not move, however, $\vec{m}_+$ and $\vec{m}_-$ exchange positions as shown in Figure 11c. This now puts the fastest moment $\vec{m}_+$ behind and the slowest $\vec{m}_-$ ahead, hence the spins will re-cluster at a time t = 2τ (Figure 11d).

The FID signal, which had decayed significantly by time τ due to the external magnetic field inhomogeneity, has now increased again, producing a "spin-echo" at time t = 2τ. If time τ is long enough such that the FID signal has completely disappeared (τ >> 1/γΔH), then an echo signal will be obtained as shown in Figure 12. This signal has the shape of two FID signals back-to-back, since the spins must rephase in the same manner in which they initially dephased.

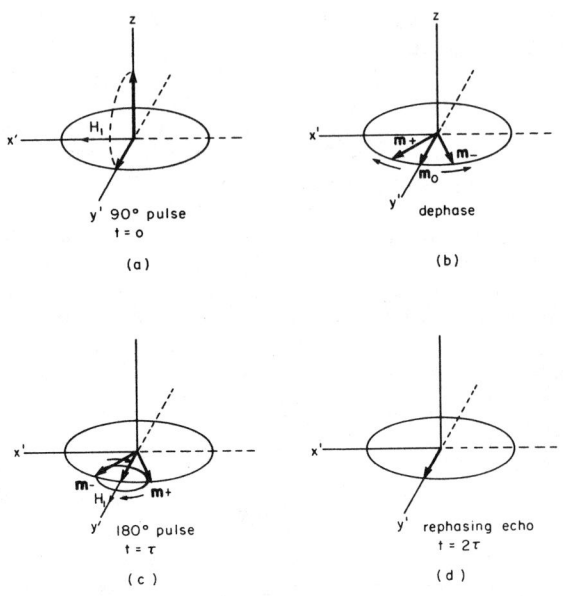

Fig. 11. CPMG spin-echo technique ($90°_{x'} - \tau - 180°_{y'}$).

The height of the echo would be the same as the original FID signal at time t = 0 if it were not for <u>true</u> T_2 relaxation. That

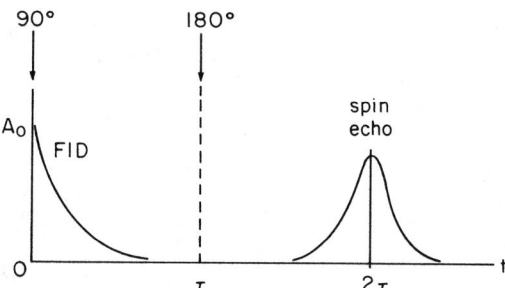

Fig. 12. Spin-echo signal produced by CPMG techique.

is, the moments $\vec{m}_+$, $\vec{m}_o$, and $\vec{m}_-$ are gradually decreasing in length due to internal field fluctuations (which cause the individual microscopic spins to dephase), but not to the external field inhomogeneity. The height of the echo at time 2τ is therefore given by

$$A(2\tau) = A_o e^{-2\tau/T_2} \qquad (34)$$

where A_o is the initial amplitude of the FID signal. If the sequence shown in Figure 12 were continued by applying another 180° pulse at time 3τ, another echo would appear at time 4τ. If the sequence is continued indefinitely, a series of echoes would be obtained as illustrated in Figure 13, the envelope of the echoes following

$$A(t) = A_o e^{-t/T_2} \qquad (35)$$

where $t = 2n\tau$. T_2 can therefore be determined from the envelope. This is called a Carr-Purcell, Meiboom-Gill (CPMG)$^{(13)}$ pulse sequence and is denoted by $90°_x\text{-}\tau\text{-}$

$180°_y\text{-}2\tau\text{-}180°_y\text{-}2\tau\text{-}$

$\text{-}180°_y\text{-}\ldots\ldots$

A similar sequence of echoes can also be generated using a Carr-Purcell (CP) pulse sequence in which all pulses have $\vec{H}_1$ along the x' axis in the rotating frame, rather than phase shifting the 180° pulses by π/2. It can be shown that the Carr-Purcell sequence also generates a similar series of echoes, however, the echoes will alternate in sign since the reclustering occurs alternately along the -y' and +y' axes due to the fact that $\vec{m}_o$ is also rotated by 180° in the CP sequence.

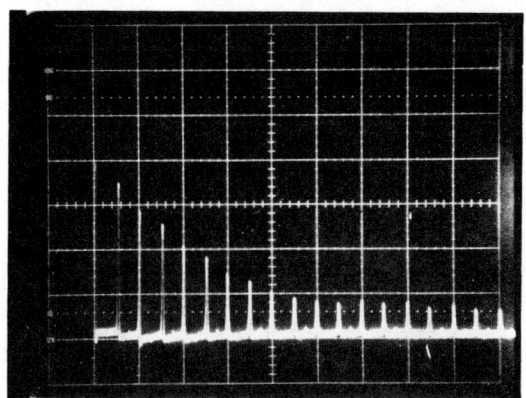

Fig. 13. CPMG repeated sequence. Multiple-spin echoes at 2τ, 4τ, 6τ,...produced by repeating the 180° pulse at intervals of τ, 3τ, 5τ,... . The echoes decrease in magnitude due to T_2 relaxation as $\exp(-2n\tau/T_2)$. The 180° pulses produce no signal, but they may be seen as blips on the baseline between the echoes.

The CPMG sequence is preferred in most instances, due to the fact that it can compensate for the fact that the 180° pulse may not be precisely 180° due to experimental uncertainty and/or non-uniformity of $\vec{H}_1$ over the sample. If the pulse were slightly less than 180°, say 180°-δ, the vectors $\vec{m}_+$ and $\vec{m}_-$ would end up slightly above and below the xy plane, respectively, resulting in an echo of reduced amplitude. After the next 180°-δ pulse, they end up back in the xy plane and the echo at t = 4τ would be a full strength echo. With CPMG the even numbered echoes are the proper strength, whereas with the CP sequence the error is cummulative and the apparent echo decay is faster than T_2.

Note that with spin echoes, we can recover the transverse magnetization which was lost by dephasing in the non-homogeneous external field, but not the magnetization lost by T_2 relaxation processes, i.e., by fluctuating internal fields. The latter is irreversible. It is also of interest to note that if a linear field gradient is purposely applied to dephase the spins, an echo can be produced merely by reversing the gradient which will cause the spins to be rephased.

VI. NMR IMAGING

Although this paper is not intended to cover imaging techniques in detail but rather basic principles, we would be remiss if we did not provide a transition to imaging for the reader, and apply the spin manipulations previously illustrated.

We will suppose initially that someone has provided us with a "slice" of tissue to image, as depicted in Figure 14 (it will be explained later how a slice of an intact body can be selected). If a 90° RF pulse is applied to the entire slice, all the spins in the slice will start precessing freely in the xy plane.

If then (after termination of the RF pulse) a small, linear magnetic field gradient is applied to the slice along the y direction, superimposed on the large field H_o along the z axis, such that the z-component of the external field varies as $H_z(y) = H_o + gy$ as shown in Figure 14; the protons will begin to precess at different frequencies depending on their location along the y-axis.

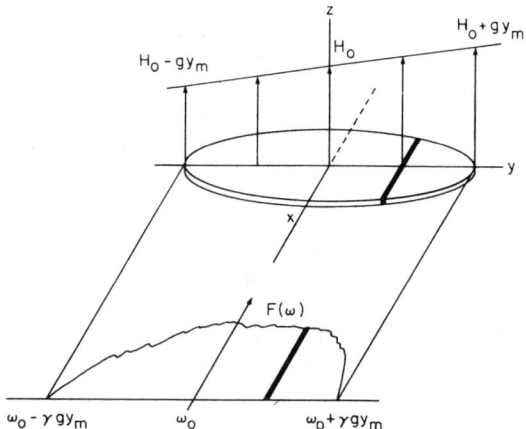

Fig. 14. Spin projection from a slice onto a line parallel to the magnetic field gradient.

The precession frequency will vary with y across the slice as

$$\omega(y) = \omega_o + \gamma gy \qquad (36)$$

where $\omega_o = \gamma H_o$, such that those protons in the shaded strip parallel to the x-axis shown in Figure 14 will all have the same precession frequency; and there exists a linear one-to-one relationship between y and precession frequency.

The shape of the FID signal from the entire slice will be complex, since it will consist of a superposition of many frequencies; however, a Fourier analysis of the signal provides information on how much of each frequency is present and thence the number of protons in each incremental strip of the slice. The Fourier transform $F(\omega)$ gives the strength of the signal from those protons precessing at frequency ω, and hence is proportional to the number of protons in the strip. Since there is a unique, linear relationship between ω and y, viz., $y = (\omega-\omega_o)/\gamma g$, $F(\omega)$ represents a spatial "projection" of proton density onto a line parallel to the gradient direction as depicted in Figure 14, i.e., $F(\omega)$ can be written as $F(y)$.

By rotating the field gradient in, say, 1° increments over 180° and repeating this sequence at each angle (90° RF pulse, gradient application and FID recording), 180 projections of the slice can be generated. CT reconstruction techniques (e.g., filtered back projection) can then be used to reconstruct from these projections the two-dimensional slice image on a display analogous to that of a CT image. That is, the slice is divided into pixels, and the proton density in each pixel is computed. The gradient can be rotated electrically [16] (a pair of gradient coils are located along the x and y axes), hence for NMR one doesn't need the mechanically rotating turret of x-ray CT.

A proton density image tends to have fairly low contrast, however, images enriched with T_1 or T_2 values can be generated in a similar fashion by using the appropriate pulse sequences. For example, the difference in proton density between grey and white brain matter is very small (< 10%), however, the difference in T_1 at 2.5 MHz is about 23%[17]. The T_1 contrast $(\Delta T_1/T_1)$ between muscle and various body tissues[18] is quite large (-25% to +40%), hence T_1 images or T_1 enriched images tend to have the highest contrast. Images based on T_2 may also have good contrast.

A. Pulse sequences

In the following, it is assumed that the width of the RF pulses is negligible compared to the interpulse delay times and relaxation times. Between RF pulses, the general solution to the Bloch equations, given by equations (27) and (29), apply. Since equation (27) assumes the initial starting time is t=0, it is convenient for the following to rewrite it for an arbitrary initial time t_o as

$$M_z(t) = M_o + [M_z(t_o)-M_o]e^{-(t-t_o)/T_1} \qquad (37)$$

All the possible pulse sequences are not covered; the emphasis here being to illustrate how the equations governing the pixel values are derived. The ACR recommended notatation for pulse sequence times is introduced into the final equations.

1. Repeated FID sequence

Some T_1 dependence can be injected by repeating the above FID sequence (another 90° pulse) before the magnetization has a chance to reach its equilibrium value M_o along the +z axis[(19)]. If the time between 90° pulses is denoted by t_R; then M_z, which is initialized to zero after the 90° pulse, will have recovered to a value given by equation (27a) at time t_R just before the next 90° pulse, and the value of the transverse component of $\vec{M}$ in the rotating frame after the repeated 90° pulse rotates M_z onto the y´ axis is

$$M_{y'} = M_o(1 - e^{-t_R/T_1}) \qquad (38)$$

This will be the value of a pixel in the image since the FID signal will be proportional to the transverse component $M_{y'}$ and the spatial encoding gradient is applied during the FID. M_o is proportional to the mobile proton density, thus if $t_R \gg T_1$, a proton density image is obtained; however, if $t_R \leq T_1$, a T_1 dependence in the image is obtained, but the FID signal strength is reduced.

2. Inversion-recovery (IR)

A method to make the image strongly dependent on T_1 is to use the T_1 measurement technique of inversion recovery (section V-C); i.e., to apply a 180° pulse to the slice to invert $\vec{M}$; apply a 90° pulse at a time t_I later in order to sample $M_z(t_I)$; apply the readout xy gradient g_{xy} after termination of the 90° pulse to spatially encode the data and record the FID; and repeat the whole sequence at a time t_w after the 90° pulse. (That is, 180° - t_I - 90° - t_w - 180°....with transverse gradient g_{xy} application and signal readout occurring during the interval t_w). The total pulse sequence repetition time is given by $t_R = t_I + t_w$. Figure 15 shows schematically the spin manipulations that occur in the rotating

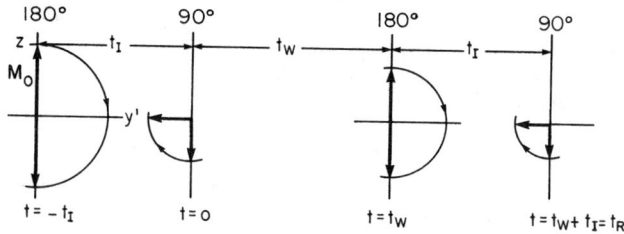

Fig. 15. Repeated inversion-recovery sequence.

frame. If $t_w \gg T_1$ such that the equilibrium magnetization recovers completely before the next 180° pulse, then the value of a pixel will be given by the previously derived equation (33), viz.

$$M_{y'} = M_o(1 - 2e^{-t_I/T_1}) \qquad (39)$$

Generally this is not a good assumption since, if one has to wait a long time ($\sim 5T_1$) between projection data collection, scan times will be quite long. If we assume that $t_w \gg T_2$ (since $T_2 \ll T_1$ for tissue) so that (as depicted in Figure 15) no transverse component of spin remains before application of the next 180° pulse, then the analysis can be simplified (we don't have to worry about spurious echoes).

After the 90° pulse, M_z is initialized to zero, hence by the time t_w just prior to the next 180° pulse it will have recovered to the value given by equation (27a).

$$M_z(t_w^-) = M_o(1 - e^{-t_w/T_1}) \qquad (40)$$

The value of M_z immediately after the 180° pulse is the negative of the above, viz.

$$M_z(t_w^+) = -M_o(1 - e^{-t_w/T_1}) \qquad (41)$$

If we solve for $M_z(t_w + t_I)$ using equation (37) with equation (41) as the initial condition (this is equivalent to integrating the Bloch equation (26) between the limits t_w^+ and $t_w^+ + t_I$), we obtain

$$M_z(t_w + t_I) = M_o[1 - 2e^{-t_I/T_1} + e^{-(t_w + t_I)/T_1}] \qquad (42)$$

Thus the value of $M_{y'}$ after the 90° pulse (the pixel value) is equal in magnitude to (42)

$$M_{y'}(IR) = M_o[1 - 2e^{-t_I/T_1} + e^{-t_R/T_1}] \qquad (43)$$

where $t_R = t_w + t_I$ is the total pulse sequence repetition period.

Typical values of t_I and t_R chosen for imaging at 6.25MHz[19] are 400 msec and 1,400 msec, respectively. In a volume element of the slice having a long T_1 (tumor or edematous tissue) where $t_I \ll T_1$ the value of $M_{y'}$ is negative since the inverted $\vec{M}$ is sampled while it is still along the -z axis. For volume elements with a short T_1 (e.g., fat), where $t_I \gg T_1$, $M_{y'}$ is positive since the magnetization has recovered onto the positive z-axis prior to the 90° sampling pulse.

3. Spin-echo Sequence (SE)

It is also possible to generate images having T_2 dependence using spin echoes. If a pulse sequence 90° - τ - 180° - τ - t_w - 90°.... is used, an echo appears at time τ after the

180° pulse (section V-D) or 2τ after the 90° pulse at the start of the sequence. The echo can be spatially encoded by applying the transverse readout gradient during its appearance. It is assumed in the following that all pulses are applied with $\vec{H}_1$ along the x´ axis. Figure 16 shows the sequence of events in the rotating frame, where the transverse (y´) and z components of the magnetization are shown separately for clarity. We will assume that the sequence period $t_R \gg T_2$ so that no transverse spin component remains when the 90° pulse at the beginning

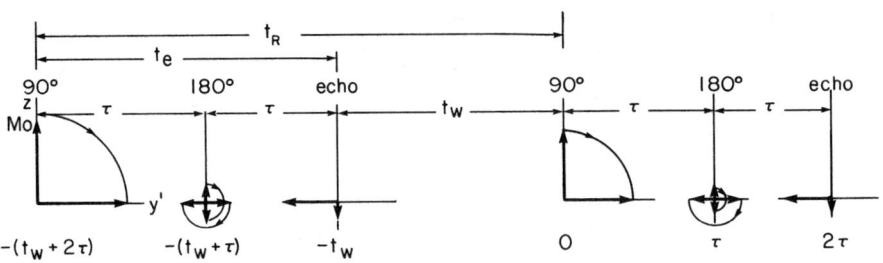

Fig. 16. Repeated spin-echo sequence.

of each sequence is applied (see fig. 16). After the initial 90° pulse at $-(t_w+2\tau)$, M_z is zeroed and will recover to a value just before the 180° pulse a time τ later, of

$$M_z(-[t_w+\tau]^-) = M_0(1 - e^{-\tau/T_1}) \qquad (44)$$

After the 180° pulse, M_z will be the negative of (44), viz,

$$M_z(-[t_w+\tau]^+) = -M_0(1 - e^{-\tau/T_1}) \qquad (45)$$

An echo will appear a time τ after the 180° pulse as the spins rephase and the transverse component regrows, however, we want the echo magnitude for the second and subsequent pulse sequences since all the other echoes will be smaller than the very first one where the z component of magnetization has its full equilibrium value. For this we need the value of M_z at the time of the next 90° pulse. Using (45) as the initial condition in (37), we obtain

$$M_z(0^-) = M_0[1 - 2e^{-(t_w+\tau)/T_1} + e^{-(t_w+2\tau)/T_1}] \qquad (46)$$

which is also the value of $M_{y´}(0^+)$ after the 90° pulse has rotated the z component onto the y´ axis. The echo magnitude at a time 2τ later is related to $M_{y´}(0^+)$ by equation (34), i.e.

$$M_{y´}(2\tau) = -M_{y´}(0^+)e^{-2\tau/T_2} \qquad (47)$$

Using $M_y(0^+) = M_z(0^-)$ and substituting (46) into (47), we obtain for the echo amplitude

$$M_y(2\tau) = -e^{-2\tau/T_2} M_o [1 - 2e^{-(t_w+\tau)/T_1} + e^{-(t_w+2\tau)/T_1}] \quad (48)$$

which is the pixel value. The exponential factor outside the bracket is the echo decay factor and the factor inside the bracket accounts for the fact that if t_w is not large compared to T_1, the z component of magnetization does not reach its full equilibrium value before the start of the next sequence.

If equation (48) is rewritten using the ACR notation where $t_E = 2\tau$ is the time from sequence start to echo and $t_R = 2\tau + t_w$ is the sequence period, we have for the pixel value

$$M_y(SE) = -e^{-t_E/T_2} M_o [1 - 2e^{-(t_R - \frac{1}{2}t_E)/T_1} + e^{-t_R/T_1}] \quad (49)$$

Typical parameters used might be $t_E = 2\tau = 80$ msec, and $t_R = 1080$ msec.

4. Modified Pulse Sequences

It is now common to produce an echo following the inversion recovery and repeated FID sequences, so that the spatial data can be collected from the echo rather than the FID. This is an advantage since the echo is well separated in time from the transmitter pulse, and its peak amplitude is well-defined. This is accomplished by applying a 180° pulse at a time τ after the 90° pulse which produces the FID. In fact, several echoes could be produced to increase the signal-to-noise ratio as in the CPMG sequence. For the inversion recovery and repeated FID, the time τ is made short compared to T_2 in order to obtain a large echo signal amplitude and to minimize the T_2 dependence injected into these sequences (i.e. $e^{-2\tau/T_2} \approx 1$); as opposed to the spin echo sequence in which 2τ is made comparable to T_2. For the repeated FID with an echo [90°-τ-180°-τ-t_w-90°...] of period $t_R = 2\tau + t_w$, the spin-echo equation (49) actually applies; however, if $t_E = 2\tau \ll T_2$, then certainly $t_E \ll t_R$, and (49) reduces to (38) with no T_2 dependence, but only in the zeroth order approximation ($e^{-t_E/T_2} = 1$).

For the inversion recovery sequence with an echo (180°-t_I-90°-τ- 180°-τ-t_w-180°...), where $t_R = t_I + 2\tau + t_w$, it can be shown using the techniques illustrated previously, that the pixel value is

$$M_y(IRSE) = M_o e^{-t_E/T_2} [1 - 2e^{-t_I/T_1} + 2e^{-(t_R-\tau)/T_1} - e^{-t_R/T_1}] \quad (50)$$

Again, if $t_E = 2\tau \ll T_2$, there is no T_2 dependence in the zeroth order approximation; that is, if $t_E \ll T_2$, then certainly $\tau \ll t_R$, and eqn (50) reduces to eqn (43) in zeroth order.

Pulse sequences will be covered later in this course and will therefore not be addressed in any greater detail here. The student should, however, be able to derive the equations for any pulse sequence based on the examples given above and the derivation of eqn (50) is a good exercise to test one's understanding.

There are more elegant methods for solving the Bloch equations; however, we believe the foregoing schematic approach leads to a better understanding of the physics.

D. Slice Selection

A slice in an intact body may be selected for imaging by applying a field gradient in the z-direction. In this case the resonant frequency will vary along the axis of the body, hence each transverse plane will have a different resonant frequency $w_o(z)$. By varying the frequency of the RF pulses, the spins in any given transverse plane may be excited. If a z-gradient g_z is applied during the 90° pulse in any of the aforementioned sequences, only the spins in a single narrow plane will be excited -- the location of the plane depending on the excitation frequency selected. Of course the slice would not be as well defined as we like (it is more like a "slice" in conventional tomography) since those protons in the top and bottom of the slice will be slightly off resonance and will not end up exactly on the y' axis in the rotating frame after the $\pi/2$ pulse. If a shaped RF pulse is used which contains a frequency spread encompassing only those protons in a rectangular slice, a better slice definition can be achieved. In addition, since the spins will dephase in the field gradient, if the z gradient is reversed for a short time after termination of the 90° RF pulse, spins will be rephased such that a maximum transverse component will be obtained.

There are many other methods of volume selection used in NMR (e.g., point, line, or plane); or, the signal from an entire 3-dimensional object can be recorded as previously described; however, discussion of these methods is beyond the scope of this paper (3).

REFERENCES

1. A. Abragam, The Principles of Nuclear Magnetism. (Oxford Univ. Press, London and New York, 1961).
2. T. C. Farrar and E.D. Becker, Pulse and Fourier Transform NMR, (Academic Press, New York, 1971).
3. E. Fukushima and S.B.W. Roeder, Experimental Pulse NMR -- a Nuts and Bolts Approach, (Addison-Wesley, Reading Mass., 1981).
4. C.P. Slichter, Principles of Magnetic Resonance, (Harper and Row, New York, 1963).
5. L. Kaufman, L.E. Crooks, and A. R. Margulis, Nuclear Magnetic ResonanceImaging in Medicine, (Igaku-Shoin, New York-Tokyo, 1981).
6. NMR Imaging, Proc. Int. Symposium, Winston-Salem, NC 1981, edited by R.L. Witcofski (Bowman Gray School of Med., Winston-Salem, NC 1982).

7. A. Messiah, Quantum Mechanics, Vol I (North Holland, Amsterdam, 1961), p. 210.
8. C.P. Slichter, Principles of Magnetic Resonance, (Harper and Row, New York, 1963), p. 14.
9. Ibid, p. 17.
10. H. Goldstein, Classical Mechanics, (Addison-Wesley, Reading Mass., 1950), p. 133.
11. J. D. Jackson, Classical Electrodynamics, (John Wiley & Sons, New York, 1962), p. 153.
12. N. Bloembergen, Nuclear Magnetic Relaxation, (W. A. Benjamin Inc., New York, 1961).
13. J. D. Jackson, Classical Electrodynamics, (John Wiley & Sons, New York, 1962), p. 143.
14. E. L. Hahn, Phys. Rev. $\underline{80}$, 580 (1950).
15. S. Meiboom and D. Gill, Rev. Sci. Instrum. $\underline{2}$, 688 (1958).
16. P. A. Bottomley, in NMR Imaging, Proc. Int. Symp., ed. R.L. Witcofski (Bowman Gray School of Med., Winston-Salem, NC, 1982) pp. 25-31.
17. C.R. Ling, M.A. Foster, and J.M.S. Hutchison, Phys. Med. Biol. $\underline{25}$, 748 (1980).
18. B. A. Coles, J. Natl. Cancer Inst. $\underline{57}$, 389 (1976).
19. I. R. Young, et al., J. Computed Tomography $\underline{6}$, 1 (1982).
20. D.I. Hoult, in NMR Imaging, Proc. Int. Symp., ed. R.L. Witcofski (Bowman Gray School of Med., Winston-Salem, NC, 1982) pp. 33-39.
21. C.P. Slichter, Principles of Magnetic Resonance, (Harper and Row, New York, 1963), p. 28.
22. D.I. Hoult and R.E. Richards, J. Magn. Reson. $\underline{36}$, 447 (1979).
23. B.L. Cohen, Concepts of Nuclear Physics, (McGraw-Hill, New York, 1971), p. 174.
24. D.M. Kramer, in Nuclear Magnetic Resonance Imaging in Medicine, ed. L. Kaufman, L.E. Crooks, and A.R. Margulis (Igaku-Shoin, New York-Tokyo, 1981), p. 184.
25. R. Damadian, Science $\underline{177}$, 1151 (1971).
26. P.C. Lauterbur, Nature $\underline{242}$, 190 (1973).
27. P. Mansfield and A.A. Maudsley, Brit. J. Radiol. $\underline{60}$, 188 (1977).
28. R. Damadian, M. Goldsmith, L. Minkoff, Physiol. Chem. Phys. $\underline{9}$, 97 (1977).

ACKNOWLEDGMENT

This paper is based on and draws heavily from the author's review article The Physics of Proton NMR, Med. Phys. $\underline{9}$(6) Nov/Dec 1982, 807-818 and large parts of the text are reproduced verbatim from that source. The author is grateful to Medical Physics and its publisher the American Institute of Physics for permission to use this material extensively for the AAPM summer school.

PHYSICAL FOUNDATIONS OF PROTON NMR: PART II -
THE MICROSCOPIC DESCRIPTION

Robert L. Dixon, Kenneth E. Ekstrand, and P.R. Moran
Department of Radiology, The Bowman Gray School of Medicine
of Wake Forest University, Winston-Salem, N.C. 27103

I. INTRODUCTION

The purpose of this part is to give medical physicists a correct picture of the quantum mechanical underpinnings of NMR in a relatively succinct fashion. The motivation was generated by many articles, papers, and commercial brochures which have appeared recently in which some of the basic physical ideas of NMR have been incorrectly stated. Since medical physicists will have to teach NMR in the immediate future, a correct understanding of basic principles is important. In part I some of these ideas were addressed, but only in a cursory fashion. Although this part contains some mathematical development, it is written such that an understanding of all of the equations is not necessary to grasp the ideas. A special effort has been made to use only elementary quantum mechanics, and to provide a treatment which is not necessarily the most elegant, but one which is easiest to understand. The reader is led through relatively simple derivations of the relaxation times T_1 and T_2 rather than simply stating the equations. In this part, the symbol $\vec{B}$ is used for the magnetic field rather than $\vec{H}$.

II. WHAT IS SPIN?

Spin angular momentum is a purely quantum mechanical quantity that has no real classical analogue. In the case of orbital angular momentum, in the limit of large quantum numbers, a classical limit is approached. For example, an earth satellite's orbits appear continuously variable since the allowed quantum orbits are so close together that they appear as a continuum. We clearly cannot approach large quantum numbers for spin (e.g. a proton has $s = \frac{1}{2}$ only). Although it is a useful analogy to consider a proton as a spinning, charged sphere, this picture should not be taken too literally since it is no doubt the internal proton structure (3 quarks surrounded by a meson cloud) which is responsible for its spin angular momentum and magnetic moment.

III. QUANTUM MECHANICAL PROTON STATES

A proton spin has a magnetic moment $\vec{\mu}$ associated with it which is proportional to its angular momentum $\vec{S}$; $\vec{\mu} = \gamma \vec{S}$.

The time dependent Schroedinger equation is written:

$$\mathcal{H}\Psi = i\hbar \frac{\partial \Psi}{\partial t} \tag{1}$$

and the Hamiltonian for a proton spin in a spatially uniform magnetic field $\vec{B}$ (or where the proton is not free to change position) is:

$$\mathcal{H} = -\vec{\mu}\cdot\vec{B} = -\gamma\vec{S}\cdot\vec{B} \tag{2}$$

where $\vec{S}$ is the angular momentum operator.

The above equations are general and apply if the magnetic field is a function of time, $\vec{B} = \vec{B}(t)$. The familiar "spin-up" and "spin-down" states are, however, stationary states of the system and can exist only in a time-independent magnetic field, i.e. if $\mathcal{H}$ is independent of time. That is, in a time-independent magnetic field we have the possibility of stationary states existing, but even in a time-independent magnetic field the proton is <u>not necessarily</u> in a stationary state.

A. Stationary States

If $\mathcal{H}$ is independent of time, then we have the possibility of stationary states since the time dependence of the wave function can be separated from the spin part as

$$\Psi(\vec{S},t) = \psi(\vec{S})e^{-i\omega t} \tag{3}$$

where ψ is independent of time and depends only on the spin components (since $\vec{B}$ is not a function of position we can ignore the spatial part of the wave function).

Using E as a separation constant and separating eqn.(1) we have:

$$\mathcal{H}\psi = E\psi \tag{4}$$

and $E = \hbar\omega$

Equation (4) is the familiar eigenvalue equation whose eigenvalues $E_n = \hbar\omega_n$ are the energy levels; and the eigenfunctions are:

$$\Psi_n = \psi_n e^{-i\omega_n t} \tag{5}$$

For a stationary state, the probability density $\Psi_n^* \Psi_n = \psi_n^* \psi_n$ is independent of time since the exponent in (5) cancels, hence there can be no time dependence (e.g. no precession of a proton spin in a stationary state); and the energy is precisely defined.

For a spin in a constant magnetic field $\vec{B}_o$ the stationary states of the system are derived as follows. If $\vec{B}_o$ is taken along the z-axis, the Hamiltonian from eqn(2) is:

$$\mathcal{H} = -\gamma B_o S_z \qquad (6)$$

Hence, the eigenstates of the system ψ_m are eigenstates of the angular momentum operator S_z (and also of $S^2 = S_x^2 + S_y^2 + S_z^2$ which commutes with S_z). That is,

$$S_z \psi_m = m\hbar \psi_m$$
$$S^2 \psi_m = s(s+1)\hbar^2 \psi_m \qquad (7)$$

with the energy levels being given by

$$E_m = -m\hbar\gamma B_o \quad , \quad -s \leq m \leq s \qquad (8)$$

For a proton $s = \frac{1}{2}$, hence only two levels are allowed, $m = \pm \frac{1}{2}$, these being the "spin-up" and "spin-down" states, respectively, depicted in fig. 1.

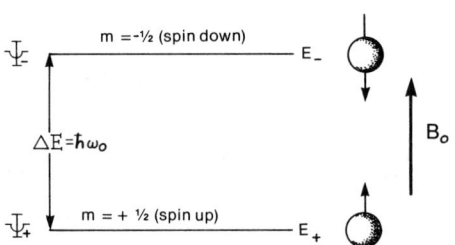

Fig. 1. Stationary states of a proton spin in a constant magnetic field $\vec{B}_o$.

If we denote the spin-up and spin-down wave functions now (and henceforth) as Ψ_+ and Ψ_-, respectively, we have:

$$\Psi_+ = \psi_+ e^{-i\omega_+ t} \quad , \quad E_+ = \hbar\omega_+ = -\tfrac{1}{2}\hbar\omega_o \quad \text{(spin up)} \qquad (9)$$
$$\Psi_- = \psi_- e^{-i\omega_- t} \quad , \quad E_- = \hbar\omega_- = +\tfrac{1}{2}\hbar\omega_o \quad \text{(spin down)}$$

Note that the Larmor frequency$^{(1)}$ $\omega_o = \gamma B_o$ is equal to the <u>difference</u> in ω_- and ω_+

$$\omega_o = \omega_- - \omega_+ \qquad (10)$$

and is proportional to the <u>difference</u> in energy levels

$$\Delta E = E_- - E_+ = \hbar \omega_o \qquad (11)$$

One point concerning these states should be made, if only because it has been belabored beyond all reason in recent NMR imaging literature. Spin-up and spin-down refer to the z-component $m\hbar$ of the angular momentum. The actual spin vector has magnitude (see eqn. 7) of $\hbar\sqrt{s(s+1)}$ which is greater than $m\hbar$, hence a quantum mechanical spin vector $\vec{S}$ cannot lie along any fixed axis in space. Since S_x, S_y, and S_z do not mutually commute, we cannot specify or measure any two simultaneously (much less all three). A measurement of any one of them must yield $\pm\frac{1}{2}\hbar$. Since we are referring to a stationary state, the spin vector should be thought of as uniformly smeared out over the surface of a cone, as depicted in Figure 2 for a spin-up

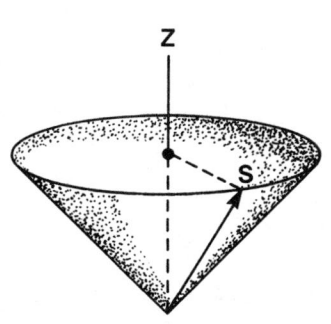

Fig. 2. Cone of constraint for the spin vector $\vec{S}$ of a proton spin in a stationary, spin-up state. The spin vector may lie anywhere on the surface of the cone with equal probability, thus it may be thought of as uniformly smeared out over the cone's surface. Only the z-component S_z and the magnitude of $\vec{S}$ are known with certainty, i.e., $S_z = 1/2\hbar$ and $S^2 = 3/4\hbar^2$.

state. That is, we cannot know either S_x or S_y simultaneously with S_z (which is precisely known in a stationary state, i.e., $S_z = m\hbar$), but we can know only $S_x^2 + S_y^2$.

If we made a series of measurements on the x, y, or z components on an ensemble of identical spin systems in, say, a spin-up state such as depicted in fig. 2 we would find, on the average, the expectation values

$$\langle S_x \rangle = \langle S_y \rangle = 0 \qquad (12)$$
$$\langle S_z \rangle = +\tfrac{1}{2}\hbar$$

Thus, any location of $\vec{S}$ around the cone is equally likely and $S_z = \tfrac{1}{2}\hbar$ with certainty. It is often incorrectly stated that $\vec{S}$ precesses around the z-axis on the surface of the cone. This cannot be the case for a pure stationary (spin-up/spin-down) state since the probability density and expectation values are independent of time. Since $\vec{S}$ is uniformly smeared out as described and cannot be specified to lie completely along any axis, then we needn't be concerned with $\vec{S}$ itself but only its components (S_x, S_y, S_z). (Of course only one component of spin can be specified with certainty at a given instant). Thus, we can really think of a spin-up state as a spin vector lying along the z axis, realizing we are dealing with a spin component only. There is no precession of a spin that exists in a stationary state and, therefore, is "parallel" (or anti-parallel) to the field direction.

B. Non-Stationary States

In non-stationary states the energy is not precisely defined and probability densities are time dependent.

A familiar example of a non-stationary state is an atom or a nucleus in an excited state. Consider a system having two stationary states ψ_1 and ψ_2 having energies E_1 and E_2 as shown in Figure 3. If coupling with the radiation field is considered,

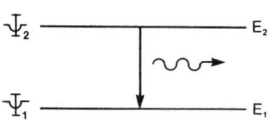

Fig. 3. Depicts a transition between states 1 and 2, where the excited state 2 is not stationary.

the upper state is not really stationary but can de-excite by spontaneous emission of a photon.

During the transition, the system exists in a non-stationary state where the wave function is a time dependent mixture of ψ_1 and ψ_2. The mean lifetime of the excited state is generally $\sim 10^{-8}$ sec for atomic transitions and $\sim 10^{-15}$ sec for nuclear transitions; however, in NMR the lifetime for spontaneous emission[2] is $\sim 10^{13}$ years in a vacuum or $\sim 10^3$ years coupled to an rf coil, due to the very small difference in the energy levels in NMR and the fact that the transition is a magnetic dipole transition. Thus, in NMR, an isolated spin may spend an appreciable amount of time in a non-stationary state consisting of a coherent mixture of spin-up and spin-down states.

Consider now the non-stationary states of a proton spin in a magnetic field. The most general solution of the Schroedinger equation (1) can be expressed as a linear combination of the spin-up and spin-down wave functions given in eqn (9); that is, as:

$$\mathcal{F} = a\mathcal{F}_+ + b\mathcal{F}_- = a(t)\psi_+ e^{-i\omega_+ t} + b(t)\psi_- e^{-i\omega_- t} \qquad (13)$$

where $|a|^2$ may be interpreted as the probability a measurement of the z-component of spin will result in spin-up ($S_z = \tfrac{1}{2}\hbar$) and $|b|^2$ the probability it will yield spin-down, thus $|a|^2 + |b|^2 = 1$.

Note that the probability density $\mathcal{F}^*\mathcal{F}$ now contains an interference term between the two states of the form:

$$e^{-i(\omega_+ - \omega_-)t} = e^{+i\omega_0 t} \qquad (14)$$

which describes a time dependence at the Larmor frequency. It is this time dependence of non-stationary states that suggests the possibility of "motion" (precession) at the Larmor frequency and the emission of radiation.

If the magnetic field is independent of time, then a and b will be constants, and the relative admixture of the spin-up and spin-down states remains constant and equal to the initial values which are determined by the initial conditions. In this case we have "free precession". If the magnetic field is time dependent, then a and b will be time dependent. That is, the relative admixture can change giving transitions between spin states.

In the following, it will be convenient to use the raising and lowering operators

$$S_+ = S_x + iS_y \qquad (15)$$
$$S_- = S_x - iS_y$$

which have the effect of raising or lowering the spin state.

$$S_+\psi_- = \hbar\psi_+ , \quad S_+\psi_+ = 0 \qquad (16)$$
$$S_-\psi_+ = \hbar\psi_- , \quad S_-\psi_- = 0$$

1. Non-stationary states in a constant magnetic field
   (free precession)

The wave function for a proton spin in an arbitrary orientation is given by equation (13).

The complex coefficients a and b can be written

$$a = Ae^{i\alpha}$$
$$b = Be^{i\beta}$$ (17)

where A and B are real and $A^2 + B^2 = 1$ since the wavefunction must be normalized with $|a|^2 + |b|^2 = 1$.

Using $S_x = \frac{1}{2}(S_+ + S_-)$ and $S_y = \frac{1}{2i}(S_+ - S_-)$ from (15) and the properties of S_+ and S_- from (16), it is straight forward to show, using the wave function in (13), that the wave function of a proton in a constant magnetic field B_o evolves in time such that the expectation values $\langle \vec{S} \rangle = (\Psi, \vec{S}\Psi)$ are given by

$$\langle S_x \rangle = \hbar AB \cos(\alpha-\beta + w_o t)$$
$$\langle S_y \rangle = -\hbar AB \sin(\alpha-\beta + w_o t) \quad (18a)$$
$$\langle S_z \rangle = \frac{1}{2}\hbar(A^2 - B^2)$$

If we make the identification $\cos \theta = A^2 - B^2$, since $A^2 + B^2 = 1$, it then follows that $\sin \theta = 2AB$, hence equations (18a) can be rewritten as:

$$\langle S_x \rangle = \frac{1}{2}\hbar \sin \theta \cos(\alpha-\beta+w_o t)$$
$$\langle S_y \rangle = -\frac{1}{2}\hbar \sin \theta \sin(\alpha-\beta+w_o t) \quad (18b)$$
$$\langle S_z \rangle = \frac{1}{2}\hbar \cos \theta$$

Equations (18) describe a precession of a vector $\langle \vec{S} \rangle$ of length $\frac{1}{2}\hbar$ about the z-axis at the Larmor frequency w_o as shown in figure 4. The angle θ is the angle of inclination from the z-axis, and $\delta = \alpha-\beta$ represents a phase shift such that δ is the initial angular offset from the x-axis at time t=0 as shown in fig. 4.

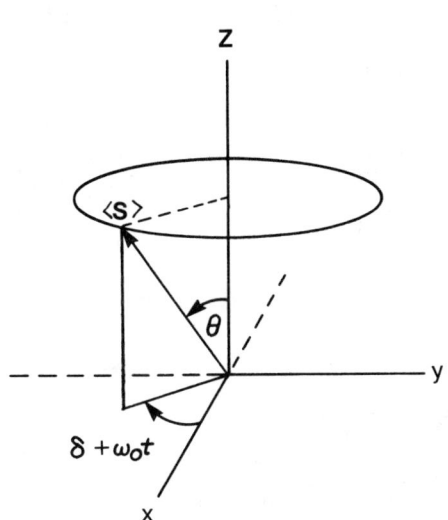

Fig. 4. Free precession in a constant magnetic field of the expectation value of the spin vector $\langle \vec{S} \rangle$ for a non-stationary proton state consisting of a coherent mixture of spin-up and spin-down states. The angle θ is determined by the relative admixture. For a pure spin-up state, $\theta = 0$; and for an equal admixture of spin-up and spin-down, $\theta = 90°$.

The phase $\delta = \alpha - \beta$ would only be determined if a measurement localized the spin at t=0. A spin can be forced into a non-stationary state by means of a measurement. For example, if a measurement of S_x at t=0 resulted in a value of $+\frac{1}{2}\hbar$ (recall such a measurement can only give $\pm\frac{1}{2}\hbar$), then from (18b), $\delta=0$, $\sin\theta = 1$, $S_z = 0$, and $A = B$, hence the wave function consists of a equal mixture of spin-up and spin-down eigenfunctions; thus it can be seen that equations (18b) in this case describe a precession of $\langle \vec{S} \rangle$ in the xy plane at the Larmor frequency. This does not imply that we know exactly where the spin vector is located after t=0. The expectation value gives only its "average" location (or the average over an ensemble of spins having the same wave function). That is, we know exactly how the wave function evolves in time after t=0, but the wave function only determines probabilities. In fact, for this example, the probability that a measurement of S_x (or S_y) will result in $\pm\frac{1}{2}\hbar$ for t>0 is given by

$$P(S_x = \pm\tfrac{1}{2}\hbar) = \tfrac{1}{2}(1 \pm \cos\omega_o t) \quad (19)$$

$$P(S_y = \pm\tfrac{1}{2}\hbar) = \tfrac{1}{2}(1 \pm \sin\omega_o t)$$

An analysis of equations (19) at $\omega_o t = 0, \pi/2, \pi$, is educational.

Thus, as previously stated, the probability density of a non-stationary state exhibits a time dependence at the Larmor frequency, i.e., we have a precessing (oscillating) magnetic dipole $\langle\vec{\mu}\rangle = \gamma \langle\vec{S}\rangle$ at the Larmor frequency.

2. <u>Non-stationary states in a time varying magnetic field.</u>

Suppose that, in addition to the static magnetic field $\vec{B}_o$ along the z-axis, we have a time varying field $\vec{B}_1(t)$ superimposed such that $\vec{B}(t) = \vec{B}_o + \vec{B}_1(t)$. The Hamiltonian can then be written $\mathcal{H} = \mathcal{H}_o + \mathcal{H}_1(t)$ where:

$$\mathcal{H}_o = -\vec{\mu}\cdot\vec{B}_o = -\gamma B_o S_z \qquad (20)$$

as before, and

$$\mathcal{H}_1 = -\gamma\vec{B}_1(t)\cdot\vec{S} \qquad (21)$$

If these are substituted in the Schroedinger equation (1) using the general wave function eqn (13), then it can be shown that $a(t)$ and $b(t)$ satisfy

$$i\hbar\frac{da}{dt} = a(\chi_+, \mathcal{H}, \chi_+) + b(\chi_+, \mathcal{H}, \chi_-)e^{-i\omega_o t} \qquad (22)$$

$$i\hbar\frac{db}{dt} = b(\chi_-, \mathcal{H}, \chi_-) + a(\chi_-, \mathcal{H}, \chi_+)e^{i\omega_o t} \qquad (23)$$

Equations (22) and (23) are equivalent to the time dependent Schroedinger equation (1) and are the usual starting point for developing time-dependent perturbation theory; however, in the foregoing we will solve them exactly without making the perturbation approximation.

We see immediately from (22) and (23) that if the magnetic field is not time varying ($\mathcal{H}_1 = 0$), then a and b are constants and remain equal to their initial values, as previously stated (free precessional case).

If $\vec{B}_1(t)$ is along the z-axis then $\mathcal{H}_1 = -\gamma B_1 S_z$, and then the second term on the right hand side of (22) and (23) vanishes by orthogonality of the wave functions and the first term produces a phase shift of a and b such that

$$a(t) = a(0)\exp\left[\tfrac{1}{2}i\gamma\int_o^t B_1(t)dt\right] \qquad (24a)$$

$$b(t) = b(0)\exp\left[-\tfrac{1}{2}i\gamma\int_o^t B_1(t)dt\right]$$

Since $|a(t)|^2 = |a(0)|^2$ and $|b(t)|^2 = |b(0)|^2$, no transitions between spin-up and spin down states are produced. A z-component of the field can only produce a phase shift of the precessing spin since the above equations (24a) have the form (17), where $\delta = \alpha-\beta$ is related to the phase of the spin, viz. it's angular offset from the x' axis in the rotating frame. Comparing (24a) to (17), the phase shift is

$$\delta(t) = \gamma \int_0^t B_{1z}(t)dt \qquad (24b)$$

It is the second term on the right hand side of (22) and (23) that can mix the two states and produce transitions. This term is non-zero only if $\vec{B}_1$ has transverse (x,y) components. Recall that $|a|^2$ and $|b|^2$ are the probabilities the spin is up or down, respectively. Thus if the spin is initially in a spin-up state at time t=0 (a(0) = 1, b(0) = 0), the transverse component of $\vec{B}_1$ through the matrix element ($\mathcal{H}_-, \mathcal{H}_1, \mathcal{H}_+$) in (23) initially feeds probability into the spin down state, and the term ($\mathcal{H}_+, \mathcal{H}_1, \mathcal{H}_-$) in (22) initially bleeds probability from the spin up state. Consider now the case of interest in NMR, i.e. an oscillating transverse magnetic field produced by a radio-frequency (RF) coil wrapped along, say, the x-axis such that

$$\vec{B}_1(t) = \hat{i} 2B_1 \cos\omega t \qquad (25)$$

where ω is the RF frequency. If $\vec{B}_1$ is resolved into two rotating components$^{(1)}$, it is only the component that rotates in the same sense as the classical Larmor precession that produces any significant effect ($B_1 << B_0$), hence $\vec{B}_1$ can be written as a rotating field

$$\vec{B}_1(t) = B_1 (\hat{i}\cos\omega t - \hat{j}\sin\omega t) \qquad (26)$$

and

$$\mathcal{H}_1 = -\gamma B_1 \cos\omega t S_x + \gamma B_1 \sin\omega t S_y \qquad (27)$$

Using (15), it is straightforward to show:

$$\mathcal{H}_1 = -\tfrac{1}{2}\gamma B_1 (e^{i\omega t}S_+ + e^{-i\omega t}S_-) \qquad (28)$$

Substituting eqn (28) in (22) and (23), it is easy to see that the first terms vanish; and it is straightforward to show, using the properites of S_+ and S_- in (16), that

$$\frac{da}{dt} = i\frac{\omega_1}{2} b e^{i(\omega-\omega_0)t}$$
$$\frac{db}{dt} = i\frac{\omega_1}{2} a e^{-i(\omega-\omega_0)t}$$
(29a)

where $\omega_1 = \gamma B_1 \ll \omega_0$, and ω is the RF frequency.

If the RF is applied at the resonant frequency, $\omega = \omega_0$, these equations become particularly simple

$$\frac{da}{dt} = i\frac{\omega_1}{2} b$$

$$\frac{db}{dt} = i\frac{\omega_1}{2} a$$
(29b)

It is easy to verify by substitution in (29b) that a solution for a proton initially in a spin-up state at t=0 ($a(0)=1$, $b(0)=0$) is:

$$a(t) = \cos\left(\frac{\omega_1 t}{2}\right)$$
$$b(t) = i \sin\left(\frac{\omega_1 t}{2}\right)$$
(30)

Recall that $|a|^2$ and $|b|^2$ are the probabilities that the spin is up or down, respectively, hence if the RF is turned on for a time t where $\omega_1 t = \pi$ (a 180° pulse), then $|a|^2=0$ and $|b|^2=1$, i.e., the spin has been inverted and a "spin flip" transition has been produced. It is readily shown using the solutions (30) in (13) that

$$\langle S_z \rangle = (\Psi, S_z \Psi) = \tfrac{1}{2}\hbar\cos\omega_1 t$$
(31)

so that the expectation value of S_z slowly turns over, and then back up again as shown in Figure 5. That is, the spin goes from

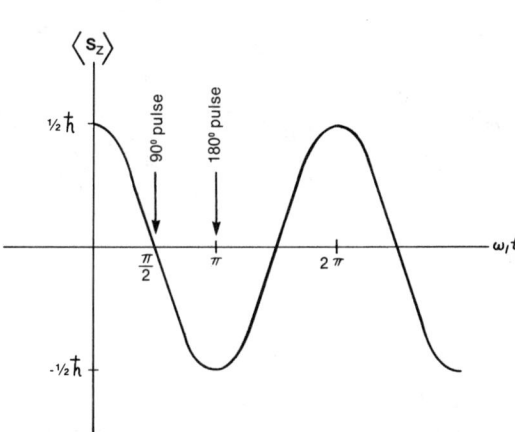

Fig. 5. Time variation of the expectation value of the z-component of spin for a proton spin initially in a spin-up state at t = 0 exposed at a RF field ($B_x = 2B_1 \cos\omega_0 t$) at the resonant frequency ω_0. For a 180° pulse ($\omega_1 t = \pi$) the spin is inverted as shown, where $\omega_1 = \gamma B_1$.

up to down and back up again, continuing this behavior for as long as the RF field is on.

The expectation value of the energy of the system is $\langle E \rangle = -\gamma B_0 \langle S_z \rangle$, hence $\langle E \rangle$ exhibits an oscillatory behavior. We can think this process as an exchange of a photon between the spin system and the RF coil as the spin turns over and then back up again. The expectation values of the other components can similarly be shown to be:

$$\langle S_x \rangle = \tfrac{1}{2}\hbar \sin\omega_1 t \, \sin\omega_0 t \qquad (32)$$

$$\langle S_y \rangle = \tfrac{1}{2}\hbar \sin\omega_1 t \, \cos\omega_0 t$$

$$\langle S_z \rangle = \tfrac{1}{2}\hbar \cos\omega_1 t$$

which describes, in the laboratory system, a spiraling down of $\langle \vec{S} \rangle$ from its initial position along the z-axis as can be seen from Figure 6. Since $\omega_1 \ll \omega_0$, $\langle \vec{S} \rangle$ makes many precessions during

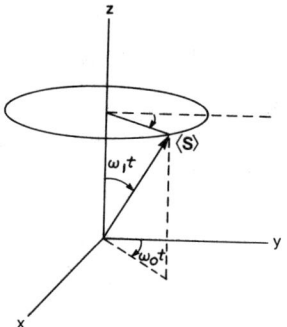

Fig. 6. Motion of the expectation value of the spin vector $\langle \vec{S} \rangle$ for a spin initially in a spin up state exposed to a RF field at the resonant frequency where $B_x = 2B_1 \cos\omega_o t$ and $\omega_1 = \gamma B_1$.

a 90° ($\omega_1 t = \pi/2$) or 180° ($\omega_1 t = \pi$) pulse. That is $\langle \vec{S} \rangle$, or $\langle \vec{\mu} \rangle = \gamma \langle \vec{S} \rangle$, obeys the classical equation of motion (part I, eqn 2).

$$\frac{d}{dt}\langle \vec{\mu} \rangle = \langle \vec{\mu} \rangle \times \gamma \vec{B} \qquad (33)$$

This can be shown more simply and elegantly using the quantum mechanical expression for the equation of motion of an operator

$$\frac{d}{dt}\langle \vec{S} \rangle = \frac{i}{\hbar}\langle [\mathcal{H}, \vec{S}] \rangle \qquad (34)$$

where $[\mathcal{H}, \vec{S}]$ is the commutator of the Hamiltonian $\mathcal{H} = -\gamma \vec{S} \cdot \vec{B}(t)$ and the operator $\vec{S}$. Using the commutation properties of the angular momentum operators (3), it is straight forward to derive (33) from (34).

For a system of N non-interacting spins, the net (macroscopic) magnetization is given by:

$$\vec{M} = N \langle \vec{\mu} \rangle \qquad (35)$$

hence, from (33) we see that $\vec{M}$ satisfies the classical equation

$$\frac{d\vec{M}}{dt} = \vec{M} \times \gamma \vec{B} \qquad (36)$$

In tissue or liquids, the relaxation times are long compared to the length of the RF pulses used, hence eqn (36) is an excellent approximation during the RF pulse. Stated differently, the RF magnetic field at resonance (B_1) is large compared to the component of the fluctuating internal magnetic field at the Larmor frequency contributed by interactions with neighboring protons - the latter being responsible for relaxation. Thus we can generally ignore the relaxation terms in the Bloch equations during the RF pulse.

IV. RELAXATION AND THERMAL EQUILIBRIUM

For a system of proton spins in a liquid or in tissue a little thought will show that the spin-up/spin-down stationary states do not exist even in the absence of applied RF power. Any given proton will feel, in addition to the externally applied static field $\vec{B}_o$, a fluctuating field $\vec{B}_1(t)$ due to the motion of neighboring protons which possess magnetic moments and therefore generate a dipolar magnetic field. The strength of this magnetic field generated by one proton in a water molecule at the position of its neighbor in the same molecule is about 4 gauss. Thus, one proton in the molecule "sees" its neighbor undergoing random changes in position as the molecule tumbles about, and this produces a fluctuating magnetic field at the position of either proton. If the motion has frequency components near the Larmor frequency, then transitions may be induced as we have seen. Protons in other molecules can, of course, contribute to this fluctuating magnetic field if they collide with, or pass by in close proximity to, the given molecule.

Thus, thermal equilibrium must be a dynamic equilibrium in which transitions are continually occurring; moreover, the protons will, in general, not exist in either a spin-up or spin-down state as these stationary states do not exist as such in a time dependent magnetic field. That is, protons will exist in states which can be described as a mixture of spin-up/spin-down states such as given by equation (13). They will therefore undergo precession at varying angles with the z-axis, with slightly more having positive than negative components of spin along z such that the net magnetization lies along z. The phases of precession will be random, such that the net xy component of magnetization vanishes.

A. Thermal Equilibrium

Equations (18a) describe a spin with a random orientation and a random phase $\delta = \alpha - \beta$ in a constant magnetic field. At thermal equilibrium we would expect a random distribution of phases δ, such that $\langle S_x \rangle$ and $\langle S_y \rangle$, when averaged over a population of spins at thermal equilibrium, will vanish. If a bar is used to denote an average over a statistical ensemble of spins at thermal equilibrium, then we know from experiment that

$$\overline{\langle S_x \rangle} = \overline{\langle S_y \rangle} = 0 \qquad (37)$$

$$\overline{\langle S_z \rangle} > 0$$

since the equilibrium magnetization $\vec{M}_0$ for a system of N protons has no transverse components and lies along the field direction (positive z-axis). Its magnitude is related to $\langle S_z \rangle$ as

$$M_0 = N \gamma \overline{\langle S_z \rangle} \qquad (38)$$

From (18a) we have

$$\langle S_z \rangle = \tfrac{1}{2}\hbar(A^2 - B^2) \qquad (39)$$

hence we expect that more spins will have A>B than the other way around.

In fact, since the system in thermal equilibrium is described by a Boltzman distribution and the system energy is proportional to $\langle S_z \rangle$, it follows that

$$\overline{B^2/A^2} = e^{-\Delta E/kT} = e^{-\hbar\omega_0/kT} \qquad (40)$$

Since $\overline{A^2 + B^2} = 1$, and $\hbar\omega_0 \gg kT$, it can be shown that

$$\overline{\langle S_z \rangle} = \tfrac{1}{2}\hbar \left(\frac{\hbar\omega_0}{2kT}\right) \qquad (41)$$

thence

$$M_0 = N\gamma \overline{\langle S_z \rangle} = N \left(\frac{\gamma\hbar}{2}\right) \left(\frac{\hbar\omega_0}{2kT}\right) \qquad (42)$$

As we have seen, at thermal equilibrium, there exists an incoherent mixture of spin states with random phases $\delta = \alpha - \beta$. Since we cannot know the individual phases, quantum statistical mechanics[4] shows that the above-described system, where the individual spins are in states consisting of a mixture of spin up and spin down states, is indistinguishable from a system consisting of a mixture of pure stationary states in which a spin is either up or down. Since $\langle S_x \rangle = \langle S_y \rangle = 0$ for a stationary state, the transverse magnetization automatically vanishes.

Relating equations (18a) to the pure system, $N\,(\overline{A^2} - \overline{B^2})$ would be interpreted as the net excess of spins in the lower (spin-up) energy state.

It is of interest to see how, by applying RF to a system of spins initially in thermal equilibrium, a coherent mixture of spin states is obtained such that a non-zero transverse component of magnetization is created. If equations (29b) for a rotating RF field at resonance are solved for an arbitrary a and b as given by equation (17) we obtain

$$a(t) = A \cos\left(\frac{\omega_1 t}{2}\right) + iBe^{-i\delta} \sin\left(\frac{\omega_1 t}{2}\right) \qquad (43)$$

$$b(t) = iA \sin\left(\frac{\omega_1 t}{2}\right) + Be^{-i\delta} \cos\left(\frac{\omega_1 t}{2}\right) \qquad (44)$$

where $\delta = \alpha - \beta$. (Since only the difference $\alpha - \beta$ appears in the expectation values we have factored out and dropped an $e^{i\alpha}$.) Using $\mathcal{F} = a\mathcal{X}_+ + b\mathcal{Y}_-$ as before, it is straightforward (but tedious) to show that the solution for a spin having arbitrary amplitudes A, B, and phase δ is

$$\langle S_x \rangle = \tfrac{1}{2}\hbar(A^2-B^2)\sin\omega_1 t \sin\omega_o t + \hbar AB[\cos\delta\cos\omega_o t - \sin\delta\cos\omega_1 t \sin\omega_o t]$$

$$\langle S_y \rangle = \tfrac{1}{2}\hbar(A^2-B^2)\sin\omega_1 t \cos\omega_o t - \hbar AB[\cos\delta\sin\omega_o t + \sin\delta\cos\omega_1 t \cos\omega_o t]$$

$$\langle S_z \rangle = \tfrac{1}{2}\hbar(A^2-B^2)\cos\omega_1 t + \hbar AB\sin\delta\sin\omega_1 t \qquad (45)$$

These equations become clearer if expressed in terms of the initial spin conditions at t=0, obtained by evaluating equations (45) at t=0, viz.

$$\langle S_x(0) \rangle = \hbar AB\cos\delta \qquad (46)$$

$$\langle S_y(0) \rangle = \hbar AB\sin\delta$$

$$\langle S_z(0) \rangle = \tfrac{1}{2}\hbar(A^2-B^2)$$

whence equations (45) are equivalent to

$$\langle S_x \rangle = \langle S_z(0) \rangle \sin\omega_1 t \sin\omega_o t + \langle S_x(0) \rangle \cos\omega_o t + \langle S_y(0) \rangle \cos\omega_1 t \sin\omega_o t$$

$$\langle S_y \rangle = \langle S_z(0) \rangle \sin\omega_1 t \cos\omega_o t - \langle S_x(0) \rangle \sin\omega_o t + \langle S_y(0) \rangle \cos\omega_1 t \cos\omega_o t$$

$$\langle S_z \rangle = \langle S_z(0) \rangle \cos\omega_1 t - \langle S_y(0) \rangle \sin\omega_1 t \qquad (48)$$

The meaning of the above equations becomes clear after a little thought if it is remembered that B_1 is along the x axis.

The next step is to average equations (48) over a population of spins initially at thermal equilibrium. It is reasonable to assume that the amplitudes (A,B) and the phases δ are statistically independent.

Since the initial distribution of spins at t=0 is a thermal equilibrium distribution, then $\overline{\langle S_x(0) \rangle} = \overline{\langle S_y(0) \rangle} = 0$ due to the random phases δ as can be seen from equations (46), and $\overline{\langle S_z(0) \rangle} = \tfrac{1}{2}\hbar\overline{(A^2 - B^2)}$ is proportional to the equilibrium magnetization and is given by (41) or (42). All but the first term in each of equations (48) vanish when the average is taken, hence

$$\overline{\langle S_x \rangle} = \overline{\langle S_z(0) \rangle} \sin\omega_1 t \sin\omega_o t \qquad (49)$$

$$\overline{\langle S_y \rangle} = \overline{\langle S_z(0) \rangle} \sin\omega_1 t \cos\omega_o t$$

$$\overline{\langle S_z \rangle} = \overline{\langle S_z(0) \rangle} \cos\omega_1 t$$

These equations have the same form as equations (32) where it was assumed that a single spin was initially in a spin up state. If we interpret $\overline{(A^2 - B^2)}$ as the fractional <u>excess</u> of spins in the spin-up state, then we see that it is only the unpaired spins that contribute to the net magnetization including the transverse component that develops after an RF pulse is applied.

The above result would be the same if we considered all spins to be initially in pure spin-up or spin downs states at equilibrium. It is clear that the spins of a pair of spin-up and spin-down protons would remain oppositely directed during the RF application as both spins rotated according to equations (32), hence paired spins would always give a net moment of zero.

B. Relaxation:

It is the internal magnetic fields that produce relaxation. If a $90°$ pulse is applied to a sample at equilibrium, a coherent mixture of spin-up/spin-down states is produced such that, after the pulse, the net magnetization $\vec{M}$ freely precesses in the equatorial plane about the magnetic field direction (z-axis) at the Larmor frequency. It we assume a perfectly uniform external magnetic field $\vec{B}_o$, then the transverse (xy) component of $\vec{M}$, which produces the free induction signal, will decay with a time constant T_2. The magnetization will also begin to grow along the z-axis toward its equilibrium value with a time constant T_1.

In the foregoing, we will assume that a spin in a uniform field $\vec{B}_o$ is subjected to a randomly fluctuating field $\vec{B}_1(t)$, due to the motion of neighboring spins. We will also assume that the x,y, and z components of the magnetic field are not correlated.

1. T_2 relaxation

Consider the transverse component of the spin vector in the rotating frame. This can be done by defining an operator S_r which is the spin projection along the x' axis in the rotating frame

$$S_r = S_x \cos\omega_o t - S_y \sin\omega_o t \tag{50}$$

It follows from eqns (18a) that

$$\langle S_r \rangle = \hbar AB \cos\delta \tag{53}$$

Note that in a static field only ($\vec{B}_1 = 0$), $\langle S_r \rangle$ remains constant as expected, i.e., the transverse spin component in the rotating frame doesn't change under "free-precession."

Since T_2 is the time constant for the disappearance of the transverse spin component $\langle S_r \rangle$, we should be able to derive this rate by taking the time derivative and putting it in the form

$$\frac{d}{dt}\langle S_r \rangle = -\frac{1}{T_2}\langle S_r \rangle \tag{54}$$

The time derivative of eqn (53) is

$$\frac{d}{dt}\langle S_r \rangle = \hbar \cos\delta \frac{d}{dt}(AB) - \hbar AB \sin\delta \frac{d\delta}{dt} \quad (55)$$

Note that the first term in equation (55) involves a change in the magnitudes of a and b which you recall can only be produced by the components of the fluctuating field $\vec{B}_1$ which are perpendicular to the static field (B_{1x} and B_{1y}), whereas the second term involves a change in the phase of a and b which is produced by the fluctuating z-component of $\vec{B}_1(t)$. The first term is related to the so-called "T_1 contribution to T_2",whereas the second term is the "secular" contribution to T_2.

In order to see the effect of the second (secular) term, consider only a fluctuating z-component, in which case A and B remain constant. (For our randomly fluctuating magnetic field, it is assumed that the x,y,z components of the field are independent and can be treated separately.) Further, we will evaluate the derivative near t=0, i.e., for small values of the phase shift δ. Then, $\sin\delta \cong \delta$, and $\langle S_r \rangle \cong \langle S_r \rangle_o = \hbar AB$, hence

$$\frac{d}{dt}\langle S_r \rangle \approx -\hbar AB \delta \frac{d\delta}{dt} = -\langle S_r \rangle_o \frac{d\delta}{dt}\delta \quad (56)$$

and $\quad \dfrac{1}{T_2'} = \delta \dfrac{d\delta}{dt} \quad (57)$

where T_2' denotes the secular component of T_2. The phase shift produced by a fluctuating z-field has already been obtained in equation (24b), viz.

$$\delta = \alpha - \beta = \gamma \int_0^t B_{1z}(t)dt \quad (58)$$

Equation (58) clearly represents the accumulation of phase shift δ of the spin away from the x' axis in the rotating frame due to an extra field $B_{1z}(t)$ superimposed on the static field $\vec{B}_o$. Substituting in eqn (57)

$$\frac{1}{T_2'} = \gamma^2 B_{1z}(t) \int_0^t B_{1z}(t')dt' = \gamma^2 \int_0^t B_{1z}(t) B_{1z}(t')dt' \quad (59)$$

where t' is a dummy integration variable. For a particular spin, $B_{1z}(t)$ will have a complex form; however, what we are actually interested in is the average over the entire population of spins. The population average of the integrand in (59) for a randomly fluctuating field is generally taken to have the form of (5-8)

$$\overline{B_{1z}(t)B_{1z}(t')} = h_z^2 e^{-(t-t')/\tau_c} \quad (60)$$

where h_z^2 is the mean square z-field, and τ_c is a time constant called the correlation time.

The form of (60) can be shown [8] to follow from the diffusion equation describing the translation or rotation of molecules, i.e., the molecules are undergoing complex Brownian motion but the average behavior can be described as a diffusion. By way of analogy, in radioactive decay individual nuclei are popping off randomly, but on average the decay is described by an exponential exp $(-\lambda t)$.

The function (60) is called a correlation function. That is, the larger the difference t-t', the less correlation there is between the fields at times t and t', thus the smaller the average product in (60). The parameter τ_c is called the correlation time, and is a measure of the time over which the intramolecular magnetic fields change appreciably (by 1/e). In water at room temperature, $\tau_c \sim 10^{-12}$ sec. If (60) is substituted in (59) and the integration is performed with the integral being taken over a time large with respect to τ_c (t>>τ_c), we obtain for the secular component of T_2

$$\frac{1}{T_2'} = \gamma^2 h_z^2 \tau_c \quad (61)$$

We will return to the non-secular component of T_2 later.

2. T_1 Relaxation

The random molecular fluctuations will generate a broadband spectrum of magnetic energy from zero frequency up to a frequently of $\sim 1/\tau_c$ where τ_c is the correlation time. We will denote the magnetic energy density in this randomly fluctuating field by $J(\omega)$.

As we have seen, it is only the transverse components B_{1x} and B_{1y} of the fluctuating field which can influence the magnitudes of a and b and thence the z-component of spin with which T_1 relaxation is concerned.

In order to determine the effect of a broadband spectrum $J(\omega)$, we need to return to equations (29a) which apply to the non-resonant condition $\omega \neq \omega_0$ for an oscillating x-component $B_{1x} = 2B_1 \cos\omega t$. If we assume the spin is initially down, $a(0) = 0$, $b(0) = 1$, and solve in the time dependent perturbation theory approximation, we have near t=0, by replacing b(t) with b(0) = 1,

$$\frac{da}{dt} \approx i\frac{\omega_1}{2} e^{i(\omega-\omega_0)t} \quad (62)$$

where $\omega_1 = \gamma B_1$

Defining $\Omega=\frac{1}{2}(\omega-\omega_0)$, and integrating (62) it results that

$$a(t) = ie^{i\Omega t}\frac{\omega_1 t}{2}\frac{\sin\Omega t}{\Omega t} \qquad (63)$$

Since $|a(t)|^2$ is the probability the spin is up, then probability flows from the spin down into the spin up state at a rate

$$w = \frac{|a(t)|^2}{t} = \frac{\omega_1^2 t}{4}\frac{\sin^2\Omega t}{(\Omega t)^2} \qquad (64)$$

which represents the transition probability per unit time (and is similar to a decay constant).

The energy density in a magnetic field is $B^2/8\pi$, thus to make the connection from the monochromatic fluctuating field $B_x=2B_1\cos\omega t$ we have been considering to the continuous spectrum, we make the replacement of the time average energy density of the monochromatic field $\overline{B_x^2}/8\pi = B_1^2/4\pi$ (the time average of $\cos^2\omega t$ is $\frac{1}{2}$) with a continuous energy spectrum $J(\omega)$, such that

$$\frac{B_1^2}{4\pi} = J(\omega)d\omega \qquad (65)$$

Replacing $\omega_1^2=\gamma^2 B_1^2$ in equation (64) with $4\pi\gamma^2 J(\omega)d\omega$ from (65) and integrating over all ω, the total transition probability per unit time becomes

$$w = \pi\gamma^2 t \int_{\omega=0}^{\infty} J(\omega)\frac{\sin^2\Omega t}{(\Omega t)^2}d\omega \qquad (66)$$

Recall that $\Omega=\frac{1}{2}(\omega-\omega_0)$, and the function

$$\frac{\sin^2\Omega t}{(\Omega t)^2} \qquad (67)$$

is only large near resonance ($\Omega=0$), thus it is the value of $J(\omega)$ at ω_0 which provides the major contribution to T_1. We can, therefore, approximate (66) by pulling $J(\omega)$ outside the integral and evaluating it at w_o. Since $dw = 2d\Omega$, and since the limits of integration on Ω of $-w_o/2$ to $+\infty$ can be replaced without error to $\pm\infty$, and since

$$\int_{-\infty}^{\infty} \frac{\sin^2 x}{x^2} dx = \pi \tag{68}$$

it follows that

$$w = 2\pi^2 \gamma^2 J(w_o) \tag{69}$$

Recall that $1/T_1$ describes the rate of change of the z-component of magnetization which is related to the net <u>excess</u> of spins in the spin up state over that in the spin down state, viz. $n = N_+ - N_-$. Since every transition described by the transition rate w produces a change of the net excess n by two, then $1/T_1$ is twice w, hence

$$\frac{1}{T_1} = 4\pi^2 \gamma^2 J(w_o) \tag{70}$$

To obtain the spectral energy density of a fluctuating magnetic field $B(t)$ it is only necessary to obtain the Fourier transform of $B^2(t)/8\pi$. The random field felt by an individual spin is quite complex; however, the time dependence for an average spin can be taken as the correlation function

$$\overline{B_x(0) B_x(t)} = h_x^2 \, e^{-|t|/\tau_c} \tag{71}$$

where h_x^2 is the mean square field fluctuation for the x-component. Taking the Fourier transform, we have

$$J'(\omega) = \frac{1}{2\pi} \int_{-\infty}^{\infty} \frac{h_x^2}{8\pi} e^{-|t|/\tau_c} e^{-i\omega t} dt = \frac{h_x^2}{8\pi^2} \frac{\tau_c}{1+\omega^2 \tau_c^2} \tag{72}$$

Since the energy density $J'(\omega)$ in (72) includes negative frequencies (due to the conventional definition of the Fourier transform) and $J(w_o)$ in (70) does not admit negative frequencies, then $J(\omega) = 2J'(\omega)$, hence

$$J(\omega) = \frac{h_x^2}{4\pi^2} \frac{\tau_c}{1+\omega^2 \tau_c^2} \tag{73}$$

We have only considered the x-component of the fluctuating field in the foregoing. The y component will also contribute equally to T_1 (the z component cannot), hence eqn (70) becomes

$$\frac{1}{T_1} = (h_x^2 + h_y^2)\gamma^2 \frac{\tau_c}{1 + \omega_0^2 \tau_c^2} \qquad (74)$$

Finally, we can obtain the other (non-secular) contribution to T_2 in a simple fashion if it is realized that $1/T_2$ is a measure of the width of the magnetic resonance line in the frequency domain. That is, the time dependence of the demodulated NMR signal which is produced by the transverse component of magnetization is $\exp(-t/T_2)$. The Fourier transform of this function gives a frequency spectrum in the form of a Lorentzian line

$$f(\omega) = \frac{T_2}{1 + (\omega - \omega_0)^2 T_2^2} \qquad (75)$$

having a full width at half maximum in the frequency domain $\Delta\omega = 2/T_2$. That is, the shorter T_2, the broader the resonance line.

Due to T_1 relaxation mechanisms (a transverse fluctuating field having frequency components at the Larmor frequency) we have seen that an excited spin-down state will have a finite lifetime Δt and hence a transition will produce a line of finite width $\Delta\omega$ given by the uncertainty relation $\Delta\omega\Delta t \sim 1$ ($\Delta E \Delta t \sim \hbar$). This is called lifetime broadening. Thus, the line width and hence T_2 will clearly have a contribution from T_1 since the state lifetime is related to T_1.

In fact, we have already derived an expression for the transition probability per unit time w of an excited spin-down state (eqn 69), and we recall that $w = 1/2T_1$. The mean lifetime of the excited state is $\Delta t = 1/w$; however, we can obtain the lifetime contribution to T_2 more directly by comparing the decay of the excited state $\exp(-wt) = \exp(-t/2T_1)$ with $\exp(-t/T_2)$ above, hence it is seen that the contribution is $1/2T_1$.

That is,

$$\frac{1}{T_2} = \frac{1}{T_2'} + \frac{1}{2T_1} \qquad (76)$$

where T_2' is the previously derived secular contribution due to a spread in the z-field (equation 61). Substituting (61) and (74) in (76), we have

$$\frac{1}{T_2} = \gamma^2 h_z^2 \tau_c + \frac{1}{2}\gamma^2 (h_x^2 + h_y^2) \frac{\tau_c}{1 + \omega_0^2 \tau_c^2} \qquad (77)$$

Since we have assumed that the x,y,z components are uncorrelated and isotropic, i.e.,

$$h_o^2 = h_x^2 = h_y^2 = h_z^2 \qquad (78)$$

we can write

$$\frac{1}{T_2} = \gamma^2 h_o^2 \tau_c + \gamma^2 h_o^2 \frac{\tau_c}{1+\omega_o^2 \tau_c^2} \qquad (79)$$

$$\frac{1}{T_1} = 2\gamma^2 h_o^2 \frac{\tau_c}{1+\omega_o^2 \tau_c^2} \qquad (80)$$

Since

$$\frac{\tau_c}{1+\omega_o^2 \tau_c^2} \leq \tau_c \qquad (81)$$

it follows from (79) and (80) that $T_2 \leq T_1$. In the case of slow molecular motion (i.e., low temperatures or viscous liquids) where $\tau_c \gg 1/\omega_o$, then there is little energy in the energy spectrum at the Larmor frequency, hence T_1 is long. On the other hand, T_2 which is dominated by the first (secular) term in (79) will be short, hence $T_2 \ll T_1$, and the line width $\Delta\omega \sim 1/T_2$ will be very broad.

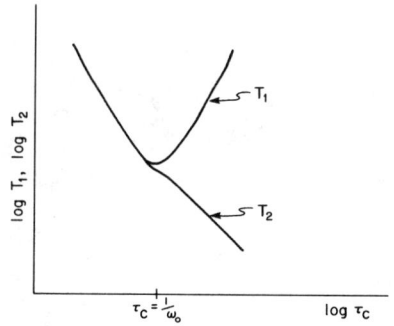

Fig. 7. Variation of relaxation times T_1 and T_2 with correlation time τ_c in a homogeneous, liquid-like medium.

As the speed of the molecules increases (τ_c decreases), T_2 will increase as shown in fig. 7, and in the limit of very rapid molecular motion where $\tau_c \ll 1/\omega_o$, $T_2 = T_1$. The line width then becomes very narrow, i.e., it is said to be "motionally narrowed." That is, in a solid, T_2 would be very short (in a way not predicted by our perturbation treatment which fails as τ_c is increased to $\tau_c \sim T_2$) due to essentially static dipolar fields dephasing the spins rapidly. For example, in ice $T_2 \sim 10$ μsec. That is, the dipole field contributed by a proton at the position of its neighbor in a rigid water molecule is $\Delta B \sim 4$ gauss. A magnetic field variation from proton to proton of $\pm \Delta B$ gives a dephasing time of $T_2 \sim 1/\gamma\Delta B = 9$μsec. If the solid is melted so that molecular tumbling is allowed, then these strong local fields are averaged out, and the line is motionally narrowed. In the case of melting ice, T_2 would jump from 10μsec to $\sim$1sec in the liquid state.

T_1 passes through a minimum at $\tau_c = 1/w_o$, as shown in fig. 7, since this correlation time produces the maximum energy density $J(w)$ at the Larmor frequency w_o. For short τ_c, T_1 is long since the total energy available in the spectrum is constant for a given temperature. That is,

$$\int_0^\infty J(\omega) d\omega = Constant$$

Since the total energy is spread out over a wider frequency range at short τ_c, there is less energy available at the Larmor frequency w_o for relaxation.

These equations have been discussed in detail elsewhere (9).

The previous simple treatment gives most of the essential features of relaxation. If a more specific model is taken, viz., the dipole-dipole coupling of the two protons in a rotating water molecule (8) where the xyz components are not independent, one obtains

$$\left(\frac{1}{T_1}\right)_{rot} = \frac{3}{10} \frac{\gamma^4 \hbar^2}{b^6} \left[j(\omega_o) + 4j(2\omega_o)\right] \quad (82)$$

$$\left(\frac{1}{T_2}\right)_{rot} = \frac{3}{20} \frac{\gamma^4 \hbar^2}{b^6} \left[3j(0) + 5j(\omega_o) + 2j(2\omega_o)\right] \quad (83)$$

where b is the proton separation distance, and $j(\omega)$ is the reduced energy density.

$$j(\omega) = \frac{\tau_c}{1 + \omega^2 \tau_c^2} \quad (84)$$

These equations are similar in form to those obtained in our previous treatment. The term $j(2w_o)$ (which is the energy density evaluated at twice the Larmor frequency) arises due to a transition in which both proton spins in the water molecular are flipped, this transition obviously requiring twice the energy of a normal single spin flip. If the rotational motion of an average molecule is described as that of a rigid sphere of radius r in a medium of viscosity η by a diffusion equation, it results that[8] the correlation time is given by $\tau_c = 4\pi\eta r^3/3kT$. There is also a translational contribution to $1/T_1$ from the spins in neighboring molecules which is of the order of one-half the rotational contribution in pure water. For further discussions of these equations, the reader is referred to references (8) and (10).

3. Relaxation in Tissues.

The preceding treatment dealt with a system in which the "sample" was microscopically homogeneous. Protons in tissue may, however, exist in a variety of environments. They may be attached to water molecules or on fat molecules or they may be bound to membranes, organelles, and other macromolecules. Protons bound in a solid-like environment such as cortical bone or on some very slowly moving macromolecules would not ordinarily be observed in an NMR experiment or image since they are not motionally narrowed and have a very short T_2, i.e., their free induction signal is gone before the receiver is active. Thus we are basically observing directly the free water component or protons in the rapidly-rotating methyl groups on some fats. The macromolecules can, however, have an effect on the relaxation of the free water molecules if there is exchange between the free and bound water components. For example, during the NMR experiment, a water molecule may briefly attach to a macromolecule where it is quickly "relaxed" and subsequently rejoin the free component to be observed again in the experiment, already "relaxed." This will have the effect of shortening the apparent relaxation time of the free water component. If the macromolecule has a correlation time τ_c closer to $1/\omega_o$ than that of the free water component, then T_1 as well as T_2 may be shortened over that of the free component alone. Relaxation in tissues has been discussed in detail in a review article by Bottomley et al.[11].

REFERENCES

1. R.L. Dixon and K.E. Ekstrand, Med. Phys. **9**, 807(1982).
2. N. Bloembergen, *Nuclear Magnetic Relaxation* (Benjamin, New York, 1961), p. 26.
3. M.E. Rose, *Elementary Theory of Angular Momentum* (Wiley, New York, 1957).
4. K. Huang, *Statistical Mechanics* (Wiley, New York, 1963) p.183.
5. Reference 1, p.81.
6. R.T. Schumacher, *Introduction to Magnetic Resonance* (Benjamin, New York, 1970) p.68.
7. C.P. Slichter, *Principles of Magnetic Resonance* (Springer-Verlag, Berlin, New York, 1980, 2nd ed.) p.166.
8. A. Abragam, *The Principles of Nuclear Magnetism* (Oxford, 1983), p.299.
9. Reference 7, p.179.

REFERENCES (Continued)

10. T.C. Farrar and E.D. Becker, <u>Pulse and Fourier Transform NMR</u> (Academic, New York, 1971) p.46.
11. P.A. Bottomley, T.H. Foster, K.E. Argersinger, and L.M. Pfeifer, Med. Phys. <u>11</u>, 425(1984).

METHODS OF RELAXATION TIME MEASUREMENTS

R. Mark Henkelman
Department of Medical Biophysics, University of Toronto
and Ontario Cancer Institute, 500 Sherbourne Street,
Toronto, Ontario Canada M4X 1K9

ABSTRACT

To understand how the signal contrast in MR imaging depends on both the relaxation times of the tissue and the pulse sequences used for the image, it is helpful to begin with an understanding of the basic pulse sequences that are used to measure relaxation times in NMR spectroscopy. This paper describes the following sequences: inversion-recovery (IR), saturation-recovery (SR), steady-state-free-precession (SSFP), Hahn spin-echo (SE), Carr-Purcell (CP), Carr-Purcell-Meiboom-Gill (CPMG), and a diffusion and motion sensitive sequence. Methods of extracting relaxation times from measured decay data are described starting with simple logarithmic plotting and increasing in complexity to analysis in terms of continuous distributions of relaxation times. The relationship of the basic sequences to MR imaging is presented. Strategies for producing T_1 and T_2 images are described and evaluated.

INTRODUCTION

Contrast in MRI is due primarily to differences in relaxation times among tissues. An exception to this generalization occurs for tissues such as cortical bone and lung where the diminished signal reflects a reduced number of protons. The brain presents a unique situation where the density of protons does not vary significantly, but the lipid protons are sufficiently tightly bound that they display T_2's which are too short to be detected by most MR imagers. Thus, it is frequently stated that there is grey-white matter contrast in the brain due to an effective decrease in proton density in the lipid-rich white material[1]. However, aside from these exceptions, most of the contrast seen in MR images arises from differences in relaxation times.

Furthermore, the signal intensity in MRI depends on the interaction between the relaxation times of the tissues and the specific parameters of the imaging process. A variety of image acquisition sequences are used in MRI to achieve different types of contrast for different clinical problems. Most of these imaging sequences are adapted from NMR spectroscopy sequences designed to measure relaxation times. Thus, a good place to begin in grasping the complexities of image contrast in MRI is to understand the basic sequences that have been used historically to measure relaxation times in NMR. This chapter provides, in a coherent manner, an introductory review of seven of the most important of these sequences.

The approach of this chapter is not intended to suggest that the purpose of MR imaging sequences is to determine tissue relaxation times. It is frequently assumed that the proton density ρ and the two relaxation times (T_1 and T_2) are the fundamental parameters that characterize the tissue under investigation, and that they represent the ultimate objective of any NMR investigation of the tissue. Such an assumption is invalid. The relaxation times and the density do represent a possible "basis set" in which differences in tissue type can be expressed. However, due to strong correlations between the relaxation times, this particular basis set is not particularly orthogonal. Differences between pathological and normal tissues are seldom optimally represented by this particular choice of basis. Furthermore, relaxation times are never measured directly in an imaging sequence, and thus they must be mathematically extracted with an associated increase in noise. The above factors all lead to the conclusion that relaxation times and proton density do not represent the most appropriate way of thinking about or characterizing contrast in clinical MRI. Nevertheless, they are a good place to start.

DEFINITIONS

For the purposes of this chapter it is appropriate to define four different relaxation times. There are more relaxation times that can be identified in different types of experiments, but this list of four is sufficient for almost all work in MRI.

T_1 - The longitudinal relaxation time.

When a spin system is at equilibrium in an external magnetic field, there is a net magnetization aligned with the external field. If this aligned magnetization is perturbed, it will recover with a time constant given by T_1. Since this recovery implies a loss of energy from the spin system - energy which is given to the material or lattice, T_1 is also referred to as the spin-lattice relaxation time.

T_2^* - The experimental transverse relaxation time.

If an aligned spin system is excited with a $\pi/2$ pulse, the net magnetization will be rotated into a plane which is transverse to the externally applied field. The transverse magnetization can be detected in this plane and will be seen to decay away in time with a time constant given by T_2^*.

Many factors contribute to this decay process:

i) return of spins to the equilibrium direction.

ii) loss of precessional coherence in the transverse plane due to chemical shifts.

iii) loss of precessional coherence due to magnetic inhomogeneities.

iv) exchange of spin excitation states within the spin system.

T_2 - The transverse relaxation time (non-recoverable).

The above description of T_2^* includes factors which are properties of the sample and also factors which are properties of the experimental technique and equipment. It is desirable, therefore, to have a transverse relaxation time which is a characteristic of the sample alone. This is designated T_2 and is sometimes called the spin-spin relaxation time. Ways to recover lost transverse magnetization due to experimental factors such as magnet inhomogeneity will be discussed in the next section.

$T_{1\rho}$ - The-spin lattice relaxation time in the rotating frame of reference.

It is often of interest to see how T_1 behaves at very low frequencies. These frequencies correspond to magnetic field strengths which are too low for direct measurements of T_1. Nonetheless, T_1 can be measured at these field strengths by applying a weak H_1 field that rotates with the Larmor frequency of the spin system. It is then possible to watch the decay of these spins locked into alignment with this H_1 field in the rotating frame of reference. The time constant associated with this relaxation is designated $T_{1\rho}$.

It needs to be appreciated that all of these relaxation times are phenomenologically introduced time constants. There is no <u>a priori</u> requirement for the decay processes to be truly exponential and thus for the time constants to be represented by a single number. This is particularly true for biological systems, as will be discussed further in this chapter.

There is a fundamental ordering between the relaxation times. T_1 is always longer than T_2 except in the case of pure liquids where it can approach T_2. This is understandable because magnetization cannot recover in the direction of the magnetic field without disappearing from the transverse plane. Similarly, T_2 is always longer than T_2^*, becoming equal only in the case of an ideal experiment.

SEQUENCES FOR MEASURING RELAXATION TIMES

Inversion-Recovery (IR)

To measure the T_1 relaxation time, the aligned magnetization is inverted using a π pulse and then, during a time TI, is allowed to recover. The amount of recovered magnetization is interrogated by tipping it into the transverse plane with a $\pi/2$ pulse and measuring the initial amplitude of the free induction decay (FID). The signal which is obtained from an IR sequence as a function of TI is initially negative for TI=0 and increases exponentially through zero to a positive asymptote for long TI values. The time constant of this recovery is T_1. The initial signal amplitude after the $\pi/2$ pulse is given by S,
$$S = M_0 [1-2 \exp(-TI/T_1)]$$

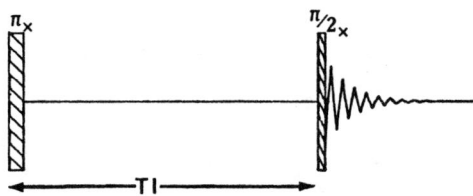

The IR sequence has twice the sensitivity range of other T_1 methods because the recovery ranges from a full negative magnetization to a full positive magnetization. The IR sequence is particularly stable with respect to imperfections in the tip angles or radiofrequency (rf) field inhomogeneities. The major disadvantage of the IR sequence is the requirement to wait at least five T_1 times between each repeat of the sequence to ensure full recovery of the aligned magnetization before the next inversion pulse. Also, the need to handle negative signals requires quadrature detection in the receiver and presents particular problems for MR imaging due to anomalous phase artifacts[2] which are encountered in most MR imagers.

Saturation-Recovery (SR)

The SR sequence avoids the requirement for full recovery between repeated experiments which makes the IR sequence so time consuming, by using the partial recovery as the method of measuring T_1. Therefore, the SR sequence is also referred to as a partial saturation (PS) sequence. $\pi/2$ pulses are repeated at a relatively short time interval TR, and the signal is proportional to the amount of spin that has recovered along the aligned position in the time TR.

$$S = M_o [1-\exp(-TR/T_1)]$$

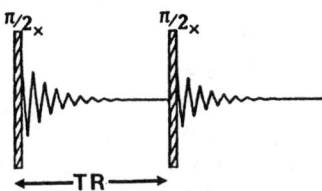

The SR sequence is attractive for MR imaging. It has a high duty cycle for data sampling and, because the signal is always positive, it avoids phase problems. The SR sequence has a factor of two less contrast range than the IR sequence, but this is often overcome by improved signal-to-noise achieved through more frequent sampling. SR is not a particularly good technique for investigating the detailed shape of the longitudinal relaxation process since it is quite sensitive to irregularities in tip angle.

Steady-State-Free-Precession (SSFP)

If the TR time in the SR sequence becomes comparable to T_2, the FID does not completely decay before the arrival of the next $\pi/2$ pulse resulting in an interference phenomenon. If a simple chain of $\pi/2$ pulses is used, the interference is destructive, but if the $\pi/2$ pulses have alternating phases, it is constructive interference. This is the SSFP sequence which allows for a very high duty cycle but gives a signal intensity which has a dependence on the ratio of T_1 and T_2.

$$S = M_o \frac{1-\exp(-TR/T_1)}{1-\exp(-TR/T_1)\exp(-TR/T_2)} \approx M_o [1+T_1/T_2]^{-1}$$

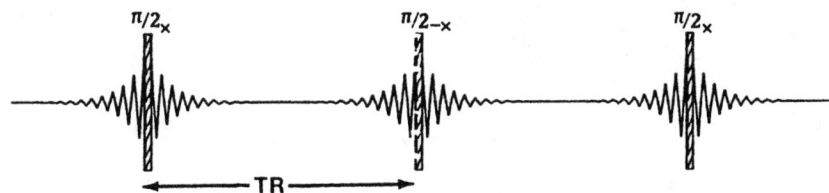

The SSFP sequence was used in some of the initial work in imaging, but because it gives poor tissue contrast it has been largely abandoned.

Hahn Spin-Echo (SE)

It was recognized early in the development of NMR that the decay time T_2^*, following a simple $\pi/2$ pulse, was shorter with greater inhomogeneity of the static magnetic field. This arises from the fact that spins in different fields have different precessional frequencies. Thus, following the $\pi/2$ pulse, the different components of the magnetization precess in phase and coherently add their contribution to the total detected magnetization. However, after a short time, the spin components get out of phase because of their different precessional frequencies, and the incoherent addition of the component magnetizations produces a zero net transverse magnetization. Thus, T_2^* is shortened by field inhomogeneities.

It was recognized by Hahn, that provided the dephasing was deterministic, the lost signal could be recovered by the formation of an echo[3]. By flipping the transverse plane over through the application of a π pulse at some time TE/2 after the initial $\pi/2$ pulse, magnetization components that had accumulated an advanced phase rotation of Φ radians with respect to some arbitary reference would then appear to be retarded by a phase angle Φ immediately following the application of the π pulse. During the next time interval TE/2, these magnetization components would recover their phase retardation because they would still be precessing faster than the reference. Therefore, at a total time TE following the $\pi/2$ pulse, all the magnetization components, whatever their phase deviation, are back in phase and contributing coherently to the total measured transverse magnetization.

Magnetization loss due to inhomogeneities or chemical shifts will be recovered by such an echo sequence provided the differing precessional frequencies remain constant over the full time interval TE. If the spins move to a different magnetic field because of flow or diffusion, or if they move to a different chemical environment through proton exchange, or even if the excited spin exchanges with the spin of a different nucleus, then the magnetization cannot be fully recovered in the echo. The decay of the echo peak amplitude due to non-recoverability, other than that due to flow or diffusion, is a measure of the T_2 relaxation time. Thus, the signal strength of the echo formed at time TE is given by

$$S = -M_0 \exp(-TE/T_2)$$

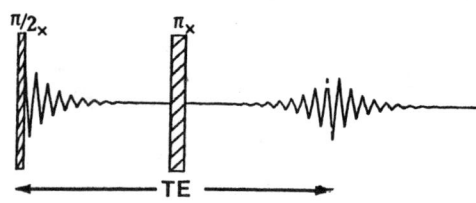

The Hahn spin-echo sequence is the basic sequence for the estimation of T_2 and it has the added advantage for imaging applications in that it allows the signal to be measured in a quiet time interval which is well removed from any high power transmitter pulse. However, there are several extensions and modifications which improve this basic SE sequence that are discussed next.

Carr-Purcell (CP)

Once it is understood how a single echo is formed, it is easy to appreciate that this process can be repeated multiple times after a single $\pi/2$ pulse producing a multi-echo sequence. This sequence was first proposed by Carr and Purcell[4] who discovered that in liquids, longer T_2 values were obtained using the CP sequence than the SE sequence. This difference arises from diffusion. In the SE sequence, movement of the spins through the inhomogeneity must be negligible over the time interval TE, which becomes unrealistic for long TE's. With the CP sequence, where long total times are produced using the nth echo and a comparatively short TE for each echo, the diffusion need only be insignificant over each TE interval. A new reference point for dephasing is established at each echo. Thus, the CP sequence gives a measure of T_2 which is less dependent on diffusional effects. The measured signal at the nth echo is given by

$$S = (-1)^n M_0 \exp(-nTE/T_2)$$

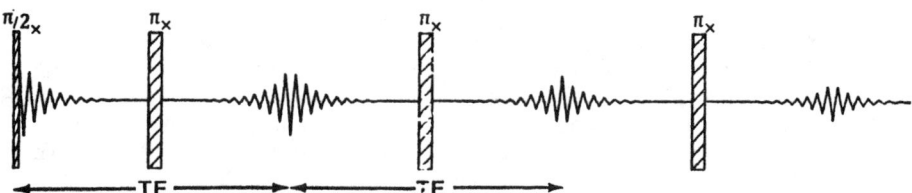

The CP sequence is much more efficient than SE for mapping the T_2 decay because a number of different time points are sampled at each repeat of the experiment. However, the sequence requires stringent accuracy of the π pulses.

Carr-Purcell-Meiboom-Gill (CPMG)

Meiboom and Gill[5] proposed a simple modification to the CP sequence which relaxes the stringency of the π pulses. In the CP sequence, if the $\pi/2$ pulse rotates the magnetization about the x axis, it is assumed that the subsequent π pulses will also rotate the magnetization further about the x axis. If there is a tip angle error in the π pulse, this error will accumulate, resulting in the magnetization being further and further out of the transverse plane. To circumvent this, the MG modification applies the π pulses along the y axis. This still flips over the transverse plane causing an echo to be formed but has two other advantages. The magnetization always rephases along +y giving a string of positive echoes. Errors in the tip angle of the π pulse cancel out with alternate echoes. The signal intensity at the nth echo is given by

$$S = M_o \exp(-nTE/T_2)$$

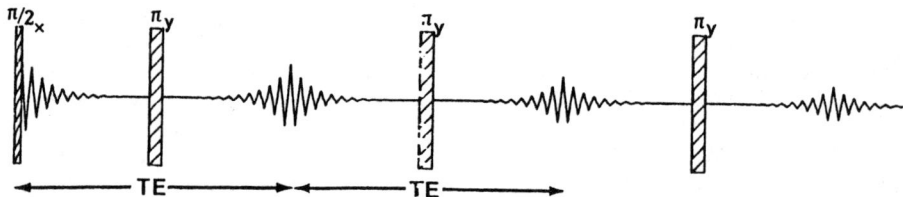

The MG modification can also be applied to the SE sequence with the effect of producing a positive echo.

CPMG is thus the sequence of choice for measuring T_2 in magnetic resonance imaging. It is not, however, without additional problems when it comes to being applied to imaging with selective pulses and gradients, some of which will be dealt with in later chapters.

A Diffusion Specific Sequence

In our discussion of NMR sequences for the measurement of relaxation times, diffusion and motion have come up several times as factors that produce an underestimate of T_2. Since diffusion and flow are important factors in MRI, we present here a sequence which specifically measures diffusion through the use of a known applied gradient. There are many possible diffusion sensitive sequences but they are variants on this basis theme.

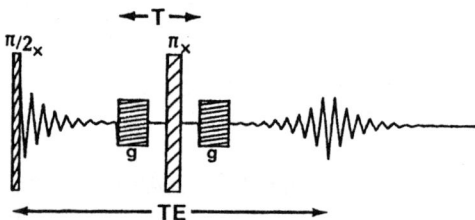

The sequence is a basic SE sequence with gradients of magnitude g applied for a duration t before and after the π pulse. Spins which do not move in the direction of the gradient will be uneffected by these gradients. However, spins which move in the direction of the gradient will be dephased, resulting in a lower signal with the gradients than when the gradients are not turned on.

The ratio of the signals in these two situations is given by

$$S(\text{gradient on})/S(\text{gradient off}) = \exp[-(\gamma gt)^2 TD]$$

where T is the time between the starts of the gradients and D is the diffusion coefficient[6].

The above section has presented a series of seven basic NMR sequences that are used for the measurement of relaxation times. Some of the relative strengths and weaknesses of each sequence have been pointed out. Many other variants of these basic sequences have been proposed but they are readily understood from the concepts described above.

ANALYSIS OF RELAXATION DATA

The sequences described in the preceding section give sets of data which describe the relaxation processes. If the decay or recovery process is exponential, a single relaxation time can be extracted from the data. There are several ways to do this. The simplest is a semi-logarithmic plot which transforms the data to a straight line that can be fit by eye. A difficulty with this approach is that the zero baseline in the case of T_2, or the equilibrium magnetization M_o in the case of T_1, must be accurately known. Obtaining accurate knowledge of the asymptotic values of a relaxation process is often the most difficult and time consuming part of an accurate relaxation experiment. An alternative graphical approach, which avoids the problem of asymptotes is that due to Mangelsdorf[7] in which the values of the magnetization at time t are plotted versus the values at a delayed time t+Δt. For exponential decays, this graph generates a straight line with a slope of exp (-Δt/T) where T is the relaxation time.

A more direct approach to obtain a relaxation time is to perform a non-linear least squares fit to the data, extracting simultaneously the time constant, the background and M_o. Most computer statistical packages provide standard programs capable of performing such fits as well as providing error estimates for the relaxation time.

In analysing relaxation data from biological tissues, it is frequently observed that a single exponential does not satisfactorily represent the data. It is then tempting to use two or more exponential components. Only those who have made serious and critical attempts to extract multi-exponential components will know what a quagmire this approach can be. In particular, the actual values of relaxation times and the magnitude of the components are usually excessively sensitive to small changes in the data, such as deletion of a few initial data points.

An alternative and much more powerful approach to the analysis of relaxation data obtained from tissue is to acknowledge right at the outset the heterogeneous nature of tissue and, therefore, anticipate continuous distributions of relaxation times.

Mathematical tools are available for such analysis[8]. Results of
this approach to analysing relaxation data are much more robust
with respect to small changes in the data. The figure shows T_1

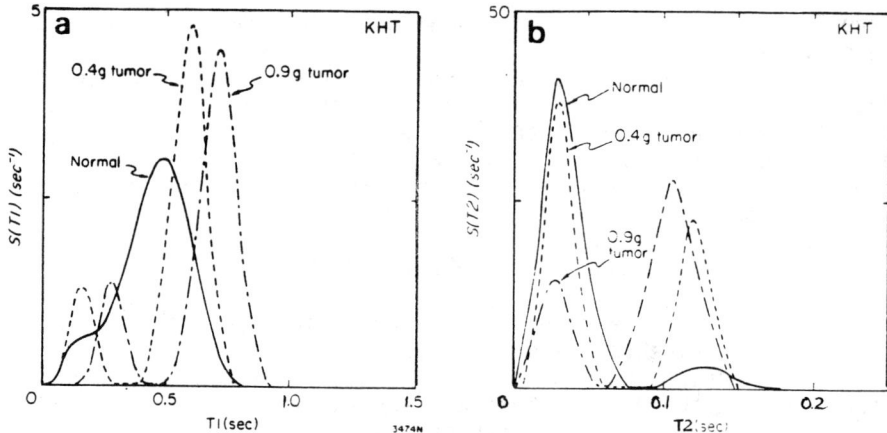

(a) Comparison of three in vivo measurements of T_1
during the course of tumour growth. Shown are
continuum analyses for a normal, healthy mouse,
and the same mouse when the tumour weighed 0.4
and 0.9 g. (b) Comparison of three in vivo
measurements of T_2 during the same course of
tumour growth.

and T_2 relaxation time distributions measured in vivo of a mouse
tumour as it grows. For both the longitudinal and transverse
relaxation times, the mean time increases as the tumour grows. For
T_1 there is an overall increase in the relaxation times of the
components, but for T_2 the increase arises from a redistribution
of spins into the longer relaxation time components. The specific
nature of these different components is still to be determined.
However, the analysis of biological relaxation data in terms of
continuous distributions of relaxation times appears to be a
fruitful field of investigation.

SEQUENCES APPLIED TO MR IMAGING

When the sequences described above are applied to imaging,
there are a number of adaptations and constraints that are imposed
by the medical application. The most serious of these constraints
is time, imposed by a requirement to have most imaging sequences
completed in a maximum of ten minutes. Most of the basic sequences
described above assume that a long time is allowed to elapse
between repeat experiments. A long time in this situation is
usually 5 to 7 times T_1 to allow complete recovery of the

magnetization to occur between experiments. Such a luxury cannot be allowed in medical imaging where any number from 128 to 512 repeated experiments are required to produce an image. Therefore, in imaging, repeat measurements are sampled with incomplete recovery causing the initial magnetization M_o to depend on the time allowed for recovery.

A second adaptation in the application to imaging is that data is almost always recorded from a spin-echo even in IR and SR sequences. As has been mentioned above, this allows the received signal to be measured during a quiet interval well away from the ringing introduced in the receiver coil by any excitation pulse.

These two adaptations limit the most popular imaging pulse sequences to a spin-echo (SE) sequence which may include multi-echoes generated from a CPMG sequence. This SE sequence is often referred to as an SR sequence when it uses a short TR even though it is implemented using an echo. The other popular sequence for imaging is an inversion spin-echo (ISE) sequence which is an IR sequence followed by an SE sequence for data acquisition. Again, the repeat time is seldom long enough to allow complete recovery of equilibrium magnetization.

The signal intensity obtained for each of these adapted imaging sequences is given by the following expressions,

$$S_{SE} = kM_o\, e^{-TE/T2}[1-2e^{-(TR-TE/2)/T1} + e^{-TR/T1}]$$

$$S_{ISE} = KM_o\, e^{-TE/T2}[1-2e^{-TI/T1}+2e^{-(TR-TE/2)/T1}-e^{-TR/T1}]$$

where k is a constant that takes into account the sensitivity, gains and normalizations of the particular imaging system. These equations differ slightly from others reported in the literature in that the longitudinal magnetization is considered to be zero immediately following the $\pi/2$ pulse rather than at the centre of the echo. These equations have been shown to hold to an accuracy of better than 10% over a realistic range of imaging and tissue parameters (9). However, systematic differences occurred under two conditions: i) SE pulse sequences with short TR showed lower signal intensity than anticipated from the equations, and ii) the apparent T_2 of the sample was reduced from its actual value as measured using CPMG in a spectrometer due to effects of the imaging gradients. Further deviations are also observed on most imaging systems when multi-slice and multi-echo options are exercised due to interference between the slices. However, the equations presented above are a sufficiently accurate description of the intensity achieved in an imager for most specific applications.

Sequences have been designed to give estimated T_1 and T_2 maps on a pixel by pixel basis. These sequences will be discussed in more detail in a later chapter, but are presented here for completeness. Sequences designed to estimate T_1 are usually based on 2-point measurements since time cannot be afforded to measure complete recovery curves. The two points are usually either an ISE and SE pair or two SE sequences with different TR times. The data could be acquired as sequential images, but it is preferable to interleave the data acquisition to minimize problems with registration. Estimated T_2 images are usually derived from CPMG sequences in which an exponential is fitted to the multi-echo decay curve. Estimates of T_2 from two echoes only are unreliable because even-numbered echoes diminish motion sensitive terms whereas odd echoes do not. Considerable care must be exercised in the use of T_1 and T_2 MR imaging sequences to determine the accuracy and applicability of the estimates. Quantitative relaxation time images in a routine and reliable manner await further refinements in MRI.

CONCLUSIONS

A series of 7 different pulse sequences or modifications that are used to measure relaxation times in NMR have been presented. Methods of analysis of the decay data obtained using these sequences have been discussed and their applications to MR imaging have been outlined.

REFERENCES

1. F.W. Wehrli, J.R. MacFall, T.H. Newton. Modern Neuroradiology Advanced Imaging Techniques. ed. T.H. Newton and D.G. Potts. Clavadel Press (1983).
2. E. McVeigh, R.M. Henkelman, M.J. Bronskill. Submitted to Medical Physics (1985).
3. E.L. Hahn. Phys. Rev. 80, 580-594 (1950).
4. H. Carr and E.M. Purcell. Phys. Rev. 94, 630-638 (1954).
5. S. Meiboom and D. Gill. Rev. Sci. Instrum. 29, 688-691 (1958).
6. J.R. Manning. Diffusion Kinetics for Atoms in Crystals. D. Van Nostrand, Princeton (1968).
7. P.C. Mangelsdorf, Jr. J. Appl. Phys. 30, 442-443 (1959).
8. S.W. Provencher. Comput. Phys. Commun. 27, 213-227 (1982).
9. P. Hardy, M.J. Bronskill, R.M. Henkelman. Medical Physics (1985) in press.

PULSE SEQUENCES FOR MAGNETIC RESONANCE IMAGING

Peter M. Joseph

University of Pennsylvania, Philadelphia, PA, 19104

ABSTRACT

The basic principle behind all NMR imaging techniques is the use of field gradients to establish a position dependence to the signal. These can be classified according to the dimensionality of the volume of space from which signals will be received; specifically, from points, lines, planes, or volumes. The larger the volume of spins which contribute to each measurement, the better is the signal to noise ratio. In medical NMR imaging, a version of the sensitive plane method using two dimensional Fourier transforms is commonly used. The plane of interest is selected by a shaped RF pulse in combination with a Z gradient. The X direction is encoded by the frequency of the received signal and the Y by its phase. A spin echo is commonly used to minimize the effects of field inhomogeneities. The standard pulse sequences can produce images whose information content is primarily proton density, T1, or T2 depending on the values of the echo time and repetition time used. Inversion recovery can also be used to provide stronger T1 contrast in the images.

INTRODUCTION

Most often, the techniques which are useful for performing magnetic resonance imaging (MRI) can be considered as an adjunct to those used to provide signals which are not localized spatially. For example, most imaging techniques can be applied to pulse sequences which are basically saturation recovery (SR), inversion recovery (IR), spin echo (SE), etc. The major way in which MRI pulse sequences differ from traditional NMR pulse sequences is the application of various field gradient pulses. Indeed, the application of gradients as a technique of spatial localization, due originally to Lauterbur[1], forms the essence of virtually all MRI techniques. The main point of this chapter is to review the various methods of doing this. For further mathematical details, the reader is referred to the excellent article by Hinshaw and Lent[2].

The usage of gradients can be analyzed into three

classes: those used in synchrony with radiofrequency (RF) pulses to selectively excite a group of spins, those used during signal acquisition (SA) as a so-called "read out" gradient, and those imposing a "spin warp" or phase shift on the spins as a function of spatial coordinates with neither RF fields nor SA operating. While there are many very different ways in which these procedures can be combined to produce MRI, they can be classified according to the dimensionality of the volume element which is initially excited by the RF pulse. That is, the spatial selectivity can be achieved through some combination of the three uses of the applied field gradients. We can therefore begin by classifying the MRI technique according to the dimensionality of the volume element excited by the RF pulse. Specifically, we can speak of a "sensitive point", "sensitive line", "sensitive plane", or "sensitive volume" as discussed by Brunner and Ernst[3].

The sensitive point method, which has been studied by Hinshaw[4], is perhaps the easiest to understand for someone without a background in image reconstruction. The idea is based on the principle that a small region of space can be selected by applying oscillating gradients in each of the three mutually perpendicular directions, X,Y,Z. This is done in such a way that the field rapidly oscillates at all points except at the particular point X_o, Y_o, Z_o. Thus, only protons located at the favored point will radiate at a unique frequency and can be selected by appropriate filtering of the received signal. This point can be considered to be a single pixel in the final image. The whole image is obtained by simply moving the sensitive point in space in such a way as to scan the desired region of the patient's anatomy.

The only situation in which the sensitive point method is advantageous is when high quality spectra are desired from a very limited region of the body [5]. As a technique for obtaining an image of an entire plane or volume of tissue, it has the serious disadvantage of great inefficiency in terms of the signal to noise ratio (SNR) obtainable per unit scan time. As we shall see later, the SNR is directly related to the volume of tissue contributing to <u>each</u> signal measurement. Hence, it is clear that the sensitive point method is the least efficient of the various methods considered, and is no longer used in clinical imaging.

SENSITIVE LINE METHODS

The sensitive line method is an improvement over the sensitive point in that signals are obtained from a line of pixels at each time rather than from just one. This method, developed by Mansfield and Maudsley[6,7], is not commonly used because the SNR is still inferior to that of the various sensitive plane methods.

SELECTIVE EXCITATION OF A PLANE

The first step in any two dimensional planar method is to selectively excite the plane of interest. Qualitatively, the concept is simple: apply a gradient g_z in the Z direction while simultaneously applying an RF pulse which has been shaped to have some desirable frequency spectrum. Thus, resonant frequency will depend on z according to

$$w(z) = g_z z \quad (1)$$

where we have for simplicity taken the gyromagnetic ratio as unity. Meanwhile, the RF pulse, whose strength at time t is $B_1(t)$, will have a spectral strength at frequency w given by

$$\tilde{B}_1(w)$$

where $\tilde{B}_1$ is the fourier transform (FT) of B_1. For nonselective pulses, the Bloch equations show that the strength of B_1 is directly proportional to the rate of turning of the magnetization vector; that is, flip angle is proportional to B_1. As proposed by Hutchison et al[8], in a selective excitation the flip angle for protons at position z should be similarly proportional to the strength of B_1 evaluated at the frequency corresponding to z. Thus using an RF waveform whose frequency components are approximately confined to a limited range of frequencies should excite only those spins within a similar range of z, whose dimensions are determined by the gradient strength and equation (1). This is approximately true as long as the flip angle is small, but fails badly when the desired flip angle is greater than 90 degrees. (See Joseph et al[5] for further discussion.) Nevertheless, since many MRI techniques call for flip angles not exceeding 90 degrees, the method is satisfactory and is widely used.

The combination of RF pulse and Z gradient pulse needed

to implement this technique is illustrated in figures 1 and 2. Figure 1 illustrates the use of a "sinc" pulse (sinc(x) is defined as sin(x)/x), whose FT is uniform across a finite bandwidth and zero outside, to achieve a uniform excitation of spins within the desired slice. Figure 2 illustrates a complete spin warp pulse sequence, in which the selective excitation can be seen as the first step. Note that it is necessary to follow the sinc pulse with a Z gradient of negative amplitude. This is needed to bring the group of excited spins into phase, since the selective excitation, even when theoretically uniform in flip angle, nevertheless induces a phase shift on the spins which is approximately proportional to the Z position[10].

Once the desired plane has been selectively excited, we can consider that the problem is essentially in two dimensions: how to determine the density of equilibrium magnetization, $M_o(x,y)$, at point (x,y). There have been two methods successfully applied to this problem: projection reconstruction (PR) and two dimensional fourier transformation (2DFT).

PROJECTION RECONSTRUCTION

The basic principle of two dimensional projection reconstruction (2DPR) is that if the NMR signal is received while a gradient G is applied whose direction lies in the X,Y plane, then the signal is proportional to the projection of M_o along the direction of G. This can be most easily seen by relating the detected signal to the phase of the magnetization, M, in a frame rotating at the Larmor frequency corresponding to no gradient. Using the usual notation in which the transverse components of M are written as a complex phasor:

$$m(x,y) = M_x(x,y) + i\, M_y(x,y), \tag{3}$$

the application of a gradient G will alter the frequency as described by:

$$m(x,y) \longrightarrow m(x,y)\, \exp(-i\, G\cdot r\, t), \tag{4}$$

that is, the frequency is altered by an amount proportional to the displacement, r, along the direction of G. The total signal received is then proportional to the spatial integral of equation (4):

$$V(t) = \int\int m(x,y)\, \exp(-i\, G\cdot r\, t)\, dx\, dy \tag{5}.$$

The essential step in most MRI techniques is to compute
the FT of the voltage V(t) and obtain its temporal
frequency distribution. It is straight forward to show
that the FT of equation (5) leads an integral projection
of m(x,y) onto the direction of G.

Projection reconstruction works by repeating the pulse
sequence N times, each time with a different set of x and
y gradient strengths such that the vector G makes
uniformly spaced steps in angle, with constant magnitude
|G|, so as to obtain a set of projections of m(x,y)
which can be reconstructed using algorithms already well
established in computed tomography [11,12]. In fact, this
was basically the method used by Lauterbur [1].

The main disadvantage of projection reconstruction for
MRI lies in its sensitivity to imperfections in the data;
relatively minor field imperfections lead to streak type
artifacts. These problems are essentially the same as
those experienced in X-ray computed tomography (CT)
scanning, where either machine imperfections or patient
motion commonly lead to streak artifacts [13].

TWO DIMENSIONAL FOURIER METHODS

Whereas in x-ray CT the physics of the problem limits us
to obtaining data which are projections of the unknown
density, in MRI it is possible by using gradients to
obtain signals which carry information about specific
spatial frequencies of the unknown m(x,y). This can be
done by applying, _before_ the signals are read out, a
gradient which will induce a phase shift on the m vector
which is a function of position. That is, equation (4)
also describes the effect of such a gradient, where the
time "t" is now considered as a fixed time interval,
unrelated to the time during signal readout.

The pulse sequence for the most common such scheme, known
as "spin warp", [14], is illustrated in figure 2. Note that
the Y gradient is pulsed before the signal is read out,
while the X gradient is turned on during SA. In the
special case where the Y gradient is zero, such data is
obviously equivalent to a projection of m(x,y) onto the X
axis. In general, the presence of a Y gradient of
strength g_y acting for time period T_y will impose a
corresponding phase shift on the m distribution, so that
the received signal will be proportional to

$$V(t) = \int \int m(x,y) \exp(-i\, g_y T_y) \exp(-i\, g_x t)\, dxdydz \quad (6).$$

Equation (6) clearly shows that the signal is proportional to the two dimensional FT of m(x,y), evaluated at the spatial frequency whose coordinates are $g_y T_y$ and $g_x t$. Note that whereas T_y is fixed for each pulse prior to readout, t is the actual time variable during readout. Thus each instant of time during readout corresponds to a specific x component <u>spatial</u> frequency of the object.

There is one subtlety which warrants discussion. Figure 2 shows that there is a second RF pulse applied, without gradients, which acts as a 180 degree pulse to produce a spin echo in the signal at a time, TE, after the 90 degree pulse. Such a spin echo technique is not necessary but does provide certain advantages. Obviously, when a delayed spin echo signal is desired so that, for biophysical reasons, a strong T2 weighting is desired in the image, such a pulse is necessary. However, even when short echo times are desired the use of a spin echo is advantageous because it tends to mitigate the effects of inhomogeneities in the main magnetic field. A second aspect is the use of a "prephasing" x gradient pulse applied before the 180 degree pulse. This has the effect of imposing a phase factor of $\exp(-i g_x T_y)$ on the distribution, which is converted to a similar phase distribution of opposite sign by the 180 degree pulse. The effect of this is that during the first half of the data readout period the signal represents <u>negative</u> x spatial frequencies. That is, as time evolves during the readout process, the x spatial frequencies evolve from a negative maximum through zero to a positive maximum. Since both positive and negative spatial frequencies are needed for image reconstruction, this trick essentially doubles the rate at which the necessary data are obtained.

In summary, the y gradient is pulsed at a different strength during each of the N pulses necessary to reconstruct an NxN pixel image, whereas all spatial frequencies are obtained in the x direction during each pulse. This asymmetry in data collection has resulted in the nomenclature of "phase encoding" for the y direction and "frequency encoding" for the x direction. In particular, any errors in data which are a function of frequency, such as the chemical shift effect [15,16], will appear as a shift in the x direction. Similarly, any errors in the relative phase of the signal between different pulses (which in practice means almost any error whatsoever which varies from pulse to pulse) will manifest as a phase error and produce streaks along the phase encoding direction. (Obviously, the role of the x and y axes could be interchanged, and scanners which use frequency encoding in the y direction and phase encoding in the x direction do exist.)

In present clinical practice, this method or a variation of it is widely employed to produce images whose resolution typically varies from 128x128 to 256x256 pixels. One popular choice of parameters is to use 256 frequency encoded measurements but only 128 phase encodings. The rationale for this asymmetric resolution is that, while the increased x resolution is "free" in terms of scanning time (requiring only a faster SA circuit), the scan time is directly proportional to the number of phase encodings. Typical scan times are a few minutes for such a scan.

With a repetition time (TR) of, say, 200 milliseconds, it is entirely possible to collect the data needed for a high resolution scan in a fraction of a minute. However, such a technique usually produces images which are too noisy for clinical diagnosis. Therefore what is commonly done is to repeat each phase encoding pulse a small number of times and average the resulting signal measurements.

THREE DIMENSIONAL SCANNING

From the theoretical point of view, the most noise efficient method of scanning is one that, during each measurement, samples useful signal from the entire volume being scanned. The reason for this is that the noise involved is purely electronic and has no relationship to the volume of nuclear spins which have been excited. In so-called "true" three dimensional methods, the 90 degree exciting pulse is non selective, i.e., is applied without any gradients and excites all of the protons within the volume of the transmitter RF coil.

There are several techniques which are capable of three dimensional scanning and reconstruction. The most obvious is a straight forward generalization of the two dimensional spin warp method; i.e., the Z direction can be phase encoded in a way identical to that used for the Y direction in the two dimensional case [17]. This is typically used with a relatively small number of Z phase encodings (in the range of 8 to 32), so as to provide data leading to that number of slices. The scanning time is obviously proportionally longer than a single scan; however, the SNR is better by a factor of the square root of the number of slices, so that no repetitions of any pulses are needed for noise reduction. In other words, while the scanner will need, say, 8 minutes to obtain 16 slices, <u>each</u> slice will have a SNR equivalent to that of a single two dimensional scan with 16 repetitions of each phase encoding pulse.

While this method has been applied in clinical MRI scanning, it is often observed that the image quality is inferior to that obtainable in 2DFT scans. The major problem is that the definition of the slice profile from a limited number of Z phase encodings does not permit a clean profile to be obtained. That is, the Gibbs phenomenon of fourier series results in considerable overlap of spillover from one slice into its neighbors. This problem can be overcome by appropriately filtering the data as a function of Z spatial frequency [17], but at the cost of doubling scanning time for a given number of slices and SNR.

A very sophisticated type of three dimensional technique, proposed by Shepp [18], involves no phase encoding but rather interprets the data obtained while the readout gradient G is applied as representing a series of measurements of proton density integrated over <u>planes</u>, as opposed to lines as in two dimensional PR. For each pulse, the direction of G is varied in the two angle coordinates of spherical coordinates, i.e., the vector G must sample the whole 4 pie of solid angle of a sphere. It can be shown that the unknown density $m(x,y,z)$ can be reconstructed from such data in a manner analogous to that used for 2DPR. This method is called "isotropic" 3D scanning because the spatial resolution obtained is necessarily the same in the x,y, and z directions. Thus it is possible to reconstruct, from a single such scan, any plane whatsoever which cuts through the sensitive volume. The method has not found wide acceptance in clinical practice, partly because it requires that a large number of scans be obtained before any image can be viewed (and therefore requires exceptional patient cooperation) and partly because such high isotropic resolution throughout the entire volume is rarely needed.

MULTIPLANAR TWO DIMENSIONAL METHODS

To date, the most popular scanning technique appears to be the so-called multiplanar two dimensional method. This is essentially a modification of the spin warp method which utilizes the time between pulses, during which the previously excited spins are relaxing toward the equilibrium M_o with time constant T1, to obtain data from spins in <u>adjacent</u> slices. The major modification to the pulse sequence shown in figure 2 is the conversion of the 180 degree spin echo RF pulse from a nonselective to a selective type. That is, a Z gradient pulse is applied together with the 180 degree RF pulse. This has the effect of causing a refocusing of only those spins lying within the Z slice selected by the 90 degree pulse. In this way, both the excitation and the spin echo production are spatially selective, so that another slice can be excited and interrogated while the first set of spins is relaxing. The method is obviously generalizable to more than two slices, and 8 to 10 slices are commonly imaged "simultaneously" in this way. This method essentially achieves the high noise reduction efficiency of the three dimensional methods without their various disadvantages.

It should be noted, however, that there are aspects to the use of a selective 180 degree pulse which have not yet been theoretically clarified. In particular, it is known that selective 180 degree pulses for spin inversion are notoriously ineffective[3]. A recent application of selective 180 degree pulses to chemical shift imaging[15] shows that linear fourier transform theory is not a reliable guide to the behavior of the spin system. It is not known at present whether these non linear effects cause significant errors in the quantitative aspects of multislice MRI scans.

ECHO PLANAR METHODS

The term "echo planar" was coined by Mansfield and Pykett[19] to describe a method for very rapidly carrying out the phase encodings necessary for 2DFT MRI. The essence of the idea is to obtain all phase encodings from a single pulse by rapidly switching the gradients between positive and negative values. Each time the x gradient is so switched, another spin echo will form. Meanwhile, the Y gradient has been allowed to increase so that a new Y spatial frequency is obtained. The clever aspect of the Mansfield and Pykett approach was their method of reducing the intrinsically two dimensional nature of the spatial frequency data to a single (large) one dimensional FT.

The most significant drawback of this approach is the requirement that the various phase encodings represent a single object; that is, any source of signal variation from the first to the last echo will be interpreted as Y spatial information. This means that the data must be obtained in a time short compared with both the T2 of the tissue and the T2* of the magnetic field. To date, it has been used to obtain low resolution images of the thorax.

NOISE AND RESOLUTION CONSIDERATIONS

For any of the MRI techniques discussed, the spatial resolution obtained is obviously proportional to the strength of the gradients used; this follows directly from the relationship

$$w = g.r \qquad (7)$$

so that a frequency change is directly translatable into a spatial displacement. From this it follows that, in principle, there is no lower limit to the size of voxel which can be resolved. However, as gradient strength is increased to improve spatial resolution, the _image_ SNR worsens (for a given SNR in the measured data). This is most easily understood by considering that the magnitude of the noise voltage is independent of the gradient strength, and therefore appears in the image as a certain noise power distributed over the number of pixels. Increasing g, by spreading a given object signal over a number of pixels proportional to g^2, thus decreases the SNR by the same factor of g^2. As we have noted, this decrease in SNR can be cancelled by increasing scanning time by a factor proportional to g^4.

In the case of spin warp imaging, it can be shown that the root mean square (rms) noise in the image is proportional to

$$\text{image noise} = \text{constant}/(\ dx \ \ dy \ dz \ /\sqrt{T(SA)}), \qquad (8)$$

where dx, dy and dz are the dimensions of the image voxels in the x, y, and z directions, and T(SA) is the _total_ time spent in signal acquisition. The constant includes such factors as receiver coil Q, filling factor, and amplifier noise figure, but is _independent_ of gradient strength and N, the number of pixels. Equation (8) shows that the fundamental parameters controlling image SNR are not N or g, but the voxel size and data acquisition time. The latter can be increased either by repeating the pulses, utilizing multiple spin echoes per pulse, or using a longer SA time on each pulse. All of these techniques are commonly used in clinical MRI scanners.

EFFECT OF RELAXATION TIMES

MRI images are commonly displayed in such a way that increased signal appears as increased brightness in the image. It is not always true, however, that the signal strength in a pixel reflects only the equilibrium magnetization, M_o, in that pixel. In fact, most clinically relevant NMR information is in the relative values of the relaxation times, T1 and T2, in the various tissues. Most commonly, the MRI pulse sequences are adjusted so as to emphasize either the T1 or T2 aspects, and are said to be "T1 weighted" or "T2 weighted".

T1 weighting is most easily produced by the so-called "partial saturation" or "saturation recovery" pulse sequence. This consists of simply repeating the basic spin warp pulses with a repetition time (TR) significantly less than T1. The magnitude of the signal so produced is, assuming that the 90 degree pulse has no error, given by

$$V = (1 - \exp(-TR/T1) \exp(-TE/T2) M_o. \qquad (9)$$

In such a scheme, shorter T1 values result in a __stronger__ signal, because the spins can more effectively recover between pulses. Such scans must be done with TE as short as possible, and certainly short compared with T2. A desirable choice might be TE = 10 ms, but few clinical scanners can achieve such short echo times; TE of 28 to 35 ms seem to be more common. It must be noted, therefore, that since the T2's of many tissues are as short as 60 to 70 ms, such "T1 weighted" scans may, in fact, contain considerable T2 weighting as well.

In some cases, it is desirable to ascertain whether an anomalous signal strength, as seen in partial saturation, is due to a change in T1 or spin density. This is easily done by increasing TR to be much longer than T1, so as to obtain a so-called "proton density" scan. The same qualifications on TE apply here, of course.

This technique is easily modified to produce T2 weighted images by simply making TR >> T1 and increasing TE to a value comparable with T2, typically about 100 ms. This technique has proved extremely useful in diagnosing pathology in the white matter of the brain, and especially for identifying the edema which often surrounds pathological tissue in that organ. By obtaining scans at 2 or more values of TE the actual value of T2 of each pixel can be obtained, using equation (9).

In situations where maximal differentiation between tissues of differing T1 is desired, such as distinguishing grey and white matter in the brain, the best choice is usually an inversion recovery pulse sequence. This is obtained by preceding the standard spin warp pulse by a 180 degree pulse, which can be either selective or non selective. A time interval TI is allowed to elapse between the inverting pulse and the subsequent (selective) 90 degree pulse. The resulting signal voltage is proportional to

$$V = (1 - 2 \exp(-TI/T1)) \exp(-TE/T2) M_o \quad (10).$$

Equation (10) is valid in the limit in which TR >> T1, so that relaxation recovery is complete between pulses. Such a scan produces excellent contrast between tissues of differing T1 and has very low noise because the long TR allows full recovery of the equilibrium M_o. However, because of the relatively long scan time needed, this technique is usually used only when accurate measurements of T1 are desired.

For further discussion of the clinical significance of the pulsing parameters, see the paper by Wehrli et. al.[20].

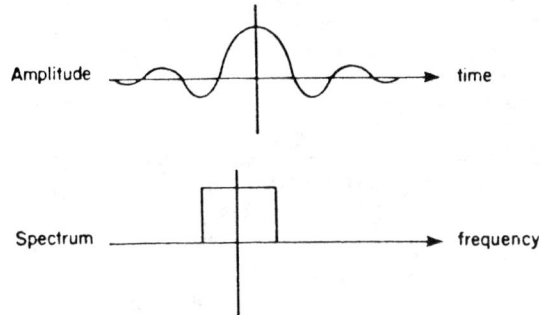

Figure 1: Amplitude waveform and spectrum of a selective excitation pulse.

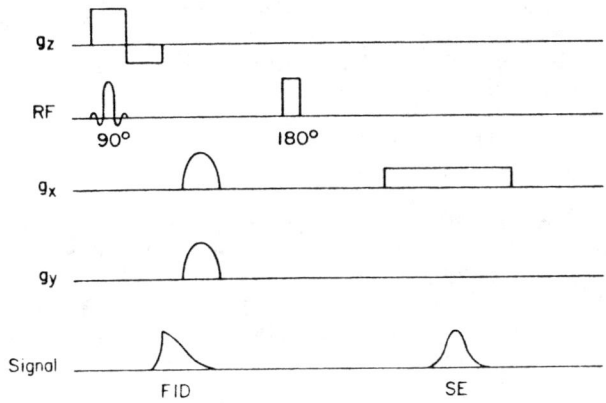

Figure 2: Pulse sequence diagram for two dimensional spin warp imaging of a transverse slice. The Y gradient, gy, varies from pulse to pulse for phase encoding.

REFERENCES

1. P.C.Lauterbur, Nature **242**, 190 (1973).
2. W.S.Hinshaw, and A.H.Lent, Proc. IEEE. **71**, 338 (1983).
3. P.Brunner, and R.R.Ernst, J. Mag. Res. **33**, 83 (1979).
4. W.S.Hinshaw, J. Applied Physics **47**, 3709 (1976).
5. K.N.Scott, H.R.Brooker, J.R.Fitzsimmons, H.F.Bennett, and R.C.Mick, J. Mag. Res. **50**, 339 (1982).
6. P.Mansfield, and A.A.Maudsley, Phys. Med. Biol. **21**, 847 (1976).
7. A.A.Maudsley, J. Mag. Res. **41**, 112 (1980).
8. J.M.S.Hutchison, R.J.Sutherland, and J.R.Mallard, J. Phys. E. **11**, 217 (1978).
9. P.M.Joseph, L.Axel, and M.O'Donnell, Med. Phys. **11**, 772 (1984).
10. C.M.Lai, and P.C.Lauterbur, J. Phys. E. **14**, 874 (1981).
11. G.T.Herman, Image reconstruction from projections. (Academic Press, New York, 1980), pp. 118-146.
12. L.A.Shepp, and B.F.Logan, IEEE Trans. Nuc. Sci. **NS-21**, 21 (1974).
13. P.M.Joseph, Artifacts in computed tomography. In: Newton TH, Potts DG (eds). Radiology of the skull and brain. (C.V.Mosby, St. Louis, 1981), pp. 3956-3992.
14. W.A.Edelstein, J.M.S.Hutchison, G.Johnson, and R.Redpath, Phys. Med. Biol. **25**, 751 (1980).
15. P.M.Joseph, J. Comp. Assist. Tomo. **9**, 651 (1985).
16. E.E.Babcock, L.Brateman, J.C.Weinreb, S.D.Horner, and R.L.Nunnally, J. Comp. Assist. Tomo. **9**, 252 (1985).
17. J.H.den Boef, C.M.J. van Uijen, and C.D.Holzscherer, Phys. Med. Biol. **29**, 857 (1984).
18. L.A.Shepp, J. Comp. Assist. Tomo. **4**, 94 (1980).
19. P.Mansfield, and I.L.Pykett, J. Mag. Reson. **29**, 355 (1978).
20. F.W.Wehrli, J.R.MacFall, D.Shutts, R.Breger, and R.J.Herfkens, J. Comp. Assist. Tomo. **8**, 369 (1984).

MAGNET DESIGN AND TECHNOLOGY FOR NMR IMAGING

K. G. Dobson
Oxford Instruments Limited, Oxford OX2 0DX, England

ABSTRACT

The development of nuclear magnetic resonance, NMR, as a powerful analytical tool for chemical analysis has been dependent upon major advances in magnet technology. The requirement for both very homogeneous and subsequently higher magnetic fields has given rise to rapid magnet developments over the last fifteen years. NMR imaging and spectroscopy have now been shown to be an important diagnostic technique employing magnetic fields for non-invasive examination of the body. Such applications require magnets with access for the human body, together with large volumes of homogeneity, presenting a new challenge to the magnet designer. The earlier advances of magnet technology for high resolution NMR have been applied to production of these new magnets for medical applications.

The objectives of this paper are to describe the design parameters and the practical realisation of a magnet suitable for imaging or spectroscopic studies. A mathematical description of a magnetic field is given and the practical achievement of a suitable homogeneous field described. This is followed by a description of specific magnet systems, superconducting, resistive and permanent, with the emphasis on superconducting magnets. Finally, the future trends in magnet technology are discussed.

MAGNET REQUIREMENTS FOR IMAGING AND SPECTROSCOPY

The important parameters in the design of a magnet for NMR imaging and spectroscopy are

1. Field Strength

2. Field Homogeneity

3. Field Stability

4. Access to the Region of Homogeneity

5. Stray Magnetic Field

All of these parameters are inter-related and govern the cost and design of a specific system. The fundamental requirements for each of these parameters is discussed below and practical achievement in a subsequent section. A summary of the technical requirements is given in table 1.

Table 1 : Magnet Requirements

	Imaging	Chemical Shift
Field Strength (T)	0.1 - 1.5	> 1.5
Homogeneous Volume (mm)		
Whole Body System	500	100
Research System	80 - 140	40 - 70
Access (mm)		
Whole Body System	1000	1000
Research System	200 - 500	200 - 500

1. Field Strength

The range of magnetic fields available for imaging and spectroscopy has increased with the development of magnet technology. Imaging systems with magnetic fields greater than 2T and utilizing superconducting magnets are now readily available. The choice of field level depends upon the differing requirements for imaging and spectroscopy.

The natural abundance and high gyromagnetic ratio of protons means that good quality proton images can be produced with moderately low magnetic fields of 0.1 -0.5 Tesla. However, the difference in the energy gap and population of nuclei in the two spin states is proportional to the applied magnetic field. Hence the number of transitions from high to low energy states increases with magnetic field. This produces a better signal to noise ratio from the NMR signal and hence better image quality with increasing magnetic field.

Conversely, it may be desirable to limit the field strength due to the problems from reduced r.f. penetration and large volume homogeneity probes operating at high frequency.

In contrast, spectroscopy and chemical shift imaging systems require high magnetic fields for optimum operation. This is a result of the lower abundance and lower gyromagnetic ratio of the nuclei observed in these systems. In the chemical shift imaging technique, the NMR frequency from a particular nucleus in a given magnetic field differs from one compound to another, the difference being the chemical shift. Also, the NMR signal is broadened due to the environment of the nuclei. Since the chemical shift is proportional to the strength of the magnetic field, working at the highest possible magnetic field will produce better resolution of the spectral lines. In order to work at fields greater than approximately 0.35T it is always necessary to use superconducting magnet systems.

The optimum magnetic field for imaging is an issue that is still unresolved. Arguments in favour of high fields are better quality images and faster imaging times. The disadvantages are those of r.f. penetration, coil design, siting and cost. The requirement for the maximum field for chemical shift imaging is not in question.

2. Field Homogeneity

In a discussion of field homogeneity requirements, it is important to clarify the definition of homogeneity. Homogeneity of a magnetic field is normally defined as the maximum deviation of the field over a given volume, measured by plotting the field at a number of points through the volume, to find the maximum and minimum values.

$$\text{Homogeneity} = \frac{B_{max} - B_{min}}{B_{central}} \quad (1)$$

This definition is of most interest to an NMR imaging experiment. An imaging magnet requires moderate homogeneity over a large volume. The imaging technique looks at the overall effects from a large volume and therefore the maximum deviation of the field is the critical parameter. For example, if a magnetic field has an inhomogeneity of 0.2 G over the imaging volume, and a pulsed gradient is applied with a strength of 2 G/cm, the field inhomogeneity leads to a spatial resolution of 1 mm.

Thus non-uniform fields can limit the spatial resolution of an imaging experiment. A typical requirement of the field homogeneity for a whole body magnet would be 40 parts per million over a 50 cm diameter spherical volume (d.s.v.).

Chemical shift imaging and spectroscopy measurements are more critically dependent upon the resolution of the NMR signal. An NMR measurement over a specific size of sample will give a signal as shown in figure 1. The important parameter is now the width of the NMR signal at half full height, that is the half-height line width (H.H.L.W.), specified over a given volume.

$$\text{H.H.L.W.} = \frac{\Delta f}{f_o} \quad (\text{ppm}) \quad (2)$$

For the example shown in figure 1, the majority of the nuclei are at the central field value corresponding to the fundamental frequency, f_o. A much smaller number of nuclei are located at field values other than the central field. In fact, the peak to peak homogeneity of the field defines the maximum spread in frequency at the base of the NMR singal, f_{max} to f_{min}. Clearly, for a given volume, the H.H.L.W. of the NMR signal (in p.p.m.) is always appreciably less than the peak to peak homogeneity (in p.p.m.) of the magnetic field. The ratio is dependent upon the magnet type.

Since the magnitude of chemical shifts is small the magnetic field must be highly uniform to ensure that the spectral lines are well resolved from each other. Chemical shift imaging requires very homogeneous magnetic fields over relatively small volumes to resolve individual lines, and the H.H.L.W. definition is more useful. A typical requirement would be 0.1 ppm H.H.L.W. over a 10 cm d.s.v. in a 100 cm bore whole body system.

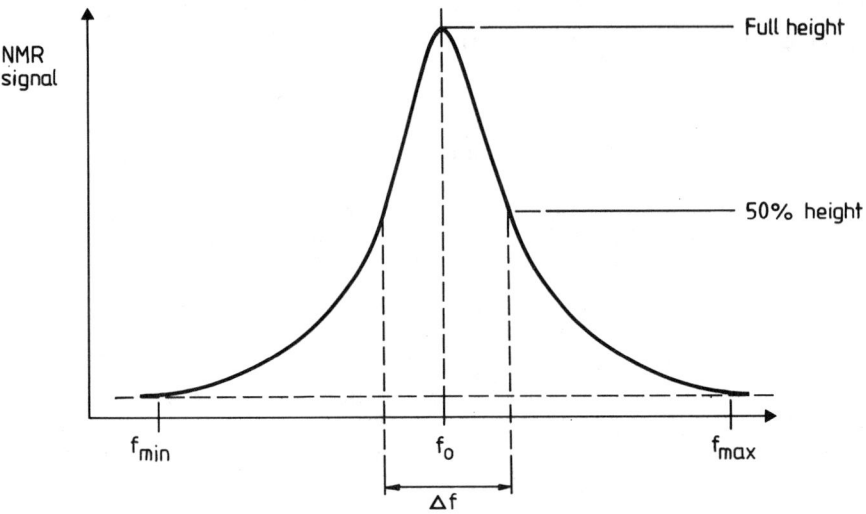

Figure 1 : NMR Resonance Signal

3. Field Stability

The nature of an imaging experiment requires repeated data acquisition cycles for improved image quality. Since signal to noise has a dependence upon magnetic field, the field stability of the magnet is very important; any noise superimposed on the D.C. field causes deterioration of the image. Stringent requirements on stability can be a problem in resistive magnets where power is continually dissipated or in a permanent magnet where temperature fluctuations lead to field drift. Superconducting systems operate in 'persistent mode' and field stability of better than 0.1 ppm per hour may be achieved.

4. Access

The access requirement for an NMR magnet system is dependent upon the application, the most common being examination of the human body. In order to provide sufficient access for a patient the clear bore of the magnet should be a minimum of 750 mm. Additional gradient coils for the imaging experiment and any correcting coils to optimize homogeneity are also located within the bore of the system, shown schematically in figure 2.

Since these coils restrict access, the bore diameter of the magnet housing must be at least 1000 mm.

Conversely, access should be minimized in order to reduce the diameter of the magnet system and hence cost. In addition to the whole body system there is a growing trend towards magnets for both paediatric studies and research applications. Typical access requirements for NMR systems are given in table 2.

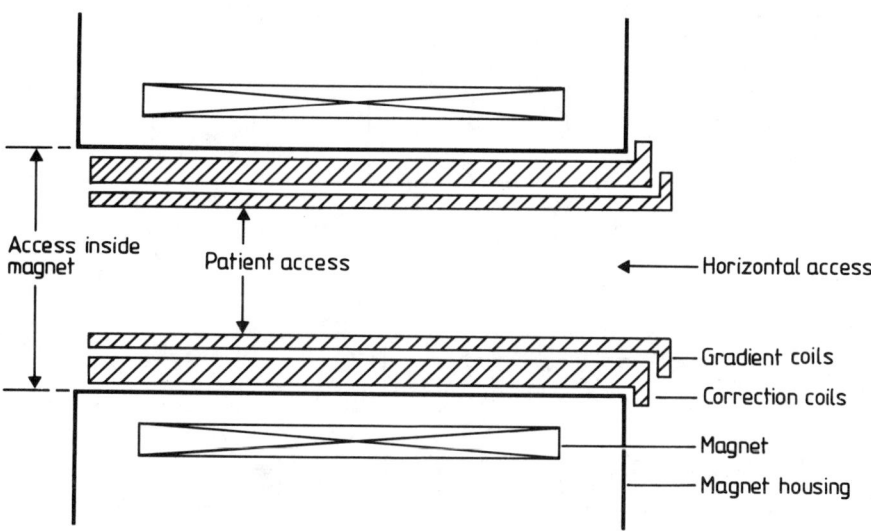

Figure 2 : Schematic of NMR Magnet System

5. Stray Field

Any magnet system will have an associated stray field extending from the magnet housing into the user environment. The extent of the stray field is dependent upon the central field and the bore. As an example, the stray field values for typical imaging magnets are given in figure 3.

This stray field can result in possible problems with day to day operation of the system. The attraction of objects into the magnet bore is a potential danger in terms of risk of injury to users and also damage to the system. Technical problems also arise since the environment may affect the homogeneity of the magnet itself. Table 3 indicates guidelines for placing objects to avoid any detrimental performance of the system from the point of view of attraction of magnetic objects.

Table 2 : Access Requirements of NMR Imaging Systems

Magnet Type	Free Access (mm)	Access Inside Magnet Housing (mm)
Whole Body	750	1000
Paediatric	390	500
Research Application	310 135	400 200

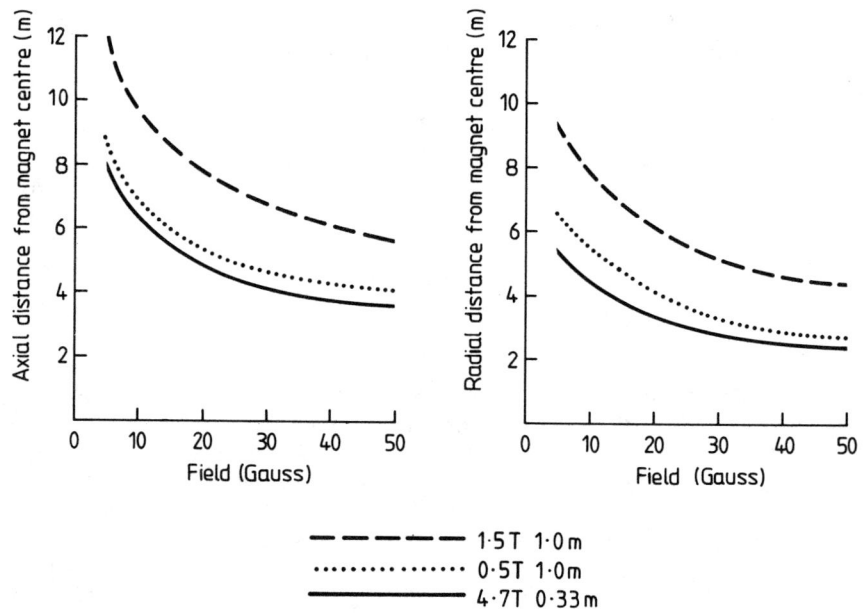

——— 1·5T 1·0m
·········· 0·5T 1·0m
——— 4·7T 0·33m

Figure 3 : Stray Fields of NMR Imaging Magnets
(Oxford Instruments Group Limited, Oxfordshire, 1985)

Table 3 : Field Limits for Devices Close to NMR Imaging Magnets

Field Limit (Gauss)	Device
5	Cathode Ray Tubes Pacemakers
10	Computers Watches Credit Cards
20	Magnetic Storage Material
50	Power Supplies Spectrometers

The table shows that careful siting of the magnet system is necessary, and from figure 3, it is clear that the problem will be aggravated for higher magnetic field. Thus siting of high field systems in restricted environments can sometimes be a problem, and critical to optimum performance of the magnet. Reduction of the stray field may be achieved using iron shielding either as a remote screen or as a closed-flux path screen.

FIELD HOMOGENEITY

The discussion in the previous section has emphasized the need for homogeneous magnetic fields for both proton and chemical shift imaging. This implies that the variation of the field must be minimized throughout the working region. A uniform or homogeneous magnetic field may be produced using an infinitely long solenoid or a uniform current density distributed over a sphere. Since these solutions are impractical or indeed impossible, it is necessary for the magnet designer to express the field within the working region due to distributions of current density. Practical current distributions are windings on circular formers with rectangular axial sections. The theory assumes a current distributed uniformly in this rectangle, perfectly circular and co-axial from which a concise mathematical description of the field variation may be obtained. The effects of non-uniform current density and of manufacturing tolerances can also be characterized in terms of this concise description, and, hence, it is also possible to design correction coil systems to optimize the homogeneity of the magnet.

The mathematical description of the spatial variation of the magnetic field from a known distribution of current density has been published in detail[1]. The discussion that follows will illustrate the techniques behind the designs of simple magnet and coil correction systems.

The fundamental procedure for designing a magnet with a spherical region of homogeneity is to describe the central field in terms of a mathematical series. The co-ordinate system for such a mathematical description is shown in figure 4, where z represents the axis of the magnet system.

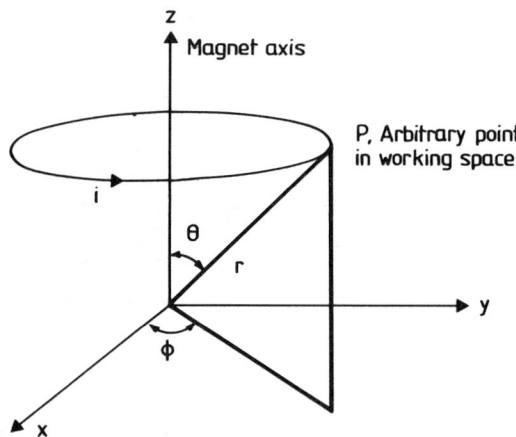

Figure 4 : Coordinate System for mathematical description of magnetic field showing co-axial current loop

The field on the axis of symmetry B(z), can be expanded as a power series of z, measured from the origin, which is also taken to be the centre of the region of homogeneity. The field is expressed as

$$B_z(z) = B_0 + B_1 \left(\frac{z}{r_0}\right) + B_2 \left(\frac{z}{r_0}\right)^2 + B_3 \left(\frac{z}{r_0}\right)^3 + \ldots$$
$$= \sum_{n=0}^{\infty} B_n \left(\frac{z}{r_0}\right)^n \qquad (3)$$

where r_0 is taken to be half the length of the region of interest. The coefficients B_n are proportional to individual currents or current densities. Since the system has axial symmetry it is also possible to extend the analysis off the axis as

$$B_z(r,\theta) = \sum_{n=0}^{\infty} \left(\frac{r}{r_0}\right)^n B_n P_n(\cos\theta) \qquad (4)$$

where $P_n(\cos\theta)$ are standard Legendre polynomials of degree n. In the absence of ferromagnetic materials the coefficients B_n are sums of contributions from individual sources about the z axis, dependent only upon the coil dimensions, axial location (shown schematically in figure 8) and proportional to the current or current density.

The principle of the design of an NMR imaging magnet is to devise a set of coils for which the variation in axial field profile is small about a particular centre. In practice, this means designing a magnet so that the B_n are zero up to a specific order.

The B_n coefficients are evaluated for rectangular coil sections using the following procedure.

1. An elementary expression for the field on the z axis is obtained from a loop, cylindrical sheet or a rectangular coil for given axial and radial locataions. These expressions are readily available in the literature[2].

2. The expression is expanded as a power series as given by equation 3, to obtain the coefficients B_n.

The details of this analysis will not be extended in the present discussion, since magnet design computer programs for the evaluation of B_n are readily available. The field variation for the B_n up to B_4 is shown schematically in figure 5.

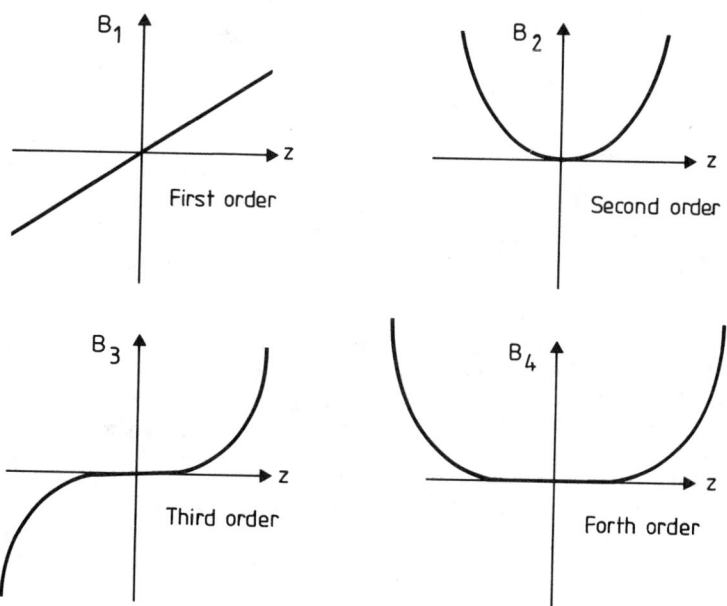

Figure 5 : Schematic Representation of Axial Field Profiles

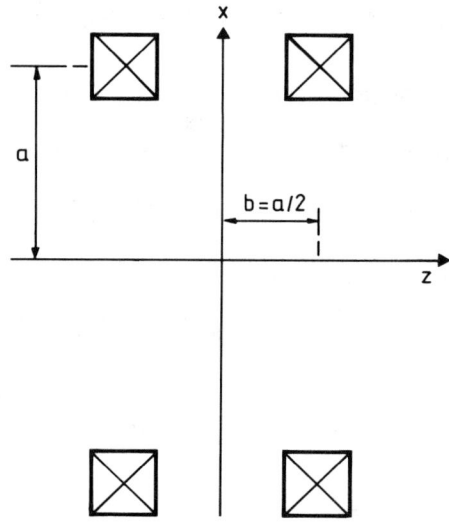

Figure 6 : Simple Two Coil Magnet

As an example of a simple magnet design, consider the two coil system shown in figure 6. This consists of two coils placed either side of the mid plane at an axial position, b, equal to half of the mean winding radius, a. Following through the analysis described above shows that the coefficient $B_2 = 0$, indicating that the axial magnetic field does not vary with z^2, that is there is no axial second order. Also since the coils are located symmetrically about the centre, odd order variations are zero. However, the first dominant impurity from such an arrangement will be B_4, which gives the field profile shown in figure 5. The high order gradients from fourth order upwards can produce a field that would not be homogeneous over a large volume. Such a profile would be unsuitable for an imaging magnet.

It is therefore necessary to include more than two coils and to include extra pairs as shown in figure 7.

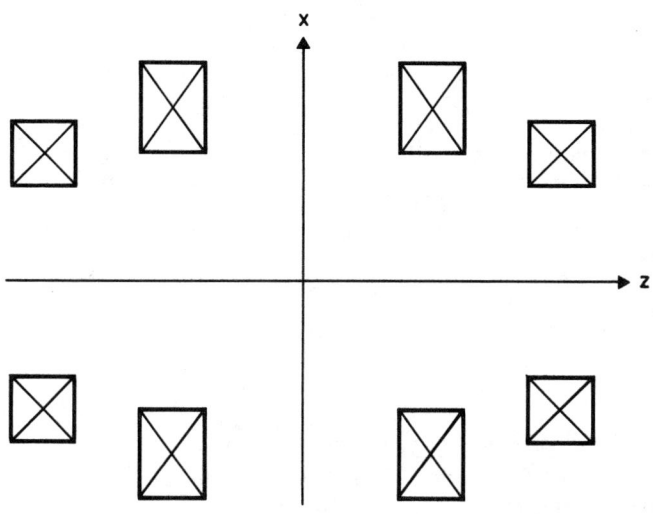

Figure 7 : Simple Four Coil Magnet Design

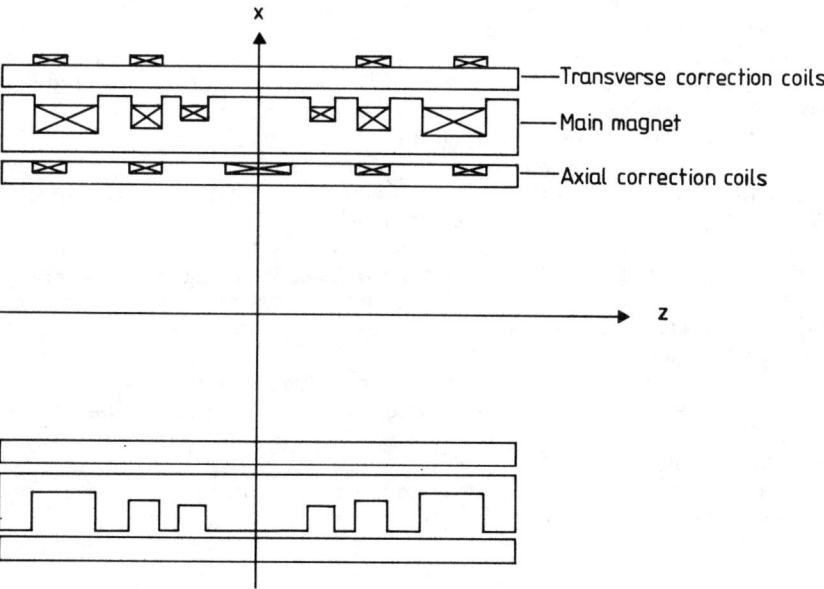

Figure 8 : Typical Six Coil Imaging Magnet

In this way the outer coils may be located axially and radially to produce B_4 of opposite sign to the inner coils. Hence, the fourth order of the combined magnet would be zero and the first non-zero gradient would be B_6, sixth order. It is possible to use four, six, eight or even more coil systems to eliminate field gradients up to any order. An imaging magnet must be designed so that the first non-zero order is eighth; such a magnet could consist of 6 coils as shown in figure 8.

The previous discussion has assumed axial symmetry and has been restricted to axial inhomogeneities. In practice the magnet will have non-axial symmetry and lead to off-axis or transverse gradients. Equation 4 may be extended to describe the magnetic field at any point in space as

$$B_z(r,\theta,\phi) = \sum_{n=0}^{\infty} \left(\frac{r}{r_o}\right)^n \{B_n P_n(\cos\theta) + \sum_{m=1}^{n} P_n^m(\cos\theta) <C_n^m \cos m\phi + S_n^m \sin m\phi>\} \quad (5)$$

where $P_n^m(\cos\theta)$ are associated Legendre polynominals of degree n and order m and the C_n^m and S_n^m are magnitudes of a particular field distortion for a particular radius r_o. This expression is a general solution of the Laplace equation $\nabla^2 V = 0$.

For the case of m = 0 the expression would reduce to equation 4 and give rise to solutions of axial symmetry. In the case of m ≠ 0, non-axial symmetry, a field gradient is produced which has a variation with ϕ. The historical notation of transverse gradients for some combinations of n and m are given in table 4.

In general, these notations are labels and for the spatial variation of a specific gradient it is necessary to refer to the spherical co-ordinate description of equation 5. For example, an X gradient would have a cos ϕ variation and a Y gradient a sin ϕ variation. In practice, it is only necessary to consider off-axis gradients up to and including third orders, to achieve the required homogeneity for an imaging magnet.

Field inhomogeneity can be generated from a number of sources; this includes non-perfect windings and incorrect (non-symmetric) positioning of the coils due to mechanical tolerances. The latter give rise to odd order gradients such as B_1 and B_3 as shown in figure 5. Winding irregularity and non-circular coils produce transverse gradients, although these may be minimized in some cases by suitable axial location of coils. In addition the environment of the magnet can also give distortions to the central field due to the presence of magnetic material.

Field inhomogeneity may be reduced using additional correction coils distributed around or inside the magnet. These coils can be of two types: movable coils connected in series with the main magnet or independently energised coils. For a moveable coil in series with the magnet the axial displacement of the coil by a distance Δb can give rise to a change in the field coefficients B_n given by

$$\Delta B_n = -(n+1) B_{n+1} \frac{\Delta b}{r_o} \quad (6)$$

Table 4 : Notation for transverse gradients

C_n^m	m=0	1	2	3
n=0	Z_0	-	-	-
1	Z_1	X	-	-
2	Z_2	ZX	X^2-Y^2	-
3	Z_3	Z^2X	$Z(X^2-Y^2)$	X^3-3XY^2
4	Z_4	Z^3X	$Z^2(X^2-Y^2)$	$Z(X^3-3XY^2)$

S_n^m	m=1	2	3
n=0	-	-	-
1	Y	-	-
2	ZY	XY	-
3	Z^2Y	ZXY	Y^3-3X^2Y
4	Z^3Y	Z^2XY	$Z(Y^3-3X^2Y)$

This equation may therefore be used to calculate a movement of a coil to produce a desired change in field profile. These coils are useful for producing axial first, second and third order corrections arising from winding irregularity. However, because they are in series with the magnet they cannot be used to correct inhomogeneity once the magnet is installed or to correct transverse gradients.

Independently energized coils are a more flexible approach. These coils may be either resistive windings located within the room temperature bore of the magnet or superconducting coils. The coils may be classified into two types: axial and transverse. An axial gradient produces gradients as described by equation 3, and consist of co-axial current loops. A transverse coil will produce a field gradient described by equation 5, and consists of a series of saddle coils. A coil correction system is shown schematically in figure 10; such correction systems are often referred to as shims.

The aim in designing a shim system is to produce a coil set with the correct field profile and necessary strength with minimum impurity. As an example, consider a shim design to produce a first order gradient Z_1. This can be achieved using the example discussed in figure 6, but with the coils on either side of the mid-plane carrying opposing currents. This system produces the most efficient Z_1 gradient but produces a large third order, Z_3, contaminant. It is possible to design a pair of coils to produce Z_1

with no Z_3 but this is an inefficient way of producing Z_1. To improve the efficiency, a coil system as shown in figure 9 must be used.

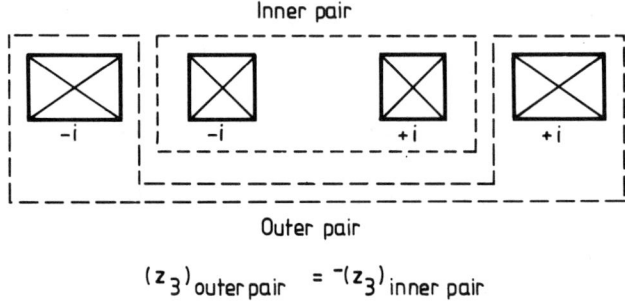

$(z_3)_{outer\,pair} = -(z_3)_{inner\,pair}$

Figure 9 : Simple Z1 Shim System

In the design of the axial shims for imaging magnets it is important that high order contaminants are minimized, since volumes of homogeniety are large. This leads to complex designs of shims as seen in figure 10, and often to reduced strength. These limitations usually limit the axial shims available to fourth or fifth order.

The transverse coils must also be designed with a minimal impurity over the large imaging volume. For such coils, contaminants are from higher order transverse gradients; thus an X shim would be contaminated by Z^2X. These are minimized in design by suitable separation of the arcs carrying opposing current. In a typical imaging magnet, transverse shims would be available up to third order.

To summarize, the homogeneity from any imaging magnet design is governed by several factors, the most critical of which is the original design. The magnet design, based upon the criteria discussed above, should have sufficient number of zero axial field coefficients, B_n, for the homgeneous volume of interest. Former manufacture must be tightly controlled to avoid introduction of axial inhomogeneity from mechanical tolerances. Transverse gradients are minimized using special winding techniques and coil designs. The inhomogeneity arising from the idealised design must be corrected with axial and transverse shim coils, the settability and availability of which will ultimately govern the homogeneity achievable from the magnet.

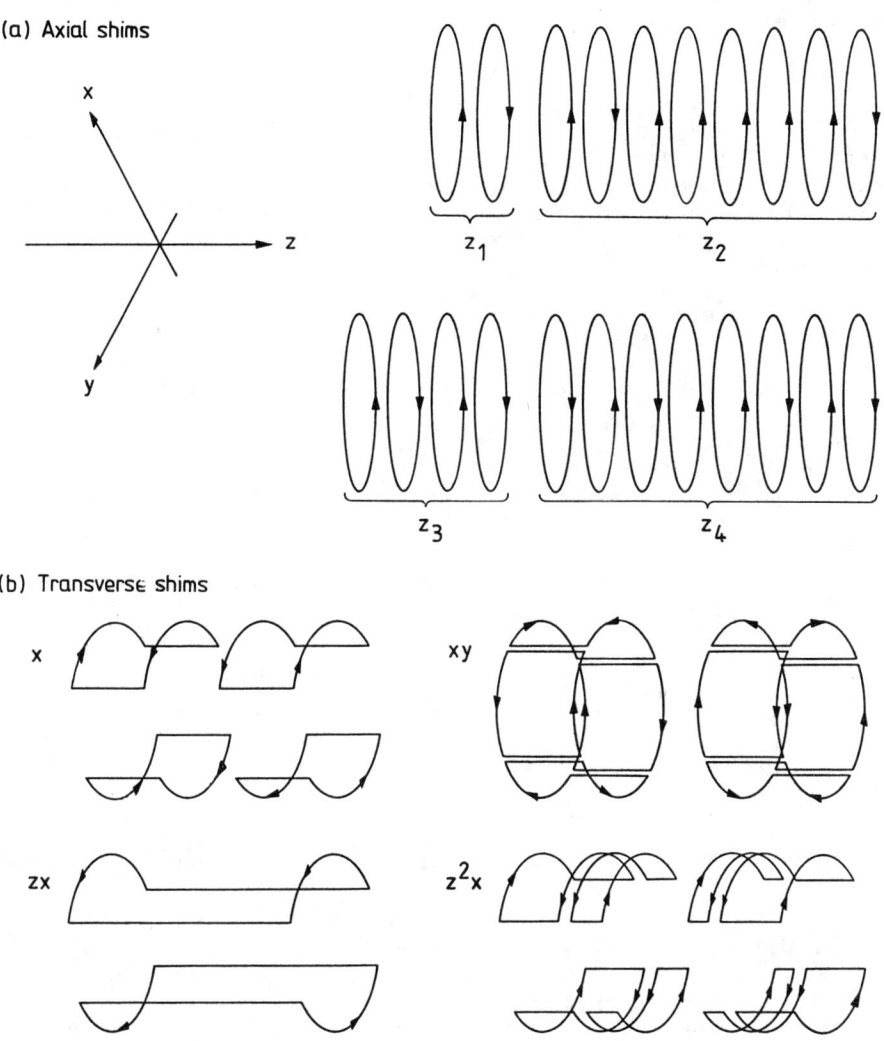

Figure 10 : Typical Shim Systems

NMR MAGNET TYPES

The following section will discuss in some detail the manufacture of superconducting and resistive imaging magnets. The emphasis of the discussion will be on superconducting systems since these are the most widely used. A very brief description of permanent magnet types is included for comparison with the superconducting and resistive systems.

1. Superconducting Magnets

Superconducting magnets are manufactured from co-axial windings of material characterised by the absence of electrical resisitivity. Superconductivity is a phenomenon, whereby when particular materials are cooled to very low temperatures, typically less than 20K, the resistivity of the material falls abruptly to zero at a characteristic critical temperature, as shown in figure 11.

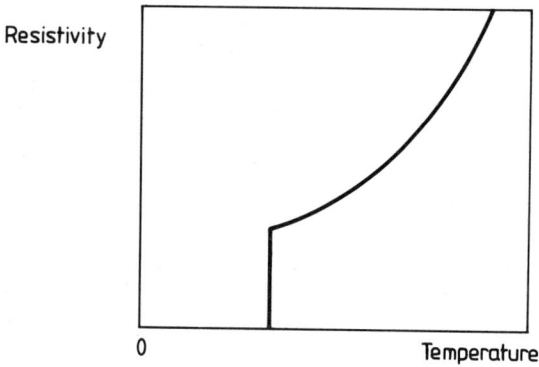

Figure 11 : Resistivity of a Superconductor as a Function of Temperature

The early discovery of superconductivity, by Kammerlingh Onnes in 1911, also showed that the material reverted to the resistive state when placed in a field of approximately 0.1 Tesla. In the late 1950's and early 1960's, so called Type II superconductors were manufactured capable of carrying current in high magnetic fields. This opened up the possibility of using such materials for the manufacture of high field magnets.

Today, Type II superconducting alloys are common place and readily available from commercial manufacturers. Superconducting material properties are illustrated in figure 12.

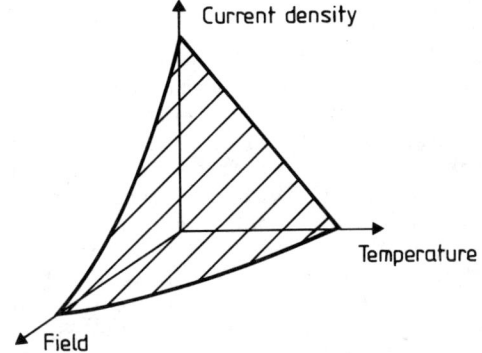

Figure 12 : Properties of Superconducting Materials

The superconducting state is represented by all points on or below the surface shown in the figure 12; points above the surface represent the conductor in the normal resistive state. The diagram clearly illustrates the relationship of the parameters important to the operation of the magnet in the superconducting state. In addition, high values of current density are achievable in a given magnetic field and at a fixed temperature, hence very high magnetic fields may be achieved from windings of such conductors. The shape of this 'critical surface' depends upon the alloy, chemical composition and manufacturers processing technique. In the following discussion it will be assumed that superconductors are available for the magnet designer as engineering materials. For a detailed discussion of superconductivity the reader is referred to reference 3.

The most important parameters affecting the design of an NMR magnet using superconductors are:

1. Superconducting material type and choice
2. Mechanical design and choice of material for magnet formers
3. Persistent mode operation
4. Quenching or training
5. Operation of the magnet at very low temperatures and hence the housing of the magnet

Each of these parameters will be discussed in more detail below. However, it should be noted that achievement of the homogeneity is dependent upon the correct location of the coils as discussed in the previous section.

Superconducting Materials

Alloys of niobium titanium are the most commonly used for magnet manufacture. In zero magnetic field Nb-Ti becomes superconducting at 9.8K and therefore the most practical operation for the conductor is at liquid helium temperature, 4.2K. There are a wide range of conductors now available and for details the reader is referred to the material specifications readily available from commercial wire manufacturers. Nb-Ti conductors consist of either one filament, single core conductor, or many fine filaments, filamentary conductor. These filaments of NbTi are embedded in a copper matrix as shown schematically in figure 13, the conductor is then varnish or cloth insulated. The choice between single core or filamentary wire depends upon the application, but for imaging magnets, the choice is usually restricted to filamentary wire.

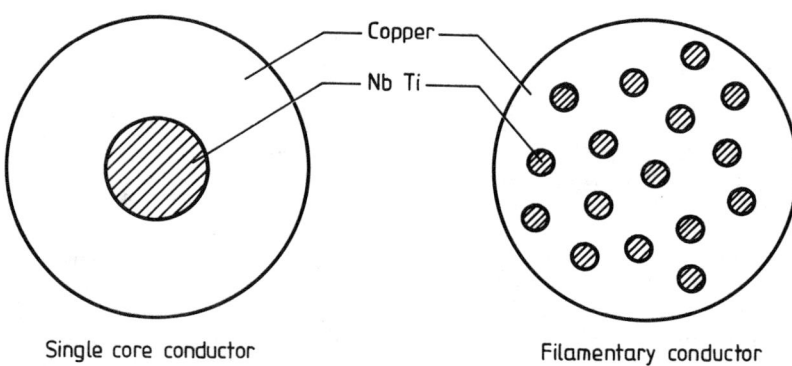

Single core conductor   Filamentary conductor

Figure 13 : Nb-Ti material types

Single core material has the advantage that perfect superconducting joints can be made, which results in excellent persistance of the magnetic field, as discussed below. The cost of single core wire is also usually significantly less than filamentary. However, the disadvantages are that critical currents, the current at which the conductor becomes resistive in a magnetic field, are limited to moderate values of the field and current. Large diameter single core conductors can also exhibit magnetic instability. In practice, therefore, the use of single core material is limited to small scale, low field magnets.

Filamentary conductors have improved magnetic stability and consequently larger diameter wires can be utilized; such conductors can carry very large critical currents in high magntic fields. Thus filamentary conductors may be used for manufacture of high field and large bore magnets.

A summary of the advantages and disadvantages of single core and filamentary wire is given in table 5.

Table 5 : Advantages and Disadvantages of Single Core and Filamentary Superconductors

	Single Core Conductor	Filamentary Conductor
Advantages	Simple Jointing	High Current Carrying Capacity
	Cheaper than Filamentary	Large Diameters Available
		Wide Range Available
Disadvantages	Low Current Carrying Capacity	Jointing Difficult
	Limited Availability	More Expensive
	Large Diameters are Magnetically unstable	

Alloys of niobium tin, Nb_3Sn and vanadium gallium, V_3Ga, are also used for superconducting magnet manufacturer. These alloys have a greater current carrying capacity than Nb-Ti alloys and consequently are used for fields greater than 10 Tesla. Since present day imaging magnets do not require such high fields, further discussion of these conductors will not be continued and the reader referred to reference 3 for more details.

Mechanical Design and Magnet Formers

For high homogeneity NMR quality magnets, the use of magnetic materials must be avoided. This is particularly important for the former on which the magnet is wound. The former must be precision machined to minimize tolerances on axial and radial location of individual coils, thereby reducing the risk of inhomogeneities as discussed previously. Also, due to forces during winding and later the Lorentz force during energisation, the former must have sufficient mechanical strength and thickness. Aluminium alloy is the most common choice for former material to achieve all of these requirements.

Persistent Mode Operation

The ability of a superconducting magnet to achieve truly persistent mode operation is one of the major advantages of this type of magnet. Figure 14 shows schematically how this is achieved.

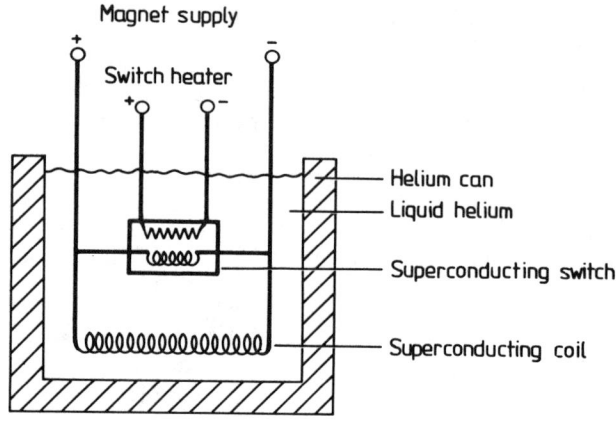

Figure 14 : Persistent Superconducting Switch

A switch, which consists of a section of superconducting wire wound in close proximity with a heater, is connected across the start and end of the magnet. Switching on the heater causes the superconducting wire to revert to the resistive state; the magnet can then be energized. Once at field the heater is turned off so that the wire becomes superconducting again. The current in the leads to the magnet is then run down. When there is no more current in the energization leads the current circulates through the switch, and the leads can be removed. Thus, after initial energization, the magnet can run without a power supply or leads in a truly persistent mode.

In practice, a magnet is wound with several lengths of conductor such that it is necessary to make a number of joints. Special jointing techniques are necessary to achieve persistent, very low resistance joints. For example, in a magnet with a typical inductance of 100 Henries, the resistance of the magnet circuit should be less than 3×10^{-9} ohms to achieve a decay of 1 part in 10^7 per hour. By means of special techniques, field stability of better than 1 part in 10^7 per hour can be achieved with magnets wound with filamentary conductor. Such techniques represent proprietory information to a commerical magnet manufacturer.

Quenching or Training

A superconducting magnet will rapidly de-energize or 'quench' when a region of the magnet windings becomes resistive. Such resistance generates heat and can propagate rapidly throughout the bulk of the windings. High voltages are generated during a quench and the magnet must be protected by the inclusion of dump resistors across each section of the coil.

The friction caused by minute movements of wire during energization can generate sufficient heat to drive the superconductor normal, this may occur at lower fields than the design field. On re-energizing, the magnet will often "train" to successively high values of field until the design field is achieved. Quenching may be avoided or at least minimized by special winding and bonding of the conductors.

Operation at Low Temperatures

In order to operate a superconducting magnet, the windings must be immersed in a bath of liquid helium which boils freely at atmospheric pressure. Liquid helium has a very low latent heat of vaporization and high cost. Hence, a small heat input gives rise to a high helium boil off. In contrast, nitrogen is cheap and has a high latent heat. The objectives of cryostat design are to minimize the heat input to the system and the liquid helium volume. A typical cryostat is shown in figure 15.

The magnet is housed in an all welded stainless steel can containing liquid helium. This is surrounded by a series of radiation shields and finally a can containing liquid nitrogen. Mechanical support of the various shields and cans is by glass fibre re-inforced struts; electrical, instrumentation and cryogen access is via one or more necks.

The heat inputs to the system are from conduction, convection and radiation. Conduction is minimized by using materials with low thermal conductivity, such as, for example, glass fibre support rods. After energization the magnet is put in persistent mode and the current leads removed. This eliminates the heat load from room temperature to the helium can down current leads. Similarly, the number of electrical access leads must be minimized. Convection is reduced by the use of vacuum techniques in the outer case of the cryostat and by designing the cryostat with minimal spacings.

The radiation load onto the helium can is given by

$$\dot{Q} = \varepsilon A \sigma (T^4 - 4.2^4) \qquad (7)$$

where ε is the emmissivity, A the surface area, σ is Stefans constant and T is the temperature of radiating surface.

In practice, the surface area is fixed by the physical size of the magnet. To reduce radiation therefore requires low values of emmissivity and a low temperature for the radiating surface. Low emmissivities are obtained using very clean polished surfaces, and layers of 'superinsulation', which consist of multiple layers of aluminium foil between the cans and shields. The largest reduction in radiation heat load is achieved using a liquid nitrogen can surrounding the helium can. The higher latent heat and low cost of nitrogen makes this approach very attractive and gives a reduction in heat load by a factor of $(300/77)^4 = 230$. In addition, intermediate gas cooled shields may be used, cooled by the enthalpy of the evaporating liquid helium and nitrogen. The use of all of these techniques results in typical boil off rates of 0.35 litres/hour for helium and 0.65 litres/hour for nitrogen for a one metre bore whole body magnet.

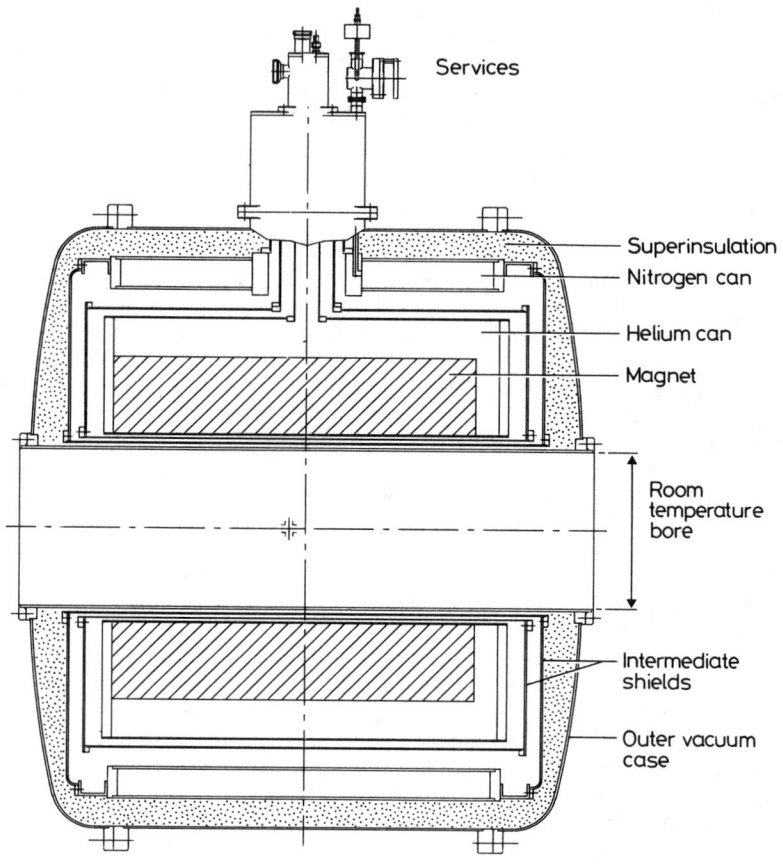

Figure 15 : Cryostat for a Superconducting Magnet

A further approach is to use a mechanical cooler to refrigerate the shields of the cryostat to very low temperatures. This has the advantage that very low helium boil off rates can be achieved, these systems are useful where helium is expensive or in short supply. However, the disadvantages are the initial cost of the cooler, reliability and service costs.

The type of commercially available superconducting NMR imaging magnets has increased significantly over the past three to four years. A typical range of systems is shown in figure 16. The figure shows that with present day technology, higher magnetic fields are only achieved with reduced bore size. The limit of magnetic field is set by the properties of presently available superconductors. Also the cost of the magnet increases rapidly with increasing magnetic field, and can present an unattractive commercial proposition.

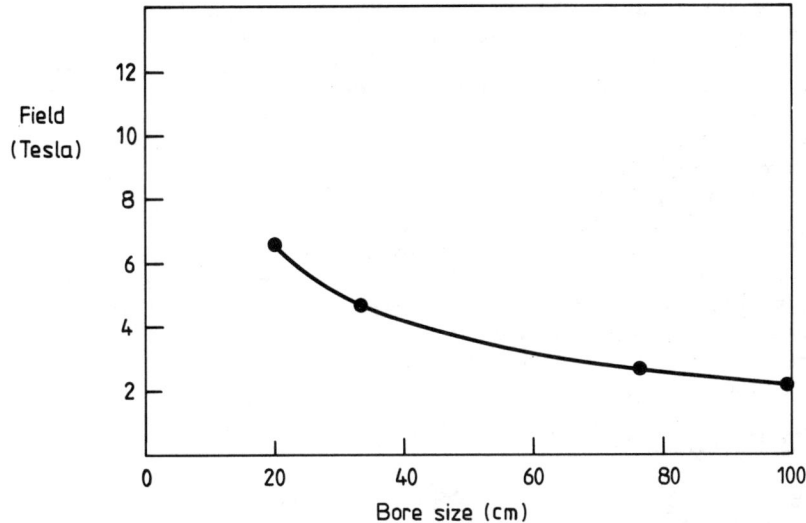

Figure 16 : Commercially available NMR Imaging Magnets
(Oxford Instruments Group Limited, Oxfordshire, 1985)

2. Resistive Magnets

The fundamental equation representing the field from a resistive magnet is given by:

$$B_o = \mu_o \, G \sqrt{\frac{W\lambda}{a\rho}} \qquad (8)$$

where G - geometry factor
       W - electrical power in watts
       λ - space factor for the winding
       a - radius in metres
       ρ - resistivity in ohms/metre

Since B_o is proportional to the square root of the power, the power requirements for very high field magnets can become unreasonable. Also the dependence of B_o on resistivity requires water cooling of the conductor to avoid temperature variation and subsequent instability of the field.

Resistive magnets are manufactured using co axial windings of copper conductor or aluminium strip carrying electrical current. Such windings can be either hollow conductors carrying water for cooling or solid conductors cooled by adjacent heat sinks. The material may be high conductivity copper insulated with polymer coating or surface oxidised aluminium. For a given power density aluminium and copper carry equal current density; however, aluminium is preferred on economic grounds.

Each main coil is wound from anodised aluminium strip conductor on an aluminium former. This provides a strong mechanical structure and the high packing factor gives excellent radial and axial heat transfer. The winding is cooled using copper tubes set into the side plates of the coil reducing the temperature uniformally through the coil and avoiding hot spots.

Each of the individual coils of the magnet are supported on an aluminium frame. Axial and lateral movement of the coils allow correction of the homogeneity. Small trim coils connected in series with the main magnet allow fine tuning of the homogeneity. A typical resistive system can produce a central field of 0.15T, for a power input of 40 - 50 kW. The quadratic dependance of power upon field strength and subsequent cooling problems limit the achievable field strength of a resistive system to approximately 0.2 Tesla. However, installation and siting is relatively simple and the ability to move individual coils allows achievement of a high level of homogeneity.

3. Permanent Magnets

The magnetic field of a permanent magnet material is generated by the valence electrons of constituent atoms. In the unmagnetized state regions of magnetization point in random directions with zero net magnetization. Upon magnetization, these regions are aligned in the same direction. This results in a large magnetic field surrounding the material.

Permanent magnet materials are classified as magnetically hard or soft, dependant upon their ability to resist demagnetization. Two of the most common permanent magnet materials are Alnico and rare earth cobalts. Alnico is an alloy of aluminium, nickel and cobalt and falls into the class of soft materials. This is normally magnetized in situ.

The most commonly used rare earth cobalt alloys are alloys of samarium and cobalt, $SmCo_5$, which are magnetically hard and can produce greater flux densities than Alnico materials. The disadvantage is the much greater cost of this material. The present paper will not discuss details of the magnet design, but will continue by comparing the advantages and disadvantages of all three types.

Comparison of NMR Magnet Types

The choice of the NMR system is often restricted to the choice of field level. If the system is required only for proton studies at low fields then the choice is between superconducting, resistive or permanent magnets. However, high field imaging systems require the use of superconducting magnets. At the end of the day, the user must decide upon a choice between high field or low field depending upon the application of the system. A comparison of the advantages and disadvantages of the three magnet systems is summarised in table 6.

Table 6 : Summary of Advantage and Disadvantage of NMR Magnet Types

	Advantages	Disadvantages
Superconducting	Fields up to 6.4T	Initial siting and installation
	Large volumes of homogeneity	High capital outlay cost
		Large stray field
	Persistent mode operation	Cryogenic refill
	Reasonable operating cost	Cryogenic costs
Resistive	Easy siting and installation	Fields up to 0.15T
	Reasonable operating cost	High power consumption
	Low capital outlay cost	Water Cooling
		Field Drift
Permanent	No electrical energy for operation	Fields up to 0.35T
		High material cost
	Low Stray field	Enormous weight, up to 100 tons
		Operating temperature must be accurately controlled

TRENDS IN MAGNET TECHNOLOGY

The future developments in magnet technology will be influenced by trends in the NMR imaging market. The current market requirement for the whole body magnets are split into low field systems, up to 1.0T, and high field systems, up to 2.0T. In addition, there is a further split into routine applications or research. At the research end of the market, there is a move towards even higher field and production of a 4T whole body system is possible in the near future. Such magnets are unlikely to become routine application systems due to the size and cost. Such a magnet involves development of new technologies and materials, hence availability must be viewed on a long timescale.

The field available from a resistive magnet must be viewed to be at the limit due to the enormous power consumptions and heating problems involved. Similarly, increased field levels from a permanent magnet can only be achieved with development of new materials with reduced cost and weight. However, the use of iron yokes in permanent magnet systems will limit the field to less than 2T due to saturation of the yoke. Therefore, any move to higher fields will only be achieved through development of superconducting systems. Expansion of the small bore imaging market for research and also paediatric work, has resulted in magnets with access less than 50 cm, but fields greater than 4T. Future developments to higher field will be dependent upon market forces.

The reduction in consumption of liquid helium and nitrogen is an important factor for the continued widespread use of superconducting magnets. This may be accomplished using coolers to cool intermediate shields of the cryostat as discussed previously. Such systems are now commercially available. Extending the technique further to produce a closed system complete with helium liquefaction would help to solve the problems of cost and supply. These systems are not yet available.

For future expansion of NMR magnets, attempts must also be made to reduce the stray field. In most cases this can be achieved by provision of an iron shield. Early initial sitings of NMR magnets involved building elaborate and expensive sites. As the number of installations has increased, this has become an impractical proposition in many cases. Future developments must aim to reduce the stray field still further, whilst minimizing the amount of iron shielding.

The requirement for mobile NMR systems has also presented the magnet designer with new challenges. These involve development of superconducting magnets which can be run to field and achieve the required field stability in as short a period of time as possible. Also, the stray field should be minimized as much as possile and the cryostat housing should withstand the rigours of transportability.

Finally, it has now been shown that NMR magnets can be used for routine medical applications and important research applications. If both of these markets are to expand significantly, the cost of the magnet must be minimized. This will require continued cost reduction of the magnet to ensure the system is as economic as possible.

REFERENCES

1. M.W. Garrett, J.Appl.Phys. $\underline{22}$, 1091 (1951)

2. D.B. Montgomery, Solenoid Magnet Design(Wiley-Interscience, NY,1969)

3. M.N. Wilson, Superconducting Magnets (Clarendon Press, Oxford, 1983)

GRADIENT COIL TECHNOLOGY

S.R. Thomas and L.J. Busse
University of Cincinnati, Cincinnati, Ohio 45267

J.F. Schenck
General Electric Company, Schenectady, New York 12301

ABSTRACT

This paper provides a review of the requirements for the gradient magnetic fields utilized in NMR imaging and presents the generalized mathematical formalism used to describe the gradient producing coils. Specific considerations are given to the various options available for design of orthogonal gradient sets. The principles of electronic circuits for driving the gradient coils are discussed with examples of typical operating parameters given. Finally, some methods for correcting gradient non-linearities are described.

INTRODUCTION

One primary function performed by the gradient coils is that of establishing the relatively weak spatially varying magnetic fields which, when superimposed on the homogeneous static main field, provide the spatial-frequency encoding required for NMR imaging techniques (1, 2, 3). Generally, the three orthogonal gradients provided are linear so that the frequency spectrum corresponds directly to a specific spatial position in a straight forward manner through the Larmor equation $\omega_i = \gamma B_i$ where, as defined elsewhere in these proceedings, ω_i is the resonance frequency associated with the field strength B_i and γ is the gyromagnetic constant for the nuclei of interest. Figure 1 provides a schematical representation of the spatial encoding properties of gradient magnetic fields. In addition, for 2-dimensional, selective irradiation techniques, the gradient fields play an integral role in determination of the plane definition and slice thickness parameters. An example of the gradient field control during selective rf excitation is shown in Figure 2. The design of the gradient coils and the associated electronic driving circuits will depend on various aspects of the imaging system including: a) the main magnet geometry (patient access axial or transverse with the static field); b) the type of investigations and pulse protocol sequences employed (rapid switching requirements versus driven equilibrium pulse sequences and oscillating gradient slice selection (4)); and, c) the intrinsic inhomogeneity of the main magnetic field.

The lower limit of the gradient magnitude required is determined by the criterion that the gradient field must be stronger than the main magnetic field inhomogeneity in order to ensure that the spatial-frequency encoding established will not be dominated by the uncontrolled nature of these intrinsic non-uniformities. This consideration has more significance for some pulse protocol sequences and image reconstruction schemes than others; for example, as shown in Figure 3, 2DFT techniques are more forgiving of inhomogeneities in the imaging plane than are projection reconstruction methods because, for the former, the nonuniformitites are manifest only as geometric distortions within the final image without an accompanying broadening of the effective system response function as is the case with projection reconstruction (5, 6). For projection reconstruction, the effect of this broadening (which would degrade spatial resolution) should be limited to less than one pixel dimension within the product image. This requires that the following relationship be satisfied: $G_m \gg \Delta B_i(N/D) = (\Delta \omega_i/\gamma)(N/D)$ where G_m is the minimum applied gradient strength, ΔB_i or $(\Delta \omega_i/\gamma)$ represents the maximum intrinsic magnetic field deviation from the central nominal value over the imaging plane field-of-view (FOV), N is the number of pixels across the image, and D is the diameter of the FOV (5, 6). Therefore, if the homogeneity specifications for a 0.15T system were 50 parts-per-million (ppm) over a 40 cm diameter volume (representing the FOV), the minimum gradient required for a 128x128 backprojection technique would be:

$$G_m \geq (50 \times 10^{-6})(0.15T)(128/0.4m) = 2.4 \text{ mT/m}$$
$$= 0.24 \text{ G/cm}$$

Typical values of the gradient field strengths used in various clinical imaging systems range from 0.01 to 1.0 G/cm. The higher value mentioned represents a change in field of only 40 G across a 40 cm FOV and illustrates the weak nature of these gradient fields relative to the static magnetic field which may range from 1000 G(0.1T) to 20,000 G(2T).

In practice, the gradient coils themselves may also be used in an offset current mode to provide additional shimming correction for first order magnetic field inhomogeneities and thus improve the effective uniformity characteristics over and above the specified intrinsic value. This function is of particular value for those systems which do not have an independent shim coil set.

Another effect, as discussed by Edelstein, et al (5), relating the minimum gradient strength necessary to the intrinsic inhomogeneity, which has significance for both projection reconstruction and Fourier transform techniques involves maximizing the signal from each voxel. This requires that T_2^* for each voxel be much larger than the signal sampling time. This statement is equivalent to the condition that $\Delta B_m \gg \Delta B_s$ where ΔB_m represents the magnetic field change in the imaging plane due to the applied gradient, and ΔB_s is the static field inhomogeneity across one pixel. Continuing with the 0.15 T system example given above, the maximum intrinsic gradient for an inhomogeneity specification of 50ppm across 40 cm would be approximately 0.02 mT/m. Thus within a slice thickness of 1 cm, the change in magnetic field, ΔB_s, would be approximately 0.2 μT; and, for a pixel dimension of 3 mm (~ 40 cm/128 pixels) under the constraint that $\Delta B_m \sim 10 \times \Delta B_s$, the minimum gradient strength required would be approximately 0.7 mT/m (0.07 G/cm).

In practice, the magnitude of the gradient employed will be limited by signal-to-noise and bandwidth considerations. It is generally undesirable to utilize gradients any larger than necessary because the frequency bandwidth required for imaging is proportional to the gradient strength. A larger bandwidth introduces more noise and increases the complexity of tuning and matching narrow band, high Q rf-coils (5).

GENERAL MATHEMATICAL DESCRIPTION OF GRADIENT FIELDS

The spin system-gradient field interaction may be expressed in terms of a second rank tensor (7) where the gradient tensor, written in Cartesian coordinates as a dyadic is:

$$\mathbf{G} = \begin{pmatrix} \vec{ii}\, \frac{\partial B_{zx}}{\partial x} & \vec{ij}\, \frac{\partial B_{zx}}{\partial y} & \vec{ik}\, \frac{\partial B_{zx}}{\partial z} \\ \vec{ji}\, \frac{\partial B_{zy}}{\partial x} & \vec{jj}\, \frac{\partial B_{zy}}{\partial y} & \vec{jk}\, \frac{\partial B_{zy}}{\partial z} \\ \vec{ki}\, \frac{\partial B_{zz}}{\partial x} & \vec{kj}\, \frac{\partial B_{zz}}{\partial y} & \vec{kk}\, \frac{\partial B_{zz}}{\partial z} \end{pmatrix}$$

The Hamiltonian for an isolated spin, $\vec{I}$, located at position $\vec{r}$ within a magnetic field including the gradient component is (7):

$$H = \hbar (\omega_o I_z + \vec{I} \cdot \mathbf{G} \cdot \vec{r})$$

where I_z is the component of the spin parallel to the static magnetic field defined in the z-direction. Under conditions of a small gradient magnetic field strength ΔB relative to a large static field B_o defining the z-axis of the spin system, the vector tensor product may be approximated as:

$$\vec{I} \cdot \mathbf{G} \simeq I_z \vec{G}$$

where the gradient vector $\vec{G}$ has 3 independent orthogonal components $G_x = \partial B_z/\partial x$, $G_y = \partial B_z/\partial y$ and $G_z = \partial B_z/\partial z$. Thus a linear, combination of these components will allow a gradient vector to be established in any arbitrary direction according to the requirements of the image plane orientation. This ability to select a plane electronically and acquire data in any readout direction without necessitating the mechanical hardware constraints of a moving gantry represents one of the positive aspects of the NMR imaging technique.

The linear gradient fields will be established by the magnetic field produced by current carrying conductors arranged in a geometrical configuration appropriate for the desired gradient orientation. The integrated magnetic field $\vec{B}(r)$ at a point $r-r_\ell$ from a wire displaced $\vec{r}_\ell$ from the origin which carries a current I is given by the Biot-Savart law (see Figure 4):

$$\vec{B}(r) = \frac{\mu_o I}{4\pi} \int_\ell \frac{(\vec{r} - \vec{r}_\ell)}{|\vec{r} - \vec{r}_\ell|^3} \times d\ell$$

where μ_o is the magnetic permeability of free space and dl is an element of the wire. The components of $\vec{B}$ may be obtained by expansion of the vector product; for example:

$$B_z(x,y,z) = \frac{\mu_o I}{4\pi} \left[\int_\ell \frac{(x-x_\ell)}{|r-r_\ell|^3} d\ell_y - \int_\ell \frac{(y-y_\ell)}{|r-r_\ell|^3} d\ell_x \right]$$

The challenge of designing linear gradient coils is then that of determining a spatial distribution for the associated conductors (wires) which will allow the desired gradient pattern to be established in an efficient manner throughout the imaging volume.

Independent coil windings to produce controlled gradient fields have been used historically with NMR spectrometers to: 1.) correct for the static field inhomogeneities in an attempt to produce as uniform a field as possible over the sample volume as required for high resolution studies, and, 2.) provide the relatively strong gradient field required for diffusion investigations. Representative papers dealing with these applications are given in references 8-13. Although the functional use of the gradient fields in NMR imaging is unique in relationship to the "classical" purposes listed above, MRI gradient coil design has as its origin these original concepts. In addition, while not the topic of this paper, shim coil configurations utilizing the same theoretical basis are often employed in MRI systems to provide correction for main magnetic field inhomogeneities (14).

In general, it is possible to expand any function $f(x,y,z)$ which satisfies Laplace's equation $\nabla^2 f = 0$ in terms of an infinite set of solid spherical harmonics. Because $\nabla^2 B_z = 0$ at all points within the image volume of interest, one may write

$$B_z = \sum_{n=0}^{\infty} \sum_{m=0}^{n} [A_{nm}^c \, r^n \, P_n^m(\cos\theta) \cos m\phi + A_{nm}^s \, r^n \, P_n^m(\cos\theta) \sin m\phi]$$

where $P_n^m(\cos\theta)$ are the associated Legendre polynomials and A_{nm}^c and A_{nm}^s are appropriate constants determined by the shape of the coils and the strength of the currents in them. In the most important case for gradient coil design consideration, the current carrying conductors will be located on a cylinder surrounding the imaging region. Under these conditions the general coefficients may be given by the simplified expressions:

$$A_{nm}^c = \frac{\mu_o}{4\pi r_o^{n+2}} \iint \lambda_\phi(\phi_o, z_o) \, f_{nm}(Z_o) \cos m\phi_o \, dA$$

and

$$A_{nm}^s = \frac{\mu_o}{4\pi r_o^{n+2}} \iint \lambda_\phi(\phi_o, z_o) \, f_{nm}(Z_o) \sin m\phi_o \, dA$$

where the normalized location of the winding along the cylinder surface (i.e. normalized axial position) is $Z_o = z_o/r_o$ with the radius of the cylinder r_o and the element of surface area given by $dA = r_o^2 d\phi_o dZ_o$. In most cases of concern, the surface current density, $\lambda_\phi(\phi_o, z_o)$ can be expressed as the product of two functions, one depending only on ϕ_o and one depending only on Z_o such that:

$$\lambda_\phi(\phi_o, z_o) = c f_\phi(\phi_o) \sigma_\phi(Z_o)$$

where c is a constant of proportionality, $f_\phi(\phi_o)$ expresses the angular variation of the surface current density and $\sigma_\phi(Z_o)$ expresses the variation along the cylindrical axis (z-direction). The task of the coil designer is to determine the shape functions $f_\phi(\phi_o)$ and $\sigma_\phi(Z_o)$ that will emphasize the coefficients of the fields desirable for the intended application and that will eliminate or minimize the coefficients of the undesirable contaminating terms. Note that although some z-directed current density (λ_z) is present, it will make no contribution to B_z.

AXIAL z-GRADIENT COILS

In general, a linear z-gradient in a defined region may be established by cylindrically symmetric coils wound on the surface of a cylinder (with the axis of the cylinder oriented along the z-direction of the magnetic field) under the constraint that the current density is antisymmetric. In this case, the surface current density which is in the ϕ direction is given by the simplified expression:

$$\lambda_\phi = c\sigma_\phi(Z_o)$$

with the antisymmetry condition that $\sigma_\phi(-Z_o) = -\sigma_\phi(Z_o)$ and $c = N_t I/r_o w_{ro}$ where N_t is the total number of turns without regard to sign and r_o is the cylinder radius. The dimensionless parameter w_{ro} involves the shape function through the relationship

$$w_{r_o} = \int_{-Z_m}^{Z_m} |\sigma_\phi(Z_o)|\, dZ_o$$

where Z_m is defined with respect to the total length of the coil (i.e., extent in the z-direction), $l_t = 2r_o Z_m$. Thus when the shape functon $\sigma_\phi(Z_o)$ (which specificies the winding density as a function of position) and the radius are fixed, c is proportional to the total number of ampere-turns on the coil. For this configuration, the magnetic field produced by the coil may be expressed as an expansion in solid spherical harmonics about the center of the coil involving only odd terms (the even terms cancel as a consequence of the antisymmetric cylindrical geometry)

$$B_z = \sum_{n=1,3,5...}^{\infty} A_n\, r^n\, P_n(\cos\theta)$$

with the expansion coefficients given by (16, 17):

$$A_n = \frac{\mu_o c}{2 r_o^n} \int_{-Z_m}^{Z_m} \sigma_\phi(Z_o)\, f_n(Z_o)\, dZ_o$$

$$= \frac{\mu_o c \gamma_n}{2 r_o^n} = \mu_o N_t I \gamma_n (2 r_o^{n+1} w_{r_o})^{-1}$$

where $\gamma_n = \int_{-Z_m}^{Z_m} \sigma_\phi(Z_o)\, f_n(Z_o)\, dZ_o$

with $f_n(Z_o) = P_{n+1}^1(\cos\theta_o)/(1+z_o^2)^{(2n+3)/2}$

One of the primary design objectives is to determine the current distribution $\sigma_\phi(Z_o)$ for a given order of homogeneity of magnetic field under the constraint that the energy stored in the coil is a minimum. It can be shown that the inductance, L, is given by:

$$L = \frac{2\mu_o N_t^2 r_o}{w_{ro}^2} S$$

and that the stored energy in the magnetic, W, field is given by:

$$W = \frac{4r_o^{2n+3}}{\mu_o} \frac{A_n^2}{2\gamma n^2} S$$

where the dimensionless factor S is defined as:

$$S = \int_{-Z_m}^{Z_m} \int_{-Z_m}^{Z_m} \frac{1}{k} [(1-\frac{k^2}{2}) K(k) - E(k)] \sigma(Z_o) \sigma(Z_o') dZ_o' dZ_o$$

with the modulus k defined by:

$k^2 = 4/(4+(Z_o-Z_o')^2)$ and $K(k)$, $E(k)$ are complete elliptical integrals of the first and second kind.

An expression for the z-gradient G_z may be obtained by differentiating the expression for B_z and setting $z = 0$,

$$G_z = (dBz/dz)|_{z=0} = A_1 = \frac{\mu_o c \gamma_1}{2r_o}$$

For $n = 1$, the stored energy would be given as:

$$W = \frac{4r_o^5}{\mu o} G_z^2 \frac{S}{\gamma_1^2}$$

Therefore, for a specified value of G_z, the stored energy can be minimized by choosing the shape function $\sigma_\phi(Z_o)$ such that S is minimized subject to the normalization constraint that $\gamma_1 = 1$. The terms γ_3, γ_5, γ_7 etc. represent contaminants that limit the gradient field linearity. Design of more sophisticated gradient coils with progressively improved linearity require additional constraints on $\sigma_\phi(Z_o)$ to achieve conditions such that

$$\gamma_3 = 0, \gamma_5 = 0, \gamma_7 = 0........etc.$$

We will now examine how some of these principles may be applied to the practical construction of z-gradient coils.

The most common design configuration for the z-gradient coils in those systems where access is oriented such that the patient axis is parallel the direction of the main magnetic field involves a Maxwell coil pair. These consist of two flat circular wire coils, each of radius r_o oriented parallel and coaxial to each other with a separation of $\sqrt{3} \, r_o$. Each carries a current of equal magnitude but opposite in direction as shown in the schematic of Figure 5. This configuration is designed to give $\gamma_3 = 0$. An ideal Maxwell coil would have a filament (coil width) of zero diameter with each coil represented by a delta function at $Z_o = \pm (\sqrt{3}/2)r_o$. Therefore, under the normalization that $\gamma_1 = 1$, the shape function for this idealized coil would be

$$\sigma_\phi(Z_o) = 0.78 \, [\delta(Z_o - \sqrt{3}/2) - \delta(Z_o + \sqrt{3}/2)]$$

For this case, the factor S, the inductance L, and the resistance R would all be infinite. In practice, real coils will have a definite width. For the example in which the width of each coil is $0.2r_o$, the shape function is given as;

$$\sigma_\phi(Z_o) = \begin{matrix} 3.945, & 0.7751 < Z_o < 0.9751 \\ 0, & \text{otherwise} \\ -3.945, & -0.9751 < Z_o < -0.7751 \end{matrix}$$

with $r_o = 0.3$ m, $G_z = 1$ G/cm, $I = 30$A and the resistance $R = 0.74\Omega$ (typical value for $N_t = 75$ and #12 AWG copperwire), $S \simeq 1.88$, $w_{ro} = 1.58$, and $L = 3.2$ mh.

Photographs of the z-gradient coils designed and constructed at the University of Cincinnati for a 6-coil, 0.15T resistive whole body imaging system (18) are shown in Figure 6a. A plot of the experimental results obtained when evaluating the z-gradient field obtained is shown in Figure 7a.

The Maxwell pair configuration as discussed above cancels the third order term in the expansion so that the initial term contributing to the nonlinearity is A_5. In order to provide a greater degree of linearity, it is necessary to cancel these higher order terms. This may be accomplished through the use of additional coil loops. Various two Maxwell pair coil designs have been described by Saint-Jalmes et. al. (19) which increase the overall efficiency by allowing equivalent field linearity with smaller coils utilizing less electrical power. This advantage is even more significant when considering switched power operation. The linearity was demonstrated to be maintained within approximately 0.2% to 0.6% over a 0.4m diameter sphere in the central region as compared to the 5% linearity deviation characteristics obtained with a single pair of the same size. To produce this same degree of linearity for the specified gradient strength, a single Maxwell pair would require a larger diameter with dc and switched power consumption 5x and 15x greater respectively.

TRANSVERSE x-and y-GRADIENT COILS

Independent, orthogonal, linear gradient fields G_x and G_y are required also in the x- and y- directions respectively as discussed in the introduction. From symmetry considerations, it is clear that any coil set assembly designed to provide G_y may be physically rotated through 90° to produce G_x. Therefore, the discussion need develop only the concepts relating to one direction. The following will address apsects of y-gradient coils.

One method of producing a transverse gradient is through the use of four straight, parallel conductors located at the corners of a rectangle each carrying a current of equal magnitude flowing in the same direction (see Figure 8a). This type of gradient coil design has been described by a number of authors (7,20) following the methods of Zupanic and Pirs (21) in which the magnetic field at a point (y,z) due to a current in a single infinite conductor oriented parallel to the x-axis at location (y_ℓ, z_ℓ) is given as the real part of the complex function representing the solution of the Biot-Savart law. For the component of the field in the z-direction, this expression would be:

$$B_z(y,z) = \frac{\mu_o I}{2\pi} \text{Re}\,[((y_\ell + iz_\ell) - (y+iz))^{-1}]$$

Letting $y + iz = \xi$ and $y_\ell + iz_\ell = ie^{i\phi}$, the above expression for B_z may be expanded as a Taylor series under the condition that $|\xi| < r_\ell$ (where r_ℓ and ϕ are the polar coordinates of the wire) giving;

$$B_z(y,z) = \frac{\mu_o I}{2\pi} \text{Re} \sum_{n=0}^{\infty} (\xi/r)^n e^{-i(n+1)\phi}$$

For the 4-conductor configuration of Figure 8a in which all currents are in the same direction, the contributions for each wire at point (y,z) combined such that all even powers of n cancel. The y-gradient is given as: $G_y = \partial B_z(y,z)/\partial y$ evaluated at z=0. The 3rd order term which would represent the first dominant contaminant and restrict the region of linearity may be made zero under the condition that $\phi = \pi(1/2 + m)/4$, m = 0, 1, 2, 3... Two angles of interest fulfilling this criteria are ϕ = 22.5° and ϕ = 67.5. If the 4 conductors lie on a circle of radius r_o with ϕ = 22.5°, the gradient up to the fourth order in the expansion coefficient will be (7);

$$Gy = \partial B(y,z)/\partial y = 1.414\mu_o I/(\pi r_o^2)$$

whereas for ϕ = 67.5° the gradient will be;

$$Gy = -1.414\mu_o I/(\pi r_o^2)$$

As discussed by Mansfield and Morris (7), these results suggest methods of addressing the requirement for providing a return current path (closed loop) for any real coil configuration. Two possible arrangements are indicated schematically in Figure 8b and c. In effect, the return path is constrained to a greater radius and would contribute a component of G_y having a smaller magnitude. In Figure 8b, this contribution is negative and the net gradient strength would be reduced, whereas in Figure 8c, the contribution is additive. In either case, the linearity characteristics would not be compromised because, with the conditions for the specified ϕ values maintained, the return conductors generate a gradient field with contaminating terms of the same order as those produced by the primary wires. In addition, for the latter option, with all four conductor pairs lying in parallel planes as shown, the field from the end connecting wires which are oriented parallel to the z-axis would not contribute to G_y. In general, however, the coil dimensions required for whole body MRI systems are somewhat too large to be practical for the latter option.

Up to this point, the discussion has been concerned with the theory for infinite parallel conductors. Obviously, in practice, coils of finite size must be employed with the appropriate return paths provided. The infinite length model may at best be used only as a guide to the optimum real world design. Bangert and Mansfield[20] described their gradient coil system which is comprised of four trapezium loops exhibiting a relatively low inductance suitable for switched field applications.

Another approach to the design of transverse gradient coils involves analysis of the spherical harmonic description under the cylindrical symmetry outlined previously in the section on z-gradient coils. To produce a transverse field, the coils must be designed such that A_{11}^s is the predominant coefficient for the y-gradient set (with A_{11}^c predominant for the x-gradient). Figure 9 shows the configuration for a single coil made from two opposed circular arcs one running from ϕ_0 to $\pi - \phi_0$ and the other from $\pi + \phi_0$ to $2\pi - \phi_0$. With the current oppositely directed in each arc, the angular variation of the surface current density $f_\phi(\phi_0)$ equals 1 for ϕ_0 to $\pi - \phi_0$, -1 for $\pi + \phi_0$ to $2\pi - \phi_0$, and 0 everywhere else. This configuration produces fields which vary only as $\cos m\phi$ with m odd. The coefficients $A_{nm}^c = 0$ for all n and m while $A_{nm}^s = 0$ for m even.

If the shape function is even such that $\sigma_\phi(-Z_o) = \sigma_\phi(Z_o)$, all coefficients A_{nm}^s with n even are made equal to zero. Thus though the use of circular arcs with the symmetry properties discussed above, a y-gradient field will be produced that has A_{11}^s as the leading term and various contaminants of the form A_{31}^s, A_{33}^s, A_{51}^s, A_{53}^s, A_{55}^s, A_{71}^s, etc.

A common design for transverse gradient coils utilizes arrays of circular arcs in the saddle coil configuration (Figure 5). Four arcs are required to provide the necessary symmetry to establish the transverse gradient with four additional arcs required for the return current paths. In addition, a total of eight interconnecting paths parallel to the z-direction are required which do not contribute to the B_z field but do substantially increase the inductance and resistance of the coil. The design considerations now center on techniques to reduce some of the contaminating terms to zero. The terms $A_{31}{}^S$ and $A_{33}{}^S$ have the most severe effect upon the linearity. They may be eliminated by the judicious selection of the coil geometry. The term $A_{33}{}^S$ which is proportional to $\cos 3(\phi_o + \pi/2)$ may be made zero by choosing $\phi_o = \pi/3$ which indicates that each arc should subtend an angle of 120°.

The term $A_{31}{}^S$ may be eliminated through the appropriate relative positioning of these arcs along the z-axis. Golay (22) showed that this condition would be satisfied if the arcs were placed at the roots of the equation $4Z_o{}^4 - 27Z_o{}^2 + 4 = 0$ which yields $Z_o = \pm 0.39$ and ± 2.57. However, coils built with these dimensions would be quite long with the total length almost three times the diameter and consequently would exhibit large values for L and R. The requirement that $A_{31}{}^S = 0$ may still be met if the outer arc is brought much closer to the origin and the inner arc is moved only slightly outward.

A photograph of the saddle coils constructed at the University of Cincinnati for the 0.15 T whole body MRI unit are shown in Figure 6 which used Z_o values of ± 0.39 and ± 1.39. An experimental plot of the y-gradient characteristics for the $z = 0$ plane is shown in Figure 7b.

Other styles of gradient coils have been utilized including those suitable for use with transverse geometry in which the main magnetic field is oriented perpendicular to the patient axis. Hutchinson has described quadrupole sets and distributed winding configurations (23). The latter consists of straight wires running on the surface of and parallel to the axis of the supporting cylinder with the density of conductors (number per radian) proportional to the sine of twice the angular position around the circumference ($\sin 2\phi$). These coils provide an acceptable linear gradient over a region extending to nearly 90% of the cylinder radius.

ELECTRONIC CIRCUITS FOR DRIVING GRADIENT COILS

As NMR imaging techniques have evolved, so too have the

complexity and capabilities of the electronics used to drive the gradient coils. The electronics required to energize the gradient coils of an NMR imaging system depend upon a number of factors: e.g., pulse protocol, type of imaging (projection or 2DFT), electrical characteristics of the gradient coils, etc. In this section, a brief overview of the evolution of gradient coil electronics is provided by discussing static, oscillating, and pulsed gradients. A more detailed description of a modern gradient drive design for arbitrary gradient manipulation is given. Examples of gradient waveforms generated and typical operating characteristics are provided.

A. <u>Static Gradients</u>

Early imaging experiments were performed using a partial saturation pulse sequence, projection reconstruction (24) and no slice selection. The gradients needed to produce a projection of an object in the xy plane are provided by a steady state current in each of the x and y gradient coils. The magnitude of these currents is related simply to the angle of the projection, ϕ, by $I_x = G\sin\phi$, and $I_y = G\cos\phi$, where G is the gradient strength. These currents are independent of time and need not be changed until data at a new projection angle is required. The circuits used to provide these currents could be as simple as a variable DC power supply; however, the circuit shown in Figure 10, more typical of those actually used, provides computer control of the gradient fields. Two digital to analog converters (DAC) are supplied with a stable voltage reference and digital data representing the sine and cosine of the projection angle ϕ. The computer or other logic source (e.g., PROMS) is used to supply the digital information. The DACs are followed by multiplying digital to analog converters (MDAC) which provide direct control of the magnitude of the gradient G. The outputs of the MDACs are buffered and routed through amplifiers capable of providing 2 to 10 amps for a typical set of saddle coils as discussed previously.

B. <u>Oscillating Gradients</u>

The first method devised for localizing the observed NMR signal to a thin slice within a three-dimensional object was based upon the use of oscillating field gradients (25). For example, to select a slice perpendicular to the z-axis, at location z_0, a field gradient of the form

$$G(z,t) = G_z(z-z_0) \sin (\Omega t)$$

can be used. The gradient is a linear function of the spatial coordinate and is an oscillatory function of time with frequency By recording the NMR signal and averaging a number of FIDs which occur at random times with respect to the period $1/\Omega$, a signal representative of the spins in the null gradient plane ($z = z_0$) is obtained. The thickness profile, $T(z,\Omega)$, of the planar region has been related to the strength of the gradient G_z and the frequency Ω (26,27).

$$T(z,\Omega) \propto J_0^2 \ (G_z(z-z_0)/\Omega)$$

where J_0 is a zero order Bessel Function. A plot of this function is shown in Figure 11. Oscillating field gradients and signal averaging therefore allow the NMR signal to be localized to a thin region in space.

An example of the electronics required to provide such oscillating field gradients is shown in Figure 12. A logic circuit (i.e., PROM or RAM) is loaded with a sine (or arbritrary) oscillatory waveform. This data is fed to a single DAC which provides the audio frequency signal. By changing the rate at which data is clocked to the DAC, the frequency of the oscillatory signal is easily adjusted. The output of the DAC is routed to MDAC's under separate computer control. The outputs are buffered and amplified with the current from each driving half of the z-gradient coil. This arrangement allows the magnitude of the gradients as well as the location of the null gradient plane ($z = z_0$) to be selected. For oscillating gradient applications, the power amplifiers must be capable of operating in a current controlled feedback mode and have a usable bandwidth greater than the maximum audio frequency (generally 500Hz).

C. Pulsed Field Gradients

More recent forms of NMR imaging make use of the spin echo phenomenon and rely on pulsed field gradients. The pulsed field gradients provide slice selection capability and are needed also for preparing the spin system for echo formation.

The early forms of pulsed field gradient circuits made use of "tuned" circuit designs. Charge storage, switching components and pulse shaping networks were used to drive the gradient coils. This approach was taken to avoid the cost of high power, wide bandwidth linear amplifier systems. Figure 13 illustrates the type of circuit used for pulsed gradient applications. Panel B shows a schematic of the circuit and panel A shows the type of waveform produced. The design details are documented elsewhere (28). This design allows the large inductive load of the gradient coil L_1 to be incorporated into the design of the driving circuit. The high transient current needed to energize the coil is provided by the charge stored on the capacitors. A modest DC power supply is sufficient to energize the entire system because of the relatively long recycle delay period.

Modern NMR imaging systems use gradient drive electronics which incorporate complete digital control of every aspect of the current waveforms to the gradient coils. The block diagram of a typical circuit is shown in Figure 14. A DAC is used to generate the analog voltage corresponding to an arbitrary gradient current waveform stored in a random access memory (RAM). This signal is buffered, amplified, and applied to the gradient coil. Normally, some type of electromagnetic interference (EMI) filtering is incorporated in the circuit so that stray radio frequency signals are not fed into the immediate vicinity of the magnet. A circuit used for EMI filtering is shown in Figure 15.

Modern imaging techniques require a gradient drive which can produce rapidly switched or shaped currents. Figure 2 shows two different pulse sequences which are commonly used in projection reconstruction and 2DFT imaging and the relation of the gradient currents to the RF pulses. Using this approach requires wide bandwidth and high current drive capability of the power amplifiers. For example, the switching needed to produce the slice selection gradient may require changes of approximately 20 amps in a 1 millisecond time interval. Power amplifiers used must have current controlled feedback, wide bandwidth, and stable operating characteristics when driving inductive loads.

Table 1. CHARACTERISTICS OF A TYPICAL SADDLE GRADIENT COIL AND DRIVE SYSTEM OF A RESISTIVE WHOLE BODY NMR IMAGING SYSTEM

Coil Impedance	
L	~10 millihenrys
R	~1 ohm
Power Amplifier	
Bandwidth	20 KHz
DC Output	4 KVA (20A @ 200V)
Output Impedance	<0.1 ohm

In most instances, gradient amplifiers can be cooled by convection or forced air cooling. In some designs, however, the gradient amplifiers may need to dissipate as much as 10 kilowatts of power. Water cooling may be required to dissipate the heat generated under these operating conditions.

METHODS FOR CORRECTING GRADIENT NON-LINEARITIES

The ideal spatial variation of field gradients used for NMR imaging encoding is thought to be linear. This results from a number of factors such as ease of signal processing and reconstruction, uniformity of resolution over the image plane, and freedom from geometric distortion. For this reason, the traditional approach for imaging system design has been to design gradient coils to produce field gradients with spatial variations as close to the linear "ideal" as possible. Any effects of residual non-linearities were either tolerated or ignored.

Recently, the mathematical formalism to correct for gradient field non-linearities has been developed for projection reconstruction (29,30) and 2DFT (6) imaging methods. The potential advantages of using these correction techniques are i) more accurate NMR images can be produced by existing imaging systems and ii) more power efficient and space efficient gradient coil designs can be developed if the requirement of perfect gradient linearity is relaxed.

In this section an overview of the correction techniques for projection and 2DFT imaging is presented. Only the two dimensional imaging case is discussed; however, both techniques are applicable to three dimensional imaging for correction of smoothly varying, minor gradient nonlinearities. For a complete description of the techniques presented, the reader is encouraged to review the original articles.

Projection Reconstruction

In conventional 2D NMR projection reconstruction, the projection P relates the object density function F(r) and the magnitude field as

$$P_\phi(\beta) = 1/\gamma \int F(\vec{r})\delta(B_g-\beta)\, d\vec{r}$$

where β is the observed angular frequency ω divided by the gyromagnetic ratio γ, δ is the dirac delta function and B_g is the functional form of the field gradients. Normally the angle ϕ of the projection is defined by a linear field gradient of magnitude G and is of the form

$$B_g(\vec{r},\vec{u}) = G\,(\vec{r}\cdot\vec{u})$$
$$= G(x\cos\phi + y\sin\phi)$$

where $\vec{u}$ is a unit vector pointing in the direction of ϕ.

Under these conditions the equation for $P_\phi(\beta)$ above can be written as a line integral of $F(\vec{r})$ over straight line paths, $\vec{r}\cdot\vec{u} = \beta/G$

$$P_\phi(\beta) = (1/\gamma) \int F(\vec{r})\,\delta\,(\vec{r}\cdot\vec{u} - \beta/G)\,d\vec{r}$$

Image reconstruction consists of inverting a series of projection measurements (either by back projection or by Fourier analysis) to estimate $F(\vec{r})$.

In the more general case of non-linear field gradients, the integral becomes a line integral of $F(\vec{r})$

over curved paths $B_g(\vec{r},\vec{u}) = \beta$. Figure 16 illustrates the effect of non-linear field gradients upon projection reconstruction. Lai (29,30) has defined a curvilinear coordinate system such that

$$q_1 = G\, b_x(x,y)$$

$$q_2 = G\, b_y(x,y)$$

This coordinate transformation is used to linearize the effect of the non-linear field gradients. In the curvilinear coordinate system the gradient field becomes

$$B_g(\vec{q},\vec{u}) = \vec{q}\cdot\vec{u}$$

$$P_\phi(\beta) = 1/\gamma \int F(\vec{r}(\vec{q}))\delta(\vec{q}\cdot\vec{u} - \beta)/|J(\vec{q})|\, d\vec{q}$$

where $J(q)$ is the Jacobian of the transformation from object coordinates (x,y) to gradient field coordinates (q_1, q_2). In this curved coordinate system, $P_\phi(\beta)$ is the "rectilinear" projection of the object

$$H(\vec{q}) = F(\vec{r}(\vec{q}))|J(\vec{q})|$$

Conventional backprojection techniques allow the image of $H(\vec{q})$ to be formed in the curvilinear coordinate system. The true image in the (x,y) coordinate system can be simply derived as

$$F(\vec{r}) = H(\vec{q}(\vec{r}))|j(\vec{r})|$$

where $j(r)$ is the inverse transformation Jacobian

$$j(\vec{r}) = \begin{vmatrix} \partial q_1/\partial x & \partial q_1/\partial y \\ \partial q_2/\partial x & \partial q_2/\partial y \end{vmatrix}$$

If the Jacobian correction is not applied, the reconstructed image is not blurred however, it will contain geometrical distortions. Lai has shown that this correction allows geometrically accurate images to be formed using non-linear field gradients. Image resolution, however, has been shown to be non-uniform and anisotropic. Resolution is better in regions of higher gradient strength.

The curvilinear coordinate system needed to perform this correction may be calculated analytically for a particular gradient coil design or may be derived numerically from an experimentally determined map of the field gradients.

2DFT Image Reconstruction

The effects of non-linear field gradients and inhomogeneous main field upon the 2DFT imaging technique have been discussed recently (6). The raw data used in this technique can be thought of as the two-dimensional Fourier transform of the desired image, sampled in a rectangular coordinate system. The coordinate system is defined by the direction u of the readout gradient and the direction v of the phase encoding gradient. The image produced can be expressed as $A(u,v)$.

The effect of gradient nonlinearities is to produce a geometric distortion of the image $A(u,v)$. The coordinate u is shifted to a new location $u + \varepsilon_u$ and the coordinate v is shifted to $v + \varepsilon_v$. The quantities ε_u and ε_v are maps of the departure from linearity of the readout and phase encoding gradient fields over the image plane:

$$\varepsilon_u(u,v) = \frac{B_u(u,v) - G_o \Delta d}{G_o \Delta d}$$

$$\varepsilon_v(u,v) = \frac{B_v(u,v) - G_o \Delta d}{G_o \Delta d}$$

In these expressions, $B_u(u,v)$ is the field produced by the readout gradient at the point (u,v), and $B_v(u,v)$ is the field produced by the maximum phase encoding gradient at the point (u,v). G_o represents the assumed linear field gradient and d is the pixel spacing. Image correction for gradient nonlinearities consists of constructing a new image $A'(u,v)$

$$A'(u,v) = K_u(u,v) \, K_v(u,v) \, A[u - \varepsilon_u(u,v), v - \varepsilon_v(u,v)]$$

The K_u and K_v factors are needed for intensity correction.

$$K_u(u,v) = 1/[1 + \partial \varepsilon_u / \partial u \Delta d]$$

and
$$K_v(u,v) = 1/[1 + \partial \varepsilon_v / \partial v \Delta d]$$

Use of non-linear field gradients with the 2DFT imaging method has no adverse effect upon resolution as long as the factors are reasonable approximations of the true nonlinearities present.

REFERENCES

1. Bottomley PA. Instrumentation for Whole-Body NMR Imaging. In NMR Imaging: Proceedings of an International Symposium on Nuclear Magnetic Resonance Imaging. Eds. R.L. Witcofski, N. Karstaedt, C.L. Partain. The Bowman Gray School of Medicine, Winston-Salem, NC. 1982. p 25-31.

2. Thomas SR, Ackerman JL. The Instrumentation of Nuclear Magnetic Resonance Imaging. In Frontiers of Engineering and Computing in Health Care, 1983. Proceedings, Fifth Annual Conference IEEE Engineering in Medicine and Biology Society. Eds. G.C. Gerhard and W.T. Miller. p 25-31. 1983.

3. Pykett IL, Buonanno FS, Brady TJ et al. Techniques and Approaches to Proton NMR Imaging of the Head. Computerized Radiol. $\underline{27}$: 1-17, 1983.

4. Holland GN. Systems Engineering of a Whole-Body Proton Magnetic Resonance Imaging System. In Nuclear Magnetic Resonance (NMR) Imaging. Editors: Partain CL, James AE, Rollo FD, Price RR. W.B. Saunders Company, Philadelphia, 1984. p 128-151.

5. Edelstein WA, Bottomley PA, Hart HR et al. NMR Imaging at 5.1 MHz: Work in Progress. In NMR Imaging: Proceedings of an International Symposium on Nuclear Magnetic Resonance Imaging. Eds. R.L. Witcofski, N. Karstaedt, C.L. Partain. The Bowman Gray School of Medicine, Winston-Salem, NC. 1982. p 139-145.

6. O'Donnell M, Edelstein WA. NMR Imaging in the Presence of Magnetic Field Inhomogeneities and Gradient Field Nonlinearities. Med. Phys. $\underline{12}$:20-26, 1985.

7. Mansfield P., Morris PG. NMR Imaging in Biomedicine. Academic Press, New York, 1982.

8. Golay MJ. Field Homogenizing Coils for Nuclear Spin Resonance Instrumentation. Rev. Sci. Inst. $\underline{29}$: 313-315, 1958.

9. Anderson WA. Electrical Current Shims for Correcting Magnetic Fields. Rev. Sci. Inst. $\underline{32}$: 241-250, 1961.

10. Tanner JE. Pulsed Field Gradients for NMR Spin-Echo Diffusion Measurements. Rev. Sci. Inst. $\underline{36}$: 1086-1087, 1965.

11. Ginsberg DM, and Melchner MJ. Optimum Geometry of Saddle Coils for Generating a Uniform Magnetic Field. Rev. Sci. Inst. $\underline{41}$: 122-123, 1970.

12. Parker RS, Zupancic I and Pirs J. Coil System to Produce Orthogonal, Linear Magnetic Field Gradients. J. Phys. E: Sci. Instrum. 6: 899-900, 1973.

13. Odbery G and Odberg L. On the Use of a Quadrupole Coil for NMR Spin-Echo Diffusion Studies. J. Magnetic Resonance 16: 342-347, 1974.

14. Romeo F and Hoult DI. Magnetic Field Profiling: Analysis and Correcting Coil Design. Magnetic Resonance in Medicine 1: 44-65, 1984.

15. Bottomley PA. A Versatile Magnetic Field Gradient Control System for NMR Imaging. J. Phys. E: Sci. Instrum. 14: 1081-1087, 1981.

16. Schenck JG, Hussain MA, Edelstein WA, Noble G. An Integral Equation for the Design of Magnetic Field Coils. Proceedings of the 1982 Army Numerical Analysis and Computers Conference. ARO Report 82-3. U.S. Army Research Office, Research Triangle Park, North Carolina. p 397-409.

17. Schenck JF, Hussain MA. Formulation of Design Rules for NMR Imaging Coils by using Symbolic Manipulation. Proceedings of the 1981 ACM Symposium on Symobolic and Algebraic Computations Association for Computing Machinery, New York, New York. p 85-93.

18. Thomas SR, Ackerman JL, and Kereiakes JG. Practical Aspects Involved in the Design and Set Up of a 0.15T, 6-Coil Resistive Magnet Whole Body NMR Imaging Facility. Mag. Res. Imaging 2: 341-348, 1984.

19. Saint-Jalmes H, Taquin J, and Barjhoux Y. Design Data for Efficient Axial Gradient Coils: Application to NMR Imaging. Magentic Resonance in Medicine 2: 245-252, 1985.

20. Bangert V and Mansfield P. Magnetic Field Gradient Coils for NMR Imaging. J. Phys. E: Sci Instrum. 15: 235-239, 1982.

21. Zupancic I and Pirs J. Coils Producing a Magnetic Field Gradient for Diffusion Measurements with NMR. J. Phys. E: Sci. Instrum. 9: 79-80, 1976.

22. Golay MJ. Homogenizing Coils for NMR Apparatus. US Patent 3,622,869, 1971.

23. Hutchison JMS. NMR Proton Imaging Techniques in Magnetic Resonance in Medicine and Biology. M.A. Foster. Pergamon Press, New York, pp 173-190.

24. Lauterbur PC. Image Formation by Induced Local Interactions: Examples Employing NMR. Nature 242:190-1, 1973.

25. Hinshaw WS. Spin Mapping: The Application of Moving Gradients to NMR. Phys. Letters A 48: 87-88, 1974.

26. Bottomley PA. Ph.D. Thesis: Nottingham, 1978.

27. Hinshaw WS. Image Formation by Nuclear Magnetic Resonance: The Sensitive Point Method. J. Appl. Phys. 47: 3709-3721, 1976.

28. Hutchinson JMS, Sutherland RJ, and Mallard JR. NMR Imaging: Image Recovery Under Magnetic Fields with Large Non-Uniformities. J. Phys. E: Sci. Instrum. 11:217-221, 1978.

29. Lai CM. Reconstructing NMR Images Under Non-linear Field Gradients. J. Phys. E: Sci. Instrum. 16: 34-38, 1983.

30. Lai CM. Reconstructing NMR Images from Projections Under Inhomogeneous Magnetic Fields and Non-Linear Field Gradients. Phys. Med. Biol. 28:925-938, 1983.

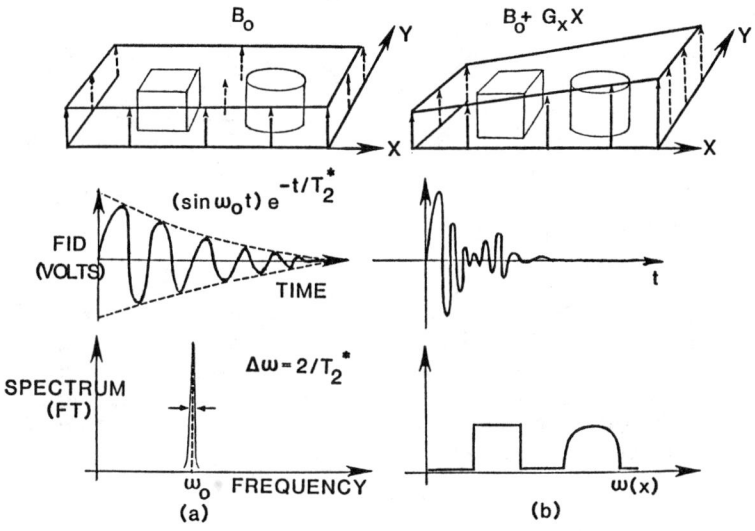

Figure 1: A schematic representation of the spatial encoding function of gradient magnetic fields (2): (a) Under a uniform magnetic field, Bo, the NMR received signal (free induction decay - FID) may be represented as a damped sine wave characterized by the effective spin-spin relaxation time T_2. The Fourier transform (FT) of this FID provides a single line spectrum centered around the resonance frequency ω_o (shown with a slightly expanded frequency axis scale to emphasize the line shape). There is no differentiation of the spatial distribution of the signal producing objects within the region of uniform field. (b) A change in the z-component of B is superimposed upon the main magnetic field here shown as a linear gradient in the x-direction, G_x. The FID is now a more complicated function as a consequence of the multiple resonance frequencies present. The resultant spectrum, which is spatially encoded through the one-to-one correspondence of frequency to x-position, represents a projection of the object space onto the x-axis.

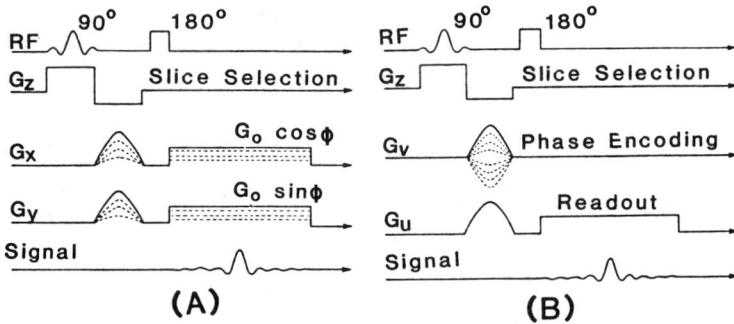

Figure 2: Pulse sequences illustrating the relationship between the gradient wave forms and the rf excitation commonly used for imaging techniques: A) Projection reconstruction; B) 2DFT. In both cases, the slice selection is provided by selective excitation in the z-direction. The time-to-echo, TE, (from the center of the 90° pulse to the center of the signal echo) is typically 30 milliseconds for T_1 weighted imaging. The text refers to the phase encoding gradient as G_v and the readout gradient as G_u. (Modified from O'Donnell and Edelstein, reference 6).

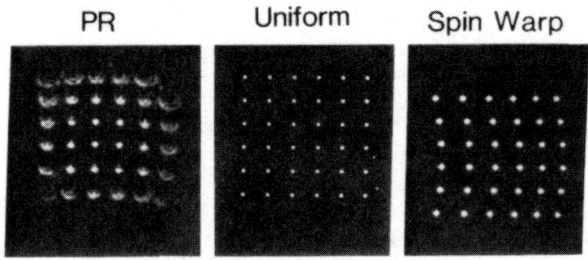

Figure 3: An example of the effect of magnetic field inhomogeneities on the reconstructed image. The center panel shows the image of a point array under conditions of uniform field. The introduction of field inhomogeneities produces blurring of the point spread function as well as geometric distortion for projection reconstruction (PR) while introducing geometric distortion only in the direction of the readout gradient for 2DFT (spin warp).

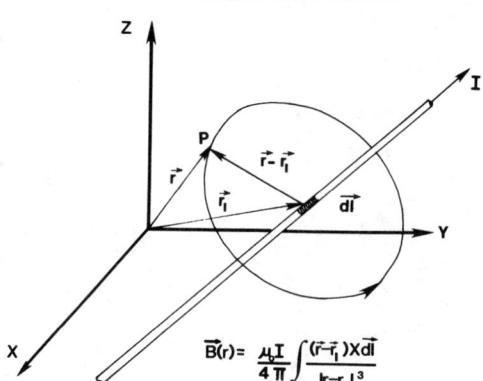

Figure 4: A schematic illustrating the use of the Biot-Savart Law for calculating the magnetic field at any point in space around a current carrying conductor.

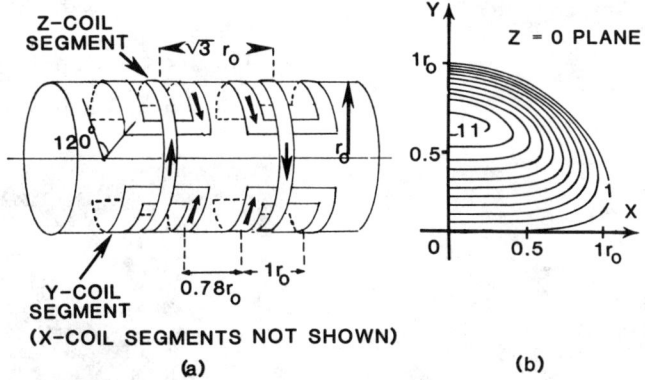

Figure 5: a) A schematic representation of the Maxwell coil pair (z-coil segment indicated) and the y-saddle coil set (one segment indicated) used to establish the z-gradient and y-gradient respectively. The x-saddle coil set is not shown; however, it would be comprised of 4 units identical to the y coils but oriented at 90° with respect to them. The direction of the current in each coil is indicated by the arrows. b) A first quadrant gradient plot in the $z = 0$ imaging plane of the gradient field generated by the y-saddle coils. The curves, as interpolated from a computer iteration of the Biot-Savart Law, would be symetrical about the x and y axes and represent intensity contour plots of the z-component of the magnetic field produced by the y-coils. Each line shown represents a different value of the gradient magnitude in arbitrary units from 1 to 11. (Modified from reference 15).

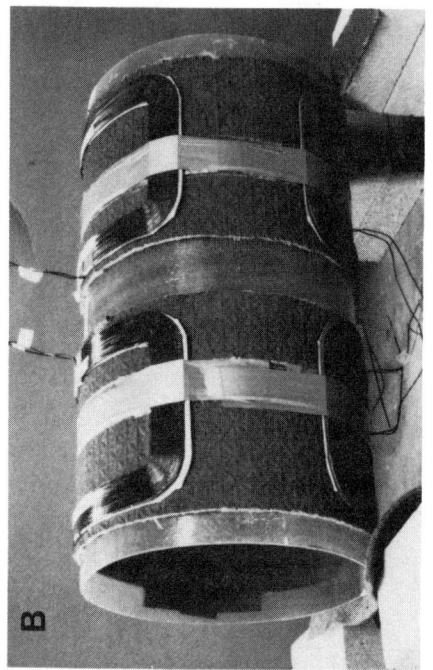
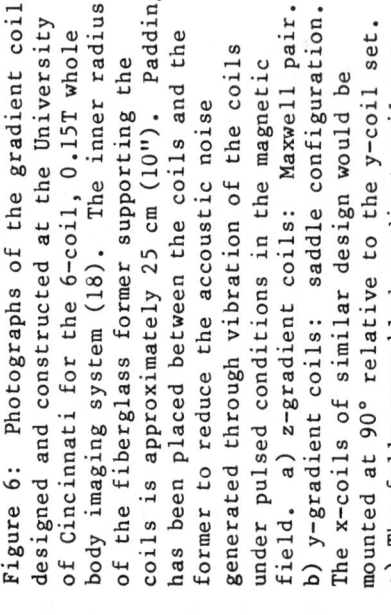
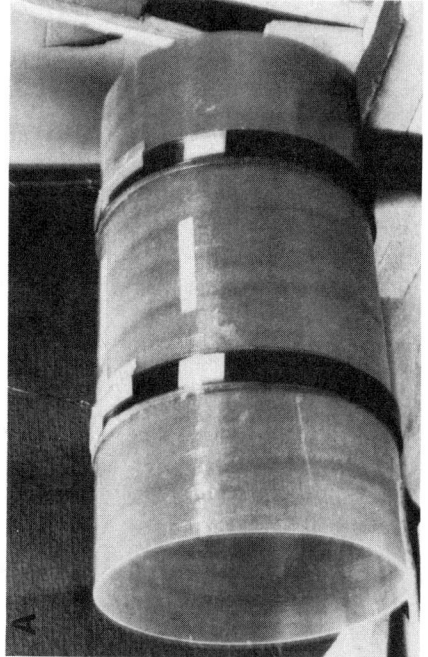
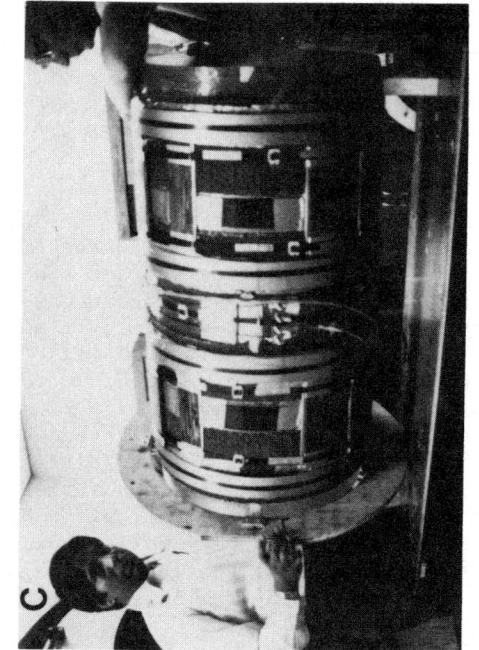

Figure 6: Photographs of the gradient coils designed and constructed at the University of Cincinnati for the 6-coil, 0.15T whole body imaging system (18). The inner radius of the fiberglass former supporting the coils is approximately 25 cm (10"). Padding has been placed between the coils and the former to reduce the accoustic noise generated through vibration of the coils under pulsed conditions in the magnetic field. a) z-gradient coils: Maxwell pair. b) y-gradient coils: saddle configuration. The x-coils of similar design would be mounted at 90° relative to the y-coil set. c) The fully assembled gradient coil set.

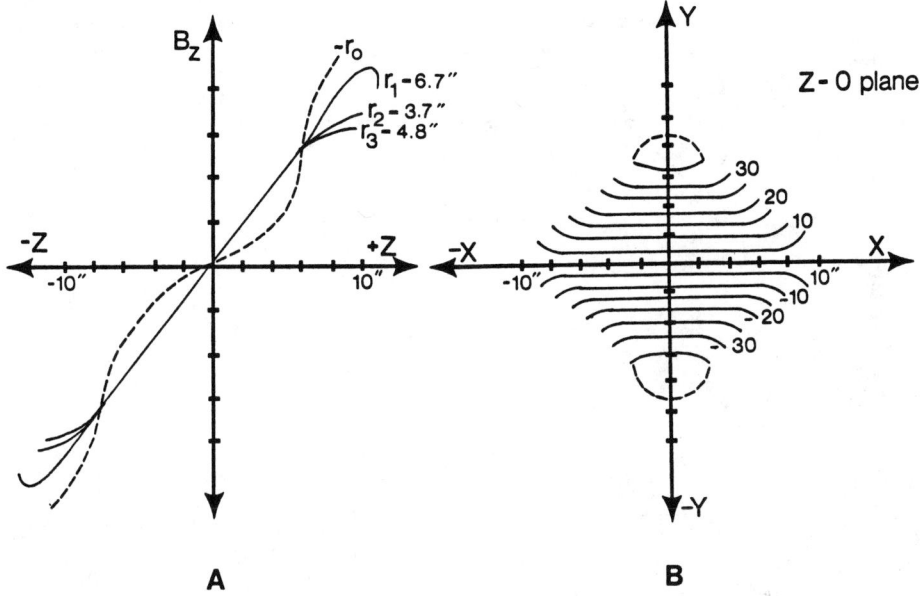

Figure 7: Experimental gradient field plots for the coil sets designed and constructed at the University of Cincinnati: a) Gradient field produced by the z-gradient coil set. b) Gradient field produced by the y-gradient coil set (z=0 plane). The curves are labeled with arbitrary relative numbers proportional to the strength of the magnetic field provided by the gradient coils.

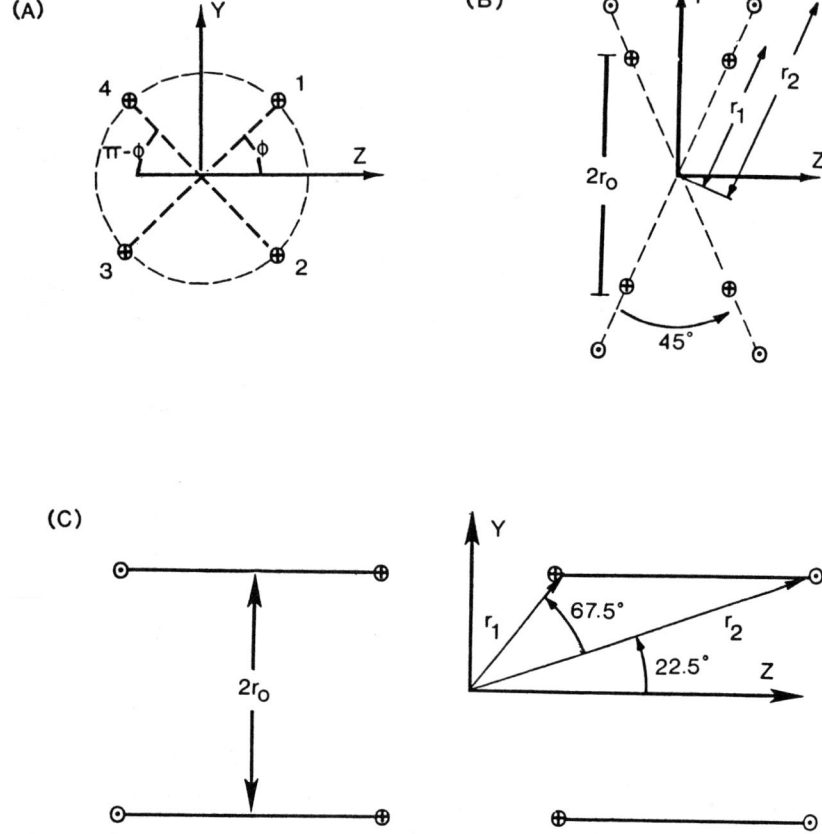

Figure 8: a) Configuration for producing a y-gradient, G_y, involving four straight conductors. b) and c) Return path options which maintain the "purity" of the gradient field. (Modified from reference 7).

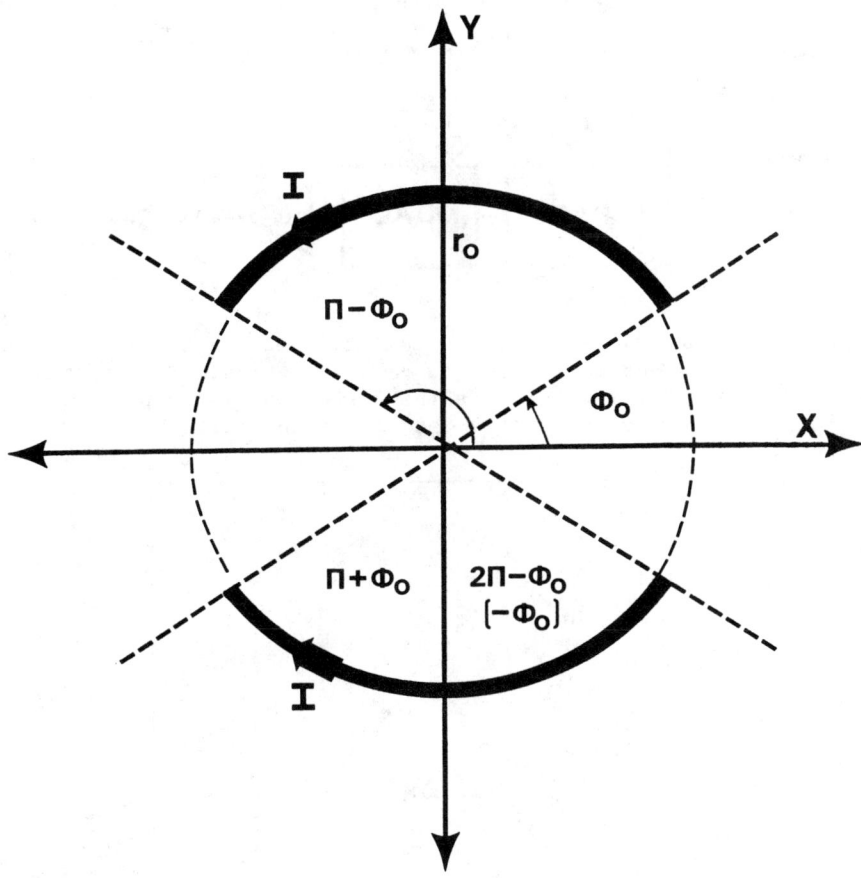

Figure 9: Two opposed arcs situated at ϕ_0 to $\pi - \phi_0$ and $\pi + \phi_0$ to $2\pi - \phi_0$ with current directions as shown. This configuration will produce a y-gradient, G_y.

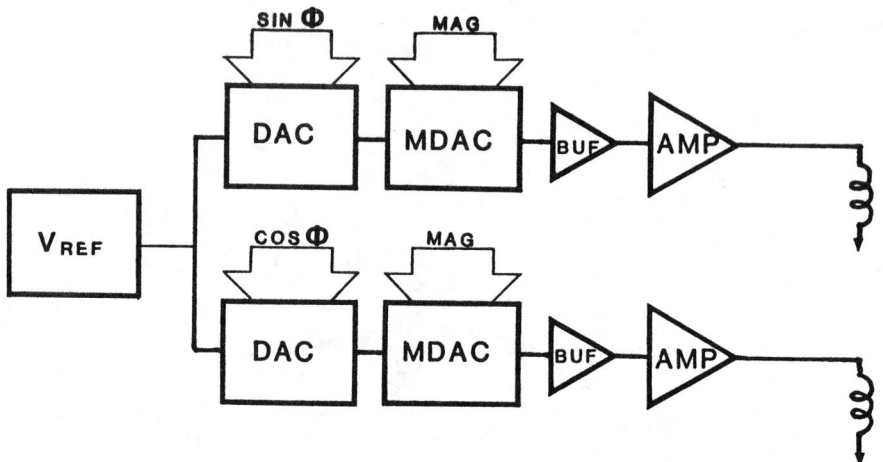

Figure 10: Block diagram of a system utilized for control of static field gradients used in projection reconstruction. The digital data controlling the DAC's determines the direction of the projection and the data controlling the MDAC's determines the strength of the gradient.

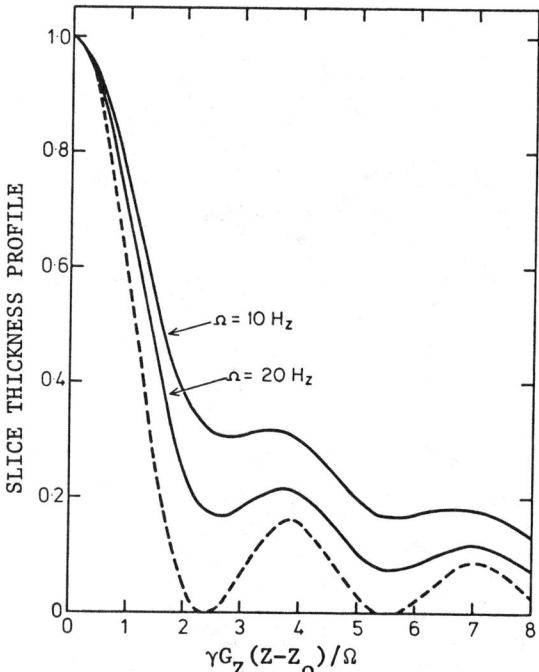

Figure 11: Plot of slice thickness profile provided by a temporally oscillating, spatially linear field gradient. Curves are parameterized for different frequencies Ω. The corresponding curves for 100 and 500 Ω would be indistinguishable from the limit represented by the dashed curve. (Modified from (7)).

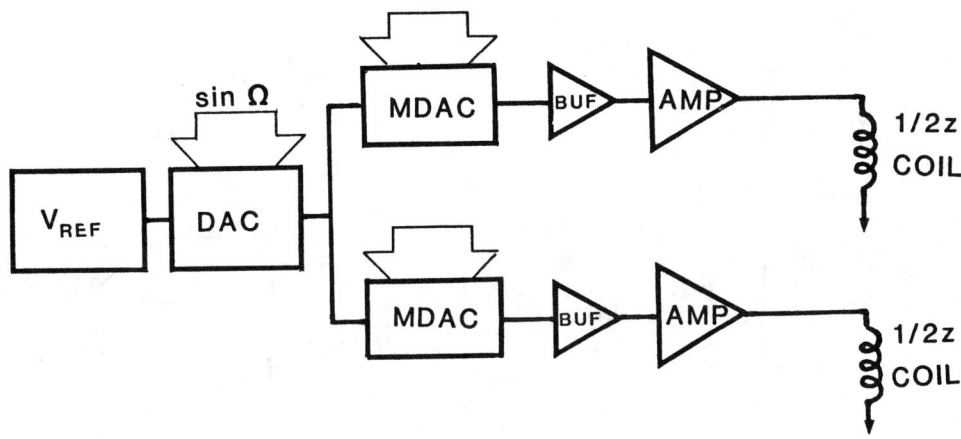

Figure 12: Block diagram of a system used for control of oscillatory field gradients which can be used for slice selection. The digital data and clock rate of the DAC controls the shape and frequency of the temporal oscillation. The data controlling the MDAC's determines the strength of the gradient and the position of the null gradient plane.

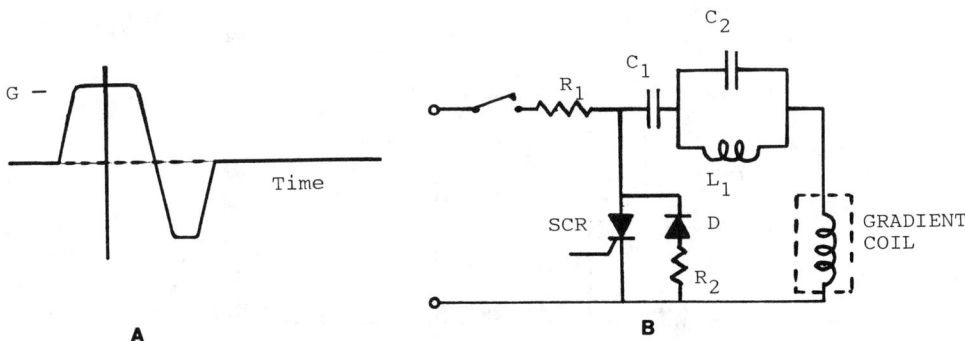

Figure 13: Pulsed field gradients used for slice selection. Panel A shows a typical waveform generated using the analog circuit in Panel B. (From reference 28).

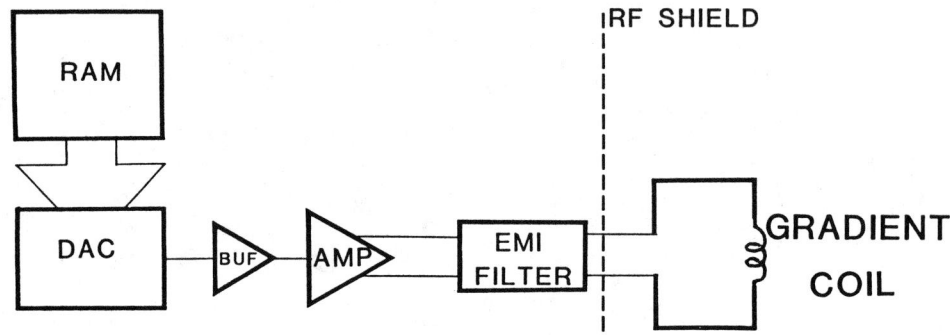

Figure 14: Block diagram of a system used to generate an arbitrarily shaped current waveform in the gradient coil. Digital information in the RAM together with the bandpass characteristics of the APM and EMI filters determine the temporal response of the gradient field.

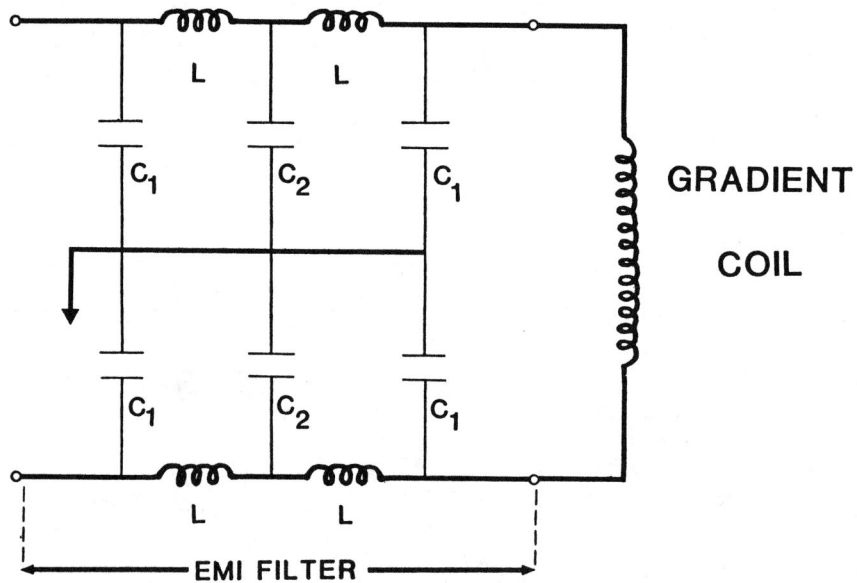

Figure 15: Detail of the multiple-pole PI filter which can be used to suppress electromagnetic interference (EMI) in the gradient fields.

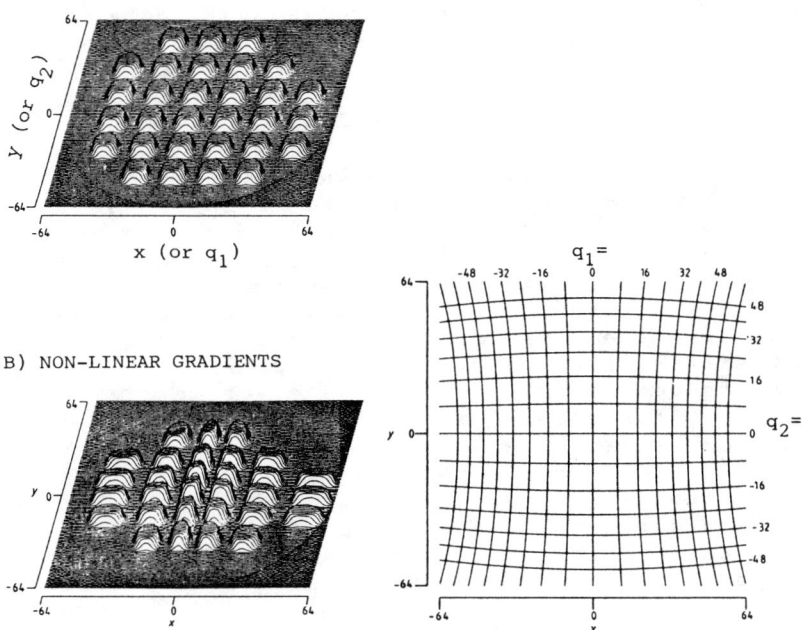

Figure 16: Schematic illustrating the effect of non-linear field gradients upon projection reconstruction. Panel A shows a phantom image reconstructed using ideal data taken with linear field gradients. Panel B shows the same phantom reconstructed from data taken with non-linear gradients. The degree of non-linearity and the curvilinear coordinate system used for image correction is shown in the plot on the right of B (from Lai 29,30).

RADIO FREQUENCY COILS

Cecil E. Hayes
General Electric Medical Systems Group,
Milwaukee, WI   53201

William A. Edelstein and John F. Schenck
GE Corporate Research & Development Center,
Schenectady, NY 12345

ABSTRACT

In this paper we provide background information needed to design and evaluate the RF coils used in biomedical applications of NMR. The emphasis is on the large structures required for head and whole body imaging. We cover briefly the fundamentals of resonant circuits followed by a more detailed treatment of the signal-to-noise performance of coils. We give a general discussion of the relevant design considerations including coil inductance, stray electric fields, shielding, quadrature excitation and reception, and RF field homogeneity. We review the principal types of imaging coils such as the solenoid, the saddle coil, the slotted tube resonator, the "birdcage" resonator, and the crossed ellipse coil. We then describe the interfacing of the rf coil to the transmitter and receiver sections of the spectrometer. We conclude with a brief discussion of surface coils.

INTRODUCTION

An NMR RF coil assembly has two primary functions: excitation of nuclear spins and detection of the resulting nuclear precession. During excitation, the RF coil serves as a transducer which converts RF power into a transverse rotating RF magnetic field B_1 in the imaging volume. High efficiency for this transmit mode of operation corresponds to maximum B_1 in the sample volume for minimum RF power. During reception, the RF coil and its associated preamplifier serve as a transducer which converts a precessing nuclear magnetization into an electrical signal suitable for further signal processing. High efficiency for this reception mode corresponds to minimal degradation of the inherent signal-to-noise ratio of the sample volume. A well designed coil can be highly efficient as both a transmitter and a receiver. For imaging it is also desirable for the excitation and reception to be spatially uniform in the imaging volume. Unfortunately spatial uniformity and high-efficiency cannot both be optimized simultaneously. Increasing the spatial uniformity will increase the required power and decrease the signal-to-noise ratio. NMR RF coils differ significantly in function from traditional antenna designs. In particular a RF transmitting antenna is designed to radiate a large fraction of its input power into its far field region. In contrast an NMR transmit coil needs to store magnetic energy temporarily in its near field region with minimal dissipation and preferably no radiation. Although the sample material may absorb significant RF energy, only a miniscule fraction of it is actually absorbed by the nuclear spins. Likewise the NMR receive coil detects the rotating nuclear magnetization without extracting any significant energy from the nuclear spins. Such a transfer of energy from the spins to the RF coil will cause a shortening of the free induction decay. Viewing the NMR RF coil as a magnetic energy storage device is a key to good coil design. Efficient energy storage optimizes both the transmit and receive performance of a coil assembly. Resonant LC circuits are a natural choice for magnetic energy storage. In the following sections we treat first the fundamentals of LCR circuits and their signal-to-noise performance. Then we enumerate some general coil design principles and apply them to a discussion of several specific coil geometries. Next we show how coils are interfaced to the RF power amplifier and the preamplifier. Finally we describe surface coils and how their design requirements differ from whole body or head coils.

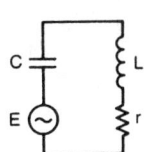

Fig. 1. Simple LCR circuit.

RESONANT CIRCUIT FUNDAMENTALS

The simple series LCR circuit of Fig. 1 can serve as an equivalent circuit for most NMR coils. If the frequency of the voltage source $E = E_o e^{i\omega t}$ is varied, the maximum peak current occurs for

$$\omega = \frac{1}{\sqrt{LC}} \qquad (1)$$

provided $r \ll \omega L$. At resonance, energy is alternately stored as magnetic energy in the inductor L and then as electrostatic energy in the capacitor C. During the transfer of this stored energy, some is dissipated in the series resistor r. The resonant circuit quality factor Q is a measure of the circuit's energy storage efficiency. Q is defined as

$$Q = \frac{\text{maximum energy stored}}{\text{average energy dissipated per radian}} \quad (2)$$

Q may be determined by measuring the resonant frequency ω and the full 3 dB bandwidth Δω:

$$Q = \frac{\omega}{\Delta\omega} \quad (3)$$

Q is also given by

$$Q = \frac{1}{r\,\omega C} = \frac{\omega L}{r} \quad (4)$$

Equating the right sides of Eqs. (3) and (4) yields

$$r = \Delta\omega L \quad (5)$$

If L is known, a rather straightforward measurement of bandwidth can be substituted for a more difficult measurement of the small, frequency-dependent quantity r. If L is not known, it can be deduced by increasing r by a known increment δr and observing the incremental change in bandwidth δω:

$$L = \frac{\delta r}{\delta\omega} \quad (6)$$

The δr must be inserted into the circuit at a point where all the current passes through it. It is often more practical to deduce the value of L from its resonant frequency when connected to a known capacitor. This procedure eliminates the lead inductance that may occur when making a direct measurement of L with an impedance meter. Resonant frequencies and bandwidths can be observed by exciting the resonance with a variable frequency signal source coupled via a small inductive loop placed on one side of the resonant circuit. The circuit's response is monitored on a scope or spectrum analyzer by way of a second small inductive loop placed on the opposite side of the resonant circuit. For high Q circuits, weak coupling must be used to prevent coil loading by the source impedance or scope's input impedance. A frequency counter may be needed to measure small bandwidths accurately.

SIGNAL-TO-NOISE CONSIDERATIONS

A precessing set of nuclear spins will induce a voltage in a RF coil which is proportional to frequency of precession, the number of spins, the degree of spin polarization, and the strength of coupling between the nuclei and the coil. The number of spins will be proportional to the sample volume V_s. The spin polarization is proportional to the static magnetic field B_o which also determines the frequency of precession ω. The degree of coupling between the spins and the coil is a function of geometry which is delineated by the Principle of Reciprocity.[1] The latter states that a time varying magnetic dipole, $\vec{m}$, induces a voltage

$$\varepsilon = -\frac{\partial}{\partial t}(\vec{m}\cdot\vec{B}_1) \qquad (7)$$

where $\vec{B}_1$ is the magnetic field at the position of $\vec{m}$ due to a unit current in the coil. Note that only the component of $\vec{B}_1$ that is parallel to the precessing component of $\vec{m}$ is important. That is, the coil sensitivity is proportional to $(B_1)_{xy}$, the component of $\vec{B}_1$ perpendicular to B_o, which is usually taken to be along the z-axis. Hence the induced signal in the coil is given by

$$\text{Signal} \propto V_s \omega^2 (B_1)_{xy} \qquad (8)$$

This signal can be represented as a series voltage source in the LCR circuit of Fig. 1.

The fluctuation-dissipation theorem indicates that there is a direct relationship between electrical resistance and noise. The thermally activated motions of the charge carriers in dissipative media produce random electric and magnetic fields which can be detected as noise. A resistance r produces an rms noise voltage V_n given by

$$V_n = \sqrt{4kTr\Delta f} \qquad (9)$$

where k is Boltzmann's constant, T is absolute temperature of the resistance, and Δf is the bandwidth set by the data acquisition system. For the LCR circuit, another series voltage source with magnitude given by Eq. (9) should be included in Fig. 1 to account for the noise voltage generated by r.

Equations (8) and (9) can be combined to obtain an expression for the signal-to-noise-ratio SNR

$$\text{SNR} \propto \frac{V_s \omega^2 (B_1)_{xy}}{\sqrt{r}} \qquad (10)$$

For the special case of small solenoidal coils used in early NMR spectrometers, Eq.(10) can be rearranged[1] to

give
$$\text{SNR} \propto \eta \, \omega^{3/2} Q^{1/2} V_c^{1/2} \tag{11}$$

where V_c is the volume of the solenoid and η is the filling factor defined as the ratio of RF magnetic energy stored in the sample volume to the total RF magnetic energy stored by the coil. Hence for conventional spectroscopy, one desired a high Q coil with good filling factor for as large a sample volume as would fit in the homogeneous region of the magnet. For <u>in vivo</u> NMR imaging, a slightly modified Eq.(10) is more applicable since coil Q and filling factor play a less direct role in SNR. The factor V_s in Eq.(10) must be divided out because imaging is concerned with SNR per unit volume or SNR for a fixed voxel size which is determined by the desired resolution and not by the total sample volume. Hoult and Lauterbur[2] extended Eq.(10) to whole body imaging by including both coil losses and patient losses in the resistance r. The patient losses may be due to dielectric effects and magnetically induced eddy currents. Magnetic losses are unavoidable since the coil responds to magnetic fields generated by the nuclear spins as well as by the random thermally activated currents in the patient. Dielectric losses arise from electric fields in the patient due to stray capacitance between patient and coil. They should be minimized because electric field effects carry no useful information. Hoult and Lauterbur[2] estimated the equivalent resistance of a patient by calculating the magnetically induced eddy current losses in a sphere of radius b with conductivity σ exposed to an RF field $(B_1)_{xy}$ due to a unit current in the coil. They found

$$r_{patient} \propto \sigma \omega^2 (B_1)_{xy} b^5 \tag{12}$$

The resistance of the coil r_{coil} is proportional to the square root of the frequency due to the RF skin effect[1]. Replacing the r in Eq. (10) with the sum of r_{coil} and $r_{patient}$ leads to the expression

$$\text{SNR}/V_s \propto \frac{\omega^2 (B_1)_{xy}}{\sqrt{\alpha \omega^{1/2} + \beta \sigma \omega^2 (B_1)_{xy}^2 b^5}} \tag{13}$$

Assuming the coil's dimensions are determined by the sample radius b, $(B_1)_{xy}$ will decrease and the coil resistance will increase with increasing sample size. However, the term for patient losses will increase more rapidly than the coil losses when either ω or b are increased. For a low-loss high Q body coil at 6.4 MHz, the coil losses r_{coil} can be approximately equal to the patient losses $r_{patient}$.[3] Hence at higher frequencies,

$$r_{patient} \gg r_{coil} \qquad (14)$$

is possible. In the limit of high frequencies, Eq.(13) reduces to

$$SNR/V_s \propto \frac{\omega}{b^{5/2}} \qquad (15)$$

Here, in contrast to Eq.(11), the signal-to-noise increases linearly with frequency and is apparently independent of filling factor η and coil Q. In fact the SNR for a fixed voxel size decreases as sample size b is increased. Due to the spatial discrimination of the imaging process, the tissue outside the voxel adds to the noise but not to the signal. The coil Q and filling factor effects have dropped out of Eq.(15) only because both are sufficiently large to satisfy Eq.(14). A high Q corresponds to a small r_{coil} and a high filling factor provides a large value of $(B_1)_{xy}$ in $r_{patient}$. The relative values of r_{coil} and $r_{patient}$ can be determined by measuring Q when the coil is empty and when it is loaded by a patient. The best indicator of coil sensitivity is the ratio

$$\frac{Q_{empty}}{Q_{loaded}} = \frac{r_{coil} + r_{patient}}{r_{coil}} \qquad (16)$$

provided dielectric losses do not contribute to $r_{patient}$. At 1.5T, this ratio can be five or more. This implies that coil losses contribute less than 11% of the observed noise voltage.

RF COIL DESIGN CONSIDERATIONS

We begin by listing some obvious and less obvious requirements for the RF coil assembly in an MR imaging system. The RF coil should resonate at the desired operating frequency, be large enough to accommodate the imaging volume, produce a homogeneous B_1 field, have a good filling factor, have minimum coil losses, be able to withstand the applied voltages, produce minimal electric fields in the sample, have minimum interaction with the rest of the system, and should permit quadrature excitation and reception. We will discuss these issues and their interrelationships in the following paragraphs.

There is a strong linkage between coil volume and its resonance frequency. Making a body-sized resonant circuit using conventional LCR circuit techniques becomes increasingly difficult as the desired resonant frequency (or static magnetic field B_o) is increased. If a simple multiple turn solenoidal coil is scaled up in size, its inductance increases proportional to its linear dimension. The capacitance needed for a given resonant frequency varies inversely with the inductance. The lower limit of capacitance is determined by the stray capacitance of the coil which also depends on its size. Hence the upper bound on operating frequency is set by the inductance and stray capacitance of the coil. Since the inductance of a simple solenoid increases as the square of its number of turns, one can obviously increase the resonant frequency by minimizing the number of turns. Unfortunately as the number of turns are decreased, the B_1 field homogeneity can also suffer. Thus for frequencies over about 15 MHz, body-sized wire wound coils are inappropriate. At high frequencies it is conceptually useful to think in terms of RF resonators instead of RF coils. This transition from lumped element circuits to distributed element resonators occurs at a much lower frequency for whole body imaging than for small sample NMR spectroscopy.

Designing high frequency resonators requires reduction of both the inductance and the stray capacitance. Using a single wide conductor in place of multiple turns of discrete wire reduces the inductance. The wider conductor permits a lower surface current density which corresponds to a lower inductance. The RF field near the conductor, which has only a tangential component, is proportional to the surface current density. Thus, the magnetic energy density, which is proportional to the field squared, is less near the surface of a wide conductor than a smaller wire. High energy storage near the conductors but outside of the sample volume degrades the filling factor. Wide sheet conductors are opaque to RF flux and can also be used to manipulate the flux distribution within the sample volume. A good filling factor requires that all inductive elements contribute to the B_1 field in the sample. Hence the capacitors should be located as close to the coil as possible to minimize extraneous magnet energy storage and energy dissipation in the capacitor leads. Similarly placing several small valued capacitors across the break in a wide conductor instead of a single larger value will reduce surface current density and lead inductance. The resonator's inductive elements should be connected in parallel rather than in series if possible.

Minimizing the inductance has two advantages in addition to permitting higher resonant frequencies. Lowering the inductance lowers the voltage developed during the transmit pulses. For a fixed magnetic flux

the voltage increases linearly with frequency and
proportional to the square root of the inductance. Hence
during transmit, higher inductances produce higher
voltages which can lead to corona discharge. Lowering
the inductance also reduces the stray electric fields in
the sample. which correspond to dielectric losses in the
sample. At low frequencies, the electric field can be
screened from the sample with a Faraday shield.[4] The
screen works on the principle of imposing a grounded
grid between the coil and the sample. The grid shunts to
ground the electric field lines that would otherwise
pass through the sample. The screen is unusable at high
frequencies for two reasons. The screen introduces a
large stray capacitance to ground which limits the
maximum resonant frequency. At high frequencies, the
self inductance of the grid prevents it from defining a
ground plane. At higher frequencies, electric fields can
be reduced by using coil symmetry to introduce virtual
ground planes.[5] For example, the balanced circuit in
Fig. 2 has a virtual ground at the center of the coil.

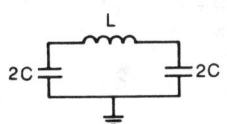

Fig. 2. Balanced circuit.

The maximum voltage in the coil with
respect to ground is one half what it
would be if one end of the coil were
grounded.

The fringe field of a coil extends
outside the coil for a distance
comparable to one or so diameters. Thus
the coil may interact strongly with the
surrounding environment. Such
interactions with the gradient or shim
coils, for example, can produce spurious resonances or
extraneous losses in the coil. The usual solution is to
surround the coil with a shield opaque to RF fields.
The shield develops image currents which concentrate the
fringe field between the coil and shield and reduce the
field strength in the sample volume. Such distortion of
the field distribution increases as the spacing between
shield and coil decreases. Thus a tightly fitted shield
can reduce the filling factor and add to the resistive
coil losses.

Another desirable design feature for an RF
resonator which should find increasing utility in the
future is the ability to implement quadrature excitation
and reception.[6] Such a structure should have two
geometrically and electrically orthogonal resonant modes
tuned to the same resonant frequency. Exciting both
modes with equal magnitudes but with phases differing by
90 degrees develops a constant magnitude B_1 rotating in
the same direction as the nuclear spin precession. It
requires half as much RF power to generate such a
rotating B_1 field compared to the more conventional
oscillating linear B_1 field. The signal received in each

of the two resonant modes can be summed after phase shifting one channel by 90°. The signal-to-noise ratio will be increased by a factor of square root of two since the two signals are coherent but the two noises are not coherent. Quadrature excitation and reception have the additional advantage of reducing RF penetration artifacts when imaging at high fields.[7] Quadrature operation will be possible in a resonator which possesses a four-fold axis of rotation along the B_o field direction, but this is not a necessary condition.

The homogeneity of the RF field $B_1(\vec{r})$ determines the spatial uniformity of the image intensity. The signal will be proportional to transverse component of magnetization $M_{xy}(\vec{r})$ developed by the transmit excitation. $M_{xy}(\vec{r})$ depends strongly on the flip angle θ which is proportional to $B_1(\vec{r})$. For a $\theta-\tau-2\theta$ spin echo pulse sequence, $M_{xy}(\vec{r})$ is proportional to $\sin^3 \theta(\vec{r})$.[6] The coupling of $M_{xy}(\vec{r})$ to the coil during signal reception is also proportional $B_1(\vec{r})$. As noted before, improvements in B_1 homogeneity will generally be accompanied by decreased signal-to-noise. The relative homogeneity of B_1 within the imaging volume can be increased by enlarging the RF coil. However, this approach increases the coil losses, decreases the filling factor, and adds extra tissue losses by including greater tissue volume within the coil. An alternative is to use separate transmit and receive coils. In this case, the transmit coil is enlarged since transmit flip angle inhomogeneity has the stronger effect on image uniformity. The receiver coil is smaller to minimize tissue losses. However, this approach precludes the use of quadrature excitation and reception. On the other hand, there are single coil designs with adequate B_1 homogeneity which also permit quadrature operation.

Whole body imaging requires a homogeneous B_1 field in a cylindrical volume. The B_1 field may be parallel or transverse to the cylinder's axis. The axial RF field is useful in iron core magnet or some air core magnets which produce a transverse B_o field. The transverse B_1 field is applicable to the more common solenoidal magnets. A perfectly homogeneous axial field can be generated in an infinitely long cylinder with a uniform surface current density directed around the cylinder. This corresponds to an infinite solenoid. A perfectly homogeneous transverse field can be generated in an infinitely long cylinder by surface currents parallel to the cylinder's axis. In this case, the current density is not uniform but is proportional to the sine (or cosine) of the azimuthal angle ϕ. For the $\sin\phi$ distribution, a positive current flows on the top of the cylinder and a negative current flows on the bottom of

the cylinder to give a horizontal transverse field. If
the two cylinders have equal non-zero surface
resistivities, then it requires twice as much power per
unit length to generate a unit transverse field as to
generate a unit axial field. The infinite solenoid may
be more efficient because it stores all its magnetic
energy within the cylinder, whereas for the transverse
field configuration, flux must also exist outside the
cylinder. Perfect homogeneity is destroyed when the two
cylinders are cut down to finite lengths. For a coil
length equal to the diameter, the field on the axis at
the end of the cylinder is about one half the strength
at the center of the coil. For the $\sin\phi$ current
distribution, conductive end rings must be added to
convey currents between the top and bottom halves of the
cylindrical surface. These end rings conduct current
proportional to $\cos\phi$. These added current paths, which
are not needed in the finite solenoid, contribute
additional coil losses for the transverse field
configuration. Thus, the nearly ideal axial field coil
is inherently less lossy than the nearly ideal
transverse field coil, but perhaps to a lesser degree
than Hoult and Richards´ findings for solenoid and
saddle coils.[1]

RF COIL REVIEW

In this section we describe a number of coil
designs which are currently being used or developed for
body and head imaging.

The multiple turn solenoid has been widely used in
lower frequency NMR spectrometers which employ an iron
core magnet. A long solenoid is a good approximation to
the ideal current distribution required for uniform
axial RF field. Hoult[8] has suggested that the length of
the optimum solenoid for imaging should be only about
80% of the coil´s diameter. Here he has sacrificed some
B_1 homogeneity to improve signal sensitivity by reducing
patient losses. He also found that increasing coil
losses due to the "proximity effect" require that space
between adjacent turns should equal about one half the
diameter of the copper tubing used to wind it. The
multiple turn solenoid´s operating frequency is limited
by its high inductance and stray capacitance. Cook and
Lowe suggest a modification which allows a solenoid to
operate at a much higher frequency.[9] They insert a
capacitor in series between each turn of a multiple turn
solenoid. Each capacitor cancels the inductive reactance
of a single turn of the solenoid. For example, an N turn
solenoid with inductance L might require a very small
capacitor C to resonate at a high frequency $\omega = 1/\sqrt{LC}$.
Instead of a single small capacitor, N capacitors of

value NC each are used; N-1 of them are inserted between turns of the solenoid and the last capacitor is connected between the end terminals of the inductor. The net effective inductance of the composite coil appears to be L/N since it resonates with an external capacitor equal to NC.

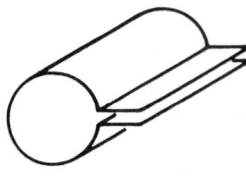

Fig. 3. Single turn solenoid.

An alternate means of reducing the inductance of a solenoid is to wind a single turn from a wide sheet of conductor. The homogeneity is maintained by making the width of the conducting sheet equal to the desired length of the solenoid. Because the sheet is opaque to RF, it forms a "flux pipe" which channels the magnetic flux in one end of the cylinder and out the other. The presence of a uniform RF magnetic field adjacent to the inner surface of the conducting sheet implies there must also be a uniform surface current flowing around the inner surface of the cylinder. To maintain this current distribution and the corresponding field homogeneity and low inductance, the tuning capacitor must be distributed evenly along the whole width of the sheet. Figure 3 shows how the conducting sheet can be extended to form the capacitor.[10]

There are a number of resonant devices for producing transverse RF fields in a cylinder. We will consider

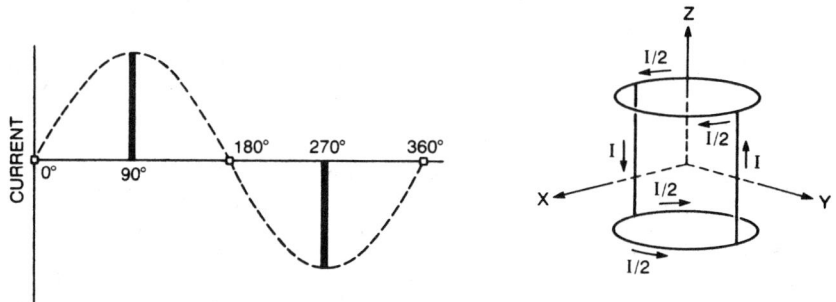

Fig. 4. Four point fit to a sinusoidal current distribution.

several in terms of how well they approximate the ideal sinusoidally weighted surface current distribution. We will deal with the case where the current density is proportional to $\sin\phi$. If $\phi=0$ corresponds to the x-axis, then the transverse field generated is parallel to the x-axis. The simplest approximation to $\sin\phi$ is a two point fit with wires running on the surface parallel to the z-axis at $\phi=90°$ and $\phi=270°$. Figure 4 shows this surface current distribution and the corresponding

coil. The two end rings complete the current path in a
symmetric manner which permits access along the
cylindrical axis. This could also be considered a four
point fit to sinϕ where the zero currents at $\phi = 0°$
and 180° require no wires. The next simplest
approximation to sinϕ is a six point fit shown in Fig.
5. This is the saddle coil configuration with two equal

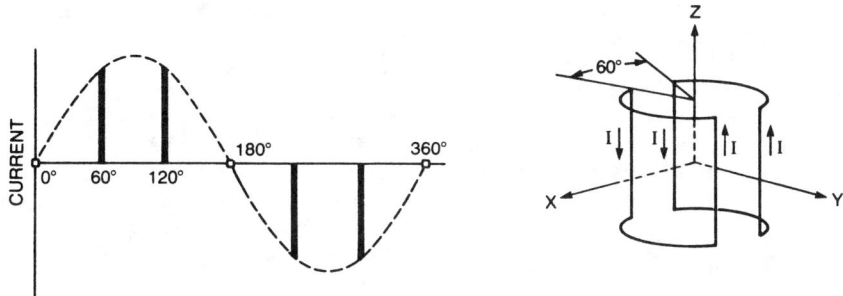

Fig. 5. Current distribution of a saddle coil.

positive currents at $\phi = 60°$ and 120° and two
equal negative currents at $\phi = 240°$ and 300°. The
wires at $\phi = 0°$ and 180° and parts of the end ring
can be omitted because they carry no current. The
inductance of the saddle coil can be reduced by
connecting both turns in parallel and by widening both
conductors until they merge along $\phi = 90°$ and
180°. In the limit of very wide conductors, the
saddle coil reduces to the topologically equivalent
single turn coil in Fig. 4. Alderman and Grant[5] used
symmetry arguments to determine preferred locations for
capacitance on the single turn coil
in Fig. 4. Assuming a single
capacitor C tunes the coil when
placed in the straight segment at
$\phi = 90°$, they found they could
replace it with capacitors equal to C
at $\phi = 0°$ and 180° on each of
the two end rings (Fig. 6). The
centers of these four capacitors
define a virtual ground plane, the
x-z plane. To shield the sample from
the electric fields developed in the
vicinity of the capacitors, they
added a guard ring inside each of the
two end rings. The guard rings float
with a ground potential at $\phi = 0°$
and 180° and develop much smaller
potentials than the voltage drop

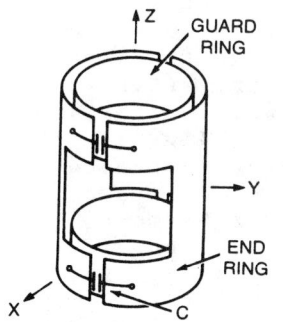

Fig. 6. Alderman-
Grant coil.

across the capacitors. The transverse midplane (Z=0) is a mirror plane of symmetry which implies it is also a virtual ground plane. Thus the sample volume is exposed to greatly reduced stray electric fields. This structure, originally intended for high frequency spectroscopy, has been extended to head imaging at 64 MHz by Bottomley et al.[11] More detailed descriptions of this coil design applied to imaging have been published recently[12,13].

The Alderman and Grant design is closely related to the slotted tube resonator of Schneider and Dullenkopf.[14] Consider a transmission line made of two parallel conductors of length ℓ separated by an air space. This line has a standing wave resonance whenever ℓ is equal to an integer number of half wave-lengths. For the one half wavelength resonance, there are high voltages at each end where electrostatic energy is stored in the capacitance between conductors and high currents in the middle region where magnetic energy is concentrated between the lines. Schneider and Dullenkopf[14] made their transmission line by cutting a slot along both sides of a conducting tube. They enclosed the slotted tube transmission line in a cylindrical conducting shield. They adjusted the angular width of the slots ϕ and the ratio of shield radius to transmission line radius b/a to optimize the RF magnetic field homogeneity (Fig. 7).

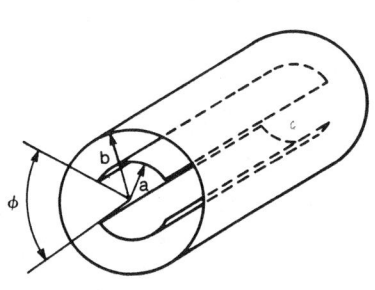

Fig. 7. Slotted tube resonator.

To avoid electric fields in the sample, the useful sample volume of a half wavelength line would have to be restricted to a small length at the center of the line. This restraint would lead to a poor filling factor since there is a large overlap of electric and magnetic energy storage volumes. At imaging frequencies, a half wavelength line would also be awkwardly long. This resonant line length can be greatly shortened if each end of the shortened line is terminated by a lumped capacitance to replace the distributed capacitance so removed. Furthermore, fitting half the terminating capacitance on each side of the cylinder produces the Alderman-Grant configuration (less the guard ring). Shorting out one end of a transmission line produces resonances corresponding to odd multiples of a quarter wavelength. The quarter wavelength resonator can likewise be reduced to a convenient length by capacitatively terminating the open end. If the slotted tube is shorted with a transverse sheet across the cylinder as Alderman has suggested,[12] field homogeneity is improved. The conducting sheet behaves as a flux mirror which effectively doubles the length of the coil. Such a coil, with access from only one end, has been built for head imaging.[12]

The slotted tube resonator develops a current distribution which is peaked near the edges of the conductors adjacent to the slots. In this respect it resembles the current distribution of the four wires of the saddle coil in Fig. 5. But there is an important difference. The conducting sheets of the slotted tube resonator are opaque to RF field and divert all the flux through the two slots. Hence the ideal slot aperture angle ϕ is significantly different from the 120° angle found in the saddle coil. A sinusoidally weighted surface current density produces optimum field homogeneity only if the cylinder's surface not only conducts current but is also transparent to RF magnetic flux. Such a surface can be approximated by a large number of parallel conductors spaced apart to allow the flux to pass between them. To improve on the saddle coil

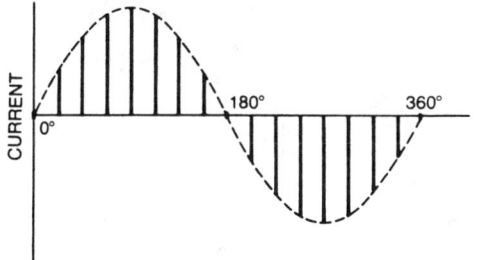

Fig.8. Multiple point fit to a sinusoidal current distribution.

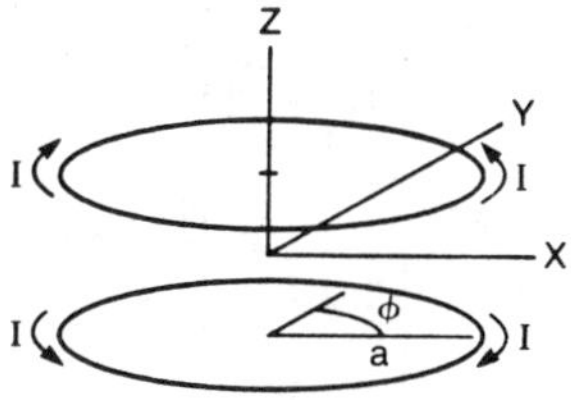

Fig. 9. Closed loop transmission line.

approximation to the ideal current distribution with more conductors requires a means of developing unequal, sinusoidally weighted currents in adjacent conductors (Fig. 8). A standing wave in a one wavelength transmission line generates the needed sinusoidal current distribution. Hinshaw and Gauss[15] wound a one wavelength coaxial cable evenly spaced onto a toroidal form. They removed the coaxial shielding from the cable lying on the inner diameter of the toroid. The exposed center conductor of the coax has the sinusoidal current weighting needed to produce a homogeneous transverse field in the inner bore of the toroid. This structure is limited to low frequencies by the need to wind a many turn toroid from a single wavelength of cable. Roeschmann[16] has built a one turn version of this concept to operate at 85 MHz by exposing the center conductor at only two places. His RF field homogeneity is similar to that of a saddle coil.

We have applied the resonant transmission line in a different way to generate a sinusoidal surface current. Consider a transmission line made from two parallel wires, each formed into a closed circle (Fig. 9). Such a transmission line closed on itself can support standing wave resonances consisting of an integer number of wavelengths. For the single wavelength resonance, if the voltage is proportional to $\sin\phi$, then the current is proportional to $\cos\phi$ in the upper circle and $-\cos\phi$ in the lower circle. This current tends to produce a transverse field along the x-axis. At 64 MHz (1.5T), the circle's diameter would be about 1.5 meters which is too large for a body or head coil. We shorten the resonant wavelength by adding many evenly spaced, equal, lumped-element capacitors between the two lines of the transmission. We call the result a "birdcage" resonator (Fig. 10).[17] The transmission line forms the two end

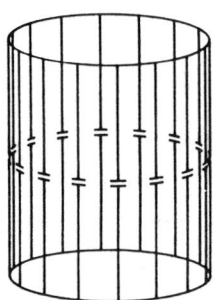

Fig. 10. Low pass birdcage resonator.

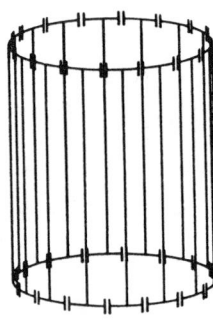

Fig. 11. High pass birdcage resonator.

rings with a voltage difference across the capacitors proportional to $\sin\phi$. Hence, the current in the capacitors is also proportional to $\sin\phi$. The long leads of the capacitors carry the desired approximation to a sinusoidal surface current density. This circuit is essentially a lumped element balanced delay line joined on itself. It can also be thought of as an N segment low pass filter. Each segment produces a phase shift of $2\pi/N$ at resonance. We have also built high pass versions of the birdcage resonator in which the capacitors are evenly spaced around both end rings and the straight segments between end rings are purely inductive (Fig. 11). We believe the birdcage resonator incorporates a number of the design guidelines discussed in the preceeding section. The large number of wires can accurately simulate the desired sinusoidal surface current. RF field homogeneity is limited only by the finite length of the structure. The multiple turns of the coil are effectively wired in parallel to reduce the inductance to that of a single turn coil or less. The distributed currents lower the coil losses and avoid developing high concentrations of magnetic field close to the conductors. Thus the uniformity of the field improves the filling factor. The lead inductance of the capacitors is fully utilized to create the desired B_1 field. The high symmetry of the resonator facilitates the use of quadrature excitation and reception. When the birdcage has four-fold symmetry, the fundamental homogeneous mode is doubly degenerate. The two modes, corresponding to surface current densities proportional to $\sin\phi$ and $\cos\phi$, are geometrically and electrically orthogonal. Both modes are excited simultaneously but with a relative phase shift of $90°$ to produce a rotating B_1 field.

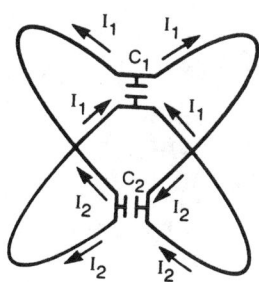

Fig. 12. Crossed ellipses coil.

The crossed-ellipse coil[18-20] also possesses a four-fold symmetry axis. The two ellipses are generated at the intersection of two orthogonal, equal radii cylinders. If each ellipse carries an equal current, the field generated is parallel to the axis of one of the cylinders. Reversing the polarity of current in only one ellipse switches the field to be parallel to the axis of the other cylinder. These two modes are orthogonal and permit quadrature operation if the static magnetic field B_o is perpendicular to the axes of both cylinders. Redpath[3] has pointed out that the two ellipses can be wired in parallel with both modes tuned and driven independently (Fig. 12). Capacitor C_1 tunes the mode corresponding to currents I_1 and C_2 tunes the mode with currents I_2. Modes 1 and 2 can be at same frequency but $90°$ out of phase for quadrature or at different frequencies for double resonance experiments.

A uniform azimuthal current density on the surface of a sphere creates a homogeneous field within a spherical volume. G.M. Bydder et al[22] fabricated spherical head coils by spiraling four or five turns of copper tube on the surface of each hemisphere. The two half coils were connected in parallel with enough space between them to provide access for the face and neck. Elsewhere there was only one or two centimeters spacing between the coil and the patient's head. The empty Q to loaded Q ratio was about four for operation at the relatively low frequency of 6.4 MHz. Hence patient induced noise is dominant even at 0.15T. The more uniform field and lower current density of the spherical configuration produced a higher filling factor and lower coil losses than a standard sized saddle coil.

INTERFACING THE RF COIL TO THE SPECTROMETER

The design requirements for connecting the RF coil to the transmitter differ somewhat from those for connecting the RF coil to the receiver. The coil serves as the load for the transmitter and as the signal source for the preamplifier. In the transmit mode, one desires to deliver power from the transmitter to the RF coil as efficiently as possible. In the receive mode, one wishes to extract a signal from the coil while minimizing the noise contribution from the preamplifier. Additional requirements are the protection of the preamplifier during the RF power pulses and the elimination of any noise contribution from the transmitter during signal acquisition.

We consider the transmitter-to-coil interface first. In general the transmitter is located some distance (tens of meters) from the RF coil and is connected to it by a RF transmission line. The transmission line conveys power most efficiently when both the source impedance and the load impedance match (or equal) the characteristic impedance Z_o of the transmission line. Typically Z_o is a real quantity in the range of 50 to 100 Ω. Transmitter circuits usually incorporate output impedance matching networks to generate the needed match to Z_o. Another matching network is needed at the interconnection of the transmission line and the RF coil. The resistance r in the LCR circuit of Fig. 1 is usually quite small compared to Z_o. For a reasonably high Q circuit, the voltage drop across L or C is substantially larger than that across r. Tapping into a fraction of this larger voltage drop is equivalent to performing an impedance transformation from r up to Z_o. The coil matching network will be most efficient if it introduces a minimum number of additional components and is located in close proximity to the coil.

Two popular capacitive matching schemes for coupling a source impedance Z_o to the coil resistances r are pictured in Fig. 13(a) and 13(b). Both circuits can be analyzed by converting the network consisting of E_{source}, Z_o, C_1, and C_2 into a series equivalent network consisting of an equivalent voltage e´, an equivalent resistor r´, and an equivalent capacitance C_{12} as shown in Fig. 13(c). Resonance occurs when $\omega^2 L C_{12} = 1$ and power matching occurs when r´=r. Note the latter condition implies that proper matching of the source impedance doubles the effective series resistance of the LC circuit and therefore halves the Q. The matching process may also be thought of as converting the whole LCR circuit into a single load resistor $R_L = Z_o$ which replaces the coil assembly (Fig. 13 (d)). The impedance matching condition and resonant frequency are given approximately by

$$Z_o \cong \frac{1}{r(\omega C_2)^2} \qquad \omega^2 \cong \frac{1}{L}\left(\frac{1}{C_1}+\frac{1}{C_2}\right) \qquad (17)$$

for the network in Fig. 13(a) and

$$Z_o \cong r\left(1+\frac{C_1}{C_2}\right)^2 \qquad \omega^2 \cong \frac{1}{L(C_1+C_2)} \qquad (18)$$

for the network in Fig. 13(b). Inductive coupling provides an alternate matching technique. A second inductor can serve as the primary winding and the RF coil as the secondary of air core transformer. Input impedance is adjusted by varying the spatial separation between the two inductors. The input impedance R_L of the coil is also its output impedance when used as a source for the preamplifier.

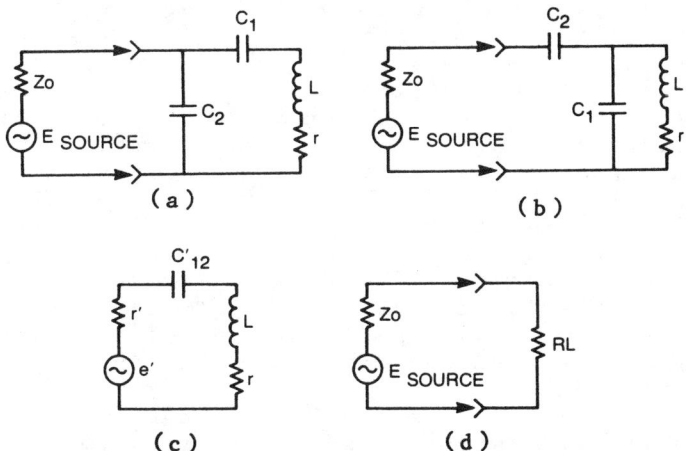

Fig. 13. Capacitive matching networks.

As stated before, the primary goal of interfacing the RF coil to the preamplifier is not optimum power transfer but optimum noise performance. The ideal preamplifier would amplify both the signal and the source noise but would add no extra noise of its own. A preamplifier is characterized by its noise figure NF which specifies how much excess noise it adds to the noise generated by a specified source impedance. An amplifier's NF, expressed in decibels, is defined by

$$NF = 10 \log \left(\frac{\text{total output noise power}}{\text{output noise power due to sources}} \right) \quad (19)$$

An equivalent definition for NF uses the ratio of square of the SNR in the coil without the preamplifier attached to the square of the SNR at the preamplifier output. Individual active components such as transistors are also characterized by a NF. The NF of a transistor is a function of the signal source impedance. There is an optimum source impedance R_{opt} which minimizes the transistor's NF. R_{opt} will not, in general, equal either the input impedance of the transistor or the source impedance of the RF coil (assumed to be Z_o). For optimum noise performance, the front end of the preamplifier must include a matching network which transforms the coil's source impedance Z_o to equal R_{opt} at the transistor. But the resulting input impedance Z_{in} at the front of the preamplifier will not, in general, equal the coil's source impedance Z_o. If Z_{in} is grossly different from Z_o, some detuning of the coil may occur during the receive mode if the coil was tuned for the transmitter's Z_o. Additional feedback network components can be added to the preamplifier to make its input impedance equal its optimum source impedance. (There are numerous vendors who supply low noise preamplifiers optimized in this manner for 50 Ω operation.) For the case $Z_{in} = Z_o$, the preamplifier loads the RF coil the same amount as the transmitter did. Hence, the preamplifier adds an effective series resistance $r'=r$ in the coil and would also double the noise power if the series resistor r' contributed the normal Johnson noise given in Eq.(9). Doubling the noise power corresponds to a NF of 3 dB for the preamplifier. For a preamplifier with NF less than 3 dB, the added series resistor r' can be thought of as cooled below room temperature. Hoult[23,24] has manipulated the preamplifier's loading of the coil to damp out ringing in high Q, low frequency RF imaging coils to increase their bandwidth and reduce their recovery time after the transmitter pulse.

The linear RF power amplifiers commonly used in MR imaging generate white noise at their output which can seriously degrade the SNR if they are connected to the RF coil during signal reception. Turning off or blanking the power amplifier during signal acquisition will eliminate this active noise source. But the long transmission line leading from the coil to the inactive amplifier must also be disconnected from the coil to prevent unnecessary loading and detuning effects on the coil during data acquisition. A simple series diode switch D_1 can be added into the transmission line where it connects to the coil input (Fig. 14). The diode switch is made of one or more pairs of crossed low-capacitance switching diodes. During the high power RF pulse, the diodes conduct with a relatively small "on" resistance. During the low-level signal acquisition, the diodes are off and exhibit a high resistance shunted by their junction capacitance. The non-linear operation of passive diodes distorts the transmitter waveform somewhat at low levels. An alternative is to replace the crossed diodes with a single pin diode which is biased on during transmit to give a low linear resistance.

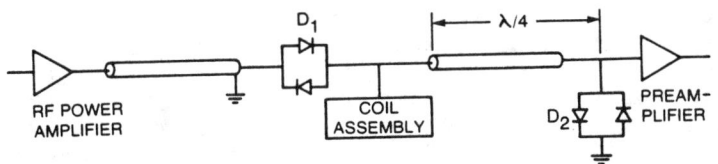

Fig. 14. Interface of coil with RF power amplifier and preamplifier.

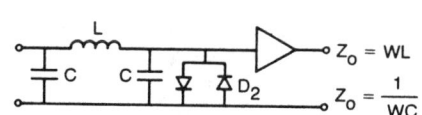

Fig. 15. Lumped element preamplifier protection.

The protection of the preamplifier during the transmit pulse is achieved in Fig. 14 by using the special properties of a quarter wavelength ($\lambda/4$) transmission line.[25] The input impedance Z_{in} of a quarter wavelength line terminated by impedance Z_L is given in terms of its characteristic impedance Z_o by $Z_{in} = Z_o^2/Z_L$. During the transmit pulse, crossed diodes D_2 have an "on" resistance small compared to Z_o so the cable's input impedance at the coil appears high. The clipping diodes D_2 limit the voltage at the preamplifier during transmit but effectively drop out of the circuit during the low level signal acquisition. If the input impedance of the preamplifier equals Z_o, the quarter wavelength line has little effect on preamplifier performance. At lower frequencies, where a quarter wavelength would be awkward, a lumped element equivalent such as in Fig. 15 can be substituted.

SURFACE COILS

Surface coils, as the name implies, do not enclose the sample but instead are placed on the surface of the sample material. Their greatest signal sensitivity is limited to a superficial region whose dimensions are comparable to the coil size. Surface coils were used initially for in vivo spectroscopy where their localized response permits acquisition of spectra predominantly from a particular organ or tissue type.[26] More recently, surface coils have been applied to imaging to achieve greatly improved signal-to-noise performance within the local region compared to whole body or head coil imaging.[27,28,29] The enhanced signal strength may be used to reduce signal averaging or to improve image resolution by decreasing the voxel size.

The simplest surface coil is a single circular loop of radius a, which has been tuned and matched for the desired operating frequency. This coil may be thought of as a very short solenoid which stores about half of its magnetic energy in the sample. Hence it has a fairly high filling factor and couples strongly to sample. Lengthening the solenoid would decrease the filling factor because additional field energy would be concentrated outside the sample. The B_1 field and the corresponding signal sensitivity for the short solenoid is highly inhomogeneous. Peak values of B_1 occur adjacent to the conductor. Along the axis of the coil (taken as the x-axis), the field per unit current varies as

$$B_1 \propto \frac{1}{a\left(1+\frac{x^2}{a^2}\right)^{3/2}} \tag{20}$$

The noise performance of this coil as a function of coil radius can be understood in terms of Eq. 13. The signal sensitivity B_1 at the center of the coil (x=0) is inversely proportional to the coil radius, a. The coil resistance will be approximately proportional to a. The tissue losses, which arise mainly from the region tightly coupled to the coil, vary approximately as a^3 (based on dimensional analysis). Hence at the sample surface, SNR for a fixed voxel size is proportional to a^{-n}, where n > 1.5. Smaller coils produce better SNR at the surface but their SNR decreases more rapidly with depth because the coil radius is also the scaling factor for the sensitivity rolloff in Eq. 20. Figure 16 illustrates the observed depth dependence of SNR at 1.5T in a lossy head-size phantom for three different surface coils and a birdcage style head coil[30]. In this case, the spins were initially excited by a uniform RF field from a body coil. The spatial dependence of SNR along the coil axis is therefore given by Eq. 20. Note that for depths greater than about 6 cm the head coil outperforms all three surface coils. The price of improving the SNR with surface coil imaging is a great loss in signal strength uniformity within the image. The surface coil is insensitive to both the signal and the noise originating from distant regions of the sample.

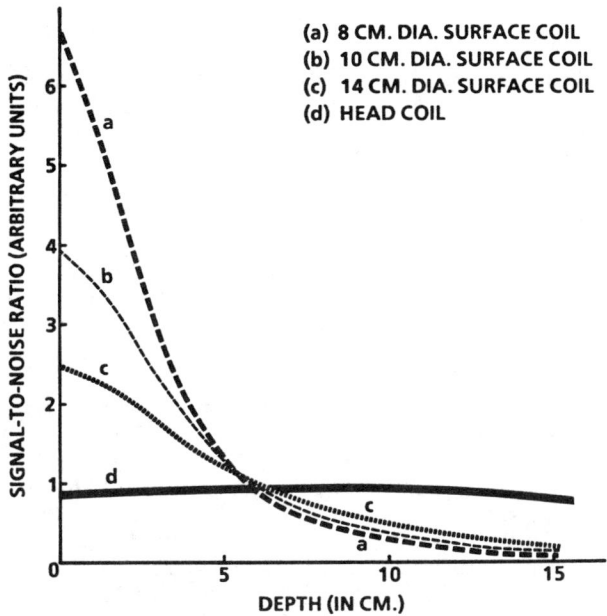

Fig. 16. SNR vs depth for surface coils and head coil.

When a surface coil is used as both transmitter and receiver coil, an even greater spatial variation in signal strength occurs.[31,32] The spin flip angle of the transmitter pulse varies with spatial position and RF power level. Different parts of the sample may be flipped 90°, 180°, 270° or more. An image would show dark bands of signal intensity corresponding to nulls created by spin flips of 180° or 360° instead of 90° or 270°. Bendall and coworkers[33] have exploited the spatial variation in flip angle to achieve spatial selectivity for in vivo spectroscopy without applying field gradients. They apply a series of pulses which cause cancellation of the signal except in a narrow zone of the sample. Grist and Hyde[34] have recently described the construction and performance of a single turn RF surface coil for P^{31} spectroscopy.

REFERENCES

1. D.I. Hoult and R.E. Richards, J. Magn. Reson. 24, 71(1976).
2. D.I. Hoult and P.C. Lauterbur, J. Magn. Reson. 34, 425(1979).
3. E. Easton, D. Flugan, W. Hinshaw, R. Salmon, J. Zinger and M.F. Floyd, 3rd Annual Meeting, Society of Magnetic Resonance in Medicine p. 200 (1984).
4. L. Pandey & D.G. Hughes, J. Magn. Reson. 56 443(1984).
5. D.W. Alderman and D.M. Grant, J. Magn. Reson. 36, 447(1979).
6. C.-N. Chen, D.I. Hoult, and V.J. Sank, J. Magn. Reson. 54, 324(1983).
7. G.H. Glover, C.E. Hayes, N.J. Pelc, W.A. Edelstein, O.M. Mueller, H.R. Hart, C.J. Hardy, M. O'Donnell & W.D. Barber, J. Magn. Reson. (in press).
8. D.I. Hoult, In: R.L. Witcofski, N. Karstaedt, C.L. Partain, eds. NMR Imaging. Winston-Salem, NC. Bowman Gray School of Medicine p. 33 (1982).
9. B. Cook and I.J. Lowe, J. Magn. Reson. 49, 346 (1982).
10. D.I. Hoult Prog. NMR Spectro. 12, 41 (1978).
11. P.A. Bottomley, H.R. Hart, W.A. Edelstein, J.F. Schenck, L.S. Smith, W.M. Leue, O.M. Mueller and R.W. Redington, Radiology 150, 441 (1984).
12. A. Leroy-Willig, L. Darrasse, J. Taquin and M. Sauzade, Magn. Reson. Med. 2 20 (1985).
13. T.A. Cross, S. Mueller, and W.P. Aue, J. Magn. Reson. 62 87(1985).
14. H.J. Schneider and P. Dullenkopf, Rev. Sci. Instrum. 48, 68 (1977).
15. W.S. Hinshaw and R.C. Gauss, U.S. Patent No. 4, 439, 733(1984).
16. P. Roeschmann, 3rd Annual Meeting, Society of Magnetic Resonance in Medicine, p. 634 (1984).
17. C.E. Hayes, W.A. Edelstein, J.F. Schenck, O.M. Mueller, and M. Eash, J. Magn. Reson. 63, 622 (1985).
18. D.I. Hoult & R. Richards, Proc. R. Soc. Lond. A 344, 311(1975).
19. W.S. Moore & G.N. Holland, Phil. Trans. R. Soc. Lond. B 289, 511 (1980).
20. T.W. Redpath & R.D. Selbie, Phys. Med. Biol. 29, 739 (1984).
21. T.W. Redpath, Third Annual Meeting, Society of Magnetic Resonance in Medicine p. 232 (1984).
22. G.M. Bydder, P.C. Butsen, R.R. Harman, D.J. Gilderdale & I.R. Young, JCAT 9 413 (1985).
23. D.I. Hoult, Rev. Sci. Instrum., 50, 193 (1979).

24. D.I. Hoult, J. Magn. Reson. <u>57</u> 394 (1984).
25. I.J. Lowe and C.E. Tarr, J. Phys. E, Ser. 2 <u>1</u>, 320 (1968).
26. J.J.H. Ackerman, G.H. Grove, G.G. Wong, D.G. Gadian, G.K. Radda, Nature <u>283</u>, 167 (1980).
27. L. Axel. J. Comput. Assist. Tomogr. <u>8</u>, 381 (1984).
28. S.J. El Yousef, R.J. Duchesneau, C.A. Hubay, J.R. Haaga, P.J. Bryan, J.P. LiPuma and A.E. Ament, J. Comput. Assist. Tomogr. <u>7</u> 215 (1983).
29. J.F. Schenck, T.H. Foster, J.L. Henkes, W.J. Adams, C.E. Hayes, H.R. Hart, W.A. Edelstein, P.A. Bottomley and F. W. Wehrli, AJNR <u>6</u>, 181 (1985).
30. C.E. Hayes and L. Axel. Med. Phys. (in press).
31. A. Haase, W. Hanicke and J. Frahm, J. Magn. Reson. <u>56</u> 401 (1984).
32. J.L. Evelhoch, M.G. Crowley and J.J.H. Ackerman, J. Magn. Reson <u>56</u> 110 (1984).
33. M.R. Bendall and R.E. Gordon, J. Magn. Reson. <u>53</u>, 365 (1983). M.R. Bendall and W.P. Aue, J. Magn. Reson. <u>54</u>, 149 (1983).
34. T.M. Grist and J.S. Hyde, J. Magn. Reson. <u>61</u>, 571 (1985).

DESIGN CONCEPTS OF PULSED FOURIER TRANSFORM NMR SPECTROMETERS

G. Neil Holland, George J. Misic
Picker International, Highland Heights, Ohio 44143

INTRODUCTION

The spectrometer of any NMR system is a key functional element. The spectrometer function here is defined as comprising an RF frequency source (eg crystal, synthesizer), a transmitter for providing modulated RF to a power amplifier and ultimately a coil or coils and a receiver which accepts the incoming RF signal from the receiver coil and preamplifier and performs a demodulation function to present the audio frequency NMR signal(s) to analog to digital converters for subsequent digital signal processing.

In this paper we explain the performance characteristics of each of the three subsystems and describe the function and purpose of RF modules such as mixers, filters, and switches used to construct a spectrometer.

Individual references have been omitted; however, a bibliography is given at the end of this paper.

FREQUENCY SYNTHESIS

The requirements for a frequency source for the spectrometer of an NMR imaging system will vary greatly dependent on design decisions for whole of the spectrometer. The simplest system is one where the DC magnetic field is fixed and the frequency source is set to the equivalent operating frequency, fo. In practice such a system is unlikely to be used since (a) the same spectrometer is likely to be used with systems operating at different field strengths, (b) imaging techniques such as multiple slice involve frequency switching during the sequence to selectively excite the various imaging planes, and (c) there are practical advantages involved in using heterodyned receivers as described in the receiver section. Therefore the ensuing discussions assume a frequency switching system is used.

The stability requirement of a frequency source is in part dictated by the magnet system and the imaging method used. The majority of imaging systems use the 2DFT phase encoding method of acquisition and reconstruction which is susceptible to temporal fluctuations. The temporal stability of the imaging system may well be dictated by the magnet system which for a cryogenic system is typically 1×10^{-7} per hour. For the frequency source not to contribute further instability a stability significantly better is required i.e typically 1×10^{-8} which predicates the use of proportional oven controlled oscillator. Commercial frequency synthesizers with the above stability characteristics and using a 10 MHz frequency reference are readily available. Furthermore, the imaging requirements of multislice techniques require phase coherent switching. In a multiple slice sequence using spin echoes both 90 and 180 degree selective pulses are applied in the presence of a gradient. The excitation frequency of these pulses determines the position where the slices are defined along the gradient axis. So that the NMR signal is demodulated "on-resonance" the frequency synthesizer has to be returned to the "zero offset" condition during the data acquisition process. Slice defining gradients used are typically 0.2 - 0.5 gauss/cm or 850 to 2130 Hz/cm. For a twenty slice multislice sequence of 10 mm slices which may be offset up to a further 10 cm the synthesizer is required to switch up to ±43 kHz from the normal center frequency. Using the 2DFT method requires that there is absolute phase coherence from view-to-view during the scan to avoid phase-encoding "ghosting". Phase coherent frequency switching is typically accomplished using digital direct synthesis where the clock rate addressing a ROM based sinewave look-up table is varied according to the required frequency. Because of logic clock rates and propagation delays, such digital synthesis schemes currently are used up to about 3 MHz. Extension to higher frequencies is accomplished by mixing with direct analog synthesis sections of the synthesizer or phase-locked-loop (PLL) circuits.

The total frequency range required of a synthesizer and the upper frequency unit is determined by magnet field strength range and the type of transmitter and receiver conversion schemes used. Covering a field strength range of 0.15 to 2.0T corresponds to a range of 6.4 to 85 MHz in Larmor frequency. Assuming single or double conversion heterodyned circuitry in the transmitter and receiver the synthesizer upper frequency may well be greater than twice the maximum Larmor frequency. More details of conversion schemes and their frequency requirements will be discussed with the transmitter and receiver sections.

THE TRANSMITTER

The primary function of the transmitter in an NMR imaging spectrometer is the formation of the various RF pulse trains required for imaging pulse sequences. Selective excitation techniques require spectrally tailored RF pulse profiles so that a modulation usually driven from a DAC has to be provided. Phase cycling techniques for artifact rejection and/or improved spatial localization require that RF pulses with the selectable phases (0, 90, 180, 270 degrees) be provided. Some recent development in selective pulses also require continuous phase modulation.

The transmitter may also be the source of reference frequencies for conversion steps within the receiver especially when phase coherence between transmission and reception is required which is generally the case.

Transmitters may be direct, single or multiple conversion depending on system requirements. Since single conversion typically offers the best compromise of versatility and simplicity the single conversion scheme is most often used. The basic principles of direct and single conversion are shown in Figure 1.

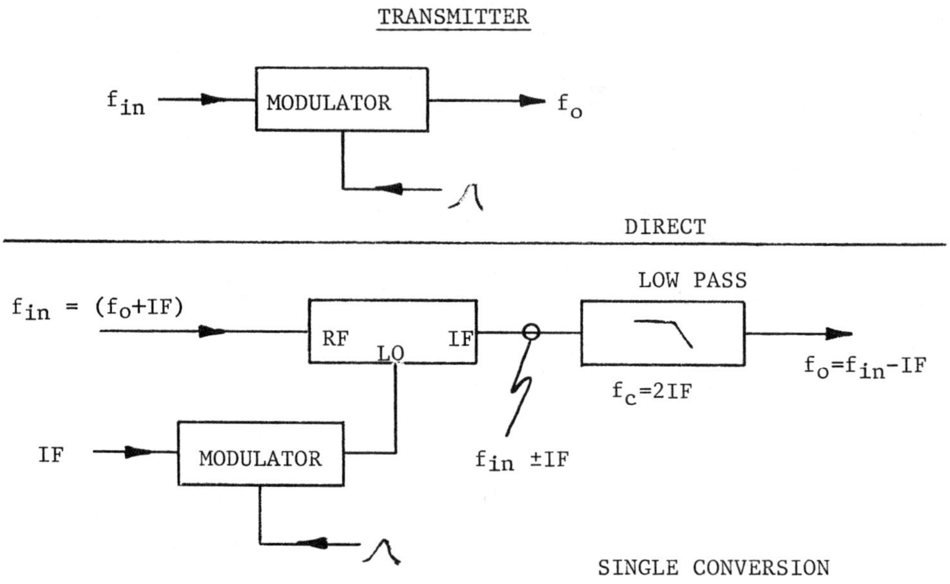

TRANSMITTER

$f_{in} \rightarrow$ MODULATOR $\rightarrow f_o$

DIRECT

$f_{in} = (f_o + IF)$ → RF/LO/IF → LOW PASS ($f_c = 2IF$) → $f_o = f_{in} - IF$

IF → MODULATOR

$f_{in} \pm IF$

SINGLE CONVERSION

FIGURE 1

A single conversion transmitter will consist of two principal signal chains - one of fixed and the other variable frequency. For reasons of accuracy the phase control and amplitude modulation will be performed on the fixed frequency section. The fixed frequency can be obtained from the synthesizer reference output either directly or by multiplication. As an example, a system with an intermediate frequency of 15 MHz will be described. The synthesizer output at 10 MHz can be converted to 15 MHz in several ways: by using a PLL circuit (multiply by three and divide by two); by using a diode tripler and filtering and dividing the output; or by using a mixing scheme. The latter probably offers the most stable method. The synthesizer 10 MHz can be converted to a TTL pulse train and divided by two using a flip-flop to give 5 MHz which can be mixed with the original 10 MHz using a double balanced mixer to give 5 and 15 MHz. The 15 MHz can be selected with a simple bandpass filter. This 15 MHz signal can also be sent to the receiver as an IF as described in the next section. If four discrete phases are to be formed, the 90° phase shift can be produced at the IF by a quadrature coupler. A quad coupler is a four port device that can be used to split an output signal into two equal isolated quadrature outputs. The fourth output is isolated (and terminated). This is shown in Figure 2. For NMR applications phase and amplitude balance of the two outputs are important parameters.

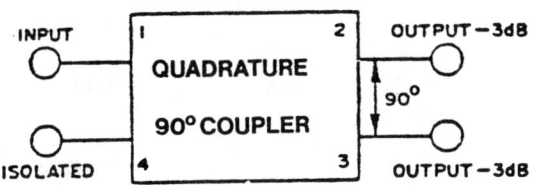

IN \ OUT	1	2	3	4
1		0°	-90°	ISO
2	0°		ISO	-90°
3	-90°	ISO		0°
4	ISO	-90°	0°	

FIGURE 2: THE QUADRATURE COUPLER

Operating at fixed frequency allows close matching of both phase and amplitude, whereas if phase selection were incorporated on the variable frequency leg a variation of 1 dB and 3° per octave in amplitude and phase would likely be experienced. Note that operation from 6.4 to 85 MHz requires coverage of over 3½ octaves. Selection of either of the two quadrature outputs of the coupler can be accomplished using RF switches such as JFET or PIN diode types with selection under logic control which will be described in more detail later.

Following the phase shift (if present) is a modulator to provide the amplitude modulation of the RF waveform required by selective excitation techniques. The modulation function is easily accomplished by using a double balanced mixer where the continuous RF waveform is applied to the LO port of the DBM and the modulation waveform is applied to the IF port. The modulated RF output is present at the RF port. It takes approximately 16 mA for full modulation without compression. This can easily be achieved by using a DAC with an op-amp buffer to convert the digital modulation envelope to an analog current modulation. Note that a double balanced mixer is capable of biphase modulation in that changing the sign of the modulation current will change the phase of the output RF by 180°. Thus a simple switch network at the DAC output can be used to change the analog output sign under logic control to give a 180° phase shift. Combined with the preceding 90° phase the four states of the two logic control lines can therefore generate the four phases of 0, 90, 180, and 270°.

If continuous phase modulation is desired, the whole of the previous arrangement can be replaced with a so called vector modulator, sometimes called a complex phasor modulator, which can be constructed from four hybrid devices. The incoming RF is fed to a quadrature coupler as before. The in-phase and quadrature outputs are fed separately to the LO ports of a pair of double balanced mixers. The RF outputs of the DBM's are combined with an in-phase power combiner. Modulating current inputs are applied to the IF ports of both DBM's. Since bipolar inputs to both ports are possible, the resultant vector can be rotated through 360° by varying amplitude and polarity of the modulation applied to each port. The concepts of biphase and quadraphase modulation are shown in Figure 3.

DOUBLE BALANCED MIXERS AS MODULATORS

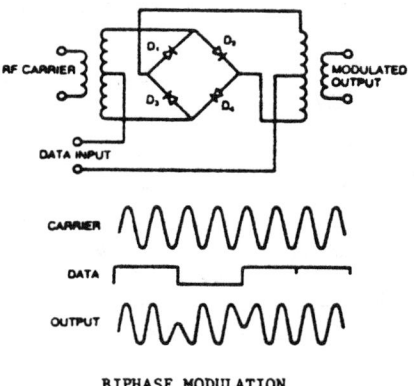

BIPHASE MODULATION

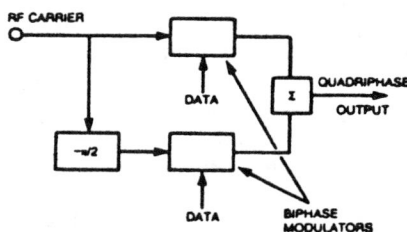

QUADRIPHASE OR CONTINUOUS PHASE MODULATION

FIGURE 3

To generate the output Larmor frequency, fo, the fixed frequency leg described above and the variable frequency synthesizer output have to be mixed together by a double balanced mixer, with the fixed frequency during the LO port of the DBM and the variable frequency feeding the RF port. The variable frequency may well come direct from the synthesizer. However, another important transmitter parameter is OFF isolation which is a measure of attenuation of the output frequency when the transmitter is gated 'off' compared to the output level when 'on'. Off isolation of > 80 dB is generally desired because of the high RF power amplification following the transmitter. Such high isolation may not be easily achieved by gating the final transmitter output alone due to leakage around the gate, so an additional gate prior to the mixer on the variable frequency leg will give increased isolation by ensuring that the output frequency, fo, is only generated when the gate is on.

Following the mixer (i.e connected to the IF port) must be a filter, usually a multiple pole low pass type, to attenuate mixer sum components since the mixer produces sum and difference of the variable frequency and IF. The filter corner frequency should be set at twice the IF with as rapid a roll off as possible for frequencies above that which allows operation to 2 IF with good attenuation of harmonics. The rapidity of the roll off of the filter determines the <u>lower</u> frequency limit of useful operation of the transmitter since for all operating frequencies below the IF the upper sideband (mixer sum) will be within one octave of the filter corner frequency.

Following the lowpass filter which derives the output frequency is a final RF gate, to allow RF pulses to be formed. The switching characteristics of RF gates in an imaging spectrometer are less stringent than in a high resolution spectrometer since (a) the RF pulses are significantly longer (hundreds of microseconds compared to microseconds) which means that risetime is less important; (b) signal sampling occurs well after the termination of RF pulse (often several milliseconds later) which means that fall time requirements are not stringent either. Nevertheless similar types of switches will be used in both types of spectrometer because of similar isolation and multioctave bandwidth requirements. Switches most often used are PIN diode types, although over the frequency range required for imaging, JFET and MOSFET switches can also be used.

PIN diode switches are typically used in small signal applications (below +10 dBm) which is consistent with the signal level in a typical transmitter. There are two basic configurations of PIN diode switches, the series and the shunt. The series switch gives good isolation at low frequencies and low insertion loss. The shunt configuration covers a wide frequency range with slightly higher insertion loss. In commercial RF switches, combination series/shunt diode arrangements are used to give isolation as high as 80 dB and insertion loss as low as 2 dB across a 5 - 500 MHz bandwidth. PIN diode switches of this form

having switching times of less than 2 usec are readily available.
PIN diode switch configurations are shown in Figure 4.

PIN DIODE SWITCHES

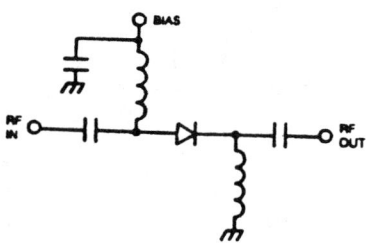

SERIES CONFIGURATION

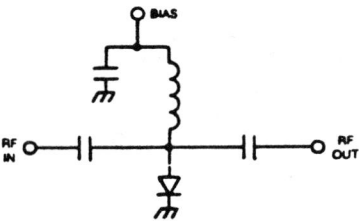

SHUNT CONFIGURATION

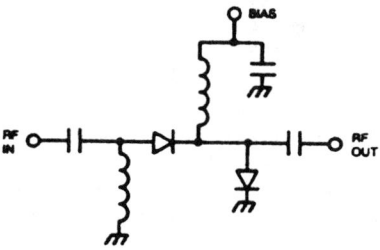

SERIES/SHUNT

FIGURE 4

The final output to drive the high power amplifier may be taken directly from the switch output or amplified and buffered as appropriate. So far no mention has been made of amplification requirements within the transmitter since in part these are a function of the detailed design - depending on the insertion losses distributed throughout the system and on the drive level requirements for the components such as mixers, combiners, etc. With present day technology there is a wide range of modular and PC mounting hybrid amplifiers available with appropriate gain bandwidth and power output capability to enable low level transmitters to be configured without resorting to designing at the transistor level. Further details will not be described here since in general the transmitter requirements are less critical than the receiver, except insofar as that any amplification provided after the modulation stage has to have good linearity so as not to limit the dynamic range of the transmitter which might affect the frequency spectra of tailored pulses.

THE RECEIVER

It is a function of the receiver of an NMR spectrometer to take the incoming NMR signal ($f_o \pm \Delta f$) from the preamplifier and demodulate it, so that the (f_o) component is removed, and the audio frequency component ($\pm \Delta f$) is presented to analog-to-digital converters for digitization and subsequent signal processing to yield an image, since the AF component contains in its frequency, amplitude and phase content the necessary spatial information for image formation.

The demodulation function can be performed in three ways, namely direct conversion, where the demodulation reference frequency is at the operating frequency, f_o, (which is also the Lamor frequency); single conversion where the demodulation to baseband occurs at a fixed frequency, but the signal at the operating frequency is mixed up or down to that intermediate frequency (IF); or mulitple conversion where two or more intermediate frequencies are present to baseband demodulation.

The signal path chosen for a spectrometer receiver will normally depend on the path chosen for the transmitter. If the transmitter is a single conversion design, the receiver will usually also be a single conversion type, using the same intermediate frequency as the transmitter carrier frequency. Typically, the reference frequencies for the receiver will be generated by the transmitter, or vice versa. This ensures that the signal phase is consistent throughout the spectrometer.

Direct conversion is the simplest scheme but is generally restricted to spectrometers operating at fixed frequency i.e with fixed magnetic field strength for evaluation of a single nuclear species.

Single conversion receivers are probably the most common. They have an operating frequency range of $2\Delta f$ to $f_{max} - (IF + 2\Delta f)$ where f_{max} is the maximum frequency of the signal source (synthesizer) with the additional dead zone of $2\Delta f$ around the IF. For discussion of the receiver we will concentrate on single conversion problems with reference to Figure 5.

Figure 5: The Receiver

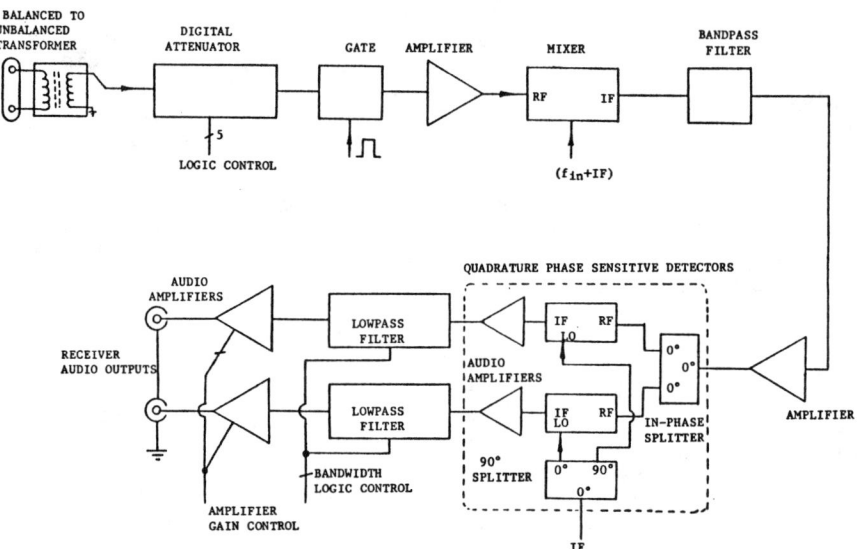

Multiple conversion types are of necessity more complex. They are used where the requirement is to cover a very wide frequency range with a variable frequency source which covers much more than that range, where there can be no dead zones or where the transmitter is also a multiple conversion type and for simplicity the same IF's are used in both transmitter and receiver.

As stated earlier the receiver function is to demodulate the incoming signal to baseband. So that the final image signal-to-noise ratio is dominated by the thermal noise of the subject and coil, the receiver must have a negligible effect on overall noise performance, and at the same time allow wide ranges of signal amplitude to be passed without significant distortion.

The first building block of the receiver is a variable attenuator, or a controllable gain amplifier. Its function is to allow sufficient variation in the system gain to optimally use the dynamic range of receiver components up to and including analog to digital converters which follow the receiver in the NMR system.

A wide signal range can be anticipated in an imaging spectrometer because of variation levels from different sequences, subjects, coils and nuclear species. This signal range variation may be as high as 40 - 50 dB although for solely proton imaging application typically will be within 30 dB.

As too much attenuation could adversely affect the noise figure of the system, and excessive gain prior to the attenuator will adversely affect the dynamic range of the system, the gain control range should not be much higher than 30 dB. Generally a digitally controllable attenuator is desirable as it is easier to interface to the scan control computer, and the size of the step of attenuation is well defined. Alternatively a dedicated RF amplifier with a remote controllable gain, such as a Plessey SL550G, may be substituted for the attenuator and the ensuing RF amplifier. This device provides low noise gain control in response to an analog voltage. A simple DAC will allow digital control of the gain of such a device (or alternatively a PIN diode attenuator). However the uniformity of gain/attenuation step size is not guaranteed. The attenuator is followed by an RF switch which prevents the receiver from receiving a very large level signal for the duration of the transmitter RF pulses in order to prevent the receiver from being desensitized for a significant period of time following the transmit pulses, and to prevent possible permanent damage to the signal handling components of the receiver from the large signal level. The switch is usually operated by the logic signal controlling the transmit enable function. The recovery time requirements, including the switching time, are much less stringent than in spectrometers for NMR of solids, since signal sampling does not generally occur until several milliseconds after the application of the last RF pulse from the transmitter. This switch might not be necessary if the preamplifier itself was gated.

The switch is followed by an RF amplifier which is required to raise signal level to the input requirements of the next stage which is the IF mixer. If the system is properly designed this amplifier will be the determinant of noise performance in the receiver. It has to have a wide bandwidth capable of covering the entire potential operating frequency range, a low noise figure of less than 3 dB and a high 1 dB compression point and high third order intercept point, probably in excess of +20 and +30 dBm respectively, since no selectivity has been introduced into the receiver at this point and intermodulation distortion (IMD) has to be prevented even in the presence of significant wideband noise, coupled with large signal amplitudes.

Following the RF amplifier is a mixer which is a three port device. The ports are labelled RF, IF, and LO. The incoming signal is fed to the RF port. The LO (local oscillator) port is fed with a reference frequency generated from the frequency synthesizer at a frequency (fo + IF). The mixer produces sum and difference frequencies of the incoming signal and LO frequency.

As an example, for a 0.5T proton imaging system, the incoming signal would be at $(21.3 \pm \Delta f)$ MHz where Δf is the signal bandwidth. If an IF of 15 MHz were selected, the mixer LO port would be fed with a frequency of (fo + IF) = 36.3 MHz. The principal mixer outputs would consist of two equal amplitude components at $(36.3 + 21.3) \pm \Delta f = 57.6 \pm \Delta f$ MHz and $(36.3 - 21.3) \pm \Delta f$ $15 \pm \Delta f$ MHz. The first of these components has to be rejected by a filter which will be described next, leaving the 15 MHz component at the desired IF.

The mixer used in the receiver is a critical component for proper operation under all conditions. To prevent undesired IMD and IF feedthrough, the port to port isolation of the mixer must be high in order to prevent the portion of the wideband noise generated by the earlier stages of the receiver falling within the IF passband being passed through the mixer and raising the noise floor of the system. Wide dynamic range is also a requirement, since the noise contribution of the mixer must be dominated by the front end noise, however, no significant IMD should occur even at the maximum signal level. To achieve these goals, a double balanced mixer consisting of a diode ring and two wideband transformers is generally used. Diode mixers provide very low noise performance along with very good large signal handling capacity. Their disadvantages are a conversion loss of typically 6 to 8 dB, and the need for a relatively large amount of local power, typically +7 to +23 dBm, the higher level being preferable to reduce IMD products.

The maximum input level to a mixer for proper operation is typically 10 dB below the LO level so that the gain of the preceding RF amplifier is determined not only by preamp gain but by mixer LO level.

Following the mixer is a bandpass filter which rejects the mixer sum components. This filter governs the overall selectivity of the NMR receiver. The bandwidth of the filter should be selected to allow sufficient passband for the widest range of frequencies required in the system. This parameter is a function of read gradient strength, in that the amount of frequency shift occurring during sampling is a direct function of the shift in the magnetic field. Since this filter is not easily changed to optimize the bandwidth for different experiments, it is selected to accommodate the widest shift requirements. Further optimization of bandwidth in experiments requiring less signal passband can be accomplished with an audio frequency filter following demodulation to baseband.

This filter needs to be very flat over the passband to within say 0.5 dB but must have a high stopband attenuation and a good shape factor. Such characteristics are available from multiple pole LC filters and from crystal filters. LC filters in general will have lower passband ripple than crystal filters which is important for signal uniformity, but higher insertion loss (as high as 10 - 12 dB) which directly affects the noise figure of the preceding RF amplifier, and hence the receiver noise figure.

Because of the combined insertion loss of mixer and IF filter there is further amplification following the filter. This stage is less critical due to its operation at fixed frequency and the narrow operating bandwidth which prevents third order intercept degradation from large off-frequency signals.

Following this last RF amplification stage are the demodulators which are universally known in the NMR world as phase sensitive detectors.

The phase sensitive detectors (PSD's) consist of two identical circuits. The incoming NMR signal has to be split equally between the PSD's. This can be accomplished with a hybrid in-phase power divider. Remembering that the NMR signal now occupies a bandwidth $\pm\Delta f$ centered around IF, the intermediate frequency, the PSD's are also fed with a reference frequency, fr, which is at the IF frequency. The references for each PSD are in phase quadrature, which can be obtained by using a quadrature hybrid, as described in the transmitter section. DBM's may be used as PSD's by feeding the incoming signal to the RF port, the reference to the LO port, and extracting the AF component from the IF port. The PSD output, Vo, is $Vo = k \cos([f_{in} - f_r]t + \emptyset)$ where k is a conversion constant (effective loss if a mixer is used); f_{in}, the frequency of the incoming signal and $\emptyset$, the phase difference between signal and ference. Maximum output occurs when the phase difference is zero (i.e $\cos\emptyset = 1$). For a second PSD with a 90° phase shifted reference, the cosine term is replaced with a sine term. Note also that, in addition to the desired audio frequency difference component, the sum component will also be produced. This is generally removed with a simple single-pole RC lowpass filter. The sum components will only cause a problem for receiver incoming signals close to the IF, since the PSD mixers will be followed by AF amplification stages which may have useful gain to a few hundred kilohertz, while subsequent filtering may remove these components, and distortion of signals within the passband may occur. The block diagram and function of a commercial phase comparator module which can be used as a pair of PSD's in NMR applications is shown in Figure 6.

For the remainder of the receiver chain following the two PSD mixer outputs, the AF signal follows two identical paths. It is critically important that amplitude, phase, and DC level balance be maintained throughout these two paths. Failure to do so can result in characteristic image artifacts. Amplitude and phase quadrature unbalance yield spurious, discrete 'ghost' images displaced from the main image. The magnitude of these ghost images is dependent on the degree of imbalance.

A qualitative specification for amplitude and phase imbalance is $\pm.1$ dB and $\pm 1°$ respectively, across the imaging bandwidth. Temporal DC fluctuations yield a characteristic center line image artefact since these fluctuations affect the zero frequency component in the first Fourier transform. Short term DC drift must be significantly less than the noise output of the receiver.

Following the PSD's are AF amplifiers generally configured using op-amp circuitry to provide fixed or switched gain. A DC nulling circuit is also usually incorporated. Following these amplifiers are pairs of matched multiple pole low-pass filters, either of the Butterworth or Bessel type and usually of four to

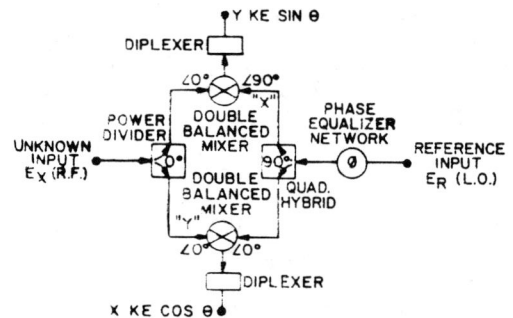

**Phase Comparator
Block Diagram**

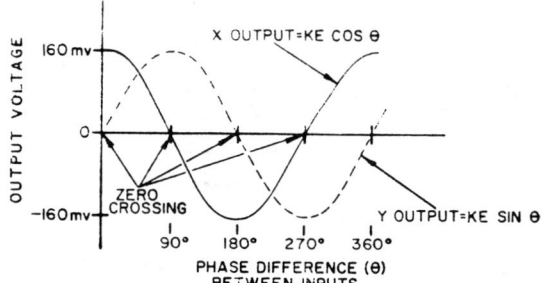

**Phase Comparator
Output Characteristics**

FIGURE 6

six poles. These filters will have a programmable bandwidth typically in the 1 – 100 kHz range – the size of step being a function of overall system (and pulse sequence) design since the function of these filters is to prevent signal and noise aliasing during the analog to digital conversion process.

Further gain may be applied at the filter outputs depending on the input level requirements of the ADC(s).

CONCLUSION

The system design requirements of a pulsed Fourier transform spectrometer for use in NMR imaging have been described. Salient design detail of a single conversion transmitter and receiver has been included to illustrate the important parameters of the RF and AF components used in an imaging spectrometer. Further details on spectrometer design as well as more information on standard RF design practices can be found in the references below.

BIBLIOGRAPHY

D.I. Hoult, Prog. NMR Spectroscopy $\underline{12}$, 41 (1978)
R.F. Karlicek and I.J. Lowe, J. Mag. Res. $\underline{32}$, 199 (1978)
D.I. Hoult and R. E. Richards, Proc. R. Soc. Lond. $\underline{344}$, 311 (1975)
E. Fukushima and S. Roeder, Experimental Pulse NMR (Addison Wesley, Reading Ma. 1981) Chapter 5.
The ARRL Handbook for the Amateur ARRL, Newington, CT, 1985)
F.E. Terman, Radio Engineers Handbook (McGraw Hill N.Y., 1943)
Reference Data for Radio Engineers (Howard W. Sams Inc., Indianapolis, IN, 1983)

Data Acquisition and Computer Requirements
for Magnetic Resonance Imaging

J. C. Hoenninger, L. E. Crooks, J. C. Watts and M. Arakawa

U. C. San Francisco - RIL, So. San Francisco, CA 94080

ABSTRACT

The nuclear magnetic resonance signal is an audio frequency voltage produced by the RF receiver. Information about the object being investigated is present in the form of variations in the spectral energy of the signal. A computer is used to convert the time domain signal into its spectral components, which may form an image, and then present the result for interpretation. For the computer to perform it's tasks, the audio voltage must be sampled and converted to digital values which are stored in the computer's memory. These general requirements are identical for both spectroscopy and imaging. However, we will concentrate on imaging. The rate at which the signal is sampled and the total number of samples in a study are determined by image resolution, image field of view, and the total number of images acquired. Selective irradiations allow multiple slices to be imaged during the magnetization recovery time of any one slice. Multiple spin echoes can be obtained from each slice and a region may be imaged additional times to change image content based on T1, diffusion, flow or chemical shift. These variously dependent images are then processed to derive the more fundamental properties. The number of these various images determines the total amount of data which the computer system must store and process. The processing, presentation and archiving of the images (both on film and magnetic tape) must be rapid so that the instrument is available to the maximum number of patients and so that physicians receive timely reports on their patients. Finally system reliability must be high and patient data should be secure.

INTRODUCTION

The approach taken to imaging has a substantial impact on signal sampling and computer system architecture. Several of the earliest sensitive point scanning techniques directly recorded the signal without need of a Fourier transform. Direct contour plot images were possible without the use of a computer at all. When the computer was used the signal from the sensitive point was measured, stored in an image matrix and then the point moved to the next location. The computer could thus be a relatively simple image processor. The next level of complexity was line scanning. Here a line volume is selected and the resulting signal is read out in the presence of a field gradient. A Fourier transform is used to divide the line into points. It is much faster and more efficient to scan a line across an object to give a planar image than to move through the plane one point at a time. Imaging speed was such that the Fourier transform could be performed during the time between signal acquisitions, and it was also possible to draw the image on the display a line at a time during the scan. These approaches have a poor signal-to-noise ratio compared to techniques that reconstruct the planar image from multiple projections of the plane. Zeugmatography, the first such reconstruction technique, is based on multiple angle projections. If the Fourier transform for each projection is performed during the imaging time, the multiple angle reconstruction can also proceed during the imaging time. Computer hardware for this task is available from the x-ray CT scanner industry.

At present the most common approach is to use Fourier transform imaging where one dimension is encoded as the phase of the spins. With this approach all the data for the phase encoded dimension must be present before the second dimension of the Fourier transform can be performed. The first dimension of the Fourier transform can proceed in parallel with the imaging. Three dimensional extensions of both these techniques are possible. If isometric resolution of an entire volume is desired the data set is very large. Using the Fourier transform technique a whole head would be imaged as at least $128 \times 128 \times 128 = 2,097,152$ voxels based on recording 16,384 projections. Imaging time for such a data set can be long but does allow the first dimension of Fourier transform to proceed in parallel. The next two dimensions of reconstruction can also be quite time consuming after the scanning is done.

For imaging a number of slices in a reasonable amount of time, multi-slice imaging with selective irradiation of the planes and a two dimensional Fourier transform in the plane is quite effective. The multi-slice approach uses sequential selective irradiation of slices so that data can be acquired from each slice while the other slices are recovering their magnetization. For example, we can excite and collect the data from each slice in 50 msec so with TR = 0.5 sec we can image 10 slices. With the data coming in from multiple slices the time available for the computer to do other tasks in parallel is severely limited. If high speed imaging techniques, such as echo planar, are implemented the requirements will again change. The data in this case are a high speed (100 msec total duration) train of spin echoes which contains all the projections for a plane. Rapid sampling and storage rates are required for this burst of data. If several seconds elapse between image acquisitions the average data rate is modest and immediate reconstruction and display of the image will be possible. If the images are repeated rapidly or if sequential slices are imaged, memory will be rapidly consumed and image reconstruction might have to wait till all the slices have been imaged.

Historically, many of the suppliers of MRI systems have experience in the x-ray CT field. They have naturally used their x-ray CT computer systems as a starting point for MRI system concepts. For single slice imaging these systems are quite effective. If three dimensional imaging is attempted, expansion of available memory is required. Reconstruction of a three dimensional data set is also slow, but could be sped up with more powerful hardware reconstructers designed with three dimensions in mind. Multi-slice imaging produces the data for all the slices together, unlike CT where slices are sequentially imaged. This again requires a different approach to storing the data during data input. Reconstruction in Fourier transform imaging is done with the aid of standard array processors performing fast Fourier transforms on the multiple slice data. This approach provides reasonable reconstruction time. Standard display systems are sufficient for viewing MRI intensity images. However, when T1, T2 or other images of fundamental properties are needed, they must be calculated from the intensity images. The host computer must support these calculations or they must be performed in a graphics subsystem.

SAMPLING CONSIDERATIONS

As you saw in the Pulsed Fourier Transform Spectrometer Design section, the NMR signal is demodulated by the RF receiver to the audio-frequency range. As such it consists of two voltages known as the in-phase (I) and quadrature (Q) components. The computer will treat these as real and imaginary inputs for the Fourier transform. Figure 1 shows the path of the I and Q signals through anti-aliasing filters to the digitizers and then to the computer. Determining the rate at which samples are taken depends on the total time available to observe the signal, the desired spatial resolution and the size of the object to be imaged (field of view). The time over which the signal is observed defines the frequency resolution of the signal's spectrum:

Frequency resolution = 1 / Observation time.

Figure 2 shows that the time available to observe the signal is fundamentally limited by T2 decay of the signal. For example, after a time equal to 3 T2s the signal has decayed to 5% of its peak value. For imaging with a train of spin echoes (Figure 3) the available time is restricted to the window between 180 deg. RF pulses with their associated pulsed gradients. Since the RF pulses last about 5 msec and gradient switching times are about 1 msec with echoes spaced every 30 msec the available signal time is about 20 msec. This is much less than the longest T2 in the body but is close to the T2 of 30 msec for muscle. Another factor in MRI is the desire to avoid the "chemical shift artifact." This develops for hydrogen where the resonant frequencies of the two strongest signal producers, water and fat, are 3 ppm different. When frequency resolution is better than 3 ppm, fat and water signals arising from the same voxel will have resolvable different frequencies and will be placed in different locations in the image. Choosing a frequency resolution wider than 3 ppm reduces this problem. One wants to choose as narrow a frequency resolution as possible since the narrower bandwidth reduces the noise content of the signal and improves signal-to-noise. This improvement is in proportion to the inverse of the square root of the frequency resolution (Figure 2). Once a frequency resolution is chosen the maximum available field gradient will set the best possible spatial resolution for the instrument. Picking a typical spatial resolution of 1 mm the required gradient with an 20 msec observation time (50.0 Hz frequency resolution) is

$$50.0 \text{ Hz}/ (0.1 \text{ cm} \times 4258 \text{ Hz/Gauss}) = 0.117 \text{ Gauss/cm}$$

where 4258 Hz/Gauss is the magnetogyric ratio of the hydrogen nucleus (Figure 3).

The maximum sized object that must be uniquely represented with this spatial resolution determines the field of view and defines the maximum frequency which must be sampled. The Nyquist sampling theory states that more than two samples must be taken for every cycle of the highest frequency to be represented by the sampled data. Since complex samples are taken the Fourier transform of the signal will contain distinct positive and negative frequencies. The imaged object may thus span a range from minus the maximum frequency, through zero frequency to the positive maximum frequency (Figure 4). If the signal is sampled 256 times during the observation time the maximum frequency is

$$\text{Frequency maximum} = (1/2) / (\text{Observation time} / 256)$$

where the 1/2 factor is due to the Nyquist condition. Since both plus and minus frequencies are imaged the frequency span is twice this amount. The field of view is then 256 times the frequency resolution, giving a space 25.6 cm wide for a 1 mm resolution . The time between samples for the example is

$$20 \text{ millisec} / 256 = 78.1 \text{ microsec.}$$

If a wider field of view suited to the body rather than the head is required at this resolution, 512 samples would be taken giving a space 51.2 cm wide.

To meet the Nyquist condition that no frequency greater than half the sampling rate (sample rate = 1/sample period) be present, a low pass filter (Figure 1) must precede the sampling system to eliminate any signal or noise frequencies above the maximum frequency. This is called an anti-aliasing filter because any frequency above the maximum frequency that passes through the filter will appear at a lower frequency in the final spectrum, ie. it is aliased to a different frequency. The filter must be dual channel since there are two signals to be sampled. The gain and phase response of the two channels must be matched to maintain the quadrature relation of the signals. If matching is poor reflected versions of the object will appear in the image. It is also desirable to have the cutoff frequency of the filter be programmable so that the field of view is easily controlled (Figure 5).

ANALOG-TO-DIGITAL CONVERSION

The dynamic range of the signal is large - the peak signal can be 16000 times the noise. There is still some signal in this noise and as systems achieve better signal-to-noise one wants to accurately quantize this signal. The quantization is done by analog-to-digital converters (ADCs). Commercial ADCs with moderate prices can perform a 14-bit (16380 levels) conversion in 15 microsec. More expensive units can provide 16-bit conversions in less than 3 microsec. Beyond 16 bits, conversion time increases and the dynamic range of the receiver becomes more of a limitation. For the following discussion we will assume that the accumulated signal can be represented by 16 bits, which is a standard word size of many mini-computers.

IMAGE DATA SIZE

We are now in a position to calculate the total amount of data which must be sampled to produce one image. With a 1 mm resolution and the 25.6 cm field of view 256 complex signal samples are taken for every line in the image. A square image done with a two dimensional Fourier transform technique will have 256 projections taken to produce the 256 lines in the second dimension of the image. The image is thus based on 256 x 256 complex signal samples. Each complex sample is two 16-bit words or a total of four bytes. This gives 262 Kbytes of data for a single image. This data, the product of sampling and analog-to-digital conversion must be transferred to a computer and stored in its memory.

SIGNAL SAMPLING CIRCUITS

So far the sampling process has been referred to as a conversion to a digital value of the low pass filtered signal voltages. If the conversion were done instantly this would be sufficient. ADCs in fact do a sequence of comparisons of the input voltage to a known set of reference voltages to determine the input voltage level (1,2). During the time taken to do this sequence of comparisons the signal voltage can change due to its dynamic nature. The converted value would not represent the signal at a precise time. This problem is eliminated by the use of a circuit known as a sample-and-hold (S/H) or track-and-hold (Figure 6). It contains several buffer amplifiers, a capacitor and a switch. During the time when no conversion is in progress a buffered version of the input voltage is applied to the capacitor via the switch. The capacitor voltage will then track the input voltage. Just before a conversion is started a signal is sent to the S/H which causes the switch to open. The capacitor voltage is now at the value of the input voltage when the switch was opened. The capacitor voltage is buffered and applied to the input of the ADC. The S/H remains in this hold state for the duration of the conversion, providing a fixed representation of the input voltage for the ADC. When the conversion is complete the switch is closed and the capacitor is charged to the new value of input voltage and tracking resumes. These units have several specifications in addition to those associated with a buffer amplifier. There is a droop rate which accounts for the charge leakage mechanisms of the capacitor and buffer. This tells how fast the capacitor voltage drops during the hold time. This voltage must be less than one bit during the ADC's conversion time. Aperture delay tells how long it takes for the switch to open after it receives the sample command. This time should pass before a conversion starts. The aperture jitter (uncertainty of this time) defines how

close to the expected time the actual sampling occurs. When fast
changing signals are being sampled this can be a significant limit to
accuracy even when the jitter is mere nanoseconds. For example, a 10
volt peak-to-peak sine wave of 10 KHz will have a maximum rate of
change such that 1 bit of a 16-bit ADC (152 microvolt) is traversed
in 0.242 nanosec. The switch is usually made of FETs so charge is
applied to the capacitor when they switch. This charge must be the
same each time they switch. Acquisition time determines how long it
takes for the capacitor to reach the input voltage after the switch
is closed. This plus the aperture time and ADC conversion time sets
the minimum time between samples and thus the maximum frequency which
can be sampled.

Two approaches can be taken to sampling the two input voltages simultaneously. Two full channels can be built, each with a S/H and an ADC
(Figure 1). The sampling and conversion of both channels is controlled by a common starting signal. Close matching of the performance of
both channels is required. The alternative is to use two S/Hs but
switch their outputs successively to one ADC. This eliminates the
matching of two ADCs and saves the cost of one ADC. It still requires matching the S/Hs, whose droop rate must be low since one S/H
has to hold for twice as long, and the switch must pass signals
equally from each S/H to the ADC. This design is also half as fast as
the first since the ADC must do two conversions for each complex
point.

DATA TRANSFER TO THE COMPUTER

Now that the data have been sampled and converted to digital values,
the values must be transferred to the computer. A direct memory
access (DMA) interface to the computer is a desirable method since it
can rapidly and independently place data into the computer's memory
in blocks whose starting locations are under program control (Figure
7a). The ADCs can be mounted on the DMA interface within the computer
enclosure (Figure 7b). This has the undesirable effect of connecting
the ADC outputs to the memory bus of the computer. These buses are
notorious sources of electronic noise from their rapidly switching
signals. Applying such noise to the output of an ADC whose input is
sensitive to sub-millivolt signals produces many problems. Another
approach is to run bundles of wires from the ADCs to the DMA, each
carrying one bit of data (Figure 8a). Buffers are usually required to
drive these cables and the computer noise still has a path to the
ADC. Optic isolation of each line will eliminate the noise path but
requires a large number of optic isolators which have a higher
failure rate than pure digital circuits. The approach we have taken
is to send the digital values over a fiber optic link from the ADCs
(mounted in the receiver) to the DMA in the mini-computer backplane
using a single fiber cable (Figure 8b). The two 16-bit values from a
conversion are loaded in parallel into a shift register, and with
appropriate start, stop and parity bits, are shifted out to the optic
transmitter. The resulting light pulses are received at the other end
of the fiber optic cable and converted to a stream of bits. These
bits are shifted into a shift register and are sent in parallel to

the DMA. The 10 MHz capacity of the optic link is sufficient to carry data as fast as the ADCs can produce them.

We use the computer for signal averaging and buffering of data as they are being written to disk memory during the imaging. Two other approaches are also possible. Since a system usually has an array processor attached to the computer for fast reconstructions the data can be directly sent to the array processor. This allows the possibility of one dimension of Fourier transformation before the data are stored to disk. With sufficient array processor accessible memory both dimensions of transformation could be done before disk storage. Since array processor interfaces and memory are usually expensive this can be a costly approach. Many modern disk memories support multiple DMA channels so it is also possible to send the data directly to the disk while the computer also has access to the disk. However, this requires an additional disk controller to write the data on the disk.

IMPACT OF IMAGING TECHNIQUE ON AMOUNT AND STRUCTURE OF DATA

Some unstated assumptions in the above discussion about how much data are handled by the computer are based on the approach we have taken to imaging. If a single slice is imaged the 262 Kbytes of data can easily reside in memory and Fourier transform processing can go on during the recovery time of the spin system. With the availability of selective irradiations this is an inefficient use of the imager. The multi-slice approach uses sequential selective irradiation of slices so that data can be acquired from each slice while the other slices are recovering their magnetization. For example, this means that for a single spin echo image, where we can excite and collect the data from each slice in 50 msec, with TR = 0.5 sec we can image 10 slices. The order of the data is thus the first projection of slice 1 then slice 2 ... slice 10, then the second projection of slice 1 then slice 2 ... slice 10, ... to the last projection. This is ten times the data of the single slice study in the same amount of time if the TRs are equal. Notice also that if one does not want to mix the data from different slices in memory the data must be placed in ten different areas. This is just the beginning when you realize that our usual imaging studies have two spin echoes from each plane (with physicians wanting more and later echoes to improve T2 contrast) and that additional studies must be done immediately with a different TR to evaluate T1 or with other variables changed to study flow, diffusion, chemical shift, etc. All these possibilities increase the total data for a single acquisition and the total number of acquisitions that must be done together to avoid patient motion. They also complicate the relation between when the data arrive in time with their source in space. This view of the data motivates our approach to attempt to write data to disk in a reasonably ordered way and do the Fourier transforms at a later time. Cost also influences us in that more processing power and/or lots of high speed memory gets around these problems.

One way storage can be saved is to take advantage of the fact that once the time domain data are transformed they need not be kept. Also, since our usual image is the magnitude of the complex Fourier transform the image occupies half the storage space of the complex data. When the phase of the image must be kept this storage advantage is lost.

MRI PULSE SEQUENCE CONTROL COMPUTER

A typical imaging procedure requires precise control of a large number of events to generate and acquire the data accurately (Figure 3). RF pulses of complex shape and various frequencies and amplitudes must be transmitted. Gradients in three directions with various timings and amplitudes must be pulsed on and off. The receiver is turned on during the spin echoes and the ADC performs sampling. The timing of these events must be repeatable and controllable to accuracies of a microsecond over total imaging times of tens of minutes. In our system this task is performed by a firmware based control computer. It is the host to an MRI Sequencer which is a custom bit slice microprocessor whose microcode is assembled, linked and loaded by a Digital Equipment Corporation (DEC) LSI-11/23 microcomputer. The MRI Sequencer uses a special counter to execute each micro-instruction for a time specified in the instruction with an accuracy of 1 microsecond. The Sequencer also has embedded registers which allow easy control of loops in the code without explicit register operations. Each microcode word has sufficient bit fields to control sequence program flow, instruction duration, three gradients, the frequency of the transmitted RF pulses, the triggering of the waveform generator and the ADC subsystem and the status of the receiver and transmitter. Control signals are sent out of the control computer thru an optic-isolator board in order to reduce noise propagated from the high speed digital circuitry. The gradient signals are converted by DACs on an optic-isolator board to bipolar analog signals. The modulating waveform which shapes the RF pulses is loaded into a programmable waveform generator by the host LSI-11/23 before the MRI Sequencer is started. The waveform generator is triggered by a field in the microcode and its output is converted to a bipolar analog signal by a DAC on a separate optic-isolator board.

The microcode is assembled from a sequence program entered using MRI sequence specific mnemonics which are supported by a full screen syntax sensitive editor in the LSI-11/23. During program entry, the control computer is accessed transparently thru the data acquisition computer console terminal. When an imaging protocol is chosen the appropriate sequence code is specified in a single command line using a special linker command syntax which allows flexible configuration of the sequence program segments which have been assembled. This code is linked and loaded into the sequencer by the LSI-11/23. The sequence is then started and image data collection begins. The pulse sequence generation is thus completely supported by the control computer once program segments have been entered and does not impact the performance of the data acquisition computer system.

MRI SYSTEM COMPUTER ARCHITECTURE

A typical multi-slice imaging procedure on our systems produces 20 two dimensional slices with two spin echo images per slice and images of 256 x 256 voxels at 0.8mm x 0.8mm x 7mm resolution (3). The size of this total time domain data set is 10.486 million bytes. Two or four data sets are collected and averaged for each spin echo, with a sampling rate of 27,800 complex samples (4 bytes each) per second (other procedures can have data rates as high as 223.2 Kbytes/sec). The four average procedure requires 31.5 min to collect data. These requirements place a significant demand on an entry level 16-bit or 32-bit mini-computer. The length of time involved in acquiring data is a severe constraint on overall system through put, in that tape archiving and image filming proceed slowly during data acquisition with either type of computer used alone. Both of the latter activities must go on in parallel with data input to provide the high through put needed to handle the large quantities of images produced by multi-slice procedures.

Our first research MRI system, designed in 1977, used a single medium performance mini-computer and had low through put for multi-slice imaging. When our first clinical system was designed in 1981, it was decided that performance enhancement would not be made by augmenting the existing computer with additional hardware. The approach chosen was to use two entry level mini-computers coupled together with an inter-processor link and thus take advantage of available hardware supported by mature software development tools.

DUAL COMPUTER ARCHITECTURE

The dual computer architecture avoids the need for large amounts of special hardware to implement an effective MRI computer system. It is efficient because it provides considerable partitioning of parallel activities (Figure 9), thus increasing system through put and reducing program and operating system scheduling complexity (4). Software need only deal with one activity at a time in either computer when managing critical resources such as CPU time, bus bandwidth and disk access. In contrast, an enhanced single computer must manage these resources carefully to support the data acquisition, display and other special subsystems supplementing it. The operator of the Data Acquisition Computer has reasonable response times in all performance areas. For example, with the PDP-11/24 used in our system, quick locator images require only 1.5 min including reconstruction. The entire 20 slice (40 image) high resolution dataset reconstruction takes only 3 min 41 sec.

During data acquisition the entire hardware resources of the PDP-11/24 are available to meet system requirements. These include direct memory access (DMA) data input, the use of large portions of memory for data buffering, data averaging by the CPU, and the disk access needed to free memory for more data. System capacity is such that no data buffering is required between the raw data input and the

Unibus DMA interface. Disk access is critical because of the large 10.4 million byte data set. This amount is far larger than the maximum 4 million bytes of physical memory that can be used in a PDP 11/24 for data buffering, so that time sensitive disk transfers must occur continuously during data acquisition. The problem is further complicated by the fact that 2048 bytes of new data are input to memory every 100 msec. We have found that a 256 kbyte physical memory combined with the use of a fixed 160 Mbyte SMD disk drive is adequate when the data acquisition task runs alone under the DEC RT-11 real time operating system. Additional disk storage is useful to temporarily store images before they are sent to the Display Computer.

In parallel with the activities above the operator of the Display Computer has rapid access to large disk areas holding images ready for display during image analysis, filming and tape archiving. High sustained levels of activity at the filming console are achieved with little difficulty because the CPU has few other demands made on it. A multi-tasking operating system allows tape archiving to be a background process in parallel with filming. Operating system tuning is simplified since no real time tasks are present.

A special consideration for the dual computer architecture is the Inter-processor Link, which allows rapid data transfer between the Acquisition and Display Computers. This DMA subsystem works with optimized software to provide very efficient transfer rates. During a transfer the Data Acquisition Computer is totally occupied with this task in our present system (future upgrades will allow multi-tasking in this computer), while the Display Computer continues to perform ongoing tasks. However, there is an impact on the filming console response time, especially if the Display Computer is performing data analysis during the transfer. Measurements of the execution times of typical floating point calculations show a 46% increase in response time at the filming console for the relatively short period (2-3 min.) of the transfer.

SECURITY

In a clinical environment, the separation of the disk file systems protects patient data which have not been archived from inadvertent corruption or loss, since data on the Acquisition Computer are saved until they are archived by the Display Computer. Otherwise, loss could occur either through hardware failure (e.g. a disk head crash) or operator error with the premature deletion of images from disk storage.

In a research setting, the partitioning of application program development onto the Display Computer (using an additional console) improves the security and integrity of the system. A good multi-tasking operating system is resistant to crashes caused by programmer activities due to it's extensive access protections and controlled privileges. Program development can go on simultaneously with image filming and archiving with little effect on system operation beyond some increases in operator response time.

Acknowledgement:

The authors gratefully acknowledge the design and execution of the dual computer illustrations by Gary Temkow.

REFERENCES

1. The Analogic Data-Conversion Systems Digest, Fourth Edition, 1981. Analogic Corporation, Audubon Road, Wakefield, Mass. 01880.

2. Analog-Digital Conversion Handbook, 1972. Analog Devices, Inc., Norwood, Mass. 02062.

3. Crooks, L.E., Hoenninger, J.C., Arakawa, M., Watts, J., McCarten, B., Sheldon, P., Kaufman, L., Mills, C.M., Davis, P.L., Margulis, A.R.. Radiology 1984; 150:163-171.

4. G.J. Myers, Advances in Computer Architecture. John Wiley and Sons, New York, N.Y., 1978.

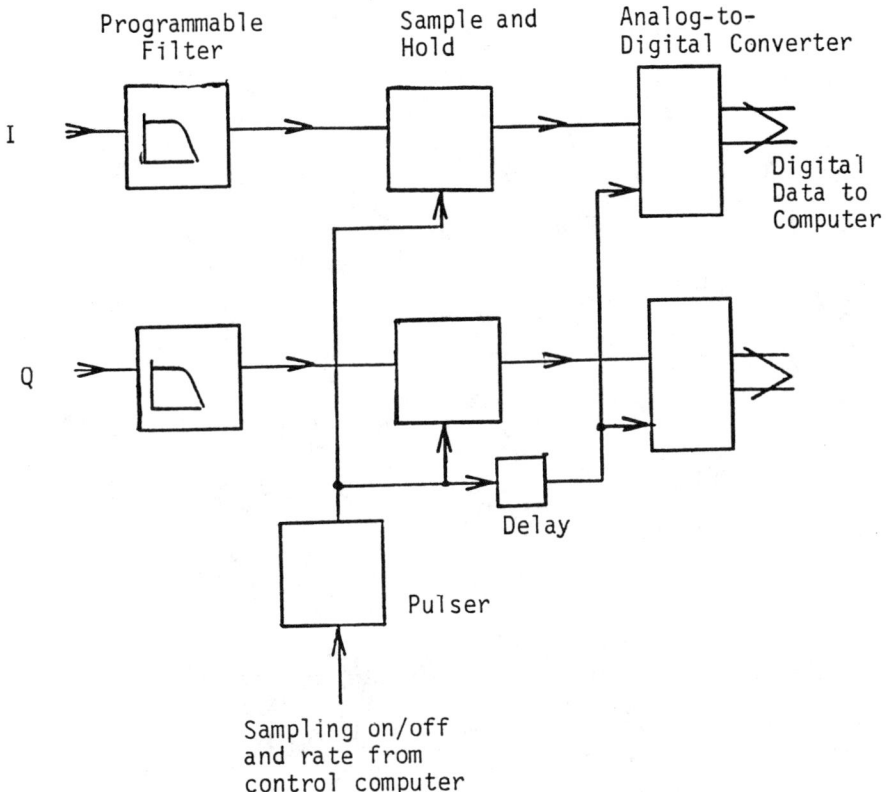

FIGURE 1. MRI signal path from the receiver to the computer. I and Q signals are low pass filtered to prevent aliasing. The filtered signals are sampled by sample and holds and are digitized by analog-to-digital converters. The digital values are transferred to the data acquisition computer. The sampling rate is set via a control computer and when sampling occurs is controlled by the imaging sequence.

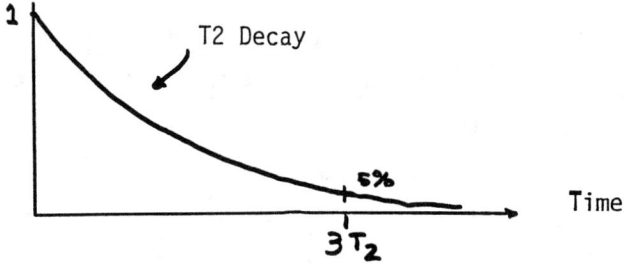

T2   CSF ≫ 200msec
      muscle ≈ 30msec

Noise $\propto \sqrt{\text{Bandwidth}} = \sqrt{1/T_0}$

spatial displacement of a chemically shifted nucleus is $\propto 1/T_0$

FIGURE 2. Frequency resolution is inversely proportional to signal observation time. The total observation time is limited by T2 decay and spatial displacement of chemically shifted nuclei. The narrower frequency resolution gives a less noisy image.

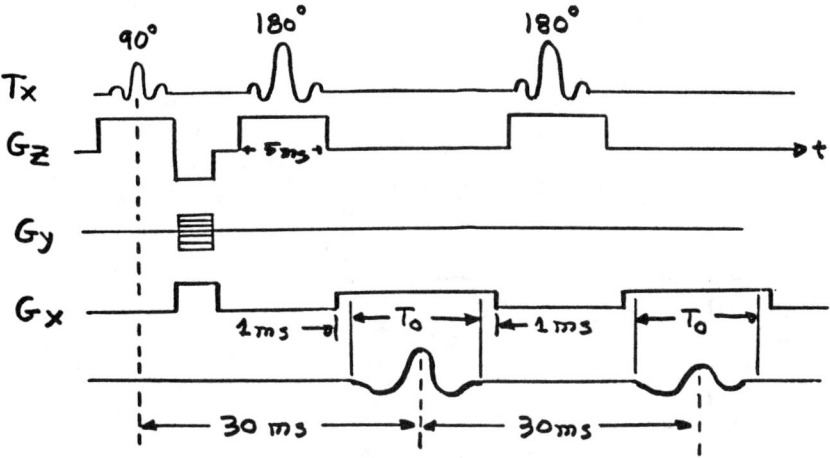

To ≃ 20 msec   A little less than muscle T2.

Gradient required for a given spatial resolution

$$\text{Grad.} = \frac{\text{Freq. Res.}}{\gamma \text{ (Spatial Res.)}}$$

γ = 4258 Hz/Gauss for protons.

$$\frac{50 \text{ Hz}}{4258 \text{ Hz/G} \cdot 0.1 \text{cm}} = 0.117 \frac{\text{Gauss}}{\text{cm}}$$

FIGURE 3. Spin echo imaging sequence. Echo signals can be observed between RF pulses. The available observation for this sequence allows a frequency resolution of 50 Hz. An 0.117 Gauss/cm gradient can provide 1mm spatial resolution in this case.

With the signal sampled every t_s seconds the maximum unique frequency is $1/2t_s$.

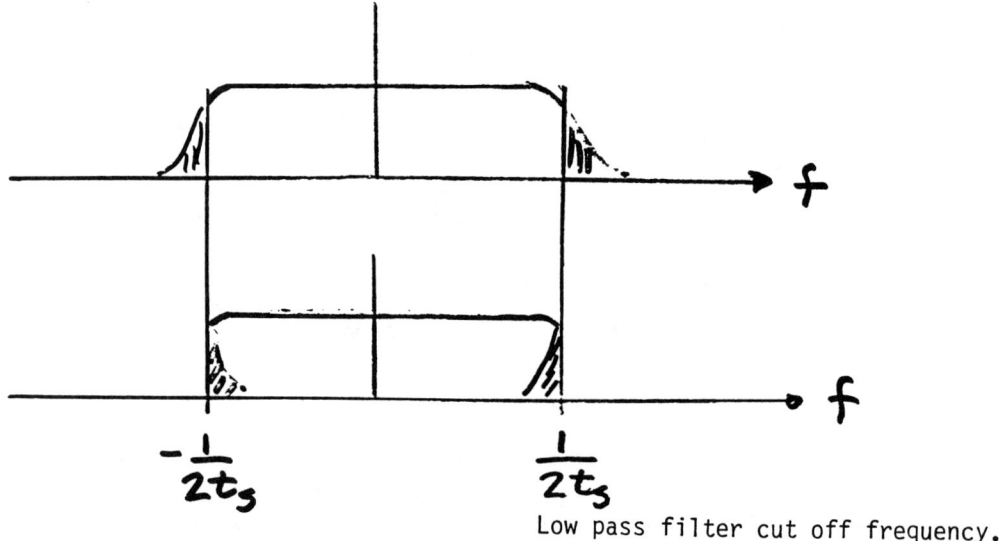

Low pass filter cut off frequency.

FIGURE 4. The maximum unique frequency which be observed is determined by the Nyquist criterion. Frequencies higher than this value must be eliminated by filtering.

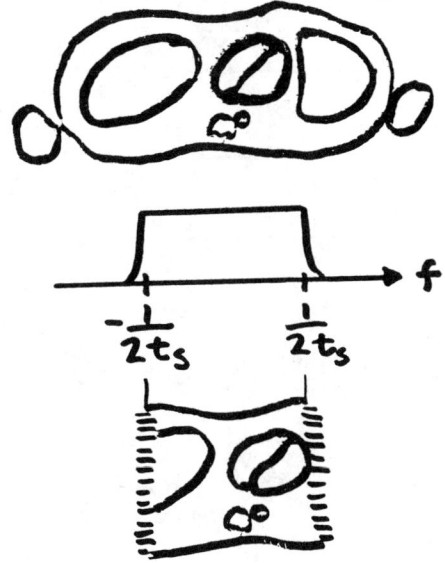

FIGURE 5. The anti-aliasing filter can be used to limit the image field of view.

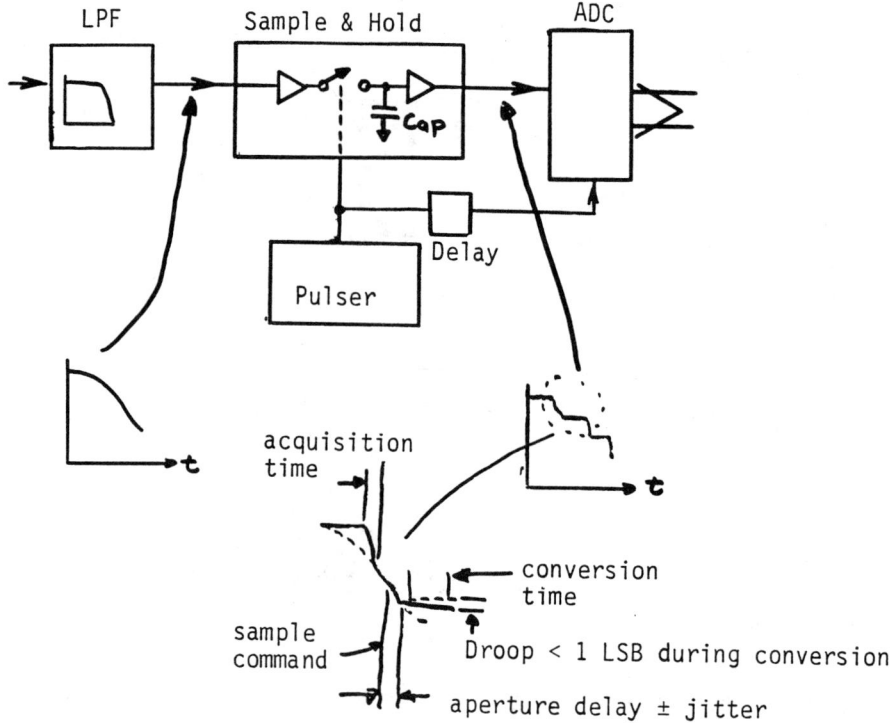

FIGURE 6. The dynamics of the signal must be frozen during the time required for the ADC to measure the signal's digital value. This function is performed by the sample and hold circuit. It uses buffer amplifiers and a switched capacitor to hold the analog value of the signal during the conversion. The dynamics of the sample and hold are important to the accuracy of the final digital value.

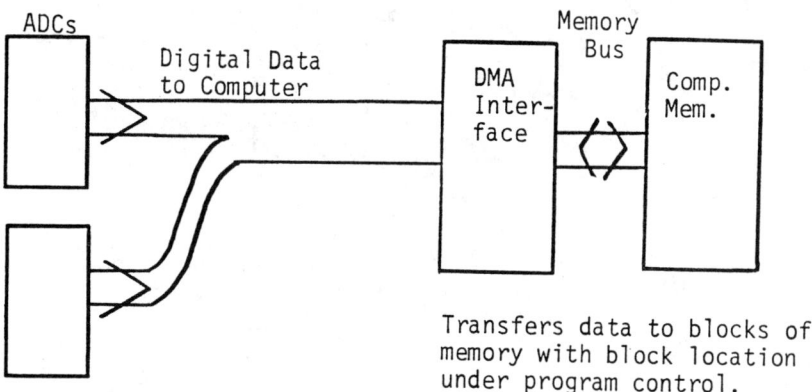

FIGURE 7a. Data path from the ADCs to the computer memory. The ADC's digital output is supplied to a Direct Memory Access (DMA) interface which will place the digital values into memory at sequential locations.

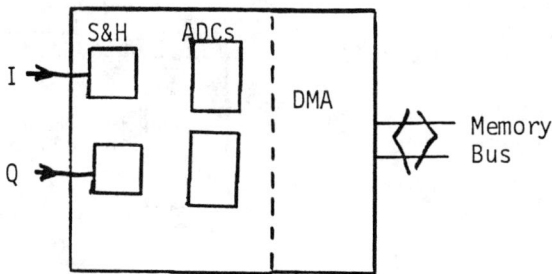

FIGURE 7b. The filtered receiver output can be routed to a circuit board containing the sample and holds, ADCs and DMA.

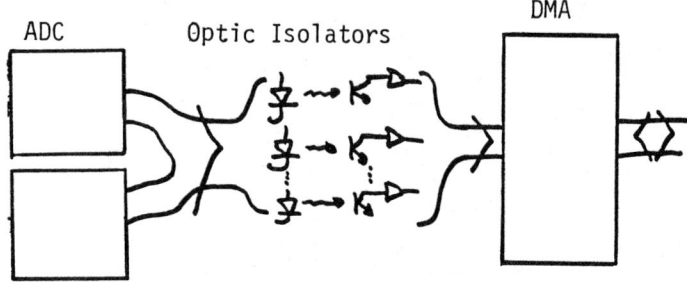

FIGURE 8a. The ADCs can be separate from the DMA and their connection can be direct through wire or isolated by optic isolators.

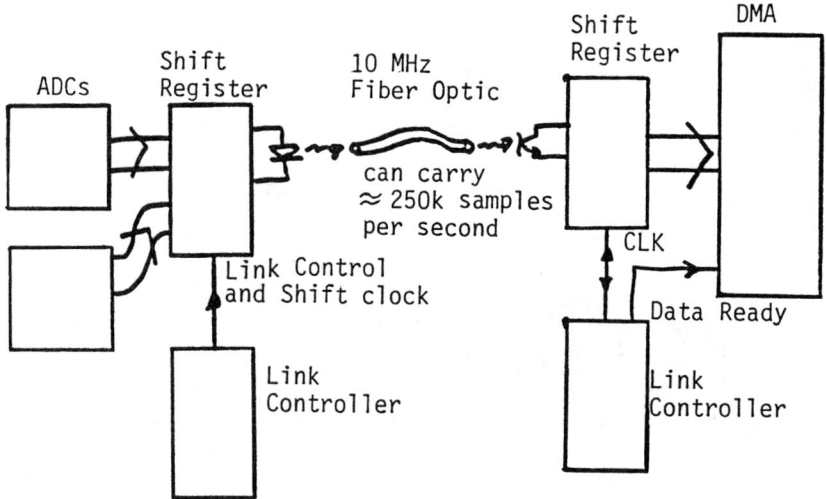

FIGURE 8b. Optic isolation can be provided by a single fiber optic cable with serial data interfaces at both ends.

199

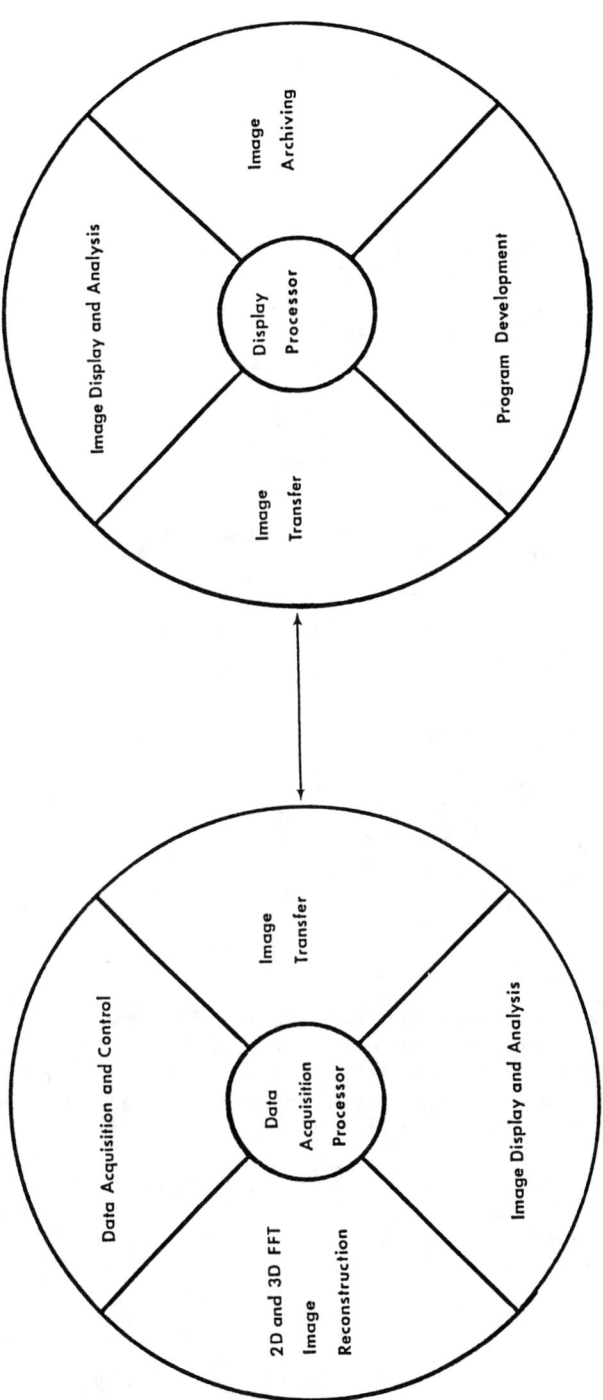

FIGURE 9a. Conceptual diagram of the dual computer architecture showing the partitioning of simultaneous tasks.

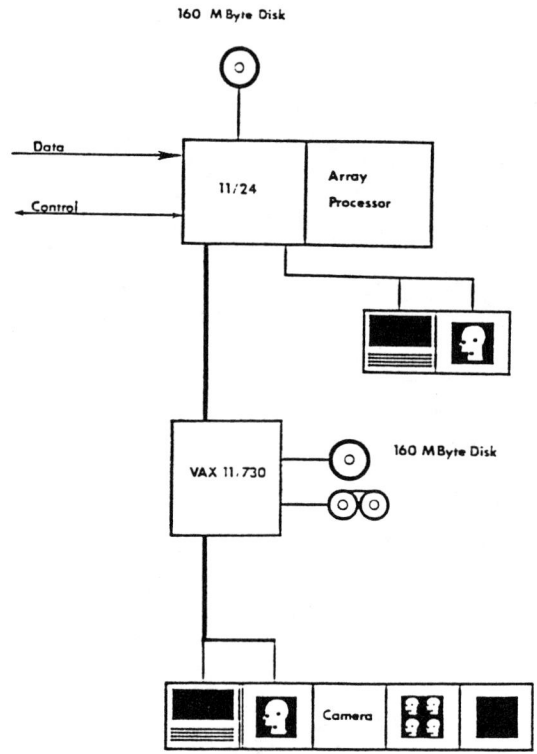

FIGURE 9b. The dual computer architecture provides two computers to perform the essentially separate tasks of data acquisition and image handling. Data acquisition must always have absolute priority use of the computer supporting it regardless of other demands made on the system, as is achieved with this design.

NMR RELAXATION IN TISSUE

M. S. Brown, J. C. Gore
Department of Diagnostic Radiology, Yale University School of Medicine, New Haven, Connecticut 06510

NMR relaxation times are primary determinants of the contrast in NMR images. They also place constraints on the speed of scanning and the design of imaging hardware, and are quantitative descriptors of tissue properties that potentially are useful parameters for in vivo tissue characterization. In this chapter we explore the underlying theory of relaxation and develop our understanding of these physical processes into a description of the behavior of protons in heterogeneous tissues. In so doing we emphasize that no adequate models have been proposed that quantitatively predict the detailed NMR behavior of whole tissues.

NMR relaxation techniques provide a powerful probe of the structure and dynamics of molecules. In liquids, relaxation is caused by non-static (time-dependent) magnetic interactions. The rapid rotational and translational motions of molecules generate fluctuating magnetic fields at the sites of relaxing nuclei which stimulate recovery of a population of spins to equilibrium. Thus, relaxation measurements are inherently measurements of the dynamic processes occuring within the molecule.

The Bloch equations[1,2] discussed in a previous chapter are empirical equations actually valid only for a system of isolated spin 1/2 particles. The simple single exponential recovery or first order process assumed in the Bloch formulation is inadequate when dealing with more complex spin systems. In general, the relaxation must be described as a sum of terms representing the contributions of different relaxation mechanisms. There are several mechanisms that can be distinguished. The most important of these are: dipole-dipole interactions, either between like spins or unlike spins (including electrons); modulation of the local magnetic field arising from chemical shift anisotropy; the coupling of the nuclear spin with the angular momentum of the molecule or spin rotation; scalar coupling fluctuations and quadrupolar effects. Each of these has a distinct physical origin but all share to some extent a common theoretical formulation.

Relaxation of protons in tissues is due almost entirely to dipole-dipole interaction with other protons (either on the same molecule or on a different molecule), and sometimes to dipolar interaction of the proton nuclear spin with the unpaired electron in paramagnetic materials.

In a system of spin 1/2 particles the wave function behavior is governed by a Hamiltonian that can be written as comprising a static term and a time-dependent component:

$$H = H_o + H(t) \tag{1}$$

The time-dependent Hamiltonian is almost always a small perturbation to the static Hamiltonian H_o so that the system may be treated using time-dependent perturbation theory or equivalently using the density matrix formalism. To introduce these consider the case of a particle of spin I interacting with a particle of spin S, such as the two protons in a water molecule. We will here be following the treatment of Solomon.[3] The static Hamiltonian of such a pair in a magnetic field B_o along the z direction is

$$H_o = -\hbar \gamma_I B_o I_z - \hbar \gamma_S B_o S_z \qquad (2)$$

Since we are interested in protons in tissue, the discussion will be limited to particles of spin 1/2. Larger values for the spin make the computations more complicated without fundamental changes.

The four eigenstates of the spins are defined as

$$\begin{aligned} I_z |+\rangle &= 1/2 \; |+\rangle, \\ I_z |-\rangle &= -1/2 \; |-\rangle, \\ S_z |+) &= +1/2 \; |+), \\ S_z |-) &= -1/2 \; |-) \end{aligned} \qquad (3)$$

so that the four unperturbed eigenstates of the pair are $|+\rangle|+)$, $|+\rangle|-)$, $|-\rangle|+)$, and $|-\rangle|-)$ with the respective occupation numbers N_{++}, N_{+-}, N_{-+}, N_{--}. These levels are shown in Fig. 1A along with the transition probabilites per unit time W_o, W_1, W_i and W_2 which are involved in longitudinal relaxation.

The transverse components of the magnetic moment can be treated in a similar fashion using the operators I_x (or I_y) and S_x (or S_y). We define four eigenstates of the spins by

$$\begin{aligned} I_x |\alpha\rangle &= +1/2 |\alpha\rangle \\ I_x |\beta\rangle &= -1/2 |\beta\rangle \\ S_x |\alpha) &= +1/2 |\alpha) \\ S_x |\beta) &= -1/2 |\beta) \end{aligned} \qquad (4)$$

The four states of the pair of spins are $|\alpha\rangle|\alpha)$, $|\alpha\rangle|\beta)$, $|\beta\rangle|\alpha)$, $|\beta\rangle|\beta)$ with occupation numbers $N_{\alpha\alpha}$, $N_{\alpha\beta}$, $N_{\beta\alpha}$, $N_{\beta\beta}$ and transition probabilities U_o, U_1, U_i and U_2, as shown in Fig 1B. It should be noted the states $|\alpha\rangle|\alpha)$, $|\alpha\rangle|\beta)$, $|\beta\rangle|\alpha)$, $|\beta\rangle|\beta)$ are not eigenstates of the energy, but they may be expanded in terms

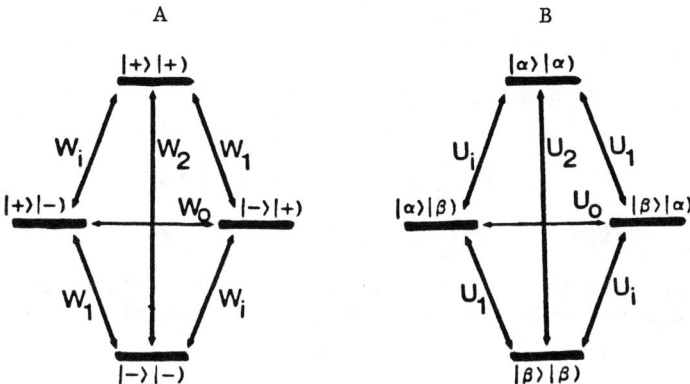

Figure 1. A) Transition probabilities between the eigenstates of the longitudinal components of the spin opertors. B) Transition probabilities between the eigenstates of the transverse components of the spin operators.

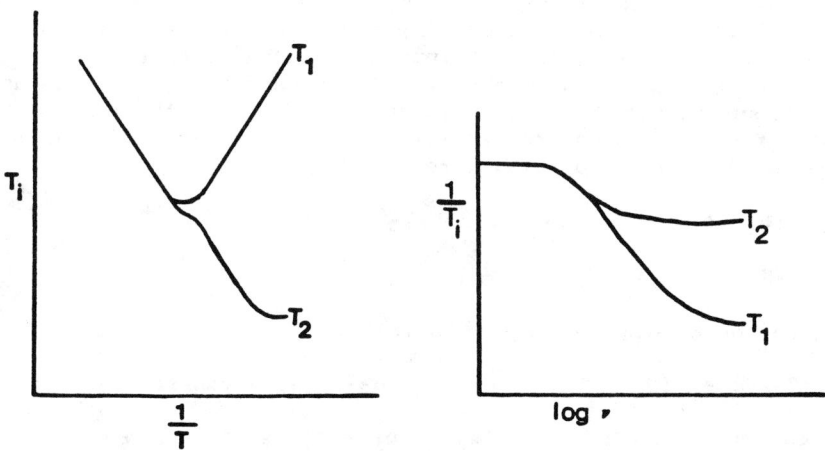

Figure 2. Schematic representation of NMR relaxation rates as a function of A. reciprocal temperature and B. magnetic field strength or Larmor frequency.

of eigenstates $|m_j\rangle$ of the energy. Two general states $|a\rangle$ and $|b\rangle$ can thus be represented

$$|a\rangle = \sum_i a_i |m_j\rangle$$

$$|b\rangle = \sum_i b_i |m_j\rangle$$

and for the case of spin 1/2, we have

$$|\alpha\rangle = (1/\sqrt{2})\ [\ |+\rangle\ +\ |-\rangle\ ]$$
$$|\beta\rangle = (1/\sqrt{2})\ [\ |+\rangle\ -\ |-\rangle\ ]. \tag{5}$$

From the definition of the transition probabilities W_s, the equations of motion for the longitudinal relaxation become

1. $dN_{++}/dt = W_i N_{+-} - (W_2 + W_1 + W_i) N_{++} + W_1 N_{-+} + W_2 N_{--} + $ constant

2. $dN_{+-}/dt = W_i N_{++} - (W_0 + W_1 + W_i) N_{+-} + W_0 N_{-+} + W_1 N_{--} + $ constant

3. $dN_{-+}/dt = W_1 N_{++} + W_0 N_{+-} - (W_0 + W_1 + W_i) N_{-+} + W_i N_{--} + $ constant

4. $dN_{--}/dt = W_2 N_{++} + W_1 N_{+-} + W_i N_{-+} - (W_1 + W_i + W_2) N_{--} + $ constant

$$(6)$$

The constants can be determined by considering the system at thermal equilibrium and inserting the proper Boltzman factor, but their precise values are not important in the computation of the relaxation times. The experimentally observable quantities are the macroscopic magnetic moments $\bar{I}_z$ and $\bar{S}_z$ which for the general case of unlike spins are distinguishable by their different Larmor frequencies and proportional to:

$$(N_{++} + N_{+-}) - (N_{-+} + N_{--}) \propto \bar{I}_z$$
$$(N_{++} + N_{-+}) - (N_{+-} + N_{--}) \propto \bar{S}_z \tag{7}$$

Insertion of equation (7) into (6) results in

$$d\bar{I}_z/dt = -(W_0 + 2W_1 + W_2)\bar{I}_z - (W_2 - W_0)\bar{S}_z + \text{constant}$$
$$d\bar{S}_z/dt = -(W_2 - W_0)\bar{I}_z - (W_0 + 2W_i + W_2)\bar{S}_z + \text{constant}$$

or

$$d\bar{I}_z/dt = -(W_0 + 2W_1 + W_2)(\bar{I}_z - I_0) - (W_2 - W_0)(\bar{S}_z - S_0)$$
$$d\bar{S}_z/dt = -(W_2 - W_0)(\bar{I}_z - I_0) - (W_0 + 2W_i + W_2)(\bar{S}_z - S_0) \tag{8}$$

I_o and S_o are the equilibrium values of the magnetic moments of spins I and S, and make the constants in eqs. (6)-(8) explicit. Identical calculations for the transverse components I_x and S_x give the results

$$d\bar{I}_x/dt = -(U_o + 2U_1 + U_2)\bar{I}_x - (U_2 - U_o)\bar{S}_x$$

$$d\bar{S}_x/dt = -(U_2 - U_o)\bar{I}_x - (U_o + 2U_i + U_2)\bar{S}_x \tag{9}$$

(Of course, the equilibrium values of I_x and S_x are zero). Notice that these equations show that in general the decay of the observed quantities is not a simple exponential but rather a linear combination of two exponentials.

Until now our discussion has been valid for the general case of two unlike spins. Now consider the case when the two spins I and S are alike (i.e. $\gamma_I = \gamma_S$), as is the case in water molecules. Then the observable quantities are $\bar{I}_z + \bar{S}_z$ and $\bar{I}_x + \bar{S}_x$ and it follows that $W_1 = W_i$ and $U_1 = U_i$. Thus, (8) and (9) become

$$\frac{d(\bar{I}_z + \bar{S}_z)}{dt} = -2(W_1 + W_2)(\bar{I}_z + \bar{S}_z - I_o - S_o)$$

and

$$\frac{d(\bar{I}_x + \bar{S}_x)}{dt} = -2(U_1 + U_2)(\bar{I}_x + \bar{S}_x) \tag{10}$$

These are exponential decays with the relaxation times defined as

$$\frac{1}{T_1} = 2(W_1 + W_2) \tag{11}$$

and

$$\frac{1}{T_2} = 2(U_1 + U_2) \tag{12}$$

Time-dependent first order perturbation theory can be used to explicitly calculate the transition probabilities per unit time between two eigenstates $|m_i\rangle$ and $|m_j\rangle$ of the unperturbed Hamiltonian with corresponding energies E_i and E_j. For the longitudinal components the relevant expression is

$$W_{ij} = \frac{1}{t\hbar^2}\left|\int_0^t \langle m_j| H(t') |m_i\rangle e^{-i\omega_{ij}t'} dt'\right|^2 \tag{13}$$

with $\omega_{ij} = (E_j - E_i)/\hbar$.
The transition probabilities per unit time between states $|a\rangle$ and $|b\rangle$ can be obtained by using the expansion in equation (5) and the orthogonality of the states ($\langle a|b\rangle = 0$). The result is

$$U_{ab} = \frac{1}{t\hbar^2}\left|\int_0^t \sum_{ij} \langle m_j| H(t') |m_i\rangle a_i b_j e^{-i\omega_{ij}t'} dt'\right|^2 \tag{14}$$

Abragam and Pound[4] have shown that in the case of rapid motion, both of these integrals result in time-independent transition probabilities per unit time.

In the case of a water molecule, the relaxation is dominated by the intramolecular magnetic dipole-dipole interaction between the two protons on the water molecule. The time-dependent Hamiltonian which describes the dipolar coupling between two spins is

$$H_D(t) = \left[\frac{\hbar^2 \gamma_I \gamma_S}{b^3}\right] [I \cdot S - 3(I \cdot r)(S \cdot r)] \qquad (15)$$

where r is the vector from spin I to spin S of length b. To first order, this simplifies to

$$H_D(t) = \frac{1}{2} \left[\frac{\hbar^2 \gamma_I \gamma_S}{b^3}\right] (1-\cos^2\theta)(3I_z S_z - I_z \cdot S_z) \qquad (16)$$

where θ is the angle between r and the z direction of the magnetic field. The rotational reorientation of the molecule changes the value of θ and causes fluctuations in the strength of the dipolar interaction which are responsible for relaxation.

This time-dependent Hamiltonian (16) may be used along with equations (13) and (14) to calculate the transition probabilities W_1, W_2, U_1, and U_2. These calculations are straightforward but lengthy, and the reader is referred to the paper by Solomon[3] for details. We merely quote the results here, which are

$$\frac{1}{T_1} = \frac{6}{20} \frac{\hbar^2 \gamma^4}{b^6} \left[\frac{\tau_c}{1+\omega^2 \tau_c^2} + \frac{4\tau_c}{1+4\omega^2 \tau_c^2}\right]$$

and

$$\frac{1}{T_2} = \frac{3}{20} \frac{\hbar^2 \gamma^4}{b^6} \left[3\tau_c + \frac{5\tau_c}{1+\omega^2 \tau_c^2} + \frac{2\tau_c}{1+4\omega^2 \tau_c^2}\right] \qquad (17)$$

Here τ_c is known as the correlation time, and is a measure of the time scale for reorientational motion of the molecule. It arises by considering the fluctuations of the local magnetic fields at the site of a nucleus. These changes may be described in terms of sets of functions $f_i(t)$ which give the time dependence of each component of the motion. The scalar product of function $f_i(t)$ with $f_j(t+\tau)$ integrated over all τ is a measure of how rapidly the local field changes in magnitude and direction and defines the correlation function G(t):

$$G(t) = \int_{-\infty}^{+\infty} f_i(\tau) \, f_j(t+\tau) \, d\tau \qquad (18)$$

If $f_i(t) = f_j(t)$, G(t) describes the correlation of one local field component with itself and is an auto-correlation function. When $f_i(t) \neq f_j(t)$, G(t) is a cross-correlation function between different local field components arising from, for example, the pairwise interactions in a 3-spin system. The correlation function can usually be considered as an exponential decay

$$G(t) = \frac{\int |f(t)|^2 dt}{|f(0)|^2} \exp(-t/\tau_c)$$

where τ_c = the correlation time discussed above.

In a pair of spins there exists an interaction energy. Since this interaction energy depends upon orientation with respect to the magnetic field, the interaction energy is time dependent and distributed in frequency and time. The frequency dependence is expressed as the power density or spectral density $J(\omega)$. The relaxation rate $1/T_1$ is directly related to the value of these functions at the Larmor precession frequency of the spin. Spectral densities are useful in the analysis of NMR relaxation because they are the Fourier transforms of time-correlation functions

$$J(\omega) = \int_{-\infty}^{+\infty} G(t) \, \exp(-i\omega t) \, dt \qquad (19)$$

Let us now return to the case of the dipole-dipole interaction between the two spins a distance r apart on the same molecule which is rotating in isotropic solutions. The spectral densities which arise from the motion of the molecule in this case are

$$J^{(0)}(\omega) = (24/15r^6) \, [\tau_c/(1+\omega^2 \tau^2_c)]$$
$$J^{(1)}(\omega) = (1/6) \, J^{(0)}(\omega) \qquad (20)$$
$$J^{(2)}(\omega) = (2/3) \, J^{(0)}(\omega)$$

The superscripts correspond to cases in which there is no net spin flip (zero quantum), one spin flip (1 quantum), and two spin flips (double quantum), respectively. Time-dependent perturbation theory and density matrix formalisms are used to give the relation between the relaxation rates and the spectral densities

$$\frac{1}{T_1} = (3/2)\, \gamma^4\, h^2\, I\,(I+1)\, [J^{(1)}(\omega) + J^{(2)}(2\omega)]$$

$$\frac{1}{T_2} = \gamma^4 h^2\, I\,(I+1)\, [(3/8)\, J^{(0)}(0) + (15/4)\, J^{(1)}(\omega) + (3/8)\, J^{(2)}(2\omega)] \tag{21}$$

Notice that these two expressions involve similar terms, except that $1/T_2$ depends on $J^{(0)}(0)$ while $1/T_1$ does not. This is because components of the local field contributing to longitudinal relaxation can also help reduce components of the magnetization in the x-y plane but the z-component of the local field can only influence magnetization components in the x-y plane, since it is collinear with the z component of magnetization.[6] Thus, the difference between T_1 and T_2 depends upon the value of the product $\omega\tau_c$. The variation of T_1 and T_2 with reciprocal temperature at constant frequency is shown in Fig. 2A. At high temperatures, τ_c is small (motion is fast), $\omega\tau_c << 1$, and $T_1 = T_2$. As temperature decreases and τ_c becomes larger (motion slows), the contribution of the $J^{(0)}(0)$ term becomes more significant, and $T_2 < T_1$. T_1 is smallest when $\omega\tau_c = 1$; this is the celebrated "T_1 minimum".

Figure 2B shows the frequency dependence (dispersion) of $1/T_1$ and $1/T_2$ at constant temperature. $T_1 = T_2$ at low frequency, but again, the values diverge as frequency increases due to the increasing contribution of $J^{(0)}(0)$.

The above discussion is valid for isotropically tumbling water molecules, relaxing via the intramolecular dipole-dipole mechanism which is modulated by the rotational tumbling of the molecules. An additional contribution to the relaxation arises from dipole-dipole interactions between the protons in a water molecule and the protons on neighboring water molecules. This intermolecular mechanism is modulated by both the rotation and translation of the water molecule. In pure water this contribution can be estimated and added to the terms described above. The spin-lattice relaxation rates for translation can be calculated using Stokes-Einstein diffusion theory:[7]

$$\left(\frac{1}{T_1}\right)_{diff} = \frac{\pi}{5} \frac{N\gamma^4 h^2}{a\,D} = \frac{6\pi^2}{5}\, \gamma^4 h^2\, \frac{N\eta}{kT}$$

Here N is the spin density, and η is the bulk viscosity. This translational contribution is added to the rotational contribution calculated above:

$$\frac{1}{T_1} = \frac{1}{T_1\ rot} + \frac{1}{T_1\ trans}$$

In magnetic field gradients, diffusion can also affect the apparent spin-spin relaxation rate. For example a standard method of measuring the translational diffusion coefficient is by using a pulsed spin echo sequence[8,9] in conjunction with pulsed field gradients.[10,11] In such a sequence, the echo amplitude after a 180° pulse at time 2τ decays as a function of the pulse spacing τ. The echo amplitude is

$$E(2\tau) = \exp(-2\tau/T_2) \exp(-2\tau^3 \gamma^2 G^2 D/3).$$

Here G is the applied field gradient, and

$$T_{2D} = 3/(\tau^2 \gamma^2 G^2 D)$$

is the effective decay time due to diffusion. G in tissue may arise from magnetic susceptibility variations at the cellular level.[11,12]

It can be seen from our discussion thus far that NMR relaxation can be dealt with in a rigorous fashion in simple systems. However, in tissue, the situation is much more complex although interactions at an atomic level must derive in similar fashion. The NMR signal in an imaging experiment may contain intensity from non-water protons such as macromolecular protons, particularly in fatty tissues with significant concentrations of triglycerides and phospholipids. These macromolecular protons relax at different rates than the water protons and are characterized by motions quite different from the isotropic fast tumbling of free water. Thus, the intrepretation of in vivo NMR relaxation as being due only to water protons may lead to erroneous conclusions. Tissue water itself may also exist in a variety of dynamical states. For example, there is a hydration layer of loosely hydrogen bonded water surrounding many macromolecular components of tissue. The degree of hydration (i.e. the thickness of the bound layer) depends upon the functional groups on the macromolecule and upon other factors such as its shape. In this layer water protons will often experience more restricted motion than in free water. Furthermore, the relaxation of water in tissue need not be due entirely to interactions with other water protons; for example, evidence has been found for magnetic cross-relaxation contributions to T_1. Protons in water molecules near the macromolecular protons may relax via <u>intermolecular</u> dipole-dipole interactions with the aliphatic protons, thereby providing another mechanism of relaxation. This should be thought of as a separate contribution to the overall relaxation rate, involving different correlation times than water intramolecular interactions. To incorporate cross-relaxation we need to represent tissue as a coupled system with three relaxation rates: those of free water, of the "solute" or macromolecular protons, and a cross-relaxation term. The contributions are not necessarily additive, however, and the system should be described using coupled differential equations like the Solomon description presented above.

Various techniques have been used to elucidate the various contributions, but overall, this is very difficult in tissue, particularly in vivo. The size of the contribution of cross relaxation in tissue is not clear at the present time. It should be noted that the dipolar interaction has a $1/r^6$ dependence, so that a water molecule close to but not in the first hydration layer of a macromolecule may not feel an intermolecular contribution, but may still move differently to free water and thus have faster relaxation.

The importance of cross-relaxation has been demonstrated by

measuring the effect of substitution of deuterated water for tissue water on tissue proton T_1.[12-16] The gyromagnetic ratio of ^2H is .15 that of ^1H, and thus the substitution reduces the strength of intermolecular proton-proton dipolar interaction. Water also undergoes rapid chemical exchange:

$$^1H_2O + {^2H_2O} \rightleftharpoons {^1HO^2H}$$

so the intramolecular proton-proton dipolar interactions are also reduced. In the absence of any cross-relaxation, T_1 should rapidly rise as the ratio $^2H_2O/H_2O$ increases. This is indeed the behavior observed in bulk water, where T_1 increases by a factor of 24 (extrapolated to full substitution). In tissue, the increase is only about 20% (extrapolated to full substitution). These results provide strong evidence that magnetic cross-exchange between macromolecular protons and hydration layer water protons dominates proton relaxation in tissues. A water proton will still interact with the same number of nearby macromolecular protons in spite of dilution with ^2H_2O and this rate should indeed be independent of deuterium dilution. The small 20% change may be due to chemical exchange of water deuterons with acidic protons on functional groups (e.g. acids, amines) found in tissues.

NMR relaxation data in tissue obviously reflects the motions of water in tissues and many studies have been performed in an attempt to elucidate the behavior of water in tissue. Experiments involving the gradual freezing of tissue water resulted in the observation of a nonfreezing water component in most tissues. The simplest model proposed to account for these observations is that tissue water exists in two environments, a "free", or unbound milieu, and an irrotationally bound layer[17]. Molecules in these two regions constantly exchange with other. If this exchange is fast compared to the relaxation rate at each site, the observed decay is still exponential and is the weighted average of the relaxation times in each environment. This is the "Fast Exchange Two Site" (FETS) model of tissue water, in which NMR relaxation times can be expressed as

$$\frac{1}{T_1} = \frac{x}{T_s} \quad \frac{1-x}{T_{H2O}}$$

where T_1 is the measured relaxation time, x is the fraction of slow moving, fast relaxing (bound) cell water, 1-x is the fraction of cell water like bulk water, T_s and T_{H2O} are their relaxation times respectively. The FETS model, however, has been found to be inadequate to explain, for example, NMR dispersion curves or the deuterium stustitution experiments described above. It requires that relaxation rates are inversely proportional to water contents, which certainly are not always related in this way. Water exists in a variety of states, some more ordered than others. Attempts to retain the conceptual simplicity of the FETS model have led to suggestions of the existence of three water fractions, hydration, vicinal, and bulk water.[18-21] The water of hydration, which is within 3 to 6 Å of the macromolecular surfaces, exhibits only rotational motion with a correlation time of about 10^{-7}s. Vicinal water, existing out to a distance of $\sim 50 Å$ from intracellular surfaces, is characterized by rotational motion and restricted translational motion with a wide range of correlation times ($10^{-7} - 10^{11}$s). The NMR relaxational properties of bulk water are similar to "free" water with a correlation time of about 10^{-12}s. Water in the free phase undergoes rapid translational and rotational motion, with a correlation time on the order of 1 ps, resulting in a rather long T_1. In addition this contribution tends to be relatively frequency independent. Bound water tends to relax faster due to its reduced motion (the slower the motion, the shorter T_1) and due to its interaction with the macromolecular hydrogen. In these molecules, rotational motion is primarily responsible for the relaxation. These correlation times are about 10 times the correlation time of the free phase. It is this component of the longitudinal relaxation which shows the most dramatic frequency dependence. Other researchers[21-23] have formulated models which incorporate distribution functions of correlation times in which parameters are empirically fitted to the data.

Another possible source of relaxation in tissues is the interaction of the nuclear spin with the unpaired electron in a paramagnetic center. This is, again, a dipolar interaction. Paramagnetic ions in solution can significantly reduce relaxation times because the mean square magnetic field at the site of a relaxing nucleus produced by an electron is about 10^6 times stronger than the field produced by other nuclei. Thus, free paramagnetic ions such as Mn^{+2} in tissue can affect relaxation times drastically. However, although the use of paramagnetic ions to increase tissue contrast has been explored, in the low concentrations found normally in tissue, it appears unlikely that there will be significant effects due to paramagnetics. Furthermore, most paramagnetic metals in tissue are bound to proteins, porphyrins or are in some other way isolated from the water environment, so that water molecules may not come close enough to interact effectively with paramagnetic centers. Exceptions may occur in some disease states, for example in the liver.

Another particularly powerful method of studying the behavior of tissue protons is to obtain the nmr relaxation rates as a function of frequency, as shown in Fig. 3. The frequency dependence of the relaxation rates is referred to as a nuclear magnetic resonance dispersion (NMRD) curve. The contribution of low frequency mechanisms is relatively independent of the Larmor frequency. NMR dispersion measurements are a method of separating the contributions of frequency dependent and non-frequency dependent components of relaxation. Several features of an NMRD curve are worthy of note. These include the inflection point in the dispersion, the magnitude of the rate at low frequency, the magnitude of the change through the dispersion, and the high frequency rate. For solutions of globular proteins, the inflection point in the dispersion seems to be correlated with the size of the protein.[24] Thus, in some way the solvent molecules report the rotational correlation time for the protein. For more complex solutions, or for tissues, the dispersion curves are not yet well understood. Koenig et. al.[25] have fitted

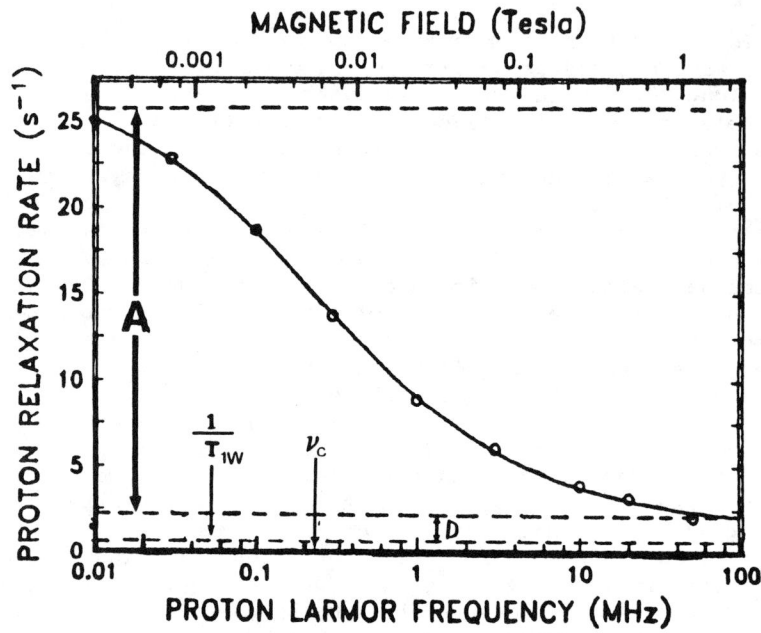

Figure 3. A fit of the Cole-Cole expression (solid curve), a heuristic four-parameter formula, to the $1/T_1$ NMRD profile of a normal rat liver. The data are thereby resolved into two components: one, the A-term, varies substantially with field and has an inflection at field ν_c; a second, the D-term, is essentially independent of field in the range illustrated. A fourth parameter β characterizes the slope of the profile at ν_c. The field-independent background contributed by the solvent to the $1/T_1$ profile is indicated by $1/T_1$. The fitted parameter values in the present case are: $A = 26.8$, $\beta = 1.08$, $\nu_c = .24$, and $D = 1.40$.[26]

the curves using the heuristic Cole-Cole expression:

$$\frac{1}{T_1} = \frac{1}{T_{1w}} + D + A \operatorname{Re}\left[\frac{1}{(1+(i\nu/\nu_c)^{\beta/2})}\right]$$

The parameters are illustrated in Fig. 3, for normal rat liver tissue.[26] A is the low-field magnitude of a dispersive component that decreases to zero at high field, D is the magnitude of a term that is independent of field, ν_c is the value of the field at which the curve inflects and β represents the slope of the curve at ν_c. The background solvent contribution is T_{1w} in protein solutions. Experiments involving deuterium substitution as described above have shown that cross-relaxation enhances the value of A without alteration of the inflection point frequency ν_c.[27]

It is clear from the above that we possess a sound theoretical and experimental understanding of relaxation in water and simple solutions. The intrinsic parameters to characterize such media are the correlation times of the local field fluctuations. However the details of relaxation in heterogeneous tissue are much more complex and our knowledge is incomplete. In tissue water samples many parts of the cellular environment by its rapid Brownian motion. In a time $T_2 \sim 100$ msecs, intracellular water will diffuse approximately 25 um. For water in a cell of diameter 10 um, therefore, each molecule will collide many times with the cell walls, so that in any NMR experiment water molecules will sample the many different microenvironments in tissue in the time they take to relax. At each encounter with a macromolecular surface, a water molecule will have its motion slowed, and the relaxation rate reflects a global average of these multiple events. Variable frequency and temperature and multinuclear studies are but three approaches to unravelling the detailed mechanisms at the atomic level. There remains however considerable uncertainty about the origin of the differences between different normal tissues and their alterations in pathological states.

References

1. Bloch F: Phys. Rev., 102:104. (1956)

2. Bloch F: Phys. Rev., 105:1206. (1957)

3. Solomon I: Phys. Rev., 99:559. (1955)

4. Abragam A, Pound RV: Phys. Rev. 92:953. (1953)

5. Slichter CA: Principles of Magnetic Resonance. Springer-Verlag, New York 1978.

6. Fukushima E, Rueder SBW: Experimental Pulse NMR. Addison-Wesley Publishing, Reading, MA (1981) p. 146.

7. Abragam A: The Principles of Nuclear Magnetism, Oxford Univ. Press, London & New York (1961).

8. Hahn EL: Phys. Rev. 80:580 (1950).

9. Carr HY, Purcell EM: Phys. Rev. 94:630 (1954).

10. Stejskal EO, Tanner JE: J. Chem. Phys. 42:288 (1965).

11. Packer KJ: J. Mag. Resonance 9:438 (1973).

12. Senftle FE: Thorpe A: Nature (London) 190:410 (1961).

13. Civan MM, Shporter M: Biophys. J. 15:299, 1975.

14. Chaughule RS, Kasturi SR, Vijayaraghavan R, Ranade SS: Ind. J. Biochem. Biophys. 11:256 (1974).

15. Fung BM: Biophys. J. 18:235 (1977).

16. Rustgi SN, Peemoeller H, Thompson RT, Pinter MM: Biophys. J. 22:439 (1978).

17. Mansfield P, Morris PG: NMR Imaging in Biomedicine, Academic Press, New York. 1982, pp. 10-32.

18. Thompson BC, Waterman MR, Cotton GL: Arch. Biochem. Biophys. 166:193 (1975).

19. Zipp A, James TL, Kuntz ID, Shihet SB: Biochim. Biophys. Acta. 428:291 (1976).

20. Clegg JS: in Biophysics of Water eds. Franks F, Mathias S. Joh Wiley, New York 365 1982.

21. Escanye JM, Canet D, Robert J: Biochim. Biophys. Acta 721:305 (1982).

22. Fung BM, McGaughy T: Biochim Biophys Acta, 343:663 (1974).

23. Held G, Noack F, Pollack V, Melton B: Z. Naturforsch. 28C 59 (1973).

24. Koenig SH, Schillinger: J. of Biol. Chem., 244:3283 (1969).

25. Hallenga K, Koenig SH: Biochemistry, 15: 4255 (1976).

26. Data from a collaboration of the authors with S.H. Koenig, IBM Watson Research.

27. Koenig SH, Bryant RG, Hallenga K, Jacob GS: Biochemistry 17:4348 (1978).

SIGNAL-TO-NOISE AND CONTRAST IN MR IMAGING

Felix W. Wehrli
General Electric Company, Medical Systems Group
Milwaukee, Wisconsin 53201

ABSTRACT

Signal-to-noise (SN) and contrast-to-noise (CN) are paramount to image quality. Both quantities are functions of four groups of parameters: (1) the imaging parameters (matrix size, field of view, slice thickness), (2) pulse sequence and timing parameters, (3) intrinsic tissue parameters (T_1, T_2, spin density), and (4) magnet field strength. The implications and interdependence of these parameters will be discussed and illustrated.

SIGNAL-TO-NOISE: DEFINITION, MEASUREMENT AND IMPLICATIONS ON IMAGE QUALITY

Noise in digital images impairs image quality. It adversely affects edge acuity and, in the extreme, renders structures of slightly different signal intensity indistinguishable. The threshold value below which an image is rated poor, doubtless, is subjective. Edelstein gives a figure of about 20:1[1].

The signal-to-noise ratio (SNR) in an image can be measured in various ways. For example, we can select a region of interest (ROI), low-frequency filter the image and subtract the thus filtered image from the original image. In this manner we obtain a figure of merit for the noise. The signal is obtained by calculating a mean pixel value from an ROI. Hence, SNR can be defined as the ratio signal/background noise amplitude. Alternatively we can place an ROI box outside the object

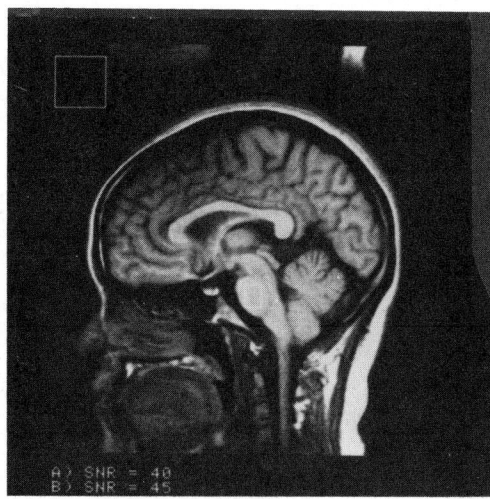

Figure 1
Noise can be measured in two different ways: (a) From the standard deviation in a signal-free ROI outside the object boundaries (upper left hand corner of image) and (b) from the ROI in which the signal is measured. In the latter case the noise is obtained by subtracting a low-pass filtered image from the original image. The two methods afforded SNR figures in the pons of the midline sagittal head image shown of 40 and 45, respectively.

boundary, and calculate the standard deviation for this pixel matrix. This method is hampered by the fact that noise often is not statistical and may vary across the field of view. <u>Figure 1</u> compares the two methods for a region of interest in a brain image.

DEPENDENCE OF SIGNAL-TO-NOISE RATIO ON IMAGING PARAMETERS

The major source of noise in MR images is the electronic noise generated in the receiver circuit and the patient[2,3]. While with today's technology, the noise of the receiver coil circuit (preamplifier, coil, etc.) can be reduced to well below 1 db, noise generated by the patient, resulting from Brownian motion of the ions in the body fluids, can be controlled only to a limited extent, for example, by confining the detection volume using local coils[4-6].

In addition, the instrument designer is faced with a variety of other noise sources, generating noise that is not statistical in nature. This includes radiofrequency transmitters and digital systems radiating at frequencies within the bandwidth of the receiver. MR imaging systems, therefore, are typically enclosed by an RF shield to minimize reception of such extraneous signals. We will not further dwell on this subject and henceforth it is assumed these extraneous noise sources are absent.

The electronic noise N_R is given by[2]

$$N_R = \xi \, \Delta\nu^{1/2} (R_c \cdot \nu^{1/2} + R_p \cdot \nu^2)^{1/2} \qquad (1)$$

In Equation (1) ξ is the coil filling factor which will be discussed elsewhere[7], ν is the resonance frequency and $\Delta\nu$ the bandwidth of the receiver. The latter is determined by the field of view D_x and the amplitude of the readout gradient G_x:

$$\Delta\nu = (\gamma/2\pi) \, G_x \, D_x \qquad (2)$$

where γ stands for the magnetogyric ratio.

R_c and R_p in Equation (1) are the resistances of coil and patient, respectively.

In an abbreviated form we may write for the signal S:

$$S \sim N(X) \cdot \Delta x \cdot \Delta y \cdot d \cdot \nu^2 \cdot f(T_i, T_1, T_2) \qquad (3)$$

In Equation (3) $N(X)$ is the nuclear density (number of nuclei X per unit volume), Δx, Δy are the pixel dimensions, d is the slice thickness. The product $N \cdot \Delta x \cdot \Delta y \cdot d$ thus corresponds to the number of nuclei per voxel that contribute to the signal; $f(T_i, T_1, T_2)$ represents the dependence of the transverse magnetization that induces the signal voltage in the receiver coil on intrinsic pulse timing parameters (T_i) and spin relaxation times (T_1, T_2). In the simplest case T_i is just the time interval between successive RF excitations.

The quantity $f(T_i, T_1, T_2)$ will be addressed with the discussion of the pulse sequence dependence of contrast. It is the principal determinant of contrast between two anatomic regions.

In two-dimensional Fourier transform (2DFT) imaging[8], we collect a free induction decay (FID) or echo which is sampled N_x times during the detection period. Each of these signals yields, upon Fourier transformation, a projection. In total N_y projections are collected to create, following a second Fourier transform, an image consisting of $N_x \cdot N_y$ pixels. If we consider further that each projection may result from averaging of n identical FID's, we obtain for the SNR (Equations 1-3):

$$SNR \sim \Delta x \cdot \Delta y \cdot d \cdot \sqrt{N_x} \cdot \sqrt{N_y} \cdot \sqrt{n} \cdot N(X) \cdot f(T_i, T_1, T_2)$$
$$\cdot 1/\sqrt{\Delta \nu} \cdot \nu^2 / \sqrt{R_c \nu^{\frac{1}{2}} + R_p \nu^2} \quad (4)$$

The term $\sqrt{N_x} \sqrt{N_y}$ in Eqn (4) results from statistical reduction of noise during data collection. Considering in addition that for the x and y dimension of the field of view (FOV), $D_x = N_x \cdot \Delta x$ and $D_y = N_y \cdot \Delta y$ holds, respectively, we can write for the SNR

$$SNR \sim \frac{D_x}{\sqrt{N_x}} \cdot \frac{D_y}{\sqrt{N_y}} \cdot d \cdot \sqrt{n} \cdot N(X) \cdot f(T_i, T_1, T_2)$$
$$\cdot 1/\sqrt{\Delta \nu} \cdot f(\nu) \quad (5)$$

where $f(\nu) = \nu^2 / \sqrt{R_c \nu^{\frac{1}{2}} + R_p \nu^2}$.

If we further take into account that the bandwidth $\Delta \nu$ is proportional to the number of samples N_x (Equation (2)) and consider only the operator-selectable imaging parameters (excluding pulse timing parameters) we obtain:

$$SNR \sim \frac{D_x}{N_x} \cdot \frac{D_y}{\sqrt{N_y}} \cdot d \cdot \sqrt{n} \quad (6)$$

Typical choices of field of view, matrix size and slice thickness are provided in Table I.

Table I Effect of FOV, matrix size and slice thickness on relative SNR

SNR	D_x (cm)	D_y (cm)	N_x	N_y	d (cm)
1	25	25	128	128	1
1/4	12.5	12.5	128	128	1
1/2	25	25	256	128	1
$1/2\sqrt{2}$	25	25	256	256	1
$1/4\sqrt{2}$	25	25	256	256	0.5

Table I shows that a twofold magnification (maintaining matrix size and reducing FOV by a factor of 2) results in a fourfold SNR degradation. The penalty paid for a twofold increase in resolution (doubling matrix size without altering FOV) results in a loss of SNR by a factor of $2\sqrt{2}$. In either of the two cases spatial resolution is the same. However, in the latter case the minimum scan time increases by a factor of 2 since we sample twice as many projections. <u>Figure 2</u> shows the effect of reducing FOV on spatial resolution and SNR.

a)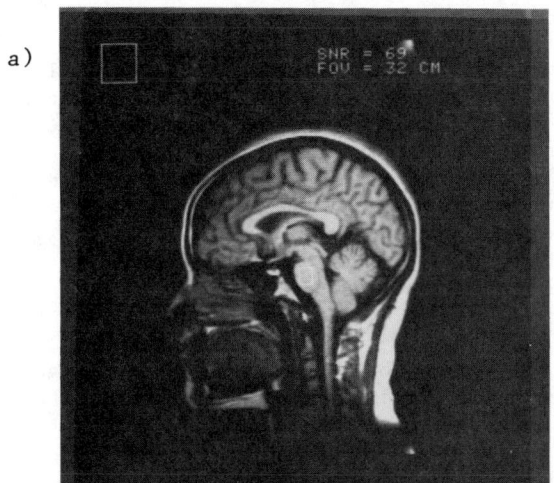

b)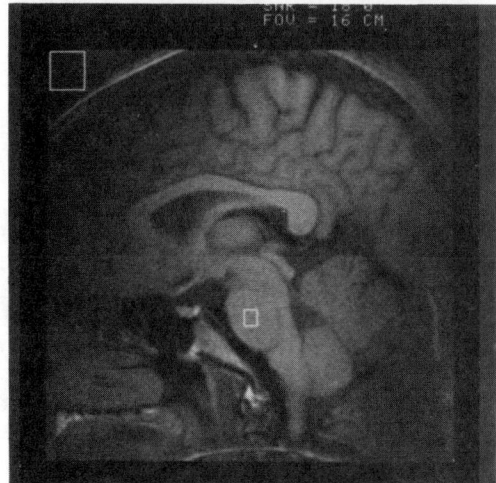

Figure 2
Effect of field of view on SNR. The two images (a and b) were obtained under identical conditions except that the field of view in image b was reduced by a factor of 2 in either dimension, resulting in an approximate reduction in SNR by a factor of 4 (SNR = 69 and 18, respectively).

If we denote the time between consecutive excitations TR and the total scan time TS,

$$n = TS/(TR \cdot N_y) \tag{7}$$

follows and, holding SNR constant, we obtain, from rearrangement of Equation (6):

$$TS \sim TR \left\{ \frac{N_x \cdot N_y}{d \cdot D_x \cdot D_y} \right\}^2 \tag{8}$$

From Equation (8) we recognize the time penalties paid for magnification, increase in matrix size and decrease in slice thickness. A simultaneous reduction, for example, by a factor of two each in field of view and slice thickness, would require a 64-fold increase in scan time to maintain SNR! Since this is totally impractical, it is important that the imager's intrinsic SNR be high enough that upon increasing spatial resolution the SNR in the image does not degrade excessively.

DEPENDENCE OF SIGNAL-TO-NOISE AND CONTRAST-TO-NOISE RATIO ON PULSE TIMING PARAMETERS

In this section we will review the dependence of the signal on pulse timing parameters and intrinsic tissue MR parameters (T_1, T_2, proton density).

The observer's ability to differentiate two regions i and j in an image depends on the differential SNR, also denoted contrast-to-noise ratio (CNR)[9]:

$$CNR(i,j) = SNR(i) - SNR(j) \tag{9}$$

The CNR therefore has the same scaling properties as the SNR as far as the basic imaging parameters, FOV, matrix size, slice thickness and number of excitations are concerned.

In 2DFT imaging, typically, the signal arises from the refocused magnetization (spin echo), following a 180° phase reversal pulse[8]. The simplest implementation of this method consists of a 90° pulse generating transverse magnetization, following TE/2 milliseconds later by the 180° pulse. The entire cycle is repeated every TR milliseconds (<u>Figure 3a</u>).

Typically, multiple echoes can be generated by applying a 180° pulse at t = TE/2, 3TE/2, 5TE/2, ..., resulting in refocusing at t = TE, 2TE, 3TE, ... (<u>Figure 3b</u>).

It can be shown that the signal for the ith echo can be expressed by the product of two terms[10]

$$S(TE_i) \sim f(TR, TE, T_1) \cdot e^{-TE_i/T_2} \tag{10}$$

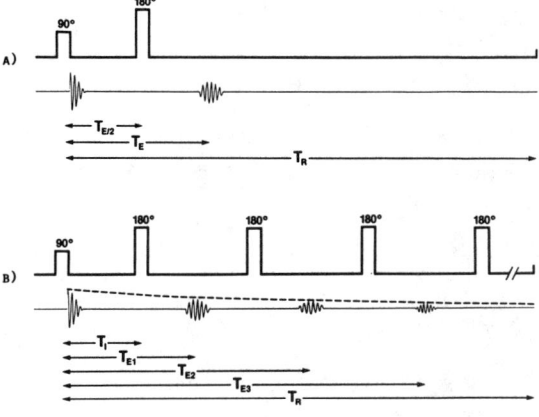

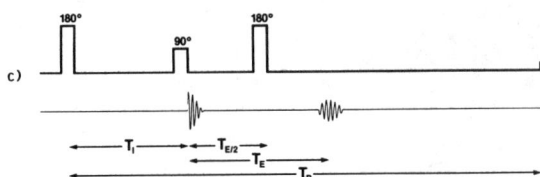

Figures 3a - c
RF pulse timing diagram for three common pulse sequences: a) spin echo, b) multiple spin echo, c) inversion recovery spin echo. Pulse timing parameters are explained in the text.

It is noteworthy that the first term in Equation (10) is independent of T_2. For a 4-echo sequence Equation (10) becomes[12]:

$$S(TE_i) \sim N(H) [1-\exp(-TR/T_1) + 2\exp(-(TR-TE/2)/T_1)$$

$$- 2\exp(-(TR-3TE/2)/T_1) + 2\exp(-(TR-5TE/2)/T_1)$$

$$- 2\exp(-(TR-7TE/2)/T_1] \exp(-iTE/T_2) \quad (11)$$

which, if $TE_{max} \ll TR$, simplifies to

$$S(TE_i) \sim (1 - e^{-TR/T_1}) \, e^{-TE_i/T_2} \quad (11a)$$

From Equation (11a) we recognize that the saturation term dictates overall signal intensity which is maximum when TR $\gg$ T_1. <u>Figure 4b</u> shows a plot of experimental signal intensity from two ROI's in multiple-echo images (<u>Figure 4a</u>), taken at the level of the kidneys.

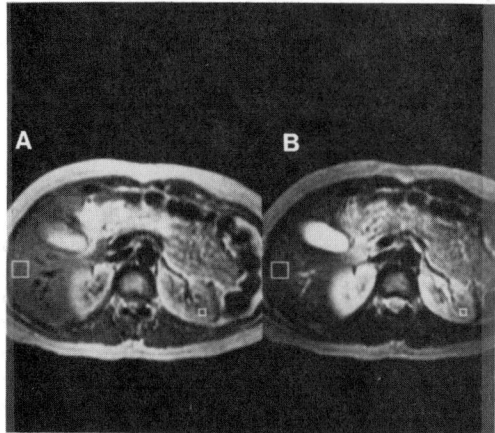
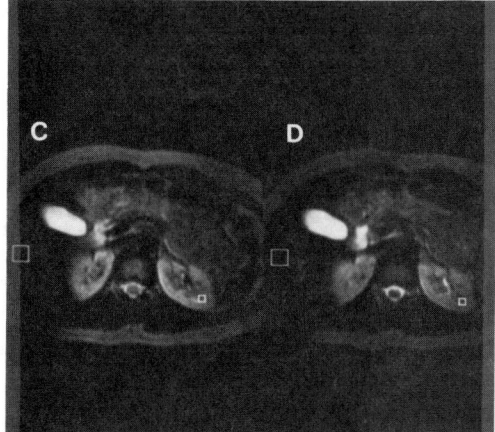
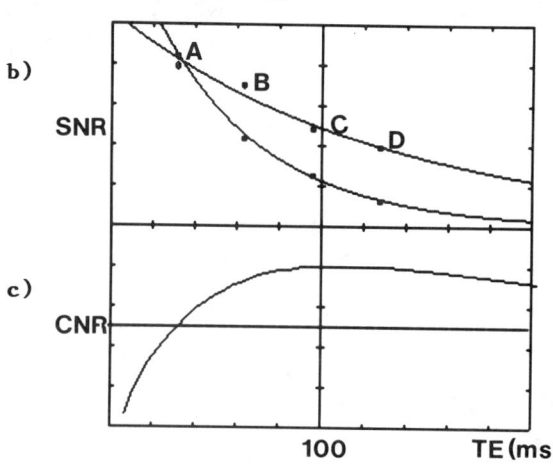

Figure 4a - c
a) 1.3T images recorded at the level of the kidneys by means of a 4-echo sequence with echo delays TE = 32, 64, 96 and 128 ms and a repetition time TR = 1.5 seconds. Note the differential decrease in signal intensity in the later echoes for liver, kidney and CSF. b) Signal intensity plotted as a function of echo delay from ROI's indicated in Figure a). Note the increase in differential signal intensity for the two tissues with increasing echo delay. c) Relative contrast-to-noise ratio for liver and kidney tissue computed from the signal intensity curves in Figure 4b, affording a broad maximum at approximately TE = 100 ms.

Whereas for short TE liver is predicted to be more intense than kidney, the reverse behavior is the case at long TE where the second term in Equation (11a) dominates. This behavior is indicative of liver possessing both shorter T_1 and shorter T_2 than kidney. The resulting CNR curve in <u>Figure 4c</u> shows that at TR = 1.5 s there is an optimum for the two tissues at TE ≃ 100 ms.

For the estimation of the global maximum of CNR for two adjoining tissues, a contour or density plot in which CNR is displayed as CNR = $f(TR,TE)$[13] is most appropriate. In doing so we have to choose between either holding scan time or number of excitations constant. We have seen previously that SNR ~ $\sqrt{n}$ and since n = $T_s/(N_y TR)$ (Equation 7), CNR for two tissues A and B can be written as[14]

$$CNR(A,B) \sim (TS/TR)^{\frac{1}{2}} (S_A - S_B) \qquad (12)$$

A CNR map for gray and white matter, calculated on the basis of the relaxation and spin density parameters, listed in Table II, assuming a fixed number of excitations, is shown in <u>Figure 5</u>[15].

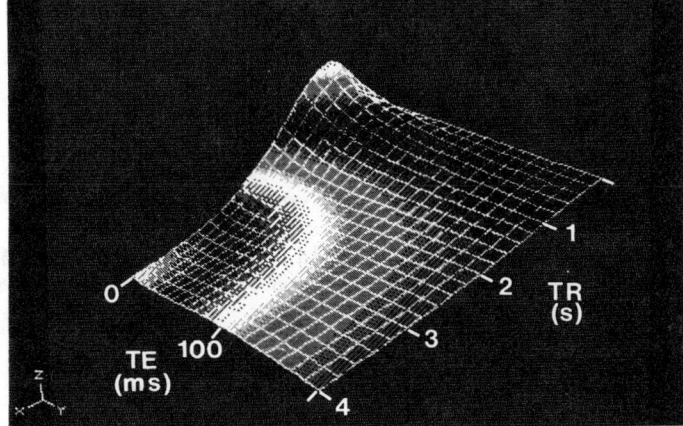

Figure 5
CNR mapped for gray and white matter, computed on the basis of the tissue parameters listed in Table II. The CNR surface was computed by assuming constant number of excitations. Note maxima at short TR, TE and long TR.

Table II Relaxation (T_1,T_2) and spin density $N(H)$ parameters used for the calculation of the CNR map in <u>Figure 5</u>[15].

	GM	WM
T_1(ms)	870	650
T_2(ms)	74	68
$N(H)$	0.93*)	0.84*)

*) relative to CSF

The CNR map for gray and white matter has two maxima, one at short TR and TE and one at long TR. In the former, contrast is caused by differentials in T_1 ($T_1^{WM} < T_1^{GM}$) whereas at long TR differences in spin density ($N^{WM} < N^{GM}$) prevail as a mechanism. However, since $T_2^{WM} \sim T_2^{GM}$, T_2 is not a mechanism of significance in this case.

Another RF pulse sequence, sketched out in **Figure 3c**, begins with a 180° inversion pulse, creating nonequilibrium magnetization which is detected TI milliseconds later by a 90° detection pulse, followed by the usual phase reversal pulse which generates an echo at time t = TI + TE.

The relaxation and pulse timing parameter dependence for the inversion-recovery spin echo signal (IRSE) is given as[14]

$$S(TI) \sim (1 - 2e^{-TI/T_1} + 2e^{-(TR-TE/2)/T_1} - e^{-TR/T_1}) e^{-TE/T_2} \quad (13)$$

If TE $\ll T_2$, TR, Equation (13) simplifies to

$$S(TI) \sim (1 - 2e^{-TI/T_1} + e^{-TR/T_1}) \quad (13a)$$

hence the TE and T_2 dependence both vanish. Peculiar to the IR sequence is that both positive and negative values are possible for the signal. If

$$0 < TI < T_1 \{ \ln 2 - \ln (1 + e^{-TR/T_1}) \} \quad (14)$$

the 90° detection pulse occurs before the longitudinal magnetization has reverted to positive values, hence creating "negative" magnetization, that is a signal that is phase-shifted 180°. Typically, however, the magnitude of the signal is displayed and sign information is discarded. The resulting CNR loss[16] occurring for the TI range encompassed by the signal zeroes for tissue A and B is evident from **Figure 6** in which SNR and CNR were computed from the tissue parameters in Table II.

FIELD DEPENDENCE OF SNR AND CNR

The field dependence of SNR and CNR has been thoroughly investigated by Hart et al[3]. It is obvious from Equation (4) that in the high-frequency approximation where $R_p \gg R_c$, SNR scales linearly with frequency. This behavior has been verified experimentally by Edelstein et al[17].

There are two complicating circumstances, however. The first is the field dependence of T_1[18] and the second the possible requirement of increased field gradient amplitudes at higher magnetic field to overcome magnetic field homogeneity and chemical shift, both scaling linearly with field strength.

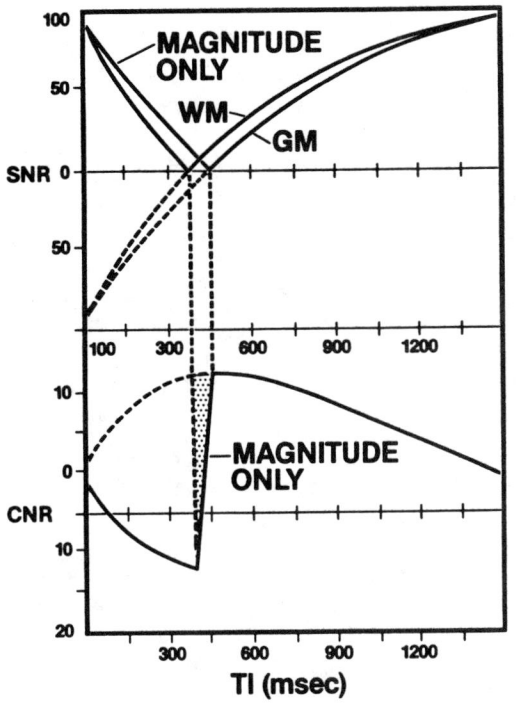

Figure 6
a) SNR for gray and white matter, calculated for an inversion recovery sequence assuming TR = 1.5 seconds and using the parameters in Table II. Dotted line shows portion of signal that is negative but is not detected as such in an amplitude display.
b) Corresponding CNR curve calculated as the difference SNR(WM)-SNR(GM). Shaded area indicates region of diminished contrast resulting from amplitude display.

In a recent survey of literature data[18] it was demonstrated that tissue relaxation data can be fitted to the empirical relationship

$$T_1 = A \cdot \nu^B \qquad (15)$$

where A and B are tissue dependent constants. T_2, by contrast, appears to be nearly independent of magnetic field strength. According to the above, the mean T_1 of muscle, for example, increases from 547 to 867 milliseconds between 0.5 and 1.5T and that for adipose tissue from 214 to 259 milliseconds. T_1^{muscle}/T_1^{fat} therefore increases from 2.56 to 3.34. Likewise we find the ratio $T_1^{muscle}/T_2^{kidney}$ to increase from 1.10 to 1.33 as field strength is increased from 0.5T to 1.5T. Table III lists the gain in CNR for various tissue interfaces between 0.5T and 1.5T assuming a linear increase of intrinsic SNR with field strength. Note that the contention of CNR loss due to the alleged convergence of T_1 at higher field cannot be upheld. However, the actual gain in CNR is, of course, highly dependent on the frequency dependence of T_1 for the tissue pair considered and the ratio of pulse repetition time to T_1 (TR/T_1).

Table III Field dependence of contrast-to-noise for various tissue interfaces

Tissue Interface	0.5T $T_1{}^a/T_1{}^b*$	C/N**	1.5T $T_1{}^a/T_1{}^b*$	C/N**
a b				
Gray Matter/White Matter	1.21	100	1.17	188
Muscle/Adipose	2.25	366	3.34	1507
Kidney/Adipose	2.56	323	2.51	1153
Kidney/Liver	1.53	182	1.32	369
Muscle/Kidney	1.10	43	1.33	354

*   From Ref. 18
**   Spin echo, TR = 1.0 s; assuming a linear increase in intrinsic S/N between 0.5T and 1.5T; normalized to gray matter/white matter contrast.

Figure 7 shows the frequency dependence of SNR and CNR for various tissues and pairs of tissues, respectively, calculated from the data in Reference 18.

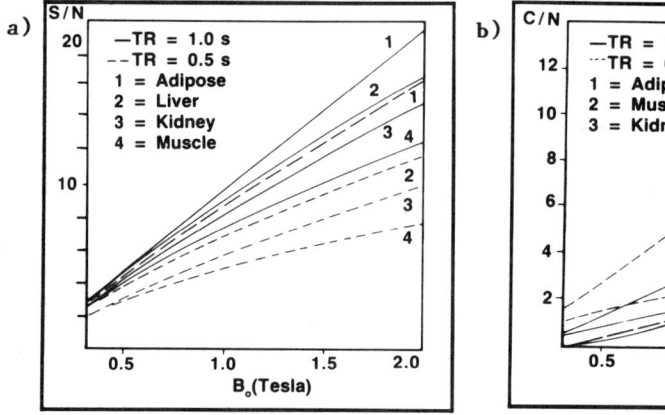
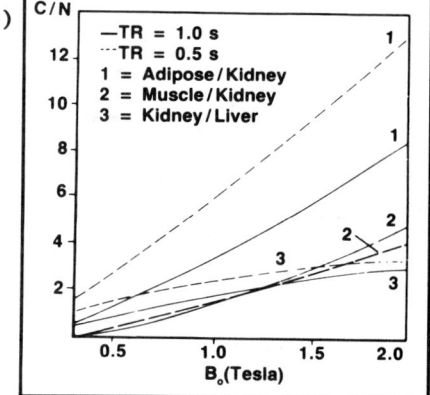

Figure 7 a, b
a) SNR dependence on field strength for skeletal muscle, liver, kidney and adipose tissue, for pulse repetition times of 1.0 s (solid lines), and 0.5 s (dotted lines), assuming a linear increase in SNR and using the empirical relationships for the field dependence of T_1, described in reference 18. b) Magnetic field dependence of CNR for the adipose/kidney, muscle/kidney and kidney/liver tissue interfaces, calculated under the assumptions given in the caption of Figure 7a.

It has been argued that in order to alleviate the fat/water chemical shift artifact[19], larger gradient amplitudes are required as the static magnetic field strength is increased. The chemical shift between water and CH_2 protons is approximately 3.5 ppm which translates into a corresponding pixel shift in readout gradient direction. At a field strength of 0.5T, assuming for example G_x = 0.2G/cm, FOV = 25 cm and N_x = 256, fat and water are shifted approximately 0.8 pixels relative to one another. At 1.5T this shift is 2.5 pixels unless gradient strength is raised by a factor of 3, in which case the pixel shift is the same as at 0.5T. It should be noted, however, that fat/water boundaries are relatively few (examples: peri-renal and retro-orbital fat) but are absent, for example, in the brain which does not contain lipid constituents. Moreover, there is no consensus among radiologists as to whether or not the chemical shift effect impairs image interpretability. For the probably exceptional cases where the effect is disturbing, methods exist for correction by creating component images[20] and exactly superimposing these to obtain an artifact-free composite image.

Another potential motivation for increasing gradient amplitudes as field strength is raised may be to overcome field inhomogeneity (unless the absolute homogeneity ΔB is maintained). Much effort therefore has been expended more recently to improve magnet field homogeneity, primarily through improved shimming technology. A relative homogeneity of $\Delta B/B_o \ll 1 \times 10^{-5}$ across the entire imaging volume can now be achieved routinely in large-bore magnets by means of computerized shimming techniques. Should, however, gradient strength be raised in proportion to field strength, this would result in a concomitant increase in receive bandwidth (Equation (2)), in which case only a $\sqrt{\nu}$ SNR gain would be realizable as the field strength is raised.

ACKNOWLEDGMENTS

The author is indebted to Ann Shimakawa, B.S.E.E. and Robert Breger, M.D. for aiding in data collection and analysis and Sue Hallchurch for preparing the manuscript.

REFERENCES

1. Edelstein WA, Society of Magnetic Resonance in Medicine, Third Annual Meeting, August 13-17, 1984, New York, Abstract p. 202.

2. Hoult DI, Lauterbur PC, J Magn Res 34, 425(1979).

3. Hart HR, Jr, Bottomley PA, Edelstein WA, et al, AJR 141, 1195 (1983).

4. Axel L, J Comput Assist Tomogr 8, 381 (1984).

5. Schenck JR, Foster TH, Henkes JL, et al, AJNR 6, 181 (1985).

6. Hayes C, Axel L, Med Phys 1985, in press.

7. Hayes C, Edelstein WA, Schenck JR, Proceedings of the American Association of Physicists in Medicine "NMR in Medicine: The Instrumentation and Clinical Applications," 1985.

8. Bottomley PA, Rev. Sci Instr 53, 1319 (1982).

9. Edelstein WA, Bottomley PA, Hart HR, Jr, Smith LS, J Comput Assist Tomogr 7, 391 (1983).

10. Wehrli FW, MacFall JR, Newton TH, Modern Neuroradiology, Volume II, Advanced Imaging Techniques, Eds. Newton TH, Potts DG, Clavadel Press, San Anselmo, CA, 1983.

11. MacFall JR, private communication.

12. Wehrli FW, Breger RK, MacFall JR, et al, Quantification of Contrast in Clinical MR Brain Imaging at High Magnetic Field. Invest Radiol 1985, in press.

13. Mitchell MR, Conturo TE, Gruber TJ, Jones JP, Investigative Radiology 19, 350 (1984).

14. Wehrli FW, MacFall JR, Shutts D, Breger RK, Herfkens RJ, J Comput Assist Tomogr 8, 369 (1984).

15. Perkins T, Wehrli FW, unpublished data

16. Hendrick RE, Nelson TR, Hendee WR, Mag Res Imaging 2, 279 (1984).

17. Edelstein WA, private communication.

18. Bottomley PA, Foster TH, Argersinger RE, Pfeifer LM, Med Phys 11, 425 (1984).

19. Babcock EE, Brateman L, Weinreb JC, et al, J Comput Assist Tomogr 9, 252 (1985).

20. Dixon WT, Radiology 153, 189 (1984).

MAGNETIC RESONANCE IMAGING OF THE BRAIN AND SPINE
CLINICAL CONSIDERATIONS

Michael T. Modic, M.D.
University Hospitals, Cleveland, Ohio 44106

ABSTRACT

This paper includes a review of the technical and clinical aspects related to proton imaging of the brain and spine. The paper outlines briefly some technical considerations of imaging as they relate to the daily clinical imaging process.

INTRODUCTION

To become a usable, effective diagnostic procedure in light of today's reimbursement policies, a new imaging modality must prove to be as accurate and cost effective in the detection of disease as routine clinical exams. As experience with MR of the brain and spine grows, it has become clear the MR is superior to conventional modalities in many situations, equivalent in some and inferior in others. The technical factors and clinical situations which determine whether MR is the appropriate test are varied and will be the basis of this review paper.

I. Technical Considerations

One of the most important considerations in clinical MR is to select the techniques that can demonstrate abnormalities in the most effective fashion. This is difficult in light of the complexities of MR and the pragmatic aspects of daily clinical imaging. Theoretical considerations are important initially for technique optimization for specific diseases but require modifications when employed to investigate an area of anatomy to cover a potential spectrum of disease states.

The major advantage of MR at this time in clinical imaging is its superior contrast sensitivity. Efforts to maximize contrast differentiation must take into consideration the influence of signal-to-noise and the spatial resolution. Clinical considerations such as subject contrast between abnormal and normal tissue and various disease processes are equally important.

In routine imaging the most common practice to improve the signal-to-noise ratio is to increase the number of averages. This, however, increases the examination time and the likelihood of patient motion. Because the ratio of signal-to-noise increases with the square root of the number of averages, the largest gain in the signal-to-noise occurs with the first few averages. Practically, more than 2 to 4 averages is rarely worth the increase in exam time because further proportionate improvement would require an exponential increase in the examination time.

Another method to improve the signal-to-noise is related to the choice of RF coils. The utilization of the head coil, body coil or various surface coils will depend on the clinical setting. Factors such as the field of view, spatial resolution needed, and patient habitus tolerance will be important.

Further improvements in the signal-to-noise can be achieved with increasing field strengths. The improvement, however, is offset to a greater or lesser degree by increases in the T1 relaxation time, RF attenuation, and chemical shift artifacts, and increases costs and difficulty with siting.

The use and overall advantages of these modifications to improve signal-to-noise will depend to a large extent on the clinical setting and will be discussed further under individual areas.

Spatial resolution is primarily controlled by voxel size and is intimately related to contrast by its relationship to signal-to-noise. The choice of voxel size will depend on the clinical setting and the overall signal. For instance, most brain pathology can be studied with a 256 x 128 matrix because contrast resolution is more important than spatial resolution. Also, improving the spatial resolution, by increasing the steps in the phase encoded direction, will increase the examination time without increasing most lesions' detectability. High resolution imaging in certain areas is mandatory such as in the orbit, sella or temporal bones, and there the increased examination time becomes a more reasonable tradeoff. The signal intensities observed and the signal-to-noise ratios will also be related to the operator selectable parameters such as TE and TR and the strength of the signal. The intrinsic characteristics of the equipment and how these images are obtained, e.g. single slice, multislice, multiecho, etc., will also interact with the overall quality of the image.

Clinical factors which require consideration include the intrinsic tissue parameters, patient tolerance, motion and in some situations, patient size. These in turn are closely related to the aforementioned technical factors. For instance, the T1 relaxation time will be affected by field strength, and the T2 values can be affected by the superimposition of the magnetic field gradients.

At the present time, there is probably no one correct way to perform a magnetic resonance study, but in fact there are probably multiple "good" ways from which to choose. Efforts to prospectively select the type of equipment and imaging parameters that will most effectively visualize an abnormality based on tissue parameters and formulated from mathematical models can be useful for suggesting a possible approach but are not often used in routine clinical practice. The major reason for this is because the nature of lesions under investigation are usually not known before the imaging study, and multiple entities are usually included in the differential diagnosis. Because of this, most clinical examinations at the present time are examples of "bet hedging." Because it is important to visualize normal anatomy and have the versatility to visualize a variety of abnormalities on a signal study, multiple acquisitions with changes in TE, TR and different RF coils are usually employed so that the widest number of abnormalities can be identified. This is also done in a way which would minimize exam time and improve patient tolerance.

What follows is a review of the clinical uses of MR in the brain and spine with an emphasis on technical modifications for disease identification.

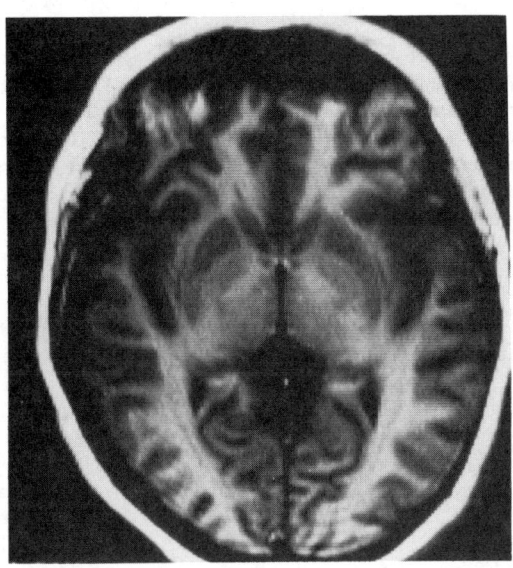

Figure 1a. Axial inversion recovery image through the level of the basal ganglia. Note the white and gray matter differentiation. In practice, short TE/TR images are usually employed for T1 contrast because of a shorter imaging time and while the contrast is not as obvious, it is adequate for most clinical imaging situations.

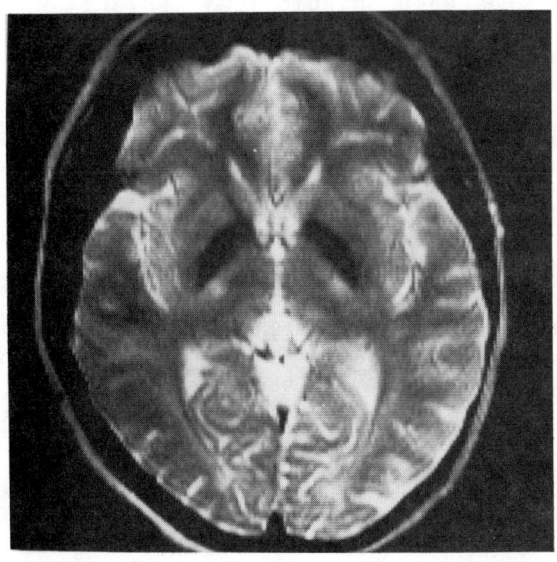

Figure 1b. Axial 120 msec TE/2 sec TR spin echo image through the level of the basal ganglia. The CSF now has a relatively higher signal intensity than the surrounding brain parenchyma. The gray white contrast is not as good as with T1 weighted images, but this technique is more sensitive to pathological processes involving the brain and this type of technique is used in most clinical situations as the initial screening sequence.

II. Clinical Imaging

To date, most brain imaging employs at least 2 spin echo sequences (Figure 1). These usually include a long TE (60-120 msec)/long TR (1.5 sec or greater) and a short TE (30 msec or less)/short TR (.5 sec or less) images. The longer TE/TR images offer superior sensitivity in most disease states when compared with conventional CT. The reason for this is most likely related to the fact that most pathological processes involving the brain result in prolongations of both the T1 and T2 relaxation times. Clinically this combination of changes can usually be identified with the best conspicuity by a process which emphasizes differences based on T2 relaxation or coherent resonance properties of the sample, and the tissues with longer T2 values will be seen as relatively high intensity regions (1,2).

Shorter TE/TR images provide excellent anatomic delineation and may be useful for characterization of lesions but lack the sensitivity for the detection of disease which is present with the longer TE/TR images. Inversion recovery images were originally the most frequently used pulse sequence. In part, this was because the original images were performed on normal volunteers and inversion recovery images provided excellent differentiation between white and gray matter would provide the best sensitivity to disease. This, however, has not proven to be true in most cases. T1 weighted images remain important for characterization, but a spin echo sequence with a short TE/TR will usually suffice for this and can be obtained in a shorter period of time.

As mentioned previously, signal-to-noise ratios increase in a linear fashion with increasing field strengths from .15 Tesla to 1.5 Tesla. At the same time, the differences in signal intensity between tissues with different T1s and T2s such as gray and white matter may decrease with increasing field strengths above approximately .5 Tesla. This could potentially result in a decrease in the difference in signal intensities between pathological lesions and surrounding normal tissues with increasing field strengths (3-6).

In routine clinical imaging (up to 1.5 Tesla), this does not appear to be a problem. This most likely is because the contrast-to-noise ratio increase, with increasing field strengths up to at least 1.5 Tesla, allows smaller signal intensity differences to be more apparent resulting in greater conspicuity of lesions. In practical terms, although the image may be more aesthetically pleasing to the eye at 1.5 Tesla, it has been our experience that there is no significant difference in lesion detection based on contrast differentiation when comparing .6 to 1.5 Tesla.

The major advantage at the present time with imaging at 1.5 Tesla as compared to lower field strengths, is that fewer averages and thinner slices can be employed without significant degradation of the image. Similar improvements, however, have also been noted with machine and coil optimization at lower field strengths.

Brain Tumors

MR has proven to be a sensitive imaging modality for neoplasms involving the central nervous system. Multiple reports have documented its accuracy as compared to computed tomography (1, 7-10). The major advantages of MR over CT at the present time are related to superior tissue contrast, reduction of bony artifacts and the ability to directly image in any plane. The disadvantages are primarily related to the acquisition time, patient motion and detection of calcium. Depending upon the pulse sequence selected, the data accumulation time with MR usually varies between 3 and 9 minutes. Between 10 and 15 sections can be accumulated during this time. Most clinical studies require at least 2 acquisitions. With CT, each section is usually obtained with a data accumulation time between 2 and 8 seconds and can be performed with an uncooperative patient more successfully.

MR has been criticized for its inability to differentiate tumor from edema and its apparent lack of specificity in distinguishing between various pathological lesions. These criticisms arise out of a comparison with CT. In a CT examination, the brain can be examined with and without contrast material so that breakdowns of the blood brain barrier can be identified as enhancement surrounding lesions. Similarly, these changes can be used to establish anatomic recognition patterns for disease states. It must be remembered that CT studies with contrast are not entirely accurate in delineating tumor margins and that with an enlarging data base in MR, similar anatomic recognition patterns should emerge.

MR appears to be as sensitive as CT for detecting supratentorial lesions secondary to either primary or metastatic disease. In some studies, MR provided a greater sensitivity (7). The superior contrast resolution of MR provides excellent differentiation of normal gray matter, white matter and CSF allowing minimal distortions of normal brain architecture to be identified.

With MR, the posterior fossa is free of bony artifacts because cortical bone does not give a detectable MR signal. An indication of the better contrast resolution of MR in the posterior fossa is that the white and gray matter of the cerebellum can be regularly visualized with MR, where it is rarely visible with CT. This lack of artifact coupled with excellent contrast resolution allows one to demonstrate the normal anatomy of the brainstem and other posterior fossa structures in any plane. MR has a sensitivity for pathological lesions in the posterior fossa equivalent to that in the supratentorial region but is clearly superior to CT for almost all disease processes because of the lack of bony artifacts (11-15).

Meningiomas may represent an exception to the rule that MR has superior sensitivity to the detection of brain neoplasms. In a recent report, meningiomas demonstrated poor contrast between the tumor and the adjacent brain on multiple pulse sequences and appeared to be better appreciated on CT (16).

Cystic lesions are usually easily identified and their contents differentiated from CSF (Figure 2). Lipid containing tumors show characteristic signal intensities. MR also appears to have advantages in the preoperative planning because of the ability to visualize the abnormality in multiple planes. Postoperatively, MR may also be more effective than CT in situations where streak artifacts related to surgical clips degrade the CT image.

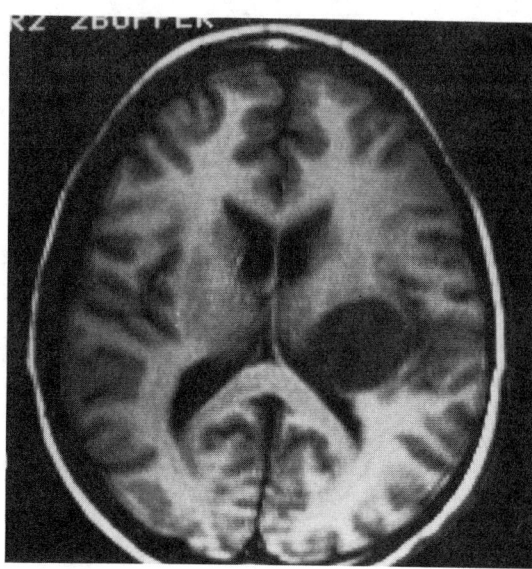

Figure 2. Cystic glioma of the brain.
Figure 2a. Axial inversion recovery image which demonstrates a large ovoid mass in the posterior aspect of the basal ganglia. Note the medial aspect of this mass has a decreased signal intensity when compared with the lateral aspect.

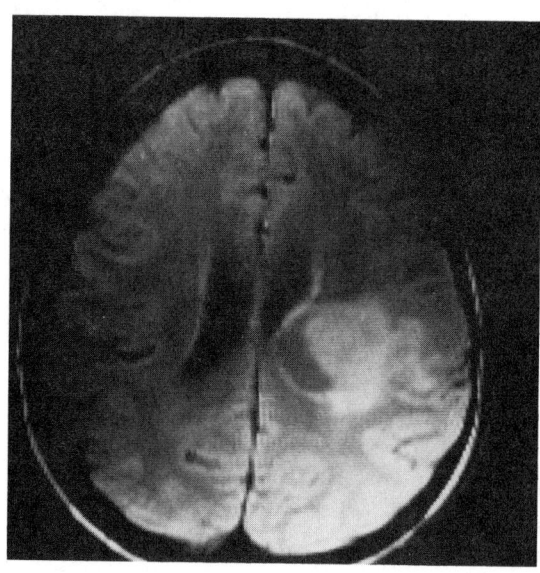

Figure 2b. Axial 30 msec TE/2 sec TR weighted image. Note now a more marked distinction between the medial and lateral aspect of this mass. The signal intensity of the medial aspect is slightly greater than that of the CSF and the adjacent ventricles but less than that of the majority of the mass. This most likely represents a cystic component.

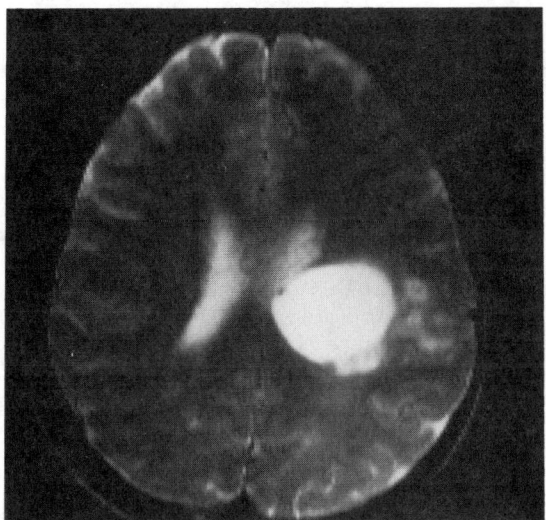

Figure 2c. Axial 120 msec TE/2 sec TR image through the same region. Note now that the entire mass has a marked increased signal intensity, but the medial portion now has a slightly greater signal intensity than the lateral aspect.

These three sequences are used for most clinical situations to characterize lesions. The inversion recovery or short TE/TR image provides T1 weighting and characterization. 30 msec TE/2 sec TR and 120 msec TE/2 sec TR provide a mixed and heavily T2 weighted image respectively.

The ultimate spatial resolution of MR with increasing field strength is yet to be determined. This will be critical for the evaluation of small tumors such as pituitary adenomas and acoustic neuromas. Spatial resolution is determined in part by matrix size and section thickness. Most CT scanners have a matrix of 512 x 512 and in some, a 1024 x 1024 matrix can be interpolated with slice thicknesses as small as 1.5 to 2 mm. At the present time, the volume elements of CT are smaller than those of MR and the spatial resolution is superior. Where a combination of contrast and spatial resolution is critical, the use of MR will depend on the clinical setting. With the currently available 4 mm slices utilizing 2-D imaging with MR, the pituitary fossa and adjacent regions are well seen on the coronal, sagittal and transverse plane, but until proven otherwise, it must be assumed that the spatial resolution of CT remains superior for the evaluation of small lesions despite the potential contrast sensitivity superiority of MR. Selective volume imaging may prove to be a way around this problem, but requires longer imaging times and is more prone to degradation by motion artifacts.

Promising results have been obtained in the evaluation of acoustic neuromas (14) and preliminary work with surface coil imaging suggests that MR may be at least equivalent to CT in the evaluation of the orbit (17).

Non-Neoplastic Abnormalities

<u>Infarct and Hemorrhage</u>. Cerebral ischemia produces early changes in the water content of tissue, changes which become more profound with the evolution of the infarction. It is these changes which appear to be detected by MR. Several animal studies have identified signal intensity changes primarily related to prolongation of the T2 relaxation time as early as 2 to 3 hours after ischemic insult. Infarctions of the brainstem and cerebellum are more clearly identified because of the absence of artifacts from the temporal bones that occur with CT.

Ischemic changes in the white matter are visualized more frequently with MR than on CT. Larger ischemic changes involving both gray and white matter are usually equally well identified. One problem with MR to date has been that small cortical gray matter infarcts may be better appreciated on a contrast enhanced CT than with MR.

Acute parenchymal bleed (less than 24 hours) may be more difficult to identify with MR than with CT. The presence of fresh blood is readily appreciated on CT. On MR images, an acute hemorrhage demonstrates an increased signal intensity on T2 weighted images and on T1 weighted images may have either a decreased signal intensity or be isointense with adjacent brain parenchyma. Because of this it may be difficult to separate an acute bleed from a non-hemorrhagic infarct. This differentiation may be critical if the use of anticoagulation is planned. In the subacute phase, MR can clearly differentiate a hemorrhagic from a non-hemorrhagic infarct because of its characteristically shortened T1 relaxation time (Figure 3). Similar problems in the identification of acute

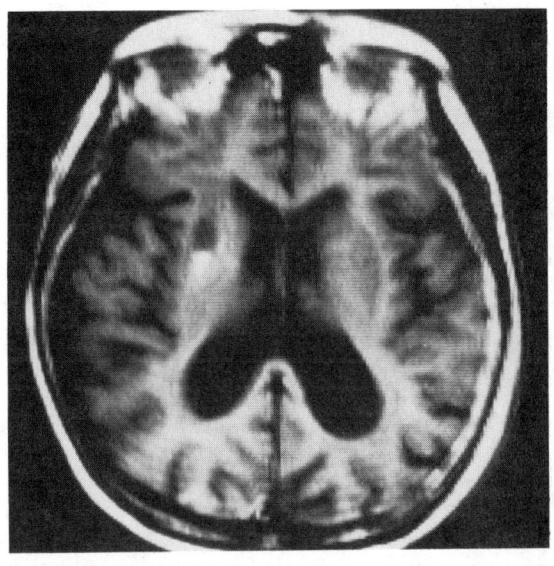

Figure 3. Hemorrhagic infarct.

Figure 3a. Axial inversion recovery image through the region of the basal ganglia. Note the area of mixed signal intensity in the right basal ganglia. The anterior portion has a decreased signal intensity and the posterior portion has an increased signal intensity when compared to adjacent brain parenchyma. There is a straight interface between the two suggesting a fluid interface. The increased signal intensity in the posterior aspect on a T1 weighted image suggests the presence of subacute blood.

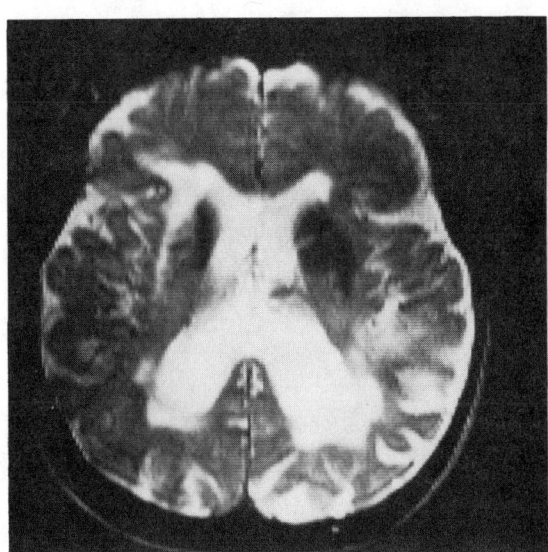

Figure 3b. Axial 120 msec TE/2 sec TR through the same region. One notes on this image an increased signal intensity throughout the entire lesion as well as abnormally increased areas of signal intensity in a paraventricular location bilaterally. The T2 weighted image itself although sensitive is inadequate for differentiating between a bland and hemorrhagic infarct as they both exhibit a prolonged T2 relaxation and an increased signal. T1 weighted images are more useful for characterizing hemorrhagic vs. bland infarcts because of the increased signal intensity on T1 weighted images noted in most subacute bleeds.

subarachnoid hemorrhage may also exist and would leave CT as the modality of choice.

In the acute phase, MR of a non-hemorrhagic acute stroke may prove to be more sensitive when the changes of edema are not sufficient to decrease x-ray attenuation on CT, but nevertheless alter the relaxation values so that the MR signal intensities are changed.

Subdural hematomas are more clearly visualized with MR than with CT because of the lack of artifacts and an isodense stage. Coronal imaging clearly delineates the size and nature of the extra-cerebral fluid collection and is very useful for surgical planning (19, 20).

One of the difficulties in the evaluation of cerebral vascular disease is that MR appears to be so sensitive to parenchymal changes. Patients with multiple infarct dementia routinely show focci of abnormal signal intensity not visualized on CT. Patients with risk factors for cerebral vascular disease often show abnormal paraventricular signal intensities which are difficult to relate to their clinical symptomatology, and multiple areas of abnormal signal intensities are seen in a high percentage of asymptomatic patients over the age of 65.

Demyelinating Disease

Although multiple sclerosis and other demyelinating disease can be identified with CT, it is usually recognized in patients in whom the diagnosis is strongly suspected on the basis of clinical features. With MR, abnormal signal intensities presumed to be MS plaques are visualized in patients with much less severe symptomatology (Figure 4). MR is often positive in the presence of a normal CT scan and will often visualize more plaques in a patient where the CT scan is positive in only one place (21, 22).

The relationship of demyelinating disease in the elderly population to the presence of abnormal signal intensities in the paraventricular area is unclear at this point and requires further study.

Congenital Abnormalities

Magnetic resonance is extremely useful in the evaluation of congenital abnormalities of the brain primarily because of its multi-dimensional imaging capability. Direct scanning in the sagittal plane clearly delineates the relationship of the suprasella region, midline structures and foramen magnum. These areas are critical in the evaluation of congenital abnormalities and are better appreciated than on CT.

The lack of artifacts coupled with excellent contrast resolution allows one to demonstrate the normal anatomy of the brainstem and other posterior fossa structures in any plane. MR is more accurate than CT in the evaluation of chiari malformations and in determining that the tonsilla herniation is not secondary to a mass lesion.

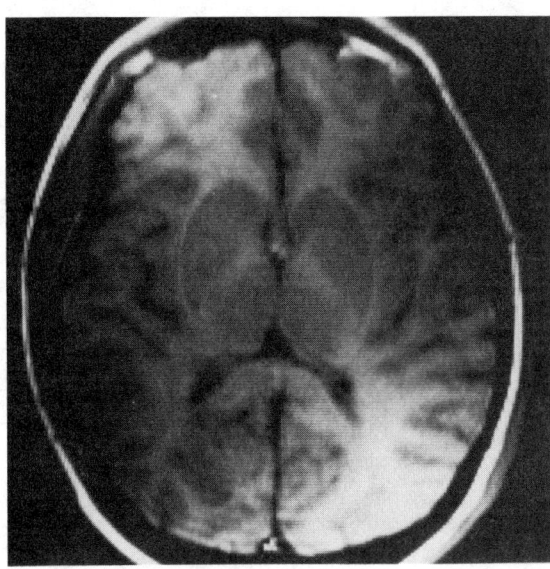

Figure 4. Multiple sclerosis.
Figure 4a. 30 msec TE/.5 sec TR axial image through the region of the basal ganglia and occipital lobes. There is a vague ill-defined area of decreased attenuation in the right occipital lobe.

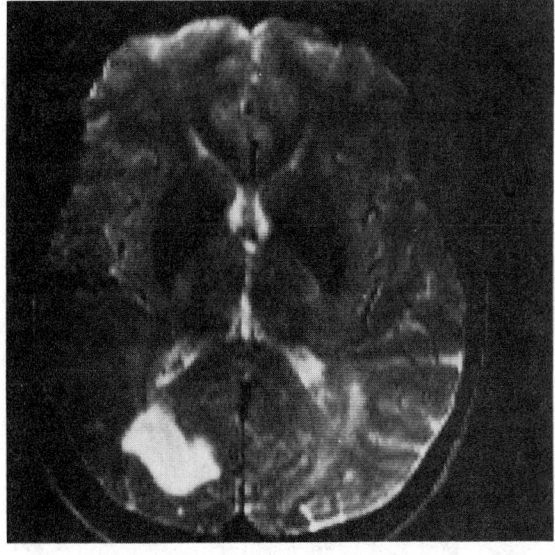

Figure 4b. 120 msec TE/2 sec TR image through the same level. On this sequence there is an obvious area of abnormality characterized by an increased signal intensity consistent with a multiple sclerosis plaque. The T2 weighted images are usually the most sensitive for the identification of demyelineating disease.

Cranial Vertebral Junction

The anterior aspects of the foramen magnum are well delineated; however, the posterior margin is less constant in appearance because of the variable amount of cortical bone present. Abnormalities of the cranial vertebral junction and congenital disorders involving the posterior fossa are better appreciated with MR than CT primarily because of the multi-dimensional imaging aspects. Abnormalities of the odontoid tip such as basal invagination and rheumatoid arthritis can be readily appreciated; however, more subtle changes may be difficult to identify because of the variable normal appearance of the structure. Plain films and CT scans may be needed for more precise definition of bony abnormalities in the region of the foramen magnum (23-24).

Syringomyelia

MR appears to be the most accurate and sensitive modality for the evaluation of syringomyelia. In most cases, a T1 weighted image can clearly identify cystic areas as sharply demarcated from the cord, and with a combination of transverse and sagittal images, its position within the cord as well as its cranial and caudal extent (Figure 5). The presence or absence of concomitant abnormalities such as chiari malformations and tumor can be determined. In the latter case, however, it may be difficult to differentiate a cystic tumor from a syrinx or small tumor causing a syrinx. Previous investigators have reported that eccentrically located cysts could be obscured by partial volume averaging. Additionally, false negative MR diagnoses are possible in syringomyelia if the cyst fluid does not have the characteristic long T1 and T2 of cerebral spinal fluid. It has been our experience that thinner sections obtained with surface coil imaging obviate the difficulty with partial volume averaging. In addition, these effects are less apparent in the axial plane. Others have demonstrated that the prolonged T1 and T2 times are not specific for syringomyelia (25-26). One case of myelomalacia was characterized by an intramedullary region of decreased signal intensity similar to cerebral spinal fluid. As experience with MR increases, other intramedullary processes that could produce a potentially false positive diagnosis of syringomyelia may be found. Despite these disadvantages, MR is the imaging modality of choice for the initial screening and follow-up of patients with syringomyelia.

Spine

The potential of magnetic resonance in the evaluation of spinal abnormalities has been well documented (27-33). In order to appreciate its role, however, a basic understanding of the importance of the pulse sequence parameters in optimizing the examination is necessary.

Previous work with MR has pointed out the importance of both T1 and T2 weighted images in the evaluation of the spinal axis (34). On the basis of in-vivo studies to optimize relative signal contrast

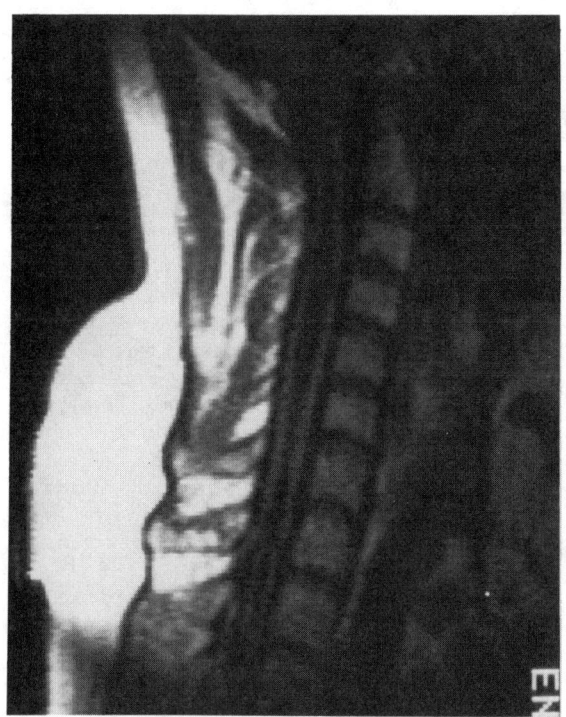

Figure 5. Syringomyelia of the cervical cord. Sagittal 30 msec TE/.5 sec TR 4 mm thick surface coil image through the cervical cord. Note the cystic area of decreased signal intensity within the cervical cord indicative of a syrinx cavity. T1 weighted images provide the most accurate depiction of syrinx cavitites secondary to the signal contrast differentiation of fluid and neural structures.

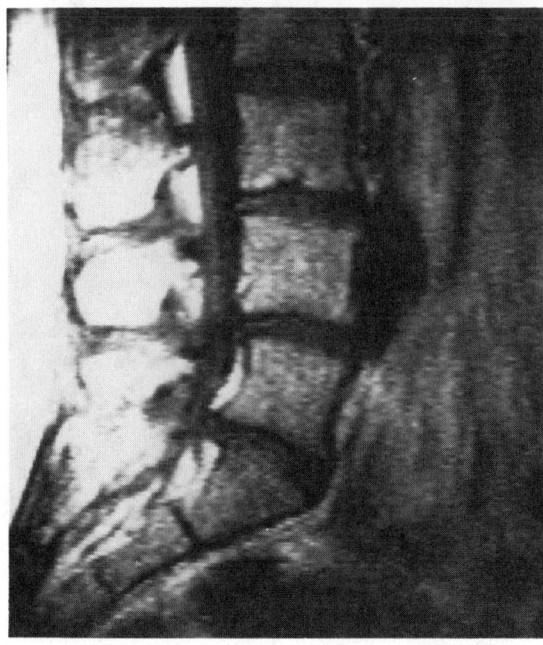

Figure 6. Herniated L5 disc. Figure 6a. Sagittal 4 mm thick 30 msec TE/.5 sec TR sagittal image through the lumbar spine. Note the protrusion of the L5 disc posteriorly.

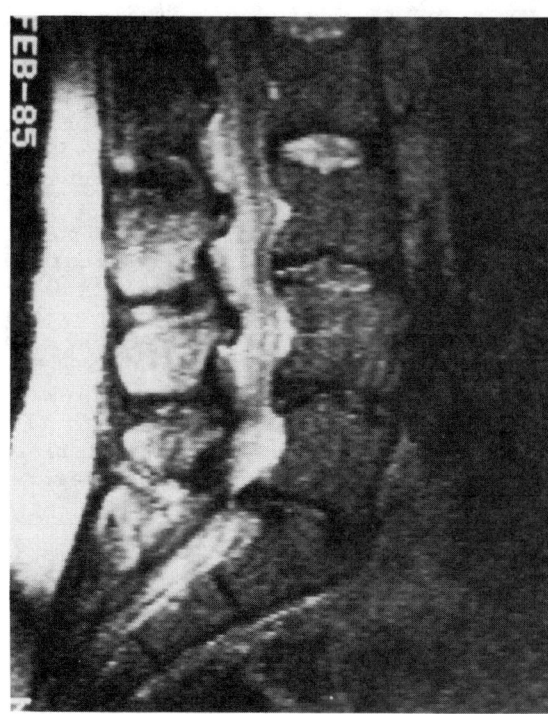

Figure 6b. 120 msec TE/2 sec TR 4 mm surface coil image through the lumbar spine. Note the decreased signal intensity of the 4th and 5th lumbar discs when compared to the 1st, 2nd, and 3rd. This decreased signal intensity is identified in degenerated discs when compared to the normal. The protrusion of the L5 disc is better appreciated by the contrast difference between the surrounding CSF and the decreased signal of the herniated disc fragment. This T2 weighted sequence produces a relative increase in the signal intensity of the CSF from the extravertebral structures.

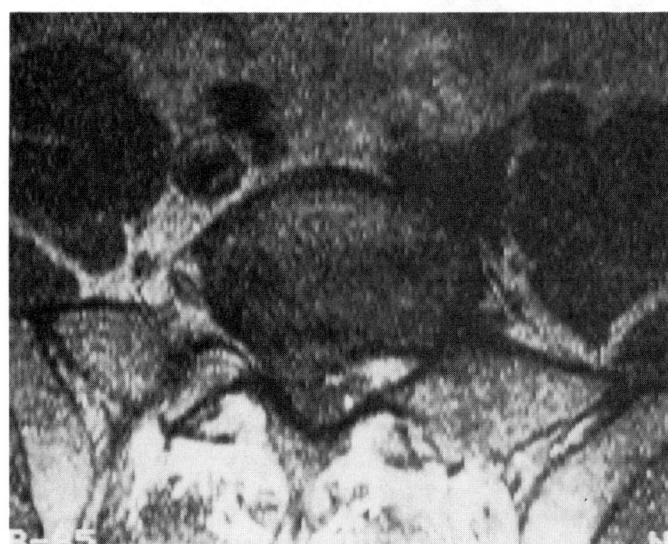

Figure 6c. 30 msec TE/2 sec TR axial 4 mm surface coil image through the L5 disc. Note the right posterolateral herniation of the disc.

differences, it appears that a combination of two spin-echo techniques provides a diagnostic examination of the spine in the vast majority of cases. First, a short spin-echo sequence (30 msec TE/.3-.5 sec TR) in the sagittal plane provides rapid localization, anatomic detail and some T1 weighting (Figure 6a). Second, a longer spin-echo sequence (60-120 msec TE/2; 3 sec TR) provides T2 and proton density weighting and allows evaluation of disc hydration, the CSF-extradural interface, and the detection of changes from tumor, infection, degeneration, trauma, and surgery (Figure 6b). In the evaluation of degenerative disease, such as herniated disc or canal stenosis, a third pulse sequence (30 msec TE/2 sec TR) in the transverse plane is routinely employed. This provides a high signal study which, when performed with surface coils, provides anatomic information comparable to a high resolution CT (Figure 6c). More intermediate pulse sequences such as 30 msec TE/2 sec TR and 60 msec TE/1 sec TR may have roles in certain circumstances.

In the vertebral bodies, changes secondary to irradiation (35) (i.e. fat replacement of marrow) and certain degenerative processes will demonstrate an increased signal intensity on the T1 weighted images.

Tumors, infection, trauma, avascular necrosis, degenerative disc, and some degenerative end plate changes demonstrate a long T1 and therefore, decreased signal when compared with normal extradural elements (Figure 7a).

Certain abnormalities, such as intradural lesions, herniated discs (depending on the degree of dehydration), infection or tumor may have a signal intensity so similar to the adjacent CSF or extradural elements on a T1 weighted pulse sequence, that they may be difficult to identify or separate. In these situations an intermediate or long TE, TR spin-echo technique is needed. This provides greater T2 weighting and sensitivity to certain disease processes involving the spine.

On the T2 weighted images, the normal nucleus pulposus has a marked increased signal intensity secondary to its hydration and stands out in sharp contrast to the decreased signal from the surrounding annulus and cortical bone. There is a cleft or notch in the nucleus pulposus created by invagination of fibrous tissue similar to the annulus into the nucleus pulposus which is a constant feature of the disc in patients greater than 30 years of age.

An additional advantage to a long TE and TR is that it produces a gray scale inversion of the CSF signal intensity because of its long T1 and T2. This produces a relatively bright image intensity of the CSF in contrast to the extradural elements. In this fashion, encroachment or filling defects in the CSF space can be appreciated in a manner similar to a contrast myelogram. Transverse images with a 30 msec TE/2 sec TR provide accurate depiction of disc herniation and canal stenosis and are useful for evaluation of the neural foramina and to lateralize defects more accurately.

Infection, trauma, most neoplasms, and certain postoperative changes demonstrate a prolonged T2 and therefore, a brighter signal (Figure 7b). The changes of disc degeneration and aging are characterized by loss of water, and therefore, decreased signal on the T2 weighted images (36, 37). Although all degenerated discs are not

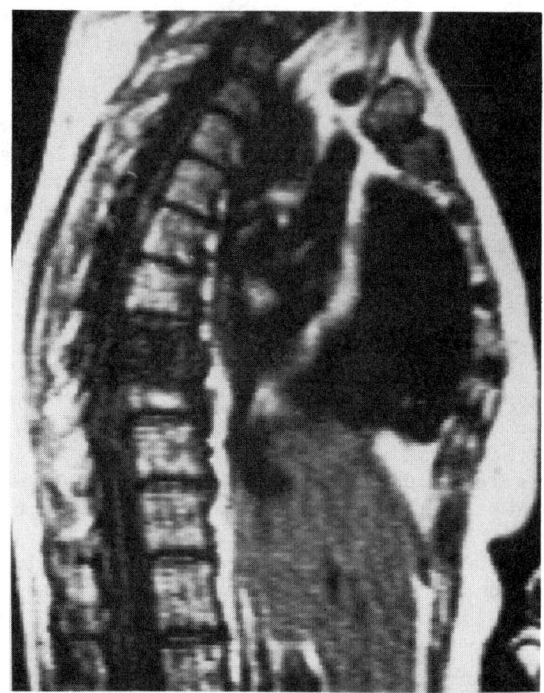

Figure 7. Thoracic vertebral osteomyelitis. Figure 7a. Sagittal midline 30 msec TE/.5 sec TR 10 mm thick body coil image through the thoracic spine. There is a marked decreased signal intensity of 2 adjacent vertebral bodies as well as the intervening disc space.

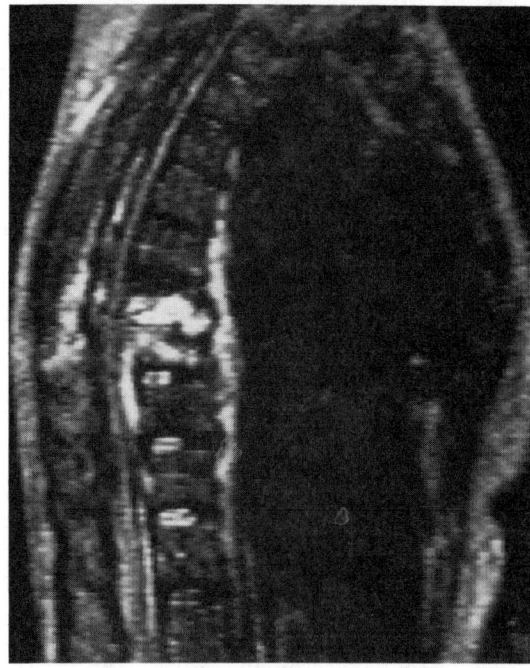

Figure 7b. Sagittal 120 msec TE/2 sec TR 10 mm thick body coil image. Note the marked increased signal intensity of the involved areas of the vertebral bodies on this T2 weighted image. The signal intensity changes in and of themselves are nonspecific and can also be identified with trauma and metastatic disease, but the morphological pattern of involvement, e.g. adjacent vertebral bodies and disc space, is characteristic of osteomyelitis.

herniated, most (if not all) herniated discs are degenerated. MR is more sensitive to the changes of degeneration than any other modality. The impingement of a herniated disc, canal stenosis, fractures, or extradural tumors can be noted.

In addition, in some patients with degenerative disc disease or following chymopapain injection, an increased signal intensity is noted in the medullary bone adjacent to the cortex which cannot be appreciated with pulse sequences with shorter TEs or TRs. These changes may reflect a more active degenerative process.

In certain situations, further pulse sequence changes such as a more intermediated T2 weighted image may be needed to identify a signal change within the cord itself, such as in multiple sclerosis (38). Scans with short TEs and long TRs (i.e. 30 msec TE/2-4 sec TR) can accurately identify the extradural-CSF interface and provide an image with increased signal. The disadvantage is that subtle vertebral body changes may not be as easily appreciated as on images with long TEs. Ideally, a multiecho sequence with both a long and short TE (30-60 msec and 120 msec) with a long TR (2-3 sec) should be obtained. A potential pitfall of the T2 weighted pulse sequences when used alone is the presence of an abnormality within or adjacent to the CSF with an equally bright signal intensity creating the situation where separation is difficult. This further emphasizes the importance of obtaining both T1 and T2 weighted images for full evaluation.

At the present time, using conventional body coil imaging, MR appears to be the superior modality for the evaluation of degeneration of the intervertebral disc and the detection of disc space infection. It appears to be superior to CT without contrast and equivalent to CT with contrast and myelography for the evaluation of patients with cervical myelopathy, tumors, trauma, postoperative changes, and congenital abnormalities. It has remained inferior to CT for evaluation of small or lateral disc herniations, neural foraminal disease, and canal stenosis and its ability to discriminate cortical bone from soft tissue. Recently, however, the introduction of surface coil technology appears to have obviated these disadvantages. Surface coils produce an improved signal-to-noise ratio over a limited distance allowing the use of thinner slices and smaller pixels with a concomitant improvement in spatial resolution. Preliminary studies indicate that trading off the increased signal-to-noise ratio for improved spatial resolution can provide MR examinations of the spine which are as accurate as myelography or CT.

REFERENCES

1. Brant-Zawadzki M, Norman D, Hans Newton T, et al: Magnetic resonance of the brain: The optimal screening technique. Radiology 1984; 152:71-77.
2. Brant-Zawadzki M, Barkowski HM, Ortendahl DA, et al: NMR in experimental cerebral edema: Value of T1 and T2 calculations. AJNR (In press).
3. Bottomley PA, Hart HR, Edelstein WA, Schenck JF, Smith LS, et al: Anatomy and metabolism of the normal human brain studies by magnetic resonance at 1.5 tesla. Radiology 1984; 150:441-446.
4. Crooks LE, Hoenninger J, Arakawa M, Watts J, McCarten B, et al: High-resolution magnetic resonance imaging. Radiology 1984; 150:163-171.
5. Crooks LE, Mills CM, Davis PL, Brant-Zawadzki M, Hoenninger J, et al: Visualization of cerebral and vascular abnormalities by NMR imaging: The effects of imaging parameters on contrast. Radiology 1984; 144:843-852.
6. Hart HR, Bottomley PA, Edelstein WA, Karr SG, Leue WM, et al: Nuclear magnetic resonance imaging: Contrast-to-noise ratio as a function of strength of magnetic field. AJR 1983; 141:1195-1201.
7. Brant-Zawadzki M, Badami JP, Mills CM, Norman B, Newton TH: Primary intracranial tumor imaging: Comparison of magnetic resonance imaging and CT. Radiology 1984; 150:435-440.
8. Brant-Zawadzki M, Davis PL, Crooks LE, et al: NMR demonstration of cerebral abnormalities: Comparison with CT. AJNR 1983; 4:117-124, AJR 1983; 140:847-854.
9. Bydder GM, Steiner RE, Young IR, et al: Clinical NMR imaging of the brain: 140 cases. AJNR 1982; 3:459-480, AJR 1982; 139:216-236.
10. Weinstein MA, Modic MT, Pavlicek W, Keyser CK: Nuclear magnetic resonance for the examination of brain tumors. Semin Roentgenol 1984; 19:139-147.
11. Bydder GM, Steiner RE, Thomas DJ, Marshall J, Gilderdale DJ, Young IR: Nuclear magnetic resonance imaging of the posterior fossa: 50 cases. Clin Radiol 1983; 20:173-188.
12. Lee BCP, Deck MDF, Kneeland JB, Cahill PT: MR imaging of the craniocervical junction. AJNR 6:2, 209-213, March/April 1985.
13. Lee BCP, Kneeland JB, Walker RW, Posner JB, Cahill PT, Deck MDF: MR imaging of brainstem tumors. AJNR 6:2, 159-163, March/April 1985.
14. New PFJ, Bachow TB, Wismer GL, Rosen BR, Brady TJ: MR imaging of the acoustic nerves and small acoustic neuomas at 0.6 T: Prospective study. AJNR 6:2, 165-170, March/April 1985.
15. Randell CP, Collins AG, Young IR, et al: Nuclear magnetic resonance imaging of posterior fossa tumors. AJNR 1983; 4:1027-1034, AJR 1983; 141:489-496.
16. Zimmerman RD, Fleming CA, Saint-Louis LA, Lee BCP, Manning JJ, Deck MDF: Magnetic resonance imaging of meningiomas. AJNR 6:2, 149-157, March/April 1985.

17. Schenck JF, Foster TH, Henkes JL, et al: High-field surface-coil MR imaging of lacalized anatomy. AJNR 6:2, 181-186, March/April 1985.
18. Spetzler RF, Zabramski JM, Kaufman B, et al: Acute NMR changes during MCA occlusion: A preliminary study in primates. Stroke 1983; 14(2):185-191.
19. Sipponen JT, Sepponen RE, Sivula A: Chronic subdural hematoma: Demonstration by magnetic resonance. Radiology 1984; 150:79-85.
20. Moon KL, Brant-Zawadzki M, Pitts LH, et al: Nuclear magnetic resonance imaging of CT-isodense subdural hematomas. AJNR 1984; 5:319-322.
21. Johnson MA, Li DKB, Bryant DK, et al: Magnetic resonance imaging: Serial observations in multiple sclerosis. AJNR 1984; 5:495-499.
22. Weinstein MA, Modic MTM: Diagnosing non-neoplastic intracranial abnormalities. Use of computed tomography and magnetic resonance imaging. Arch Clin Imaging 1985; 1:94-101.
23. Spinos E, Laster DW, Moody DM, Ball MR, Witcofski RL, Kelley DL: MR evaluation of Chiari I malformations at 0.15T. AJNR 6:2, 203-208, March/April 1985.
24. Lee BCP, Deck MDF, Kneeland JB, Cahill PT: MR imaging of the craniocervical junction. AJNR 6:2, 209-213, March/April 1985.
25. Pojunas K, Williams AL, Daniels DL, Haughton VM: Syringomyelia and hydromyelia: Magnetic resonance evaluation. Radiology 1984; 153:679-683.
26. Lee BCP, Zimmerman RD, Manning JJ, Deck MDF: MR imaging of syringomyelia and hydromyelia. AJNR 6:2, 221-228, March/April 1985.
27. Chafetz NI, Genant HK, Moon KL, Helms CA, Morris JM: Recognition of lumbar disk herniation with NMR. AJR 1983; 1153-1156.
28. Hyman RA, Edwards JH, Vacirca SJ, Stein HL: 0.6 T MR imaging of the cervical spine: Multislice and multiecho techniques. AJNR 6:2, 229-236, March/April 1985.
29. Maravilla KR, Lesh P, Weinreb JC, Selby DK, Mooney V: Magnetic resonance imaging of the lumbar spine with CT correlation. AJNR 6:2, 237-245, March/April 1985.
30. Modic MT, Pavlicek W, Weinstein MA, Starnes D, Duchesneau PM, Boumphrey F, Hardy RW: Nuclear magnetic resonance imaging of the spine. Radiology 1983; 148:757-762.
31. Modic MT, Weinstein MA, Pavlicek W, Boumphrey F, Starnes D, Duchesneau PM: Magnetic resonance imaging of the cervical spine: Technical and clinical observations. AJNR 1983; 141:1129-1136.
32. Moon KL, Genant HK, Helms CA, Chafetz NI, Crooks LE, Kaufman L: Musculoskeletal applications of nuclear magnetic resonance. Radiology 1983; 147:161-171.
33. Norman D, Mills CM, Brant-Zawadzki M, Yeates A, Crooks LE, Kaufman L: Magnetic resonance imaging of the spinal cord and canal: Potentials and limitations. AJR 1983; 141 1147-1152.
34. Modic MT, Pavlicek W, Weinstein MA, et al: Magnetic resonance imaging of intervertebral disc disease. Radiology 1984; 152:103-111.

35. Ramsey RG, Zacharias CE: MR imaging of the spine after radiation therapy: Easily recognizable effects. AJNR 6:2, 247-251, March/April 1985.
36. Lipson SJ, Muir H: Experimental intervertebral disc degeneration: Morphologic and proteoglycan changes over time. Arthritis and Rheumatism 1981; 24:12-21.
37. Lipson SJ, Muir H: 1980 Volve award in basic science. Proteoglycans in experimental intervertebral disc degeneration. Spine 1981; 6:194-210.
38. Maravilla KR, Weinreb JC, Suss R, Nunnally RL: Magnetic resonance demonstration of multiple sclerosis plaques in the cervical cord. AJNR 1984; 5:685-689.

NMR SPECTROSCOPY FOR IN VIVO DETERMINATION OF METABOLISM: AN OVERVIEW

Ray L. Nunnally, Ph.D.
The University of Texas Health Science Center at Dallas
Dallas, Texas 75235

INTRODUCTION

METABOLISM. The ability of living cells and tissues to function properly is directly linked to basic biochemical events. The term metabolism is used to describe the integrated, concerted cellular biochemical processes that support cell and organ functions. Metabolism is the fundamental basis for understanding function and physiology in living systems. Therefore, any method or methods that provide localized metabolic information for clinical diagnostic use would be of significant value. A central issue in the study of most disease states is the correlation between the pathophysiology and the metabolic competence of the region incurring injury or disease. This problem is particularly important for conditions that involve compromised blood flow and oxygenation to an organ or part of an organ having obligatory requirements for these two components. Myocardial infarction and cerebrovascular occlusion (stroke) are two prominent examples. Important elements in the clinical treatment of infarction and stroke are determinations of the location, size, and extent of the injury, and a knowledge of the time course of metabolic impairment and the onset of irreversible damage. Although there are techniques which use x-rays, ultrasound, and radionuclides (nuclear medicine) for determining the size and location of injury, to date there is no clinically proven method of directly and noninvasively assessing the metabolic competence of an injured site. Thus, the noninvasive determination of metabolic function for characterizing the extent of deterioration and for the periodic monitoring of the efficacy of therapies on impaired regions would be extremely useful.

Initial studies of tissue metabolism with phosphorus nuclear magnetic resonance (^{31}P NMR) were reported about 10 years ago[1]. Such studies have now been extended to the measurement of metabolism in human skeletal muscle[2,3] and brain[4]. Human tumors have also been analyzed directly[5]. Should progress in the field of *in vivo* NMR spectroscopy continue at its present rate, it is apparent that the routine clinical use of NMR as a means of evaluating tissue and organ metabolism will occur in the near future.

The most commonly observed nuclide for organ and tissue metabolism is ^{31}P. Enumeration of the most relevant reasons for this is as follows: 1) Virtually all cells derive their free energy from adenosine triphosphate (ATP). This compound is present in most cells at levels which are detectable by ^{31}P NMR. 2) Other key phosphorylated compounds and inorganic phosphate (P_i) are observable by ^{31}P NMR also. Using the chemical and NMR properties of P_i it is also practical to measure intracellular pH. 3) The bioenergetic information from ^{31}P NMR measurements has significant potential and relevance for evaluation of cell function.

Carbon-13 (^{13}C) NMR has also been used to study intermediary metabolism[6-8]. Since virtually all intermediary metabolites (except for sugar phosphates) are not phosphorylated, it is not possible to observe these compounds except with ^{13}C-enrichment. It may be possible to use ^1H NMR under certain circumstances to observe some specific metabolites present in sufficient quantity (3-5mM). This will require the use of specialized complex pulse sequences to eliminate the water resonance and other broad signals in order to directly observe the narrow lines associated with small molecular species inside cells. Still, the limited range of chemical shifts (~10ppm) for ^1H causes problems with separating poorly resolved signals. The ^{13}C isotope is only 1% naturally abundant, whereas ^{31}P and ^1H are 100% abundant. There are a number of disadvantages to the application of ^{13}C NMR. Briefly these are: 1) the cost of synthesized substrates incorporating specific ^{13}C-labeling is high; 2) the strong coupling between ^{13}C and ^1H requires that heteronuclear proton decoupling be used to simplify the spectrum and to enhance sensitivity. This not only makes the experiment more complex, it introduces a complication of potential local tissue heating by absorption of the ^1H decoupling rf energy. 3) The inherently low sensitivity of ^{13}C requires even longer signal averaging times to obtain usable signal-to-noise of the data.

Hydrogen (^1H) or proton NMR spectroscopy has become increasingly more interesting and useful for the study of cellular and organ function. The principal attractions for ^1H NMR spectroscopy is its inherent sensitivity and the ubiquity of protons on almost all compounds of physiological and biochemical importance. The primary difficulties with in vivo ^1H NMR are the strong signals from water and fat which must be eliminated or suppressed, the small range of chemical shifts for protons, and presence of a large number of overlapping resonances.

Nevertheless, these three nuclides are the most likely candidates for future research and clinical use of NMR spectroscopy. Examples for each will be given and the utility of each discussed in Section III.

NMR SPECTROSCOPY. A brief introduction to the key elements of spectroscopy is needed to provide some familiarity with the theory and terminology of NMR techniques. For a more complete discussion of the basics of NMR spectroscopy, the book of David Gadian[9] and the review article by Meyer, et al.[10] are recommended. Briefly, the atomic nuclei of various elements possess a physical property that is analogous to "spin." The determinant for nuclear spin is conferred by the composition of neutrons and protons in a given elemental species. Thus, an odd number of protons (eg, the hydrogen nucleus) or an odd number of protons and neutrons (eg, deuterium) or an even number of protons and odd number of neutrons (eg, fluorine-19) produces a condition of a nonuniform distribution of charge in the nucleus. This nonuniform charge can be treated as a circulating current (although it is circulating over a very small distance) and therefore has associated with it a magnetic moment. The placement of bulk material having atomic nuclei with spin into a strong, uniform magnetic field causes the nuclei to attempt to align with the magnetic field. This is analogous to the alignment of a compass needle with the earth's small magnetic field. This simple picture is complicated by the fact that the nuclei are not statically oriented in the applied magnetic field, but actually precess at a known frequency as a consequence of the torque experienced by the nonuniform charge in the magnetic field. A simple equation describing such a precession phenomenon was postulated by Larmor (equation 1):

$$\omega_0 = \gamma B_0 \quad (1),$$

where ω_0 is the rate of precession in radians per second, γ is a constant characteristic of the nuclear species termed the gyromagnetic ratio, and B_0 is the external or applied magnetic field. In principle, the ω_0 of all the hydrogen nuclei should be identical for a constant B_0, ω_0 of all phosphorus nuclei should be identical, as well (but ω_0 of $^{31}P \neq \omega_0$ of ^1H, since $\gamma\, ^1H \neq \gamma\, ^{31}P$). The key to NMR spectroscopy is that the distribution of electrons about any given nucleus provides some shielding to the nucleus from the B_0 field. Since the distribution of electrons is a function of the molecular structure in which the atoms (and their nuclei) are located, the actual field experienced by the nucleus differs from the B_0 field by some small amount. Thus, equation 1 can be modified to

$$\omega = \gamma B_0 (1 - \sigma) \quad (2),$$

where σ is the shielding constant for the nuclei in a specific molecular environment. The difference or shift in the precession frequency is called the chemical shift. These shifts (σ) are typically on the order of 10^{-6} to 10^{-5}, σ is independent of B_0 and the precession (or resonant) frequencies are reported as parts per million (ppm) relative to a standard reference frequency. Figure 1 shows the information obtainable with NMR spectroscopy. The frequency scale is normalized by the convention of reporting chemical shifts in ppm.

The NMR experiment consists of applying an oscillating frequency identical to the precession frequency of the nucleus of interest. This application of such an external frequency identical to the Larmor frequency constitutes a condition of resonance; hence the name of the method. At resonance, the nuclei absorb energy and are forced away from a state of equilibrium. As the nuclear spins realign with the B_0 field after this perturbation, the absorbed energy is released and this can be detected. The time required for the nuclei to return to the original equilibrium condition is the so-called spin lattice ("T_1") relaxation time. The resultant signal intensities detected by the NMR experiment are proportional to the concentration of the nuclei in given environments when acquired under conditions which allow for full T_1 relaxation to occur. This also assumes no additional complications such as nuclear Overhauser effects or chemical exchange which may alter signal intensity to different extents for a given spin in a specific molecular environment.

INSTRUMENTATION AND TECHNIQUES

BASIC NMR SYSTEMS. There are three basic elements of any NMR instrument. These are: the magnet and associated shim and imaging gradients, the rf transmit and receive system, and the data acquisition and data processing system. The fundamental differences for NMR spectroscopy compared to MRI are the requirement for much greater field uniformity (homogeneity) in the region sampled and high field strengths. It is not unusual to desire field uniformity to better than one part in 10^7, particularly for proton spectroscopy applications. There are at least two other additional capabilities which are normally required for doing the complete range of NMR spectroscopy experiments. The first capability is that of heteronuclear and homonuclear narrow band and broadband decoupling. This typically requires the incorporation of a second rf signal generating system into the spectrometer. This system may work specifically for proton decoupling, or may be a broadband unit capable of providing a range of frequencies. The second important aspect is that of multi-nuclear observe capabilities. This is typically implemented by the use of a broadband signal generating system coupled to a broadband rf radiofrequency amplifier to provide fairly uniform power output over a broad range of rf frequencies.

Most NMR spectroscopy systems incorporate a field frequency locking system capable of providing excellent stability for compensation of small drifts in either the main magnetic field or the rf signal generating unit. The "lock unit" may also be used to optimize the magnetic field homogeneity, although most researchers use a simple scheme of detecting the water and fat proton signal from the object in a simple "one pulse" experiment. By integrating the free induction decay signal so obtained, it is possible to adjust the room temperature resistive shim sets to optimize field uniformity in the sampled region. This is routinely done for each and every experiment for spectroscopy, as opposed to magnetic resonance imaging systems which may only adjust homogeneity very infrequently (once every several months, or once per year).

The systems which are currently available commercially for NMR spectroscopy can be divided into three basic types based upon the bore size and magnetic field strength available. Small bore systems can be arbitrarily divided into those magnets having a 9 to 13cm diameter clear bore, operating at magnetic field strengths of from 4.2 to 9.4T. These may be either vertical or horizontal bore systems, although the vertical bore orientation is the most prevalent at this time. Medium sized systems are those having a clear bore of 20 to 50cm in diameter and operating at magnetic field strengths from 1.9 to 4.7T. Large size systems comprise those having a clear bore of 76 to 100cm in diameter and operating at magnetic field strengths of 1.5 to 2T. There is some interest in obtaining one meter bore magnets operating at fields to 4T, and there are proto-type development projects for such magnets underway at this time although no meter bore 4T magnet having requisite field homogeneity has been produced to date.

RADIO FREQUENCY COILS. Possibly the most important element for in vivo spectroscopy, other than the basic instrumentation, is the rf coil used for transmission and detection of the NMR signals. The radio frequency coil is the first step in the chain of detection of the nuclear spins. As a consequence of this key role this subject is worthy of considerable attention. It is not the purpose of this review to develop the theory and engineering behind appropriate coil design. It is worth noting that coil size and shape can be used to enhance the effective application of NMR spectroscopy to the study of organ and tumor metabolism. This is an important area of research and engineering development for improved signal detection by NMR techniques.

Complications can arise for rf coil use in spectroscopy which are not encountered in normal MRI applications. First, it may be desirable to have an rf coil tuned to resonance over a broad range of frequencies, thus obviating the need for a number of different NMR coil assemblies with associated tuning and matching capacitors. Second, it is often advantageous to have a single coil which operates at two resonance frequencies simultaneously. For example, it may be desirable to observe both phosphorus and protons in a time-shared manner. This will require a more complex tuning scheme to obtain a double resonant condition in the coil. And, of course, there are always trade-offs in coil performance when multiple tuning is implemented.

SPATIAL LOCALIZATION. A number of techniques have been proposed and tested for providing spatial localization of the detected NMR signal for spectroscopy. In the case of ^{31}P and ^{13}C spectroscopy it is highly unlikely that multi-dimensional imaging will ever be practical. This is due to the low sensitivity and relatively low concentrations of these nuclides as compared with protons. The prospects of doing chemical shift imaging of small protonated compounds is far more likely. Consequently, it will be necessary to employ methods which provide well-defined and reproducible spatial localization for acquiring NMR spectroscopic information. The three methods which appear to be most promising at this time are: 1) rotating frame spatially resolved NMR spectroscopy, 2) composite pulse sequences which yield a "depth" discrimination, and 3) one-dimensional line scanning techniques which will yield an NMR spectrum along a single projection through an object. For methods 2 and 3 above, a number of different approaches have been suggested and tested. The fundamental drawback to any spatially localized technique is that all methods produce an effective reduction in sample filling factor which translates into reduced signal-to-noise for the given voxel. In addition, all methods proposed to date suffer from the drawback that sample noise remains constant but the volume selected for data acquisition is reduced, thereby yielding a degradation in sensitivity because the noise from the entire sample volume is still present in the detection of the NMR signal.

A description of the rotating frame magnetic resonance method has been provided by Garwood, et al.[11] While this method has some good attributes it also has two features which reduces potential for a number of applications. A primary deficiency of the method is the need to apply a presaturation pulse to effectively reduce the magnetization along the Z (B_0) axis to zero. This must be done to eliminate a smearing along the axial direction of the rf coil due to phase differences which arise from the non-linear B_1 field. The second problem is that the uncertainty in the width, shape, and location of the plane sampled is potentially large. Despite these problems, the technique is very promising.

Bendal has recently provided a comprehensive review of the composite pulse sequences which he has devised for providing spatial localization using surface coils[12]. In general, the depth pulsing sequence approach appears to be the most flexible and offer the most convenient method for obtaining NMR spectra from selected volumes sub-tended by the B_1 field generated in a surface coil. A problem inherent to both rotating frame and depth sequences is the inability to know precisely where NMR data is coming from in the absence of a method which provides direct imaging for anatomic correlation. Even the line scan technique will suffer from this problem and, furthermore, has the additional complication of obtaining signal along an entire plane which may be contaminated with many different tissue types. Haselgrove, et al., presented the first one-dimensional line scanning results[13].

IN VIVO SPECTROSCOPY

TECHNIQUES. Upon initial consideration, it would seem that obtaining in vivo NMR spectra is no different from acquiring MRI data. In fact, this should be true, but in practice there are a number of things which can markedly affect the quality of data and the time necessary to acquire data for spectroscopy measurements. The first consideration is that of the magnetic field strengths used as compared to imaging. With the present generation of magnets, operating a system at 1.9T is at the lower end of the scale for spectroscopy work. With the availability of horizontal bore magnets operating to 4.7T, the problems caused by strong fringing fields and the hazards related to the rapid acceleration that magnetic objects can undergo when attracted to the magnet represent major safety and equipment concerns. Additionally, small ferromagnetic items such as paper clips and staples which might normally go completely unnoticed when trapped in the bore of a magnet used for imaging, become significant perturbations on the magnetic field when one is trying to maintain a few parts in 10^7 homogeneity over a 4 to 6cm volume. These are, however, practical issues which can be effectively dealt with by proper planning and simple checking of the NMR system.

A group of problems which are typically more difficult to solve are those related to the problems presented by actual sample or subject which is placed in the magnet for study. Many research systems are sited in facilities that lack radio frequency shielding. The large, open bore of 30cm and larger size magnets does not provide effective shielding of external rf signals. Furthermore, animals and humans serve as good antennas because of their conductivity properties and tend to cause further signal detection problems when any part of the body sticks out either end of the magnet. As a consequence, proper rf shielding and/or careful attention to rf grounding become important aspects for making successful NMR measurements in vivo. Additional problems often arise from respiratory and other involuntary motion, cardiac motion, and the presence of large bone structures (such as the skull). All of these factors tend to contribute to degradation in the apparent homogeneity and the average sensitivity of the NMR measurement which is caused to fluctuate by motion effects. Bone and other connective tissues can cause problems because they can contribute very broad NMR signals as well as presenting an additional barrier for detection of the NMR signal from the region desired. One final difficulty may be that of restraining the subject for studies. This can be particularly difficult in studies where no anesthetic is desirable or appropriate, or where exercise is even part of the actual protocol.

To briefly summarize the above, there are a number of impediments which arise routinely in trying to perform <u>in vivo</u> spectroscopic measurements. Most if not all of these complications can be managed with careful attention to the design and construction of the rf coil assembly and support and restraint devices used in patient and subject handling. In many cases, it may be necessary to devote funds to proper site preparation, including installation of a rf shielded room, for example.

The techniques required for spectroscopic studies vary from a very simple "one pulse" sequence for most ^{31}P studies to more complex pre-saturation schemes and composite pulse sequences for depth selection. ^{13}C NMR studies are generally made more complex by the requirement for proton decoupling. As one wants the most effective proton decoupling with the least amount of deposited rf power, this typically requires a more complex decoupling scheme such as MLEV or a WALTZ sequence[14]. Proton spectra require the use of presaturation schemes also enhanced by a solvent suppression sequence (typically, a 1,3,3,1 sequence[15]) and T_2 discrimination to detect the narrow line resonances which arise from small molecules in the cells and which effectively eliminate the water and fat peaks which tend to dominate the proton spectrum because of their much higher concentrations. Figure 2 shows a series of diagrams depicting some of the different types of pulse sequences which are commonly used for all of the above described techniques. More recently, even more complex schemes have been proposed for spectral editing and elimination of unwanted peaks by multiple quantum transition NMR. A number of these newer schemes hold significant promise, but will not be discussed in this overview.

One additional area which is now becoming of greater interest and practical application is that of multinuclear NMR studies utilizing multiple tuned resonant coils. For example, the ability to monitor ^{31}P and proton spectra in a time-shared, near simultaneous or sequential fashion offers the additional benefits of obtaining more information in essentially the same time as needed to acquire a single spectrum of one nucleus. Numerous developments in this area are underway and this promises to be a very important field of application for a number of research and clinical studies.

RESULTS AND TYPES OF INFORMATION AVAILABLE BY SPECTROSCOPY. The potential value of noninvasive, metabolic determinations within the human body is evident to those who understand the relationships between physiological function and biochemistry. A brief overview of the utility of phosphorus NMR spectroscopy in assessing metabolism will be given as one example of the potential power of NMR spectroscopy. As an aside, the basic elements of ^{31}P NMR also apply to the use of ^{13}C NMR, with two major exceptions. First, the ^{31}P

nuclide is 100% naturally abundant; ^{13}C is only 1% naturally abundant. This means that in comparison with phosphorus where all nuclei contribute to the NMR measurement, only 1% of the carbon atoms are detectable by NMR. To enhance the sensitivity of a ^{13}C measurement it is often necessary to give substrate compounds of interest that have specific carbon sites selectively enriched with ^{13}C (to 80%-90% ^{13}C enrichment). There is an additional benefit of ^{13}C - namely, it permits labeling studies for determining the uptake and distribution of label within tissues. This could not be done if the natural abundance of ^{13}C was 100%, for example. Second, because of a strong interaction ("coupling") between the carbon nucleus and the hydrogen nucleus which results in a splitting of the ^{13}C signal into multiple peaks (all at a reduced intensity) it is often necessary to eliminate such interactions by the application of energy at the frequency of the hydrogen resonances ("decoupling"). For the types of metabolic studies in humans which will be done with ^{13}C, this decoupling method is apt to produce potentially dangerous heating within the body.

Why is the phosphorus nucleus of such potential importance for metabolic studies? There are four principal attributes which recommend ^{31}P NMR: 1) the major chemical sources of free energy for cellular functions contain phosphorus, 2) the ability of cells to maintain adequate levels of high energy phosphates such as adenosine triphosphate (ATP) and phosphocreatine (PCr) is a clear indication of metabolic function, 3) cellular high energy phosphates can reflect metabolic alterations associated with either genetic defects or with cell transformations resulting from cancer, and 4) the intracellular hydrogen ion concentration (pH) can be measured using the precise frequency of the inorganic phosphate signal in the ^{31}P NMR spectrum. Figure 3 depicts in a diagrammatic manner the key role of phosphorus in cellular metabolism and some of the possible alterations that can occur with cellular injury and diseases.

As an _in vivo_ example of ^{31}P NMR evaluations of metabolism, Figure 4 shows the effects of isoproterenol stimulation on myocardial high energy phosphates in an _in vivo_ rabbit model and the subsequent recovery when the animal resumed normal breathing. The sequence of spectra shows the depression of the PCr level during maximal stimulation when compared with the control myocardium. As well as the mild acidosis that occurs, the sequence also demonstrates the recovery of PCr and loss of inorganic phosphate (Pi) with recovery. One of the points clearly shown is that of the ability to make repeated, sequential metabolic measurements noninvasively with NMR.

Figure 5 shows results of a regional infarction in a dog model. For both cases a surface coil was employed to give the desired spatial localization. Conditions for the measurements are given in the figure legend. The model of ischemia involves the use of an inflatable balloon occluder placed around the left anterior descending (LAD) coronary artery. The first set of spectra indicate the stability of the preparation and the second set show the alteration in phosphorylate substrates in the myocardium after a 2.5 hour ischemic insult.

Some preliminary results in human studies are shown in Figures 6 and 7. Figure 6 is a series of ^{31}P NMR spectra from the human forearm (palmaris longus muscle group) during the course of exercise. Figure 7 is a natural abundance ^{13}C spectrum demonstrating the ability to obtain good quality ^{13}C NMR data from the tissue of the forearm. The ^{13}C spectrum was obtained without hydrogen decoupling.

Brain metabolism can be examined using both ^{1}H and ^{31}P NMR spectroscopy[16,17]. Typical results from dog, rabbit, and neonatal pig models are shown in Figure 8 (a,b,c). These spectra were obtained using a 1.9T, 30cm horizontal clear bore (25cm usable bore) magnet interfaced to a multinuclear spectrometer. A 4cm (O.D.) surface coil was used for all measurements. The high field homogeneity was optimized in all cases by observing the proton signal obtained with the surface coil singly tuned to the ^{31}P resonant frequency. There is ample sensitivity to ^{1}H even without a tuned circuit, although the efficiency of energy transmission is very poor at the ^{1}H frequency. The peak width at half height for the water signal was always between 10-20Hz (no exponential line broadening was used). Note that, whereas there are some small differences in the spectra, the overall character of the spectra are remarkably similar.

It is now possible to routinely obtain NMR spectroscopic data from selected regions with the body of live animals and humans. ^{31}P NMR spectra from selected regions of the adult and neonatal human brain have been obtained by a number of different laboratories[18,19]. Clearly, as magnet technology advances to the point where stable, high field magnets having large homogeneous volumes can be routinely manufactured, NMR spectroscopy is destined to become an important tool in medical practice.

REFERENCES

1. D. I. Hoult, S. J. W. Busby, D. G. Gadian, et al.: Observations of tissue metabolites using ^{31}P nuclear magnetic resonance. Nature 252, pp. 285-287 (1974).
2. R. H. T. Edwards, M. J. Dawson, D. R. Wilkie, et al.: Clinical use of nuclear magnetic resonance in the investigation of myopathy. Lancet, pp. 725-731 (March 27, 1982).
3. M. J. Dawson, R. E. Edwards, D. R. Wilkie, et al.: ^{31}P NMR studies of metabolites in the human forearm. Physiol Soc (in press).
4. E. B. Cady, M. J. Dawson, P. L. Hope, et al.: Non-invasive investigation of cerebral metabolism in newborn infants by phosphorus nuclear magnetic resonance spectroscopy. Lancet, pp. 1059-1062 (May 14, 1983).
5. R. A. Zimmerman, P. A. Bottomley, W. A. Edelstein, H. R. Hart, et al. Amer J Radiol 6, pp. 109-110 (1985).
6. A. D. Sherry, R. L. Nunnally, and R. M. Peshock: Metabolic studies of pyruvate and lactate in perfused guinea pig hearts by ^{13}C NMR: Determination of substrate preference by glutamate isotopomer distrubtion. J Biol Chem (1985) in press.
7. S. M. Cohen, P. Glynn, and R. G. Shulman. Proc Nat'l Acad Sci 78, pp. 60-64 (1981).
8. K. J. Neurohr, E. J. Barrett, and R. G. Shulman. Proc Nat'l Acad Sci 80, pp. 1603-1607 (1983).
9. D. G. Gadian: NMR and Its Application to Living Systems. Oxford University Press, Oxford, pp. 14-18, 29-34, 37, 122-1252 (1982).
10. R. A. Meyer, M. J. Kushmerick, T. R. Brown: Application of ^{31}P NMR spectroscopy to the study of striated muscle metabolism. Am J Physiol 242, pp. C1-C11 (1982).
11. M. Garwood, T. Schleich, G. B. Matson, and G. Acosta. J Mag Reson 60, pp. 268-279 (1984).
12. M. R. Bendall: Chapter 8 in **Biomedical Magnetic Resonance** (T. L. James and A. Margulis, eds.). Radiology Postgraduate Education, University of California, San Francisco, 1985.
13. J. C. Haselgrove, U. H. Subramanian, J. S. Leigh, Jr., et al.: In vivo one-dimensional imaging of phosphorus metabolites by phosphorus-31 nuclear magnetic resonance. Science, 220, pp. 1170-1173 (1983).
14. A. J. Shaka, J. Keeler, T. Frenkeil, and R. Freeman. J Mag Res 52, pp. 335-338 (1983)
15. P. J. Hore. J Mag Res 55, pp. 283-300 (1983)
16. K. L. Behar, D. L. Rothman, R. G. Shulman, O. A. C. Petroff, J. W. Prichard. Proc Nat'l Acad Sci 81, pp. 2517-2519 (1984).
17. M. Hilberman, U. H. Subramanian, J. Haselgrove, J. B. Cone, et al. J Cereb Blood Flow Metab 4, pp. 334-342 (1984).
18. K. M. Brindle, M. B. Smith, B. Rajagapalan, G. K. Radda. J Mag Res 61, pp. 559-563 (1985)
19. P. L. Hope, E. B. Cady, P. S. Tofts, et al. Lancet, pp. 360-369 (August, 1984).

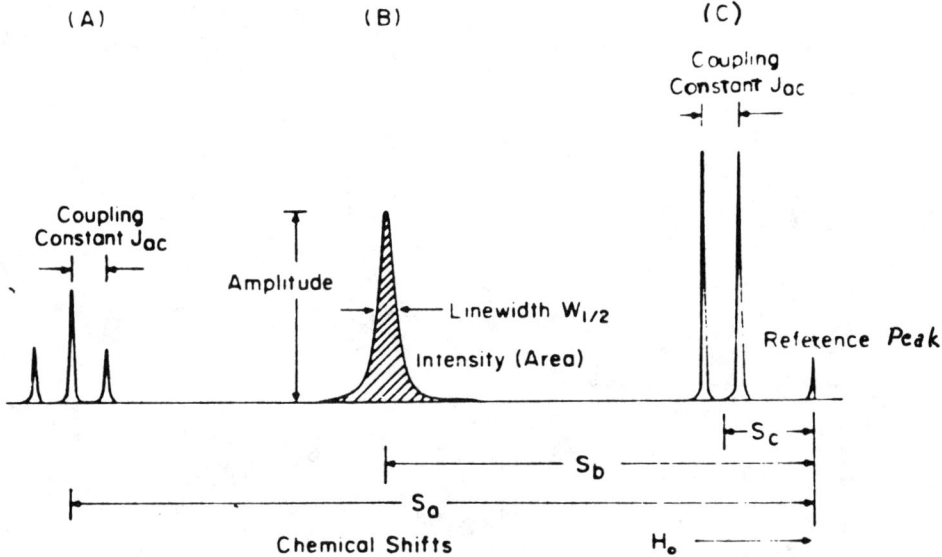

Figure 1. Nuclear magnetic resonance spectral parameters.

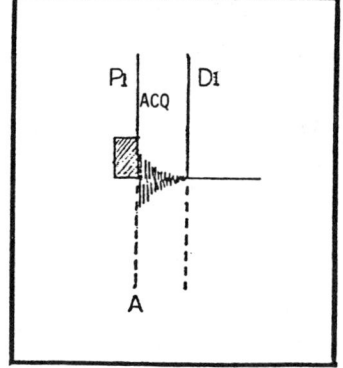
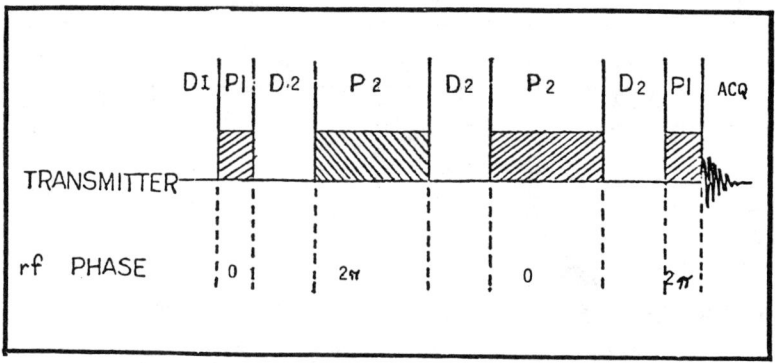

Figure 2. Two linear diagrams of simple NMR experiments demonstrating the key parameters used and one approach to a graphic representation of the experiments.

Figure 3 (next page). The top panel (A) shows a very simplified scheme of the requirements for oxygen and substrate delivery to cells in order to support normal generation of adenosine triphosphate (ATP). The ATP is then utilized to support a number of functions in the normal maintenance and function of specific cell types. As ATP is used, it liberates its free energy and forms break-down products which can then be resynthesized to form ATP. The bottom panel (B) indicates how a number of changes in either the delivery of oxygen, substrate, or the alteration of intracellular pH as well as the removal of break-down products can lead to impairment of the normal generation of ATP. Virtually all of the consequences of these failures can be monitored using phosphorus NMR.

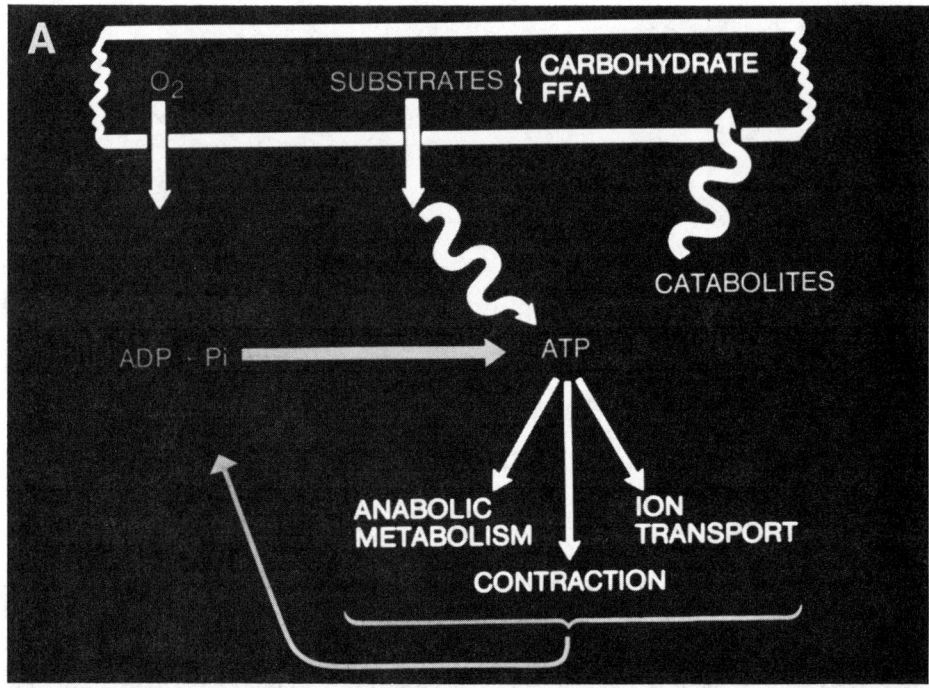
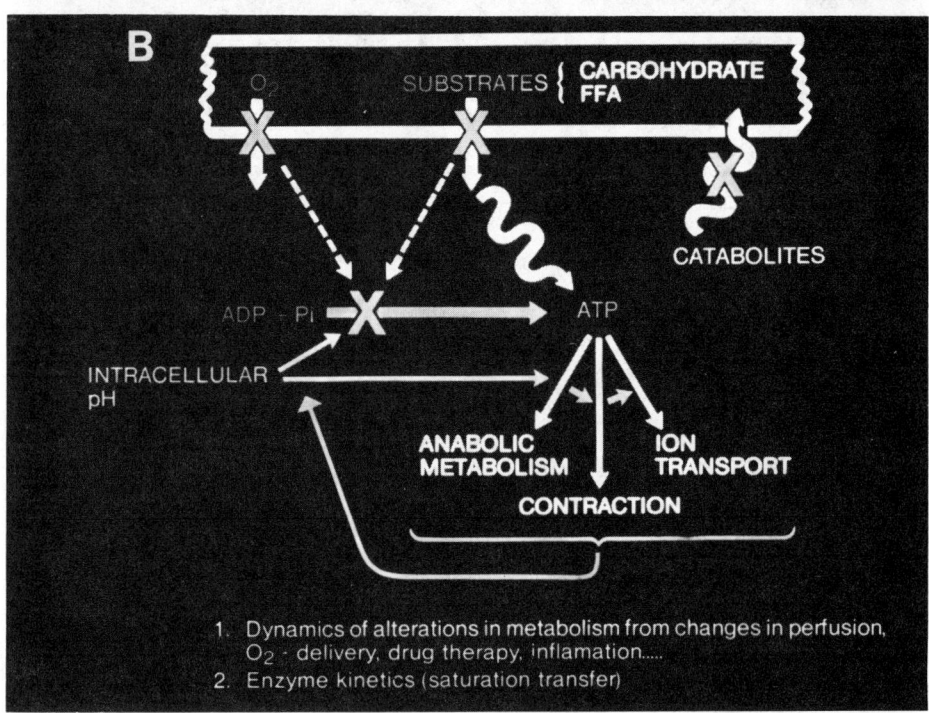

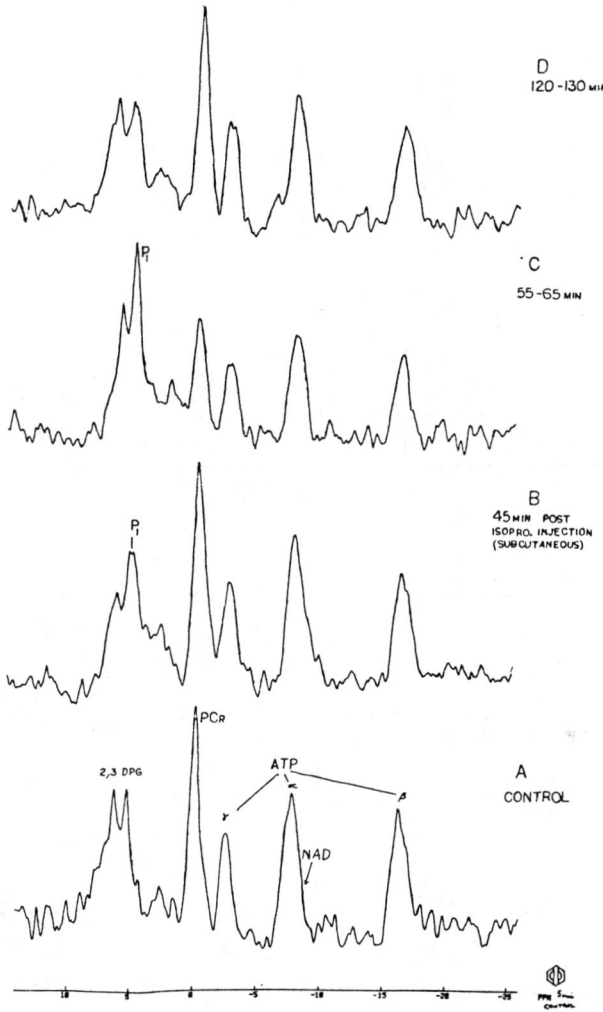

Figure 4. Sequential P-31 TMR spectra from a live rabbit. A surface coil was placed over the left upper thorax and the magnetic field profiled to a sensitive volume of 2 cm (diameter). The control spectrum shows a representative P-31 result from the region of the heart (note the large 2,3 DPG peaks). The animal was subsequently challenged with isoproterenol and increases in [P_i] and reductions in [PCr] and [ATP] were detected in spectra B and C. The heart returned to normal two hours after isoproterenol administration as shown in D.

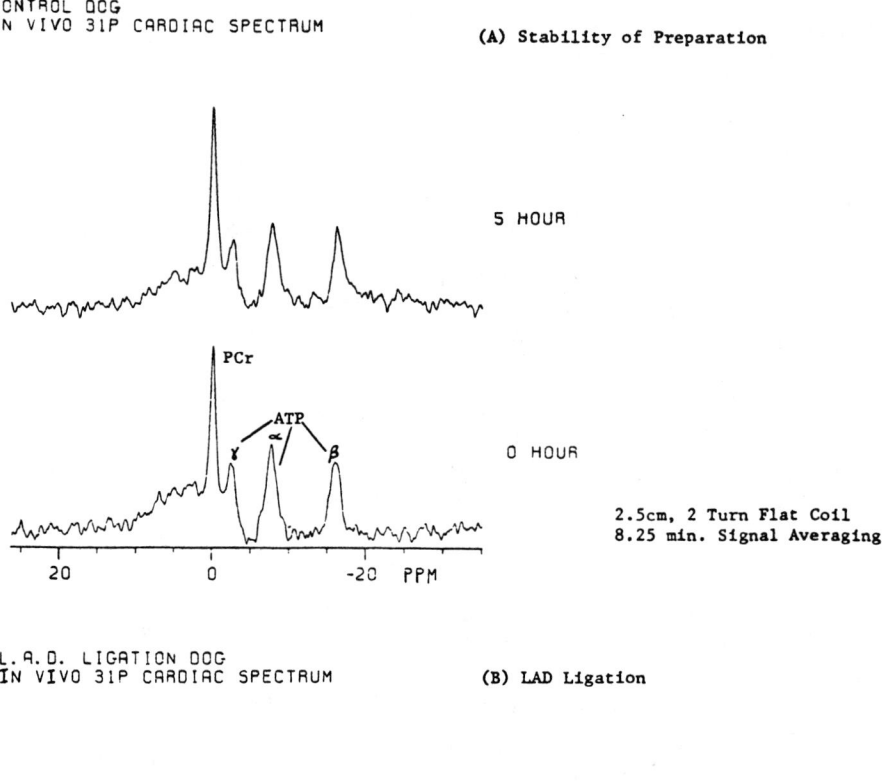

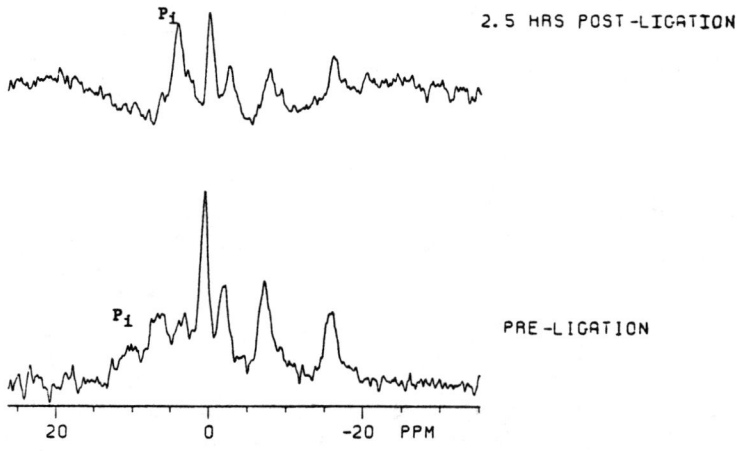

Figure 5. Regional infarction in a dog model. (A) Control dog representing preparation stability. (B) Alteration in phosphorylate substrates in the myocardium after a 2.5 hour ischemic insult.

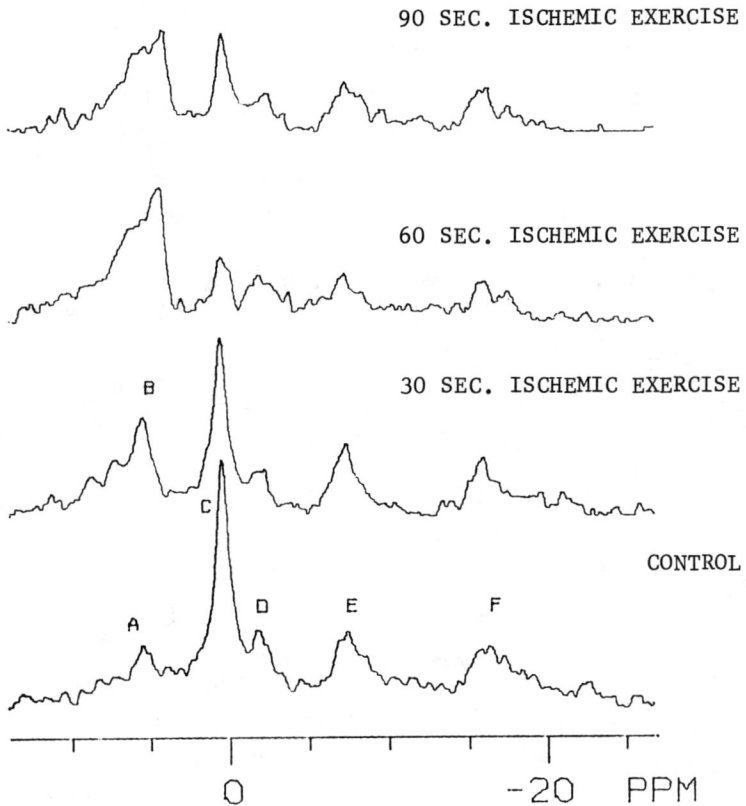

Figure 6. A series of P-31 NMR spectra from the forearm of a normal adult. Peak assignments are as follows: A, B, inorganic phosphate (pi); C, phosphocreatine; D, E, and F, the three phosphate signals of ATP. Each spectrum is the result of 12 transients acquired over a 30 second interval.

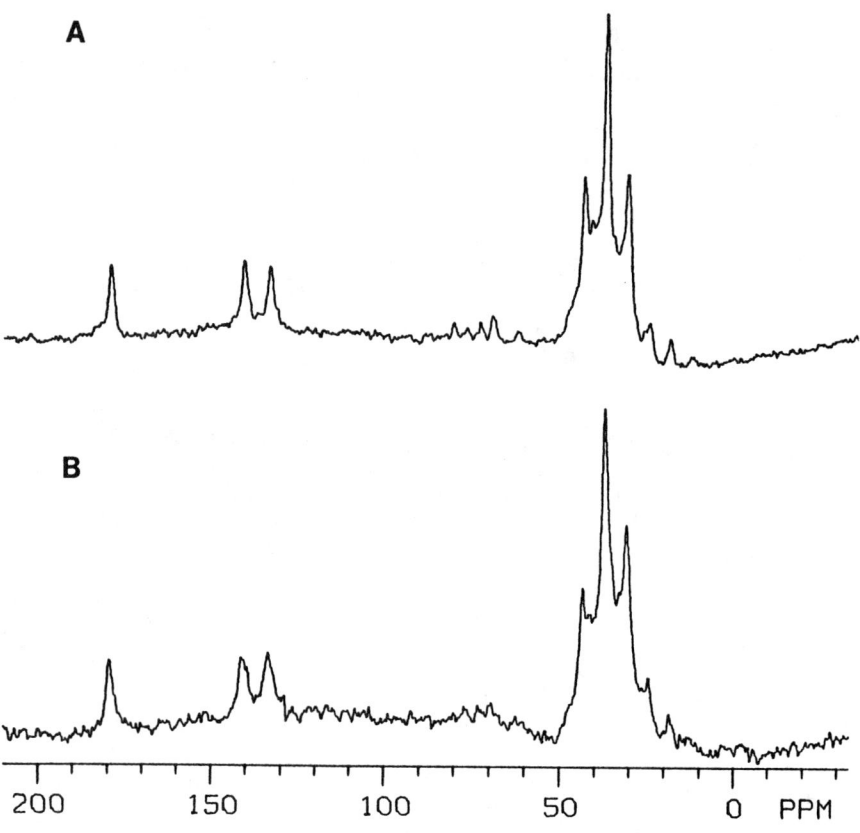

Figure 7. Typical C-13 NMR spectra from the human forearm of two different individuals. The spectra (6 minutes each, natural abundance C-13) arise primarily from subcutaneous fat. No proton decoupling was used.

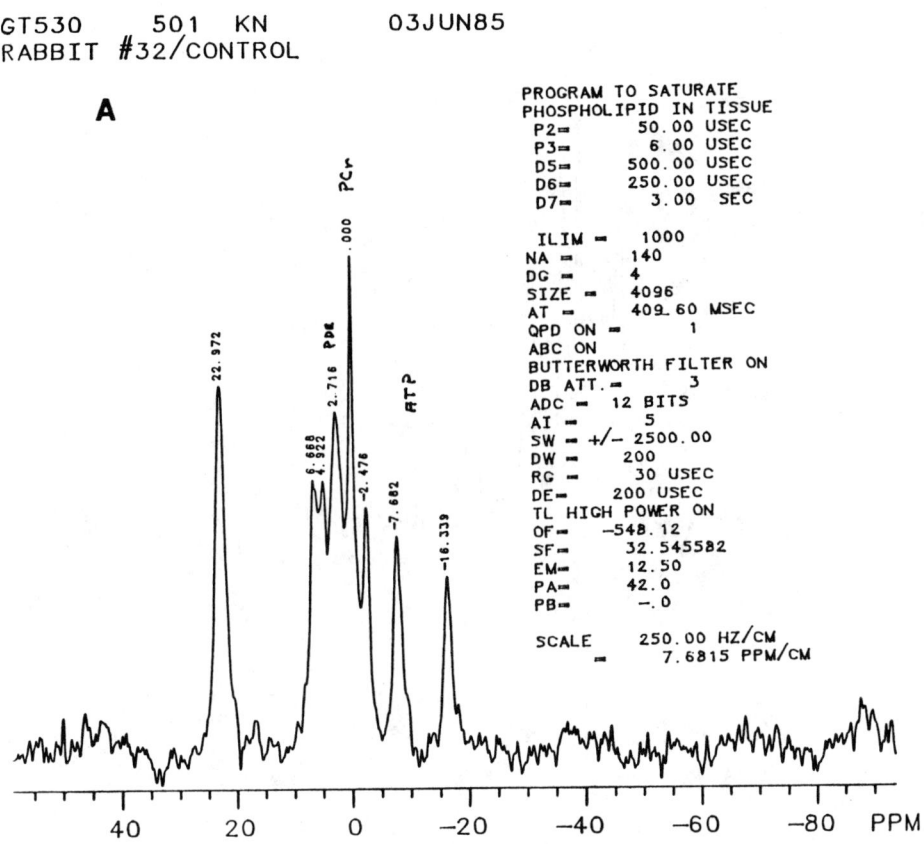

Figure 8. A series of three spectra showing the typical results obtained from the brain of three different animal species. The first spectrum (A) was obtained from a live rabbit using a 4cm surface coil. The second spectrum (B) was obtained in a similar fashion from a beagle dog, and the third spectrum (C) was obtained from a newborn pig (age 7 days). The peak which arises at 22.9ppm is that obtained from a reference compound for purposes of chemical shift and integration. The signal which arises in the 2.7 to 2.9ppm is that associated with the phosphodiester region. A presaturation pulse sequence has been used to minimize a broad phosphate signal which underlies the area to the left (downfield) side of phosphocreatine.

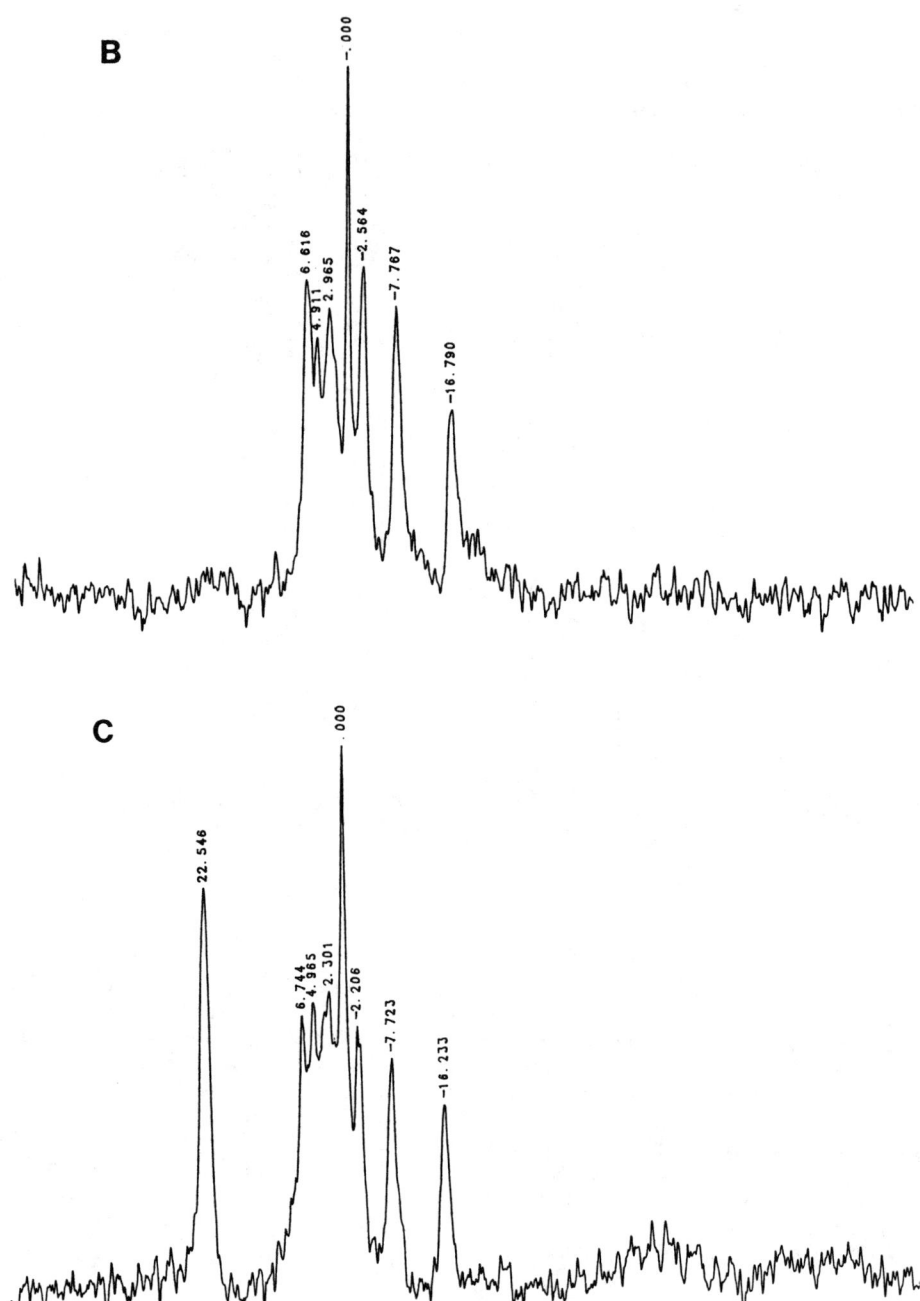

Figure 8 (continued).

APPLICATIONS OF FLUORINE IMAGING

S.R. Thomas

University of Cincinnati, Cincinnati, Ohio 45267

ABSTRACT

The potential application and utilization of ^{19}F-NMR techniques in medicine are discussed. The possibilities considered include use of various fluorine labeled substrates, perfluorocarbon compounds, fluorinated gasses and anesthetics.

INTRODUCTION

The characteristics of ^{19}F which make this nucleus uniquely suited for high contrast NMR imaging <u>in vivo</u> are well recognized and include: a high gyromagnetic ratio (40.05 MHz/T), spin 1/2, a sensitivity relative to protons of 0.83, 100% natural isotopic abundance, and an extremely low biological occurrence. The high sensitivity provides a signal-to-noise ratio on a nucleus-per-nucleus basis comparable to that of protons, while the high gyromagnetic ratio, representing a resonant frequency approximately only 6% lower than that for protons (42.58 MHz/T), allows the use of existing proton NMR instrumentation with a minimum of component adjustments and tuning procedural difficulties.

Aspects concerning the intrinsic total body occurrence of fluorine in man relevant to ^{19}F tracer imaging possibilities have been discussed by Thomas, et. al. (1). Under the conservative assumption that 2.6g of fluorine per the standard 70kg man (2) is distributed uniformly throughout the body, the intrinsic concentration would be less than 2 mM. In fact, the actual soft tissue concentration would be much less because most of the ^{19}F is likely to be incorporated into bone minerals (fluoroapatite). Any resonance arising from such motionally hindered ^{19}F will be broadened and/or have so long a longitudinal relaxation time as to be unsuitable for standard imaging methods. (The development of solid-state imaging techniques, however, might hold some promise for visualizing nuclei confined within a rigid matrix.) The above estimates are on the order of the endogenous fluorine levels reported for canine myocardium of 1 to 2 mM(3). However, other investigators put the concentration of ^{19}F in biological tissue at much lower levels, namely, in the sub-micromolar range (4). Nevertheless, even for the upper estimate, these levels of intrinsic concentration are too small to give any detectable ^{19}F signal under practical imaging protocols. Thus, these facts set the stage for high contrast ^{19}F tracer imaging if suitable biocompatible fluorine compounds can be developed for introduction into living systems. This paper will review some of the ongoing research and diagnostic potentials for <u>in vivo</u> ^{19}F NMR techniques.

FLUORODEOXYGLUCOSE (FDG)

Nuclear medicine PET procedures (Positron Emission Tomography) using positron emitting ^{18}F are well documented and include extensive clinical research with ^{18}F-FDG for investigations of brain and myocardial metabolism and infarct detection (5,6,7). The potential for NMR imaging of stable ^{19}F-FDG has been considered by Thomas, et. al. (1). It was estimated that the concentrations required for imaging would be several orders of magnitude greater than the intrinsic biological levels or in the 0.1 to 1.0 M range. A 0.1M solution of FDG represents a fluorine concentration approximately 1/1000 that of hydrogen in water and, since the time required to achieve a given signal-to-noise ratio is inversely proportional to the square of the concentration, severe sensitivity losses would be encountered which must be overcome. Attempts to increase the quantity of this tracer introduced in vivo must analyze existing uptake and toxicity data. As summarized in reference 1, two principal forms of FDG have been utilized, 2-deoxy-2-fluoro-D-glucose (2-FDG) and 3-deoxy-3-fluoro-D-glucose (3 FDG). These two compounds differ only in the position of the single fluorine atom within the molecule. The biokinetic characteristics involving trapping within the metabolic pathways of the brain have been studied through PET techniques more extensively for 2-FDG than for 3-FDG. Work with rhesus monkeys has demonstrated that 3-FDG exhibits behavior identical to that of glucose in passing the blood brain barrier (8) and thus also may be useful in the measurement of glucose metabolism in the brain (although the optimal time for imaging may be shorter than that for 2-FDG due to the slightly different biokinetic properties observed). The toxicity data analysis would indicate that 2-FDG with a relatively high lethal dose in rats (LD_{50} = 600 mg/kg) will be an unlikely candidate for a human in vivo ^{19}F NMR imaging agent, whereas 3-FDG, which is considerably less toxic (non-toxic in rats at levels of 5g/kg), offers considerable greater promise for NMR applications in the study of glucose metabolism.

A high resolution fluorine spectrum of 2-FDG at 2.1T (84.7 MHz for fluorine) is shown in Figure 1. The spectrum exhibits a doublet of triplets due to spin-spin couplings. There are several difficulties associated with NMR imaging studies involving complicated spectra resulting from non-equivalent chemical environments for the individual atoms within the molecule, namely: (a) the potential for generating chemical shift artifacts (9,10), and (b) a loss of spatial resolution in the image through the blurring associated with reconstruction utilizing a line broadened due to unresolved spin-spin and/or chemical shift peaks as the system response function. A concentric cylinder (annulus) phantom image shown in reference 1 consisting of a 0.68 M solution of 2-^{19}F-FDG taken at 0.75 T (30 MHz for fluorine) exhibited several of the problems encountered. Even at a concentration of 0.68M, the signal-to-noise ratio in the image was relatively low for the pulse protocol used (partial saturation, TR = 0.625s, 50 averages, filtered back projection, 18 projections). In addition, there was

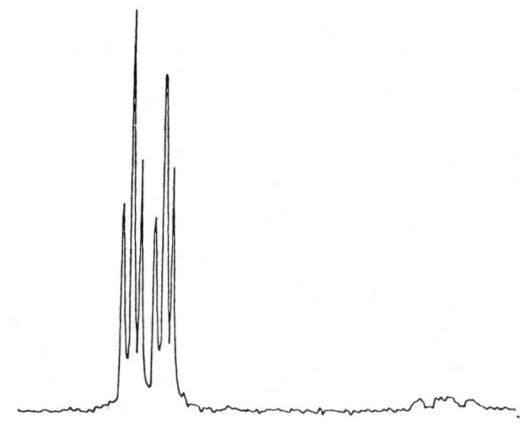

Figure 1: NMR fluorine spectrum of 2-FDG at 2.1 T (84.7 MHz). The doublet and triplet splittings are approximately 49 Hz and 13 Hz respectively. The chemical shift is -33 ppm with respect to an external reference of C_6F_6.

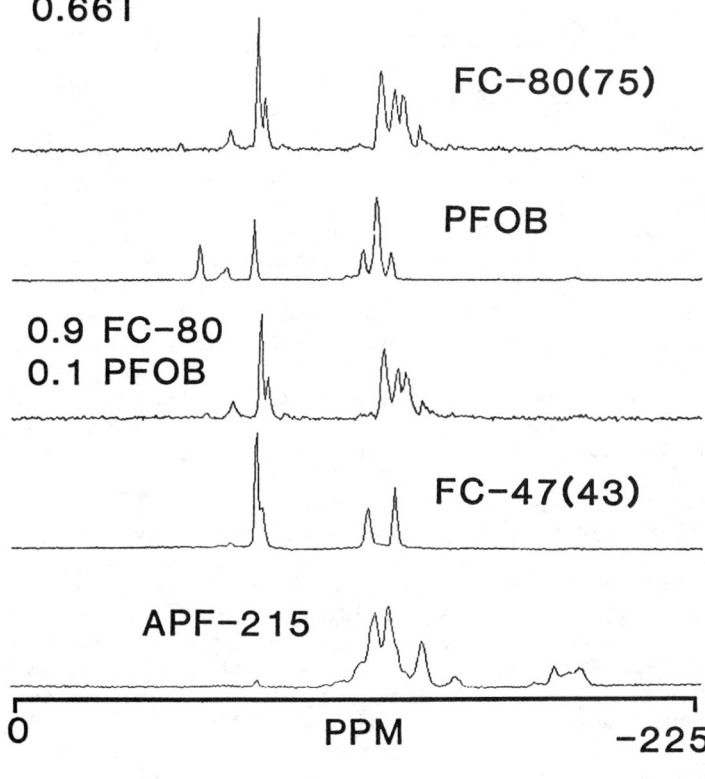

Figure 2: The chemical shift spectra of some perfluorocarbon compounds taken at 0.66T (26.4 MHz for fluorine). a) F-propylfuran, FC-80 (or FC-75) $[C_8F_{16}O]$; b) F-octyl bromide, PFOB $[CF_3(CF_2)_7Br]$; c) F-tributylamine, FC-47 (or FC-43) $[(CF_3CF_2CF_2CF_2)_3N]$; d) F-phenathrene, APF-215 $[C_{14}F_{24}]$. Of note is the fact that PFOB is radiopaque as a result of the single bromine atom incorporated at the end of the CF chain.

a loss of resolution manifested as a rounding of the edge characteristics due to the broadened spectral line (a weakly defined doublet with the triplet lines shown in Figure 1 not resolved at the lower field of 0.75T). This fact illustrates the desirability of deconvolving the broad, relatively complicated spectral line shape during the image reconstruction process. Deconvolution techniques have been developed for removing the effects of chemical shift and improving spatial resolution in the NMR imaging of perfluorocarbon compounds (10).

Recently there has been a report by Berkowitz and Ackerman (11) describing in vivo spectroscopic investigations of 2-FDG at 4.7 T (~188 MHz for fluorine) using a double resonance proton decoupled surface coil placed on the head of an anesthetized, intact rat. Spectra were shown as a function of different times post bolus intravenous injection of 50 mg 2FDG. The spectrum taken at later times exhibited additional resonances not seen at earlier times. The authors comment that this result indicates the potential of using such fluorine labeled substrates to study metabolism in vivo. Other investigators also have initiated research involving 2-FDG and NMR techniques (12,13,14).

PERFLUOROCARBON COMPOUNDS

As discussed above, the signal-to-noise ratio (S/N) provided by the fluorine tracer is of prime importance when considering its application in NMR imaging. If, instead of a single fluorine atom within the molecule as in the case for FDG, there were N equivalent fluorine nuclei, an advantage in averaging time of N^2 would be realized on a mole for mole basis neglecting relaxation time differences. (That is, to obtain the same S/N with a single fluorine atom per molecule as for a one pulse experiment using the N-atom mocule, N^2 averages would be required). This point leads naturally to the consideration of using a highly fluorinated group attached to a biologically significant substrate which would confer minimal toxicity at the concentrations required for imaging.

One such possibility, the perfluorocarbon (PFC) compounds, are beginning to show increased utility as emulsions in biological and clinical applications (15,16). In 1966, Clark et. al. (17) demonstrated that certain perfluorocarbon liquids could be breathed with survival which initiated the use of highly fluorinated organic compounds for respiration and artificial blood (popularly known as "blood substitutes"). The suitability of the perfluorocarbons for these applications was based on the properties of chemical and biological inertness combined with the ability to dissolve up to 60 volume % of oxygen and 120 volume % of CO_2 (18). Initial research focused on the oxygen and carbon dioxide transport capability in an effort to identify fluorocarbons with the best molecular structure to form emulsions for intravascular use while confining body retention to the period of functional usefulness (19). The potential of ^{19}F NMR imaging (1,20) and spectroscopic techniques has now opened significant new avenues for highly sensitive investigations of the in vivo properties and diagnostic capabilities of the perfluorocarbon compounds. Recent work has demonstrated the feasibility of NMR imaging of PFC emulsions and neat liquids (21, 22, 23, 4). The ^{19}F NMR spectra of some PFCs are shown in Figure 2. As evident from this figure, the PFCs have complex spectra which result from the non-equivalent chemical environments for the individual fluorine atoms within the molecular configuration. These characteristics give rise to potential complications as discussed above including degradation of the signal-to-noise ratio and introduction of chemical shift artifacts which must be addressed in the NMR imaging phase (10).

One unique application for the PFCs is the potential for monitoring the oxygen tension (pO_2) in tissue and organs (21,22,23,25). This possibility is based upon the intrinsic paramagnetism of O_2 which significantly affects the spin-lattice relaxation time T_1 of the PFC. The relaxation rate T_1^{-1} has been found to increase linearly with pO_2 (21,22,26,27,28). This inverse relationship between T_1 and pO_2 is shown in Figure 3. Preliminary investigations involving PFC accumulation in rat liver have demonstrated that, for certain PFCs, clinically significant pO_2 differentials may be determined in vivo with an eventual quantitative precision projected to be 10 Torr over the physiologically important pO_2 range for the liver of 0 to 100 Torr (26). In addition, regional differences in tissue oxygenation in organs concentrating the PFCs may be monitored qualitatively as well as quantitatively through the contrast enhancement provided in the image for those areas experiencing a higher pO_2 level. The enhancement is derived from the increased signal due to a reduced T_1 value. Aspects of this application were demonstrated by Thomas et. al. for liquid breathing of PFC neat liquids (24,25). Figures 4 and 5 show some examples of this lung imaging research. General possible future uses of PFCs in the pulmonary system include diagnosis of a variety of lung diseases (ventilation defects, pulmonary carcinoma, etc.), monitoring neonatal lung mechanics, and in possibly devising new treatments for cystic fibrosis and pulmonary emphysema. In addition, as evident in Figure 5, there are real possibilities for the use of PFCs as NMR gastrointestinal contrast agents.

Another area of interest representing potential utility for NMR PFC investigations centers on the temperature dependent properties of some of these compounds (29). The relative magnitude and shape of various spectral lines for a given PFC as a function of temperature possibly may be used to monitor temperature gradients in vivo. The nature of the different coupling mechanisms between non-equivalent fluorine atoms gives rise to intensity variations reflecting the relative rates of chemical exchange which are directly related to the temperature. The eventual development of thermal imaging is postulated.

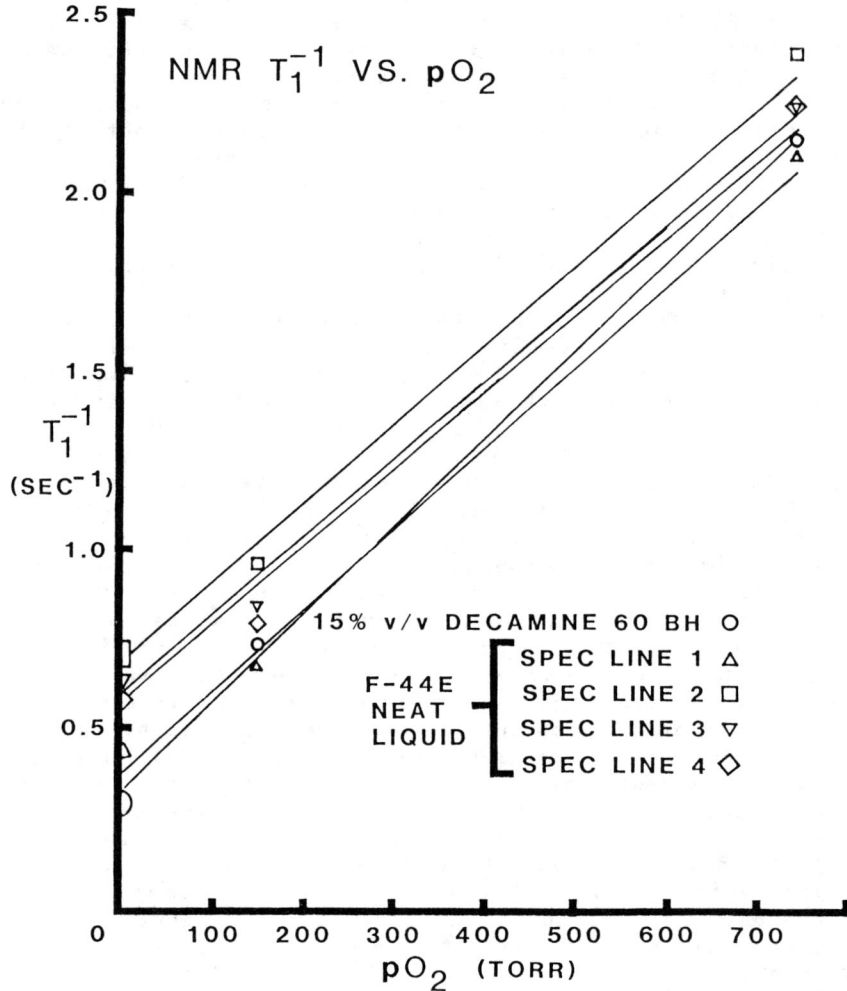

Figure 3: Data illustrating the linear relationship between the relaxation rate $(T1)^{-1}$ and the partial pressure of oxygen (pO_2) for several PFCs. The response of the four spectral lines of F-44E (F-di-n-butyldihydroethylene) are shown as well as the bridge head fluorines in F-decalin. (From reference 19.)

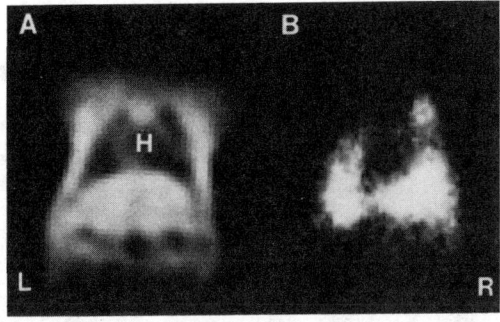

Figure 4: A) The coronal proton image through the thorax of a rat. The lung field is demarcated as a low signal area. Although ungated, the heart wall (H) is visible. NMR technique: 0.14T (6.0 MHz for protons), 2DFT, TE=34 ms, TR=500 ms, 8 averages, 64 phase amplitudes, slice thickness ~4mm.
B) The coronal image of APF-215 in the lungs of the same rat taken immediately following the proton image. NMR technique: 0.14T (5.7 MHz for fluorine), partial saturation, TR=500 ms, 64 averages, 72 projections, no slice selection. (From reference 25.)

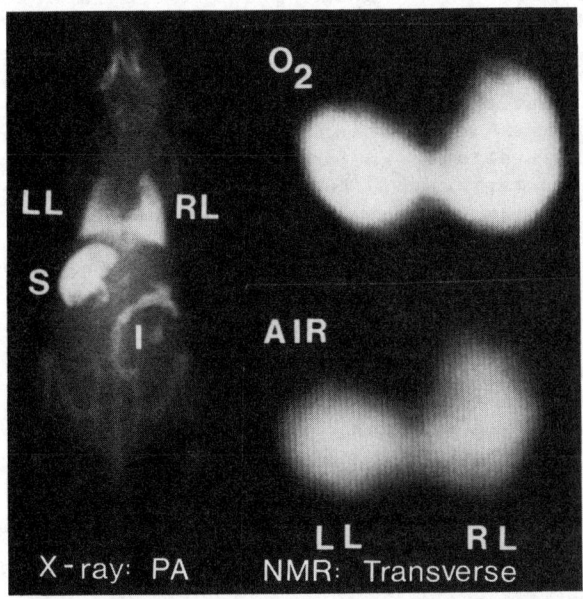

Figure 5: Radiograph and transverse NMR images of a mouse following liquid breathing of a 2-to-1 FC-75/PFOB mixture. The x-ray opacity of PFOB is the result of the single bromine atom incorporated at the end of the CF chain. Some of the PFC mixture had been swallowed by the mouse during the liquid breathing procedure and can be seen in the stomach (S) and intestines (I). This illustrates the potential of using the PFCs as gastrointestinal contrast agents. The transverse NMR images were taken without slice selection with only the lung field within the sensitive volume of the rf coil (left lung LL, right lung RL). The signal enhancement (approximately 10%) as the result of breathing pure oxygen is evident. NMR technique: 0.63T (25.1 MHz for fluorine), partial saturation, TR=150 ms, 128 averages, 72 projections. (From reference 25.)

OTHER ^{19}F NMR INVESTIGATIONS

Gas phase ^{19}F NMR imaging has been reported by Heidelberger and Lauterbur (30) who proposed that this technique could be used for ventilation imaging to visualize the distribution and exchange of gases within the lungs. Images of CF_4 were shown for various concentrations of the gas in phantom cylinders and within an excised pair of rabbit lungs.

The retention of fluorinated anesthetics has been studied spectroscopically in rabbit brains using surface coil ^{19}F-NMR methods by Wyrwicz, et. al. (31,32). The additional resonances observed as a function of time following administration for both 1% halothane and 1.5% isoflurane provide direct evidence of the kinetics associated with the formation of bound species or other molecular environment changes for these anesthetics. Recent additional investigations also have reported on the research aspects of NMR techniques applied to the study of inhaled anesthetics (33,34).

Horner et. al. (35) have evaluated the use of ^{19}F NMR imaging in the study of tissue perfusion. A water soluable ^{19}F labeled compound (Mallinckrodt MP-312: a meglumine salt of trifluoromethyl sulfonic acid) was used to demonstrate a decrease in myocardial perfusion in a rabbit heart model involving coronary arterial ligation. It was proposed that these techniques would find future applications in diagnosis and evaluation of general perfusion defects including clinical situations exhibiting enhanced as well as decreased perfusion characteristics. Nunnally et. al. (36) have studied the uptake and metabolism of fluorinated anti-tumor agents (5-fluorouracil) with F-19 NMR spectroscopy. They postulate the nearly simultaneous observation of ^{19}F and ^{31}P utilizing a double tuned coil which would represent a significant application of _in vivo_ NMR in the evaluation of tumor therapy.

Acknowledgments: The author would like to acknowledge the other members of the group at the University of Cincinnati involved in ^{19}F-NMR research: Jerome L. Ackerman, Leland C. Clark, Jr., Lawrence J. Busse, Ronald G. Pratt, R. Samaratunga, Richard E. Hoffman, and Stephen L. Dieckman.

REFERENCES

1. Thomas SR, Ackerman JL, Gobel JR, et. al. Nuclear Magnetic Resonance Imaging Techniques as Developed Modestly Within a University Medical Center Environment: What Can The Small System Contribute at This Point? Magnetic Resonance Imaging, 1: 11-21, 1982.

2. Standard Man - Total Body Content For Some Elements. Radiological Health Handbook (Revised Edition): 214, U.S. Government Printing Office, 1970.

3. Goldman MR, Fossel ET, Ingwall T, et. al. Feasibility of ^{19}F as an Agent for NMR Imaging of Myocardial Infarction: An In Vivo Study. (Abstract) J. Nucl. Med. 20: 604, 1979.

4. McFarland E, Koutcher JA, Rosen BR, et. al. In Vivo ^{19}F NMR Imaging. J. Comp. Asst. Tomography, 9: 8-15, 1985.

5. Gallagher BM, Ansari A, Atkins H, et. al. ^{18}F Labeled 2-FDG as a Radiopharmaceutical for Measuring Regional Myocardial Glucose Metabolims In Vivo: Tissue Distribution and Imaging Studies in Animals. J. Nucl. Med. 18: 990-996, 1977.

6. Phelps ME, Hoffman EJ, Selin C, et. al. Investigation of ^{18}F 2-FDG for the Measure of Myocardial Glucose Metabolism. J. Nucl. Med. 19: 1311-1319, 1978.

7. Phelps ME, Mazziotta JC. Positron Emission Tomography: Human Brain Function and Biochemistry. Science 228: 799-809, 17 May 1985.

8. Tewson TJ, Welsh MJ, Raichle JE, et. al. ^{18}F Labeled 3-FDG; Synthesis and Preliminary Biodistribution Data. J. Nucl. Med. 19: 1339-1345, 1978.

9. Dwyer AJ, Knopp RH, Hoult DI. Frequency Shift Artifacts in MR Imaging. J. Comp. Asst. Tomography, 9: 16-18, 1985.

10. Busse LJ, Thomas SR, Pratt RG, et. al. Deconvolution Techniques for Removing the Effects of Chemical Shift in NMR Imaging of Perfluorocarbon Compounds. (Abstract.) Med. Phys. 12: 516, 1985.

11. Berkowitz BA and Ackerman JJH. 2-Fluoro-2-Deoxy-D-Glucose (2FDG) Metabolism In Vivo: A ^{19}F-(^{1}H) NMR Study. (Abstract.) The Society of Magnetic Resonance in Medicine - 4th Annual Meeting, August 19-23, 1985. London. 759-760.

12. Babcock EE and Nunnally RL. In Vivo and In Vitro Determination of 2-Fluoro-deoxyglucose by F-19 NMR Imaging and Spectroscopy. (Abstract.) The Society of Magnetic Resonance in Medicine - 4th Annual Meeting, August 19-23, 1985. London. 751-752.

13. Nakada T and Kwee IL. Non-Invasive Demonstraton of In Vivo 2-Fluoro-2-Deoxy-D-Glucose Metabolism in Rat Brain by F-19 NMR Spectroscopy. (Abstract.) The Society of Magnetic Resonance in Medicine - 4th Annual Meeting, August 19-23, 1985. London. 806-807.

14. Wyrwica AM, Murphy R, Prakash I, et. al., 2-Fluoro-2-Deoxy-D-Glucose Metabolism in the Rat Brain. The Society of Magnetic Resonance in Medicine - 4th Annual Meeting, August 19-23, 1985. London. 827-828.

15. Ohyanagi H, Toshima K, Sekita M, et. al. Clinical Studies of Perfluorochemical Whole Blood Substitutes: Safety of Fluosol-DA (20%) in Normal Human Volunteers. Clinical Therapeutic 2: 306-312, 1979.

16. Perfluorochemical Oxygen Transport. International Anesthesiology Clinics: Spring, 1985: Vol 23, No. 1. Little Brown and Company, Boston, 1985.

17. Clark LC, Jr., Gollan F. Survival of Mammals Breathing Organic Liquids Equilibrated with Oxygen at Atmospheric Pressure. Science 152: 1755-1756, 1966.

18. Wessler EP, Iltis R, Clark LC, Jr. The Solubility of Oxygen in Highly Fluorinated Liquids. J. Fluorine Chemistry 9: 137-146, 1977.

19. Clark LC, Jr., Becattini F, Kaplan S, et. al. Perfluorocarbons Having a Short Dwell Time in the Liver. Science 181: 680-682, 1973.

20. Holland GN, Bottomley PA, Hinshaw WS. ^{19}F Magnetic Resonance Imaging. J. Magn. Reson. 28: 133-136, 1977.

21. Clark LC, Jr., Ackerman JL, Thomas SR, et. al. Perfluorinated Organic Liquids and Emulsions as Biocompatible NMR Imaging Agents for 19-F and Dissolved Oxygen. In: Advances in Experimental Medicine and Biology, Volume 180: Oxygen Transport to Tissue-VI. Editors: D. Bruley, H.I. Bicher, D. Reneau. Plenum Publishing Corporation. PP. 835-845.

22. Clark LC, Jr., Ackerman JL, Thomas SR. et. al. High Contrast Tissue and Blood Oxygen Imaging Based on Fluorocarbon ^{19}F NMR Relaxation Times. (Abstract.) J. Mag. Res. Med. 1: 135-136, 1984.

23. Joseph PM, Yusasa Y, Kundel H, et. al. In Vivo Imaging of a Fluorinated Blood Substitute at Low Fields. (Abstract.) Med. Phys. 11: 375-376, 1984.

24. Thomas SR, Clark LC, Jr., Ackerman JL, et. al. NMR Imaging of Lung Using Liquid Perfluorocarbon. (Abstract.) Society of Magnetic Resonance in Medicine, 3rd Annual Meeting. New York, New York. August 13-17, 1984. PP. 717-718.

25. Thomas SR, Clark LC, Jr., Ackerman JL, et. al. NMR Imaging of the Lung Using Liquid Perfluorocarbons. Journal of Computer Assisted Tomography 10: 1-9, 1986.

26. Lai CS, Stain SJ, Miziorko H, et. al. Effect of Oxygen and Lipispin Label TEMPO-paurate on Fluorine-19 and Proton Relaxation Rates of the Perfluorochemical Blood Substitute, FC-43 Emulsion. J. Mag. Res. 57: 447-452, 1984.

27. Kong, CF, Holloway GM, Parhami P, et. al. Carbon-13 and Fluorine-19 NMR Study of Perfluorochemical Emulsions. J. Phys. Chem., 88: 6308-6311, 1984.

28. Clark LC, Jr., Thomas SR, Pratt RG, et. al. NMR determination of Liver pO_2 In Vivo Using Perfluorocarbon Emulsions. (Abstract.) Society of Magnetic Resonance in Medicine. 4th Annual Meeting. London, England. August 19-23, 1985. 40-41.

29. Ackerman, JL, Clark LC, Jr., Thomas SR, et. al. NMR Thermal Imaging. (Abstract.) The Society of Magnetic Resonance in Medicine - 3rd Annual Meeting. New York, New York. August 13-17, 1984. 1-2.

30. Heidelberger E, Lauterbur PC. Gas Phase ^{19}F-NMR Zeugmatography: A new Approach to Lung Ventilation Imaging. (Abstract.) 1st Annual Meeting. The Society of Magnetic Resonance in Medicine. August 16-18, 1982. Boston, MA. PP. 70-71.

31. Wyrwicz AM, Pszenny MH, Schofield JC, et. al. Noninvasive Observation of Fluorinated Anesthetics in Rabbit Brain by Fluorine-19 Nuclear Magnetic Resonance. Science 222: 429-430, 1983.

32. Wyrwicz AM, Ryback K, Pszenny MH. In Vivo ^{19}F NMR Study of Fluorinated Anesthetics Elimination From a Rabbit Brain. (Abstract) - 3rd Annual Meeting. The Society of Magnetic Resonance in Medicine. New York, New York. August 13-17, 1984. 763-764.

33. Conboy CB and Wyrwicz AM. Localization of Halothane in a Rat Brain with 19-F NMR Rotating Frame Zeugnatography. (Abstract.) of Magnetic Resonance in Medicine - 4th Annual Meeting. London. August 19-23, 1985.

34. Higuchi T, Naruse S, Horikawa Y, et. al. *In Vivo* 19-F NMR Spectroscopic Study of Normal and Pathological Brains. (Abstract.) The Society of Magnetic Resonance in Medicine - 4th Annual Meeting. London. August 19-23, 1985. 795-796.

35. Horner SD, Babcock EE, Nunnally RL. Evaluation of Myocardial Perfusion by ^{19}F NMR Imaging. (Abstract.) The Society of Magnetic Resonance in Medicine - 3rd Annual Meeting. New York, New York. August 13-17, 1984. 338-339.

36. Nunnally RL, Babcock EE, Antich P. The Direct Observation of 5-Fluorouracil Metabolism by the Liver in the Intact Rabbit: A 19-F NMR Study. (Abstract.) The Society of Magnetic Resonance in Medicine - 4th Annual Meeting. London. August 19-23, 1985. 810-811.

CHEMICAL SHIFT IMAGING

Ian L. Pykett, Ph.D.
Advanced NMR Systems, Inc. Woburn, MA 01801

ABSTRACT

An outline of the methods proposed and utilized for Chemical Shift Imaging is given, together with a summary of experimental and early clinical data thus obtained. The prospects of the wide-scale utilization of such techniques in clinical diagnosis and magnetic resonance research are discussed.

INTRODUCTION

Until recently, the techniques of clinical magnetic resonance imaging (MRI) and biological magnetic resonance spectroscopy (MRS) have developed somewhat independently. The former methods have utilized virtually exclusively the proton (^1H) resonance, to yield spatially-resolved images in which there is no discrimination among signals arising from hydrogen nuclei existing in different chemical groups; that is, no chemical shift resolution is obtained. In contrast, biological MRS studies have traditionally yielded nuclear magnetic resonance (NMR) spectra (rather than images) in which chemical shift resolution is of paramount importance. Such spectra contain no spatial information; they usually represent the integral of the signal from the entire sample enclosed within the receiver coil. Furthermore, the large majority of studies have been conducted using non-proton resonances, especially phosphorus (^{31}P) and (^{13}C), since these are of special importance in studies of metabolism.

Despite their rather contrary emphasis, MRI and MRS both have provided information of great biological and clinical significance. Furthermore the information obtained in each case, although emphasizing distinctly different aspects of the NMR phenomenon, has been entirely complementary.

Thus it has long been desirable to obtain both spectrally and spatially-resolved information in a single study. The principal barrier to practical implementation of such techniques of "spectroscopic imaging" or "chemical shift imaging" (CSI) has been related less to the lack of development of an appropriate theoretical solution than to the development of the appropriate technology. Spectroscopic applications, for instance, typically demand magnetic fields of both high uniformity (in order to obtain the requisite chemical shift resolution) and strength (in order to maximize spectral dispersion, and also to obtain adequate signal-to-noise ratios from nuclei of relatively low physiological abundance and NMR sensitivity). These requirements have been realizable for MRS research because the samples typically used (and, hence, the magnets required,) are relatively small; studies are usually performed on excised tissue, or small animals such as mice and rabbits. MRI, on the other hand, does not demand such a high-field strength because the signal obtained from the highly abundant and sensitive nucleus ^1H is relatively large. It has therefore been possible to develop low - and medium-field magnets sufficiently large that they can accommodate the whole human body.

The smaller, high-field system required for MRS and the larger, lower-field MRI systems have therefore tended to encourage mutual exclusivity. However, the development within the last two years of whole-body superconducting magnets with field strengths as high as 2.0 tesla, together with the addition of imaging capabilities on smaller, research-oriented spectroscopy systems, has led to substantial growth in the area of combined imaging and spectroscopy. The convergence of the disciplines has been helped also by the development and implementation in both MRI and MRS, of surface coil technology.

The following sections outline briefly the variety of techniques which have been utilized in spectroscopic imaging, and review the data thus obtained.

METHODS OF CHEMICAL SHIFT IMAGING

The development of "surface coils[1]" and localized magnetic resonance ("FONAR[2]" and "Topical Magnetic Resonance[3] (TMR)) enabled NMR spectra to be acquired noninvasively from a small localized volume ("sensitive point") within intact biological samples. In surface coil techniques, a small radiofrequency (RF) coil is used to acquire the resonance signal only from the tissue adjacent to, or close to[4], the coil. Localized NMR techniques employ high-order static magnetic field gradients to create a small region of homogeneous field deep within the object. This method of magnetic field profiling is often used in conjunction with surface coils, such that the combined spatial selectivity of the two methods yields an increased definition of the region of interest.

A simplistic approach to true chemical shift imaging, in which spectral information is obtained independently from many locations within a selected volume, would involve scanning a sensitive point step by step throughout the desired region or, alternatively, would involve moving the object periodically throughout the sensitive region, thus obtaining an NMR spectrum at any number of points. This approach, however, suffers from the low sensitivity common to all point-imaging methods[5]. Of the techniques thus far proposed for electronic control of the location of the sensitive point[6,9], three[6,8] utilize RF pulse and field gradient control sequences that render the amplitudes of the spectral lines a complicated function of the relaxation times, making quantitative studies difficult[10].

Several techniques have been proposed or demonstrated in which the increased sensitivity of line, plane, or whole-volume imaging is combined with chemical shift spectroscopy measurements [11-17]. Such approaches in general allow NMR spectra to be extracted from all points within the image matrix or, alternatively, separate images corresponding to each of the chemically shifted peaks may be displayed. A number of these reports[13,17] utilize various extensions of the original Fourier imaging technique[18] or its rotating frame analog[19]. Many variations on the basic "Fourier CSI" theme are possible. Thus, for example, most frequently a three-dimensional Fourier technique has been used, in which two dimensions encode for spatial information within a pre-selected plane, and the third dimension provides chemical shift resolution. However, this may be extended to a four-dimensional CSI experiment in order to obtain three resolved spatial dimensions at the expense of an increased data acquisition time. Spatial information is most often obtained via the usual method of applying phase-encoding gradients after RF excitation but prior to signal sampling, as in non-chemical-shift-resolved Fourier Imaging[20]. Spectral resolution is then obtained by sampling the signal in the absence of magnetic field gradients. In the case of Fourier techniques applied in the rotating frame, the NMR spin system is excited with a non-uniform RF field. Specifically, the RF field distribution applied is in the form of a linear RF field gradient, such that the angle of tip of the magnetization vectors varies linearly in the direction of the gradient. By analogy with Fourier imaging methods in which a series of data acquisitions is obtained while successively increasing the magnitude of the phase-encoding gradient, in the case of rotating frame CSI, the NMR signal is sampled following successive increases of RF field intensity. Rotating frame CSI has been demonstrated thus far only for one-dimensional spectroscopic imaging[13]. It is straightforward to adapt this method for spectroscopic imaging using surface coils, for which a non-uniform (and also, non-linear) RF field distribution is inherent [21,23].

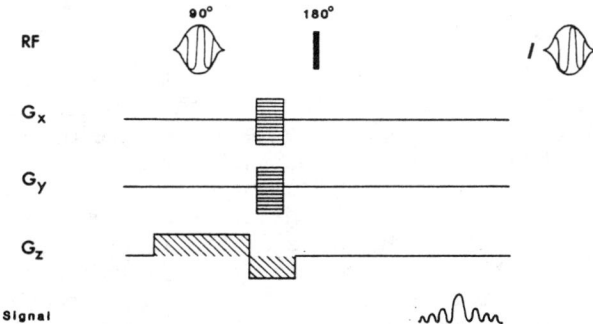

Fig. 1. Schematic representation of a generalized pulse sequence used to perform three-dimensional CSI. (Reprinted from Rosen BR, Pykett IL, and Brady TJ, In: Biomedical Magnetic (Resonance (ed. James TL and Margulis A), Radiology Research and Education Foundation, San Francisco (1984) by permission).

Figures 1 and 2 give a schematic representation of a generalized RF pulse and magnetic field gradient timing diagram, and consequent data matrix, for a three-dimensional Fourier CSI experiment.

The pulse sequence in Figure 1 utilizes phase encoding gradients for spatial localization in the x and y axes, following selection of a tomographic plane in the z axis. The signal, elicited as a spin-echo, is sampled in the absence of any field gradient.

Following successive applications of the pulse sequence of Figure 1, during which the magnitudes of the phase-encoding gradients G_x and G_y are progressively increased, a three-dimensional data set is generated. Following Fourier-transformation, the data matrix will be as shown in Figure 2.

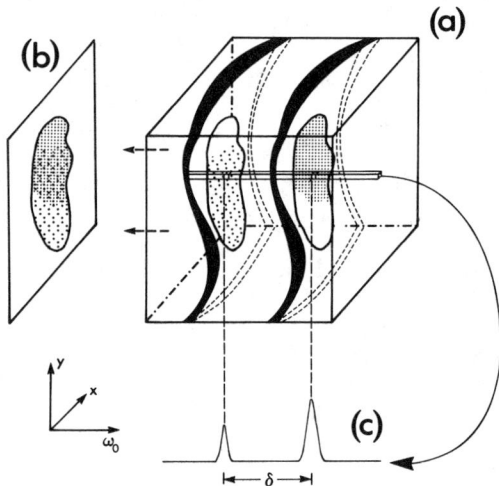

Fig. 2 Sketch of the three dimensional array (a) obtained following Fourier Transformation of the time data. The spatial coordinate axes are denoted x and y, and ω_0 defines the chemical shift axis. Each chemical shift-resolved image is distributed about a curved surface; in this sketch the varying "thickness" of the image data demonstrates schematically the way in which the line width of a particular peak may alter depending on the local field heterogeneity. The more usual, nonchemical shift-resolved image (b) is obtained by integrating the data along the ω_0 axis. An NMR spectrum (c) may be retrieved from any x,y coordinate. (Reprinted from Pykett IL et al., Radiology, 149 (1983) by permission).

Image data corresponding to each of the spectral peaks (a "δ-image") is distributed about a curved surface; the precise shape of the surface is defined by the static field non-uniformities within the selected section. The width of the distribution of data on either side of the surface will depend on the line width of the particular peak, which may arbitrarily be defined as $f_{\frac{1}{2}}$ the full width at half maximum height. As in conventional NMR spectroscopy, both intrinsic (sample-related) line broadening mechanisms and static magnetic field heterogeneities (ΔB_0) define $f_{\frac{1}{2}}$. Note, however, that in this case the line-broadening contribution from ΔB_0 depends only on the magnetic field non-uniformity over any given voxel which, since the voxels may be made almost arbitrarily small, will usually be very much less than the nonuniformity in B_0 extant over the whole imaging volume. The effect of this latter heterogeneity is only to shift the NMR spectra arising from each of the voxels relative to one another. Indeed, this provides a convenient method for mapping the magnetic field distribution.[24] When more than one resolved peak exists in the NMR spectrum, the separate δ-images will each be distributed about similar curved surfaces, parallel to one another, and separated by their chemical shift differences.

The more usual proton NMR image may be derived by integrating the NMR spectrum at each voxel location. This corresponds to the projection of all the various δ-images onto a plane orthogonal to the chemical shift axis, and may be obtained simply by summing all of the reconstructed image data planes.

Spectroscopic variants of the "echo-planar" imaging method have also recently been proposed[25]. In echo-planar imaging, a completely resolved spatial image is obtained in a single data acquisition sequence[26,27]. In the spectroscopic variant, four-cycle data sequences are proposed which again would enable very rapid and efficient data collection. However, application of these methods is likely to be less appropriate for imaging of nuclei other than ^{1}H, since the required signal averaging would tend to vitiate the advantages gained by the much more technically complex rapid acquisition schemes.

In the event that there exists <u>a-priori</u> knowledge of the NMR spectrum of the object of interest, and it is required simply to measure the amplitudes of the constituent peaks (whose chemical shift positions are assumed to remain fixed relative to one another), then it is possible to perform one of a variety of other spectroscopic imaging methods in which images of only specific peaks are generated. For example, techniques of selective saturation or selective excitation may be employed to suppress or independently excite specific spectral resonances [28,29]. Such methods may be utilized to obtain images of moieties present only at low concentrations, against a background of normally high signal arising from similar nuclei in much more abundant (but chemically-shifted) compounds. Thus, a selective saturation pulse at the frequency of the ($-CH_2-$) lipid resonance in a biological sample, applied immediately prior to each pulse sequence in a standard imaging experiment, will greatly reduce the contribution of lipid signals to the overall proton response.

Another method, especially simple to implement in practice,

requires sampling of the NMR signal in the presence of a magnetic field gradient. In this case, chemical shift information is encoded by altering the pulse sequence timing parameters and detecting the consequent phase changes in the acquired signals. This has been demonstrated for the special case of just two spectral peaks[30] (the ^{1}H resonances from lipid and from water) in which, for one image denoted the "opposed" image, the pulse sequence timing parameters are chosen so that the signals from water and from fat are sampled exactly 180-degrees out of phase with each other. For a second image, denoted the "in-phase" image, the parameters are adjusted as for normal imaging such that the water and lipid resonances are in phase. Subtraction and addition of the two resultant images yields images of fat only and water only, respectively. This method permits resolution of chemical shift information even at low field strengths. Furthermore, magnetic field non-uniformities are manifested as phase errors, which can effectively be removed by using the magnitude of the Fourier transformed data. However, negative signals in the opposed image then cannot be distinguished from positive signals of equal magnitude, resulting in possible interpretational ambiguities.

The method of encoding chemical shift information via altering the pulse sequence timing parameters can be extended to obtain chemical shift images when the spectral distribution is not known a priori[31].

EARLY EXPERIMENTAL DATA

The first NMR Chemical Shift Images obtained in-vivo exhibited resolved resonances from lipid and water protons in a cat-head and in a human forearm.[16] In addition to demonstration of the technique itself, these data showed that no lipid signal was observed from the brain, indicating that the discrimination between grey and white matter tissue observed on clinical NMR head images is probably due to local modifications of water proton relaxation times rather than to direct observation of myelin lipids per se. This finding has since been corroborated for human brain tissue[32].

Subsequent studies, using fatty liver model in rats, evaluated the potential of the technique for investigation and diagnosis of fatty liver disease[33,34], which had not been diagnosable in earlier studies performed without the benefit of chemical shift resolution[35]. Relaxation times of each of the two principal peaks in the spectrum were also determined, demonstrating two distinct populations of non-exchanging protons. An excellent correlation between lipid signal amplitudes obtained in-vivo, and liver triglyceride levels subsequently obtained in vitro, was found. The technique has recently been extended to determine the feasibility of studying less abundant metabolites (specifically, lactates) using solvent suppression (selective saturation) methods[29].

The method of spectroscopic imaging noted above, based on observation of phase shifts introduced as a result of differences in resonance frequencies between two spectral peaks, has also been applied to the study of fatty infiltration of the liver[36], in this case in humans. Again, increased sensitivity of detection to this class of disease was observed when spectroscopic discrimination was used. An abnormal fat-to-water ratio in the bone marrow of a patient with a relapse of chronic myeloid leukemia has also been demonstrated by CSI[31].

Three-dimensional Fourier CSI techniques have been utilized to obtain spectroscopically-resolved in-vivo ^{31}P images of the cat brain[37], indicating the potential to monitor local metabolic events in this manner. Similar methods have also been used to obtain ^{19}F images of a variety of clinically-safe fluorinated compounds, for use as potential contrast agents or probes of physiological function (e.g.: anesthetic perfusion and phagocytic activity in the liver)[38].

Finally, it has been brought to the attention of the MRI community[39,40] that in conventional proton imaging procedures, where spectral resolution is not explicitly required, the chemical shift phenomenon can nevertheless manifest itself as an asymmetric boundary artefact. This is observed at interfaces between tissues having different chemically shifted resonances. The artefact is especially evident at the junction of peri-renal fat and renal parenchyma; its existence could potentially lead to erroneous diagnosis.

SUMMARY

Proton chemical shift imaging is already becoming an accepted adjunct to standard magnetic resonance imaging procedures for some diseases. The potential clinical or biological utility of spectroscopic imaging of other nuclei remains to be evaluated; the primary problem is related to the very long imaging times typically required for completely resolved chemical shift images. The techniques most likely to become useful are those in which adequate signal-to-noise ratio and spatial resolution can be obtained in a reasonable period of time. Surface coil technology, which maximizes sensitivity by virtue of an increased filling factor, used together with one of the wide variety of chemical shift imaging methods, might therefore become one such class of methods.

Via chemical shift imaging, the physician and the research scientist are able to glean information of a truly chemical and biochemical nature in a completely non-invasive manner. Such information may not be available through any other procedure.

REFERENCES

1. Ackerman, J.J.H., et al: Nature 283, 167 (1980).
2. Damadian, R., et al: Science 194, 1430 (1976).
3. Gordon, R.E., et al: Nature 287, 736 (1980).
4. Ng, T.C., Glickson, J.D., Bendall, M.R.: Mag. Res. in Med. 1, 450 (1984).

REFERENCES (Cont.)

5. Brunner, P., Ernst, R.R.: J. Mag. Res. 33, 83 (1979).
6. Hinshaw, W.S.: J. Appl. Phys. 47, 3709 (1976).
7. Bottomley, P.A.: J. Mag. Res. 50, 335 (1982).
8. Scott, K.N., et al: J. Mag. Res. 50, 339 (1982).
9. Aue, W.P., et al: J. Mag. Res. 56, 350 (1984).
10. Meire, F.T., Thatcher, F.C.: J. Appl. Phys. 50, 4491 (1979).
11. Lauterbur, P.C., et al: J. Amer. Chem. Soc. 97, 6866 (1975).
12. Bendel, P., Lai, C-M, Lauterbur, P.C.: J. Mag. Res. 38, 343 (1980).
13. Cox, S.J., Styles, P.: J. Mag. Res. 40, 209 (1980).
14. Brown, T.R., Kincaid, B.M., Ugurbil, K.: Proc. Natl. Acad. Sci. USA 79, 3523 (1982).
15. Maudsley, A.A., et al: J. Mag. Res. 51, 147 (1983).
16. Pykett, I.L., Rosen, B.R.: Radiology 149, 197 (1983).
17. Hall, L.D., Sukumar, S.: J. Mag. Res. 56, 314 (1984).
18. Kumar, A., Welti, D., Ernst, R.R.: J. Mag. Res. 18, 69 (1975).
19. Hoult, D.I.: J. Mag. Res. 33, 183 (1979).
20. Edelstein, W.A., et al: Phys. Med. Biol. 25, 751 (1980).
21. Haase, A., Malloy, C., Radda, G.K.: J. Mag. Res. 55, 164 (1983).
22. Schleich, T., et al: Proceedings of the Third Ann. Mtg., Soc. Mag. Res. in Med., p.661 (1984).
23. Clarke, G.D., Nunnally, R.L.: Proceedings of the Third Ann. Mtg., Soc. Mag. Res. in Med., p.161 (1984).
24. Maudsley, A.A., Simon, H.E., Hilal, S.K.: J. Phys. E17, 216 (1984).
25. Mansfield, P.: Mag. Res. in Med. 1, 370 (1984).
26. Mansfield, P., Pykett, I.L.: J. Mag. Res. 29, 355 (1978).
27. Rzedzian, R., et al: Lancet, p. 1281 (December 1983).
28. Hall, L.D., Sukumar, S., Talagala, S.L.: J. Mag. Res. 56, 275 (1984).
29. Rosen, B.R., Wedeen, V.J., Brady, T.J.: J. Comput. Assist. Tomogr. 8, 813 (1984).
30. Dixon, W.T.: Radiology 153, 189 (1984).
31. Sepponen, R.E., Sipponen, J.T., Tanttu, J.I. J. Comput. Assist. Tomogr., 8, 585 (1984).
32. Bottomley, P.A., et al: Radiology 150, 441 (1984).
33. Rosen, B.R., et al: Radiology 154, 469 (1985).
34. Rosen, B.R., Pykett, I.L., Brady,T.J., In: James,T.L. and Margulis, A.R. (eds) Biomedical Magnetic Resonance (Radiology Research and Education Foundation, San Francisco) p.257, (1984).
35. Stark, D.D. et al: Radiology 148, 743 (1983).
36. Lee, J.K.T. et al: Radiology 153, 195 (1984).
37. Maudsley, AA et al: Radiology 153, 745 (1984).
38. McFarland, E. et al: J. Comput. Assist. Tomogr., 9, 8 (1985).
39. Soila, K., Viamonte M., Jr and Starewicz,P.M.: Radiology 153, 819 (1984).
40. Babcock E.E. et al: H, Comput. Assist. Tomogr. 9, 252 (1985).

PARAMAGNETIC PHARMACEUTICALS IN BIOMEDICAL MAGNETIC RESONANCE

George E. Wesbey

University of Washington, School of Medicine

Seattle, WA 98195

INTRODUCTION

The ultimate value of diagnostic pharmaceuticals in magnetic resonance imaging (MRI) and spectroscopy is presently uncertain. With regard to MRI, we begin with the premise that there are stages or types of diseases for which the sensitivity or specificity of lesion diagnosis can be increased by pharmacologically altering image contrast. This premise has held true for all imaging modalities studied to date. With this in mind, the issue is not whether diagnostic pharmaceuticals will be incorporated into routine MRI, but rather under what circumstances and by what mechanisms they will be clinically useful. The ultimate role of diagnostic paramagnetic pharmaceuticals for in vivo magnetic resonance spectroscopy is unclear because they are still in the embryonic stage of clinical development and therefore will not be discussed in detail in this chapter.

In MRI, with the wide variety of sequences of operator-selected radio-frequency (RF) and magnetic gradient pulse sequences available to manipulate image contrast, instances of "isointense" lesions are rare. This totally noninvasive way to show MRI contrast between normal and abnormal tissues is by operator-manipulation of the various and gradient pulse sequences, such as altering the RF pulse repetition time (TR), the inversion-delay time (TI), and the spin-echo delay time (TE). The pulsed magnetic gradient sequence also affects the MRI signal intensity and can be manipulated (Wesbey et al., 1984a). These nonpharmaceutical manipulations may well be sufficient for detecting disease with MRI. However, the search for the optimum MRI pulse sequence to detect a lesion is a time-consuming process, and patient evaluation is prolonged. Use of paramagnetic pharmaceuticals to hasten identification of isointense lesions may come to be an economic necessity in MRI. Most diagnostic imaging studies have instances of limited sensitivity or specificity, or both. MRI is currently very sensitive to the detection of abnormality, but not often helpful in distinguishing among the various possible causes for the abnormality. Tissue-, organ-, or tumor-specific paramagnetic pharmaceuticals could prove a useful supplement to the routine practice of MRI in lesion detection and characterization. Another use for MRI paramagnetic pharmaceuticals is for assessing organ perfusion at the capillary level; for example, the assessment of the functional integrity of the kidney (Brasch et al., 1983a).

Other manipulations of MRI signal intensity for contrast purposes can be accomplished by using strategies other than paramagnetic enhancement of nuclear relaxation. Alterations of nuclear spin-density or tissue temperature or viscosity may be utilized as alternative pharmacological or physical methods of contrast enhancement. For instance, alteration of temperature in biological systems to change MRI signal intensity is presently impractical in the clinical setting. Reduction of water viscosity to decrease T1 (spin-lattice) and T2 (spin-spin) relaxation times can be achieved by use of ethanol (Dornbluth, et al., 1982). However, patients could not drive home after administration of ethanol. Proposed "spin-density" modifying agents, such as furosemide, olive oil or clomiphene (Beall, 1984), would be poorly tolerated by most patients at the doses studied in animals for alteration of relaxation rates in normal tissue adjacent to neoplastic tissue. Caille et al. (1982) have proposed glucose as a spin-density modifying agent. A drawback to spin-density modifying agents is that the best contrast between tissues of differing mobile spin density is observed at time-consuming long RF pulse repetition times (TR greater than four times T1, asymptotic imaging) (Wehrli et al., 1983). In contrast, paramagnetic shortening of T1 relaxation times, in our experience, achieved optimal lesion-to-background contrast with short TR values (0.5 sec or less), thereby reducing imaging time.

Paramagnetic pharmaceuticals are the most promising group of diagnostic MRI pharmaceuticals; they can demonstrate temporal profiles of proton relaxation enhancement, depending on pharmaceutical biodistribution. Unlike electron-absorbing contrast agents used in radiography, or radioactive isotopes used in nuclear medicine, the paramagnetic agents used in MRI are not directly displayed on the image. Rather, it is their indirect effect on water-proton relaxation rates that is displayed in the images as changes in MRI signal intensity.

MRI METHODS

Unless otherwise noted, all MRI studies with paramagnetic pharmaceuticals discussed hereafter were investigated on a 3.5 Kgauss spin-echo MRI system. Two such MRI units at the University of California, San Francisco were employed for these studies (Crooks et al., 1980; Crooks et al., 1982). The first is a .35 T resistive magnet system with a 6.5 cm effective aperture for imaging of small animals and in-vitro samples. Spatial resolution was 0.5 mm by 1 mm in the X and Y dimensions with a slice thickness of 4.2 mm. The second MRI unit was a 0.35 Tesla superconducting magnet with a 55 cm effective aperture for imaging. Slice thickness was 7 mm. On each MRI system, 2 Carr-Purcell spin-echo's were routinely obtained at 28 and 56 msec after the selective 90° radiofrequency pulse. (TE, time to echo, 28 and 56 msec.) Pulse repetition times (TR) chosen ranged from 0.5 to 2 sec. Four averages of the RF signal were routinely utilized. Images were acquired by interleaved multisection 2D-Fourier transformation with phase encoding (spin-warp imaging).

With the radiofrequency pulse sequence employed at our institution, MRI signal intensity can be expressed by the approximation: $I = N(H)f(v)(exp-TE/T2)[1-exp(-TR/T1)]$. $N(H)$ is the density of mobile hydrogen nuclei; $f(v)$ is the proton velocity function; the other variables have been defined. The assumptions underlying this approximation for MRI signal intensity are discussed by Herfkens et al., (1981). As one can deduce from this formula, signal intensity increases with a shorter T1 and/or a long T2 relaxation time. Conversely, with long T1s and/or short T2s, signal intensity decreases. Intensity also increases with increasing mobile spin concentration. Flowing hydrogen nuclei also affect the MRI signal intensity. Molecular self-diffusion of water protons through pulsed magnetic gradients used in MRI can reduce the observed T2 relaxation time and thus reduce signal intensity (Wesbey, et al., 1984a).

PARAMAGNETISM

Enhancement of water proton relaxation times by addition of paramagnetic ions is as old as the discovery of the proton resonance signal (Bloch et al., 1946). Thus, introducing paramagnetic pharmaceuticals into biological fluids or tissues can alter signal intensity contrast between tissues because of proton relaxation enhancement, namely shortening of T1 and/or T2.

The idea of incorporating paramagnetic agents into biological systems for in vivo MRI, to change tissue contrast by reduction of T1 and T2 relaxation times, was first proposed by Lauterbur (1978). In this article, the use of intravenously administered manganese ion as a potential myocardial perfusion agent was first introduced to the early MRI literature. Hollis et al. (1978) initially proposed the use of the manganese ion for in vivo relaxation enhancement of phosphorus-31 chemical shift resonances of myocardial phosphorylated metabolites.

Three types of magnetic properties are of interest in MRI: paramagnetic, diamagnetic, and ferromagnetic. Paramagnetic substances are characterized by unpaired protons or electrons. These spinning charged particles generate a local magnetic field. Since the magnetic moment of the electron is 658 times greater than the proton (Weast et al., 1981), the magnetic moments of free radicals or ions with unpaired electrons will be much greater than molecules with only unpaired nuclei, and will hereafter be referred to as paramagnetic. Paramagnetics develop a magnetic field, and those with unpaired electrons can be spectroscopically analyzed by a magnetic resonance technique called electron spin resonance (ESR; also called electron paramagnetic resonance, or EPR). Diamagnetic substances repel an applied magnetic field. 99.5% of biological tissue constituents are diamagnetic whereas only 0.5% are paramagnetic (Swartz, 1982). Ferromagnetic substances develop such a large magnetic polarization when placed in a weak magnetic field (Pauling, 1960), that with removal of the magnetic field, many ferromagnets (such as metallic iron) retain their magnetization. Since ferromagnetism is a "domain" phenomenon, metal ion complexes or free radicals in solution can be either paramagnetic or diamagnetic but not ferromagnetic. No human tissues or fluids are known to be ferromagnetic (Brittenham et al., 1982).

Effect on Nuclear Relaxation Rates

In the absence of a paramagnetic solute, the principal relaxation mechanism of solvent nuclei is related to random Brownian motion and the viscous or frictional forces involved in such motion (Poole et al., 1971). How does the presence of a paramagnetic substance, such as a metal ion complex, effect T1 and T2 relaxation of neighboring water protons in solution? This is best explained by first looking at T1, or the growth towards equilibrium magnetization. Nuclear spins align parallel (lower energy state) or antiparallel (higher energy state) to an applied static magnetic field (Fukushima et al., 1981). Growth towards equilibrium magnetization of the sample (T1 relaxation) takes place as high energy spins give up energy to become low energy spins. In the classical NMR experiment, this growth is initiated by the RF pulse at the nuclear precessional frequency. The paramagnetic, with its very large magnetic moment relative to that of the proton, tumbles randomly in solution. This creates randomly varying fields at the hyrdrogen nucleus distributed in frequency and time. The time distribution and frequency distribution of the local fields are Fourier transform pairs. The frequency dependence of the carrying magnetic fields is called the spectral density. The fluctuating magnetic field from the tumbling paramagnets have a frequency component of its spectral density that fluctuates at the proton Larmor precessional frequency. The amplitude of this local magnetic field at the Larmor nuclear frequency is determined by the dynamics of the electron-nuclear interaction. Thus, a magnetic field interaction (similar to the RF pulse in the NMR experiment) between the electron magnetic dipole and the nuclear magnetic dipole induces a transition of the higher energy nuclear spins (antiparallel to the applied static magnetic field) to the lower energy nuclear spins (parallel to the field). This mechanism is termed an electron-nuclear dipolar interaction. The tumbling paramagnetic ions can be thought of as multiple additional RF pulse transmitters which hasten these nuclear spin energy transitions. T1 is thus shortened by paramagnetic ions that "broadcast" at the protons' Larmor frequency.

T2 proton relaxation is observed at the termination of the 90° RF pulse. The RF pulse synchronized the protons' precession in phase at a uniform Larmor frequency in the X-Y (transverse) plane of the rotating frame of reference. At termination of the RF pulse, differing local magnetic environments within the sample cause precessing protons to lose their synchrony and phase, since their Larmor frequencies become more heterogenous. T2 measures the decay process of the bulk magnetization vector in the transverse (X-Y) plane as magnetic energy is distributed within the spin system. Tumbling paramagnetic ions, with their large magnetic moments, act to augment the variations in local magnetic fields experienced by the protons and make them dephase faster. Thus, T2 decay is enhanced.

Relaxation times (T1 and T2) are often expressed as relaxation rates (1/T1, 1/T2). Thus paramagnetic relaxation-enhancers decrease relaxation times and increase relaxation rates.

Scalar (also called contact or hyperfine) contributions to proton relaxation enhancement are also important for a few paramagnetics, such as the Mn^{+2} aquoion. The unpaired electron is sufficiently delocalized so that much of its local magnetic field is exerted on adjacent water protons in the immediate hydration shell surrounding the aquoion.

Paramagnetic agents can exhibit different relaxation-rate enhancement of water protons with the different static magnetic field strengths proposed for human MRI (Engelstad et al., 1983; Brown et al., 1985). This complicated phenomenon of dispersion of relaxation rates suggests that the "ideal" paramagnetic relaxation-enhancer should have field-independent relaxivity characteristics. Such an "ideal" paramagnetic may well be difficult to find. Relaxation rate dispersion can be due to the paramagnetic correlation time, T_c. This variable reflects the time-scale of the important electron-nuclear dipolar interaction that modulates relaxation rate enhancement. Another variable that affects paramagnetic proton relaxation is the magnetic moment (μ). The relationship between μ and the relaxation rate enhancement is [$1/T1$, $1/T2 \propto \mu$]. However, one cannot generalize from this relationship that with greater magnetic moments, one always sees greater proton relaxation enhancement. It is the effective magnetic moment (μ_{eff}) which better predicts the relaxivity characteristics of a paramagnetic. The cations with the strongest absolute magnetic moment in the atomic table, Dysprosium $^{+3}$, and Holmium^{+3} (10.5 Bohr magnetons) (Kyker et al., 1956) are poor proton relaxers (Pople et al., 1959), due to a weaker μ_{eff}. A very important variable affecting relaxation rate enhancement is the distance, r, from the water proton to the paramagnetic center. The relaxation rates are directly proportional to r^{-6} (Dwek, 1973). Relaxation rates increase linearly with the coordination number of the metal ion or metal complexes due to a greater number of inner sphere coordination sites available for water proton access to the unpaired electron(s).

It should be noted that all of the aforementioned discussions on paramagnetic effects on proton relaxation apply to other NMR sensitive nuclei of biological interest, including ^{13}C, ^{19}F, ^{23}Na, and ^{31}P. Not all paramagnetics effectively enhance proton relaxation. Those paramagnetics with strong magnetic moments without strong proton relaxation effects are often excellent chemical shift reagents for NMR spectroscopy studies. Such an example is the previously mentioned Dy^{+3} cation. Chemical shift reagents cause upfield or downfield displacement in the Larmor resonance frequency of molecules containing a particular nucleus, providing potentially valuable biomolecular information. Thus both intravenously administered paramagnetic "shift reagents" or relaxation-enhancers may one day be used in human NMR spectroscopy studies. In addition, in vivo ^{13}C and ^{19}F imaging or spectroscopy will probably occur with exogenously administered pharmaceuticals containing ^{13}C enriched foodstuffs, or perfluorocarbon emulsions with ^{19}F.

Paramagnetic Effects on the MRI Signal

As previously noted, paramagnetic relaxation-enhancers shorten T1 and T2 relaxation times of neighboring hydrogen nuclei. This dual effect creates very complex changes in the MRI signal, which further depends on the RF pulse sequence chosen (saturation-recovery, inversion-recovery, or spin-echo). T1 shortening by paramagnetics acts to increase signal intensity; T2 shortening acts to decrease intensity. The concentration of the paramagnetic also affects the relative changes in T1 and T2 shortening. MRI estimates of in vivo relaxation time decreases induced by paramagnetics may be of diagnostic utility, rather than complex intensity changes.

DESIRED PHARMACEUTICAL PROPERTIES OF PARAMAGNETICS

As with all diagnostic pharmaceuticals in radiology and nuclear medicine today, paramagnetic pharmaceuticals should be pure, stable, nontoxic, readily available, and inexpensive. They should have the potential to be conjugable to tissue or organspecific biomolecules and should undergo efficient renal excretion. Most proposed paramagnetic pharmaceuticals for MRI to date have not had prior toxicity studies in biological systems. Those proposed agents that have had extensive toxicity studies, such as manganese and other metal or rare earth ions, are unsuitable for consideration of usage in human patients in an unaltered state (Christensen, 1972). Metal ions complexed to ligands retain their paramagnetic behavior and have greater likelihood of tolerance in biological systems (Wesbey et al., 1983b).

PARAMAGNETIC AGENTS

Paramagnetic agents have been delivered to biological systems in MRI by three routes of administration: oral, intravenous, and inhalational. The following review of paramagnetic MRI studies will be organized into these three categories.

Oral Gastrointestinal Agents

Currently, several problems face abdominal MRI. Unless one performs sagittal, coronal, and axial imaging on all patients, sectional imaging in general is not ideal for identification of segments of gut. Variability exists in the anatomic position of the gut from patient to patient; motion of the gut by peristalsis changes the contour and position of the gut. Despite generally superior soft tissue contrast in MRI, the gut wall can be isointense with adjacent abdominal organs (Wesbey et al., 1983a) (Figure 1).

Several paramagnetic and nonparamagnetic agents have been proposed as potential GI labeling agents. The first proposed agent was mineral oil. Newhouse et al. (1981) injected 30 cc of mineral oil by esophagogastric intubation into guinea pigs, and found resultant high signal intensity within the stomach and small bowel in animal MRI experiments. However, the required volume of mineral oil necessary to opacify the GI tract in humans would quite likely lead to undesirable side effects, such as diarrhea. Young et al. (1981) administered 300 ml of 2% ferric chloride solution to an adult volunteer. Opacification of the fundus of the stomach was found on inversion recovery NMR imaging. However, aqueous ferric chloride is toxic, as manifested by marked GI irritation (Spector, 1956), (Christensen, 1972). Water has also been proposed as a GI labeling agent (Hutchison, Smith, 1983). These investigators found that the MRI intensity of water within the GI tract on their imagers was desirable for pancreatic delineation. Clinton et al. (1983) have studied 3 potential GI contrast agents for MRI. The first is gadolinium-oxalate, an insoluble suspension of gadolinium, the most powerful proton relaxer in the atomic table (Pople, 1959). The other proposed GI labeling agents by this group have been chromium-EDTA and chromium acetylacetonate. Contrast-opacification of the GI tract has been demonstrated with both chromium-EDTA and gadolinium-oxalate. Investigations at the University of California, San Francisco, have centered on the use of paramagnetic ferric ammonium citrate, a commonly available iron compound found in nonprescription pharmaceuticals (Wesbey et al., 1983a, 1985).

Ferric ammonium citrate (FAC) is the major ingredient in liquid Geritol R (J.B. Williams Co.) (Baker, 1982). From in-vitro and animal imaging studies of aqueous FAC in dilute concentrations, a prototype human GI dose of 500 ml of 1 millimolar (mM) FAC was formulated. Dilute iron solutions shorten the T1 of water protons, increasing MRI signal intensity. This

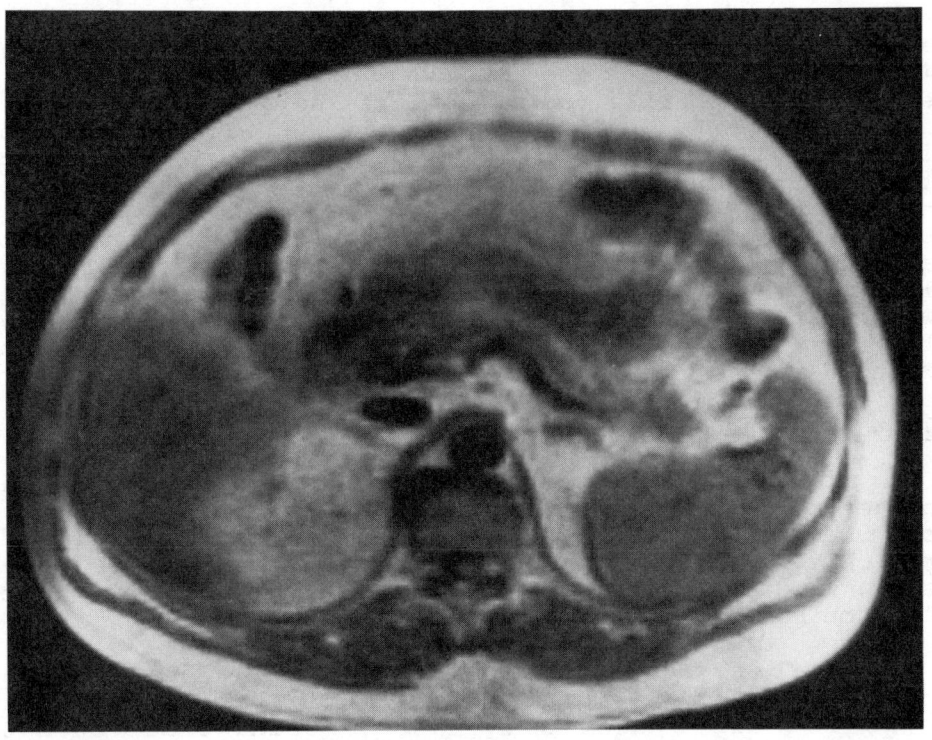

Figure 1. Transaxial magnetic resonance (MR) image (TR = 1.0 sec; TE = 28 msec) of the upper abdomen in a supine adult patient. Notice the inability to distinguish the duodenal portion of the gastrointestinal tract from the immediately adjacent head of pancreas. No paramagnetic oral agent was given. (Reprinted with permission from Wesbey GE, Brasch RC, Engelstad BL, et al. Radiology 149:174-180, 1983.)

dose of 500 ml of 1 mM ferric ammonium citrate amounts to 49% of the dose recommended for daily supplementation and 16% of the dose recommended for the treatment of iron deficiency anemia. Representative examples of contrast-enhancement of the stomach and duodenum in various human volunteers are illustrated in Figures 2 - 3.

An unresolved question is whether GI labeling agents are more useful by producing increased or decreased image intensity, i.e. positive versus negative contrast enhancement. Unlike radiographic techniques, MRI depicts fat as very high signal intensity. The problem of isointensity of iron or other paramagnetic agents with fat may be overcome by proper selection of the RF or gradient pulse sequences. However, the simple utilization of negative contrast agents, such as water or air may well turn out to be the optimal method for GI labeling in MRI. Preliminary results in our department with the use of water have been disappointing because of the isointensity of water with adjacent visceral organs with TR ranging from 1.0 to 2.0 seconds (Figure 4).

Intravenous Agents

There are two major categories of intravenous paramagnetic agents potentially suitable as diagnostic pharmaceuticals in MRI. The first is organic free radicals, in particular the nitroxide spin labels. The second is transition metal and rare earth complexes, such as iron, manganese, and gadolinium.

Nitroxide spin labels (NSL) are stable free radicals that have been widely used in molecular biophysical research since the early 1960s. Using electron spin resonance (ESR) spectroscopy, NSL have proven to be valuable in the study of molecular motion particularly within cell membranes. NSL are readily combined chemically with a variety of biomolecules and pharmaceuticals and thus serve as paramagnetic labeling

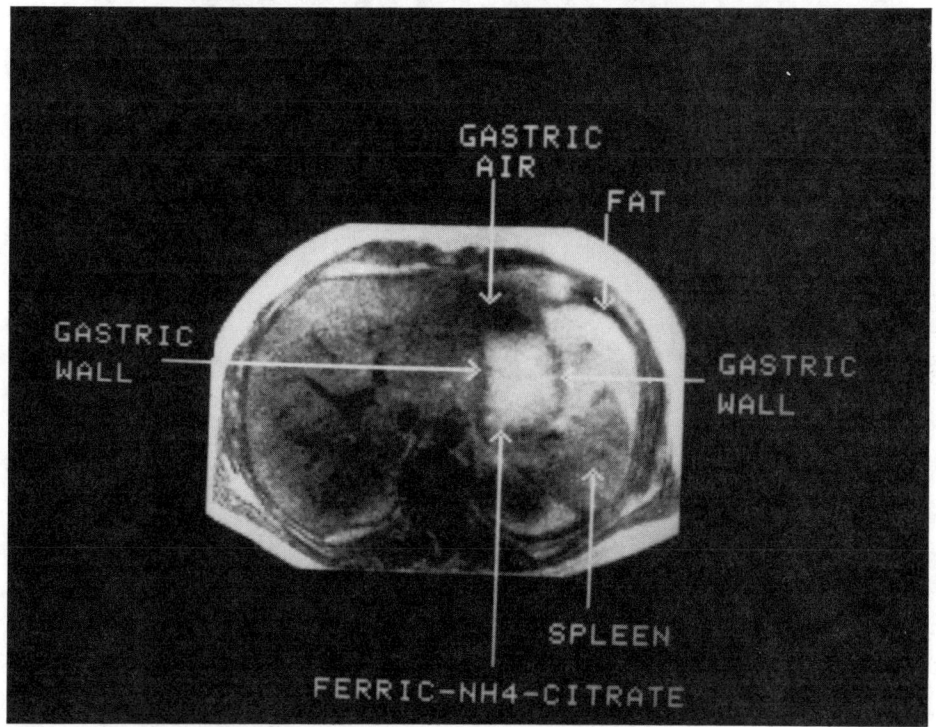

Figure 2. Transaxial MR image (TR = 1.0 sec; TE = 28 msec) of the upper abdomen of a supine adult volunteer ten minutes after oral ingestion of 500 ml of 1 mmol/L ferric ammonium citrate demonstrates high signal intensity from the lumen of the stomach, with definition of the gastric wall. (Reprinted with permission from Wesbey GE, Brasch RC, Engelstad BL, et al. Radiology 149:174-180, 1983.)

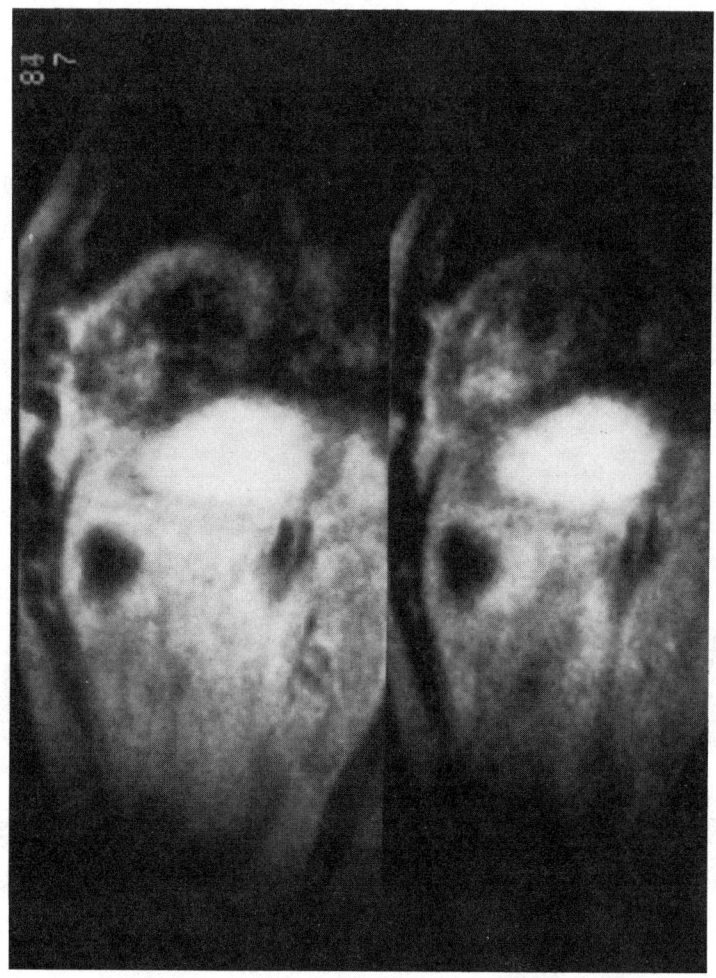

Figure 3. Parasagittal MR images (left, TR = 1.0 sec, TE = 28 msec; right, TR = 1.0 sec, TE = 56 msec) of the lower thorax and upper abdomen of a supine adult volunteer 15 minutes after oral ingestion of 500 ml of 1 mmol/L ferric ammonium citrate shows conspicuous high signal intensity from the lumen of the fundus of the stomach at the thoracoabdominal junction.

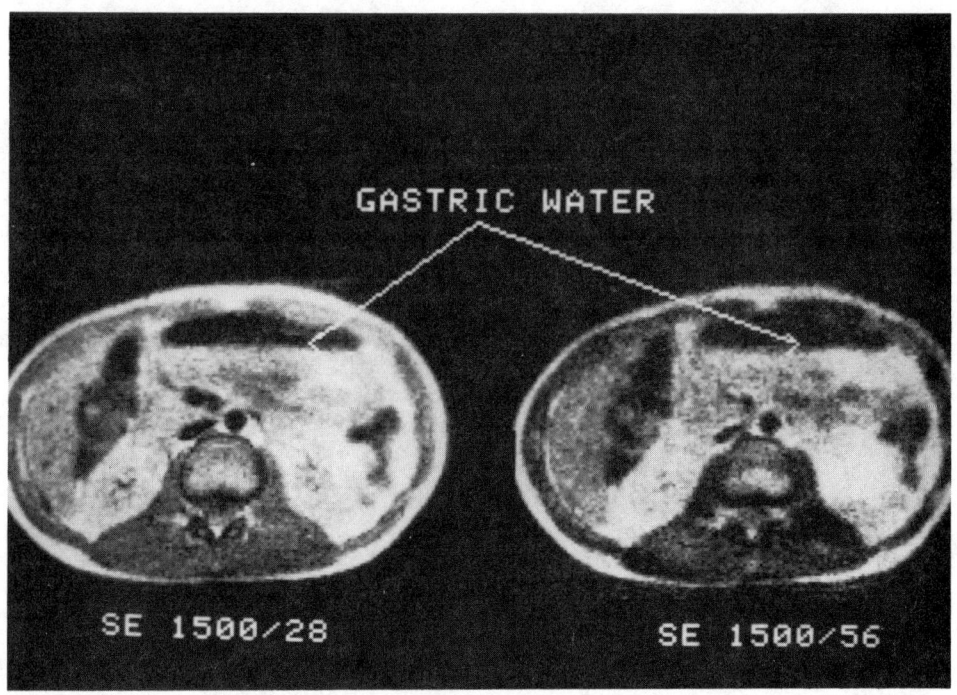

Figure 4. Transaxial MR images (left, TR= 1.5 sec, TE = 28 msec; right, TR = 1.5 sec, TE = 56 msec) of the upper abdomen of a supine adult volunteer 15 minutes after oral ingestion of water illustrates isointensity of the MR signal from water in the stomach compared to the adjacent liver. The gastric wall is not defined.

agents, for example spin-labeled propanolol (Rauckman et al., 1976).

This unique group of synthetic organic chemicals containsan unpaired electron which is sterically shielded from certain chemical reactions; for example, the compounds are stable in water for months. Two major classes of NSL tested as MRI contrast enhancing agents are the piperidinyl compounds (saturated six-membered rings) and the pyrrolidinyl compounds (saturated five-membered rings).

The concept of using NSL as in vivo diagnostic agents to enhance contrast on proton MRI images is relatively new; only recent information is available on the biodistribution, in vivo metabolism, and potential toxicity of these compounds used as pharmaceuticals (Couet et. al., 1984, 1985) (Afzal, 1984).

Several applications of NSL employed as diagnostic contrast enhancing agents have been successfully demonstrated in experimental animals. MRI images obtained after intravenous injection of NSL have yielded information on the functional status of the kidneys in various disease states (Brasch et al., 1983a); with renal insufficiency (Figure 5) the kidney does not change in MRI appearance but for normal kidneys the excretion of NSL leads to an observable increase in MRI signal. Similarly, relaxation enhancement produced by NSL has been observed with implanted renal cell carcinoma, acutely infarcted myocardium (Ehman et. al., 1985; McNamara et. al., 1985) and focal disruption of the blood brain barrier by infection and radiation (Figure 6) (Brasch et. al., 1983b).

The tolerance of animals, and particularly humans, for NSL is largely unstudied. The acute LD 50 in rats of a piperdinyl compound used for MRI contrast enhancement in our laboratory (TES) is 15.1 mM/Kg (Afzal, et. al., 1984). A minimally useful dose for MRI is 0.04 mM/Kg (Brasch et. al., 1983a).

Because certain nonstable free radicals are involved as intermediates in many forms of carcinogenesis, it was mandatory to test for any mutagenic effect (Afzal et. al., 1984). It should be noted that the body normally contains a variety of free radical compounds (eg. melanin). Sister chromatid exchanges and Ames assays for mutagenesis were performed using two NSL compounds in concentration up to 10^{-3}M. The tested compounds were those shown to be useful in MRI, TES and TPC. TPC is a pyrrolidinyl NSL. Also tested were the hydroxylamine and

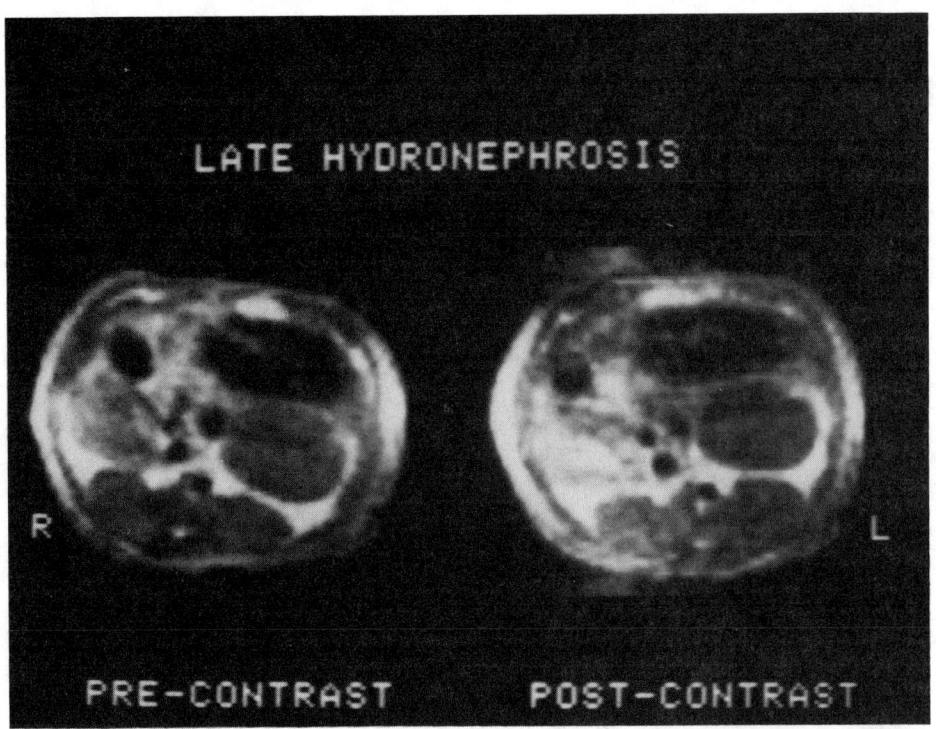

Figure 5. Transaxial MR images (TR = 0.5 sec; TE = 28 msec) through the midabdomen of a supine rat with a surgically ligated left ureter causing hydronephrosis of the left kidney. Prior to intravenous administration of the paramagnetic nitroxide spin label "TES" (1g/kg), a normal right kidney and an enlarged left kidney are seen. The post-contrast MR image shows easily observable high signal intensity in the urine of the right renal pelvis, indicating normal urinary excretion. However, the hydronephrotic left kidney shows no observable intensification after administration of "TES" reflecting a poorly excreting left kidney. (Reprinted with pemission from Brasch RC, London DL, Wesbey GE, et al. Radiology 147:773-779, 1983.)

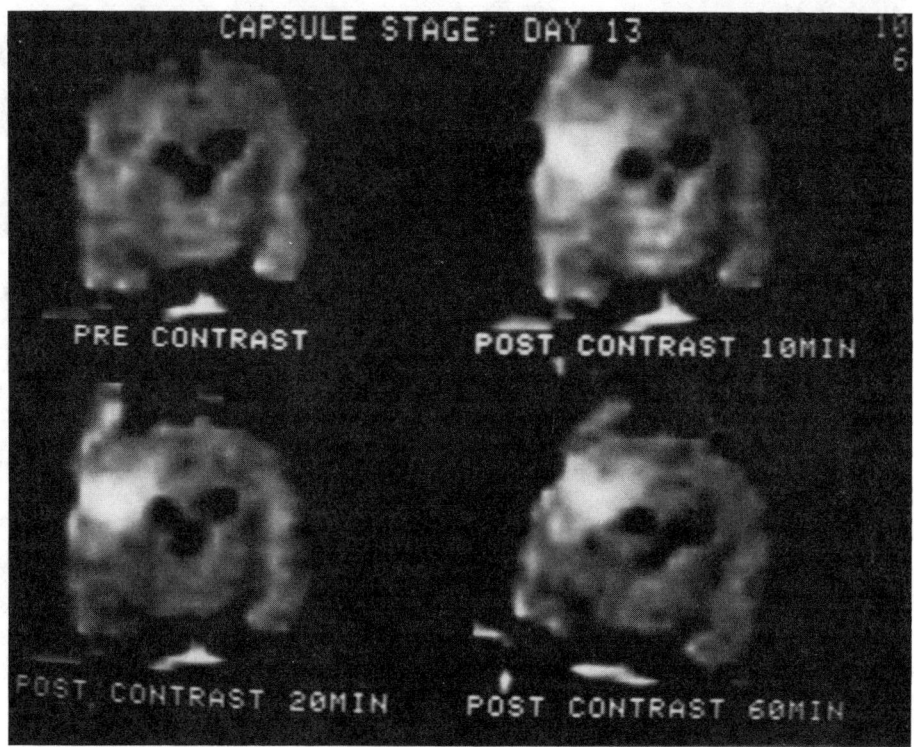

Figure 6. Coronal MR brain images before and after intravenous administration of the NSL "TES" to a dog with an implanted left hemispheric pyogenic cerebral abscess. Dramatic contrast-enhancement is seen, identifying the focal breakdown in the blood-brain-barrier. (Reprinted with permission from Brasch RC, Nitecki DE, Brant-Zawadski MN. <u>AJR</u> 141:1019-1024, 1983.)

amine derivates of these NSL, which are potential metabolites in vivo. All assays showed no mutagenic effect of the NSL compounds or their metabolites. The sister chromatid exchange assay is the most sensitive indicator of chemical carcinogenic, mutagenic behavior. Further toxicologic studies of NSL are required before clinical trials can be considered.

Pharmacokinetic studies in animals using NSL (Couet et. al., 1984; Griffeth et al., 1984) indicate that intravenously injected NSL are subject to in vivo reduction to yield a nonparamagnetic hydroxylamine derivative of the parent compound. This reduction occurs in vivo with ascorbic acid, but a separate enzymatic reduction is also likely. the in vivo reduction of NSL appears to be saturable (Griffeth et. al., 1984), and with sufficient doses of NSL (over 0.04mM/Kg) enough of the paramagnetic persists to obtain diagnostic information. As a class, pyrrolidine NSL are more resistant to reduction than piperidine NSL (McNamara et. al., 1984a).

In summary, NSL have been shown to be diagnostically useful in animals as contrast-enhancing agents for MRI. More studies of the metabolism, pharrmacokinetics, and toxicity are needed before clinical trials can commence. A new nonionic NSL called "NAT" which is well-tolerated (LD50 25mM/Kg) and demonstrates resistance to in vivo reduction has recently been reported (Grodd et. al., 1985).

Transition Metal and Rare-Earth Complexes

The cations of the transition metal series contain anywhere from 0 to 5 unpaired electrons, conferring magnetic moments ranging from 0 to 5.9 Bohr magnetons (Pauling, 1960). For the lanthanons (rare earths) the number of unpaired electrons varies from 0 to 7, with variations in the magnetic moments of the lanthanons from 0 to 10.5 Bohr magnetons (Kyker et. al., 1956). As previously discussed, the presence of a strong magnetic moment (from many unpaired electrons or significant spin-orbit coupling) does not guarantee efficient proton relaxation enhancement capabilities by a paramagnetic.

As mentioned earlier, the first metal cation proposed as a paramagnetic pharmaceutical for proton MRI was the bivalent manganese ion Mn^{+2}. Several early studies (Lauterbur et. al., 1978; Brady et. al., 1982) indicated promising relaxation rate enhancement by in-vitro NMR spectrometry and imaging experiments. However, even at the minimum dose necessary to achieve in vivo tissue relaxation rate enhancement, Mn^{+2} has been shown to be unacceptably toxic to the cardiovascular system. In a study by Wolf and Baum (1983), injected doses of Mn^{+2} as low as 10 micromoles per kilogram demonstrated hypotensive effects as well as electrocardiographic effects in experimental animals. In fact, for all transition metal and rare earth cations, known toxicity at doses necessary to effect tissue relaxation probably precludes any serious consideration of using a pharmaceutical composed of these uncomplexed cations for human imaging. Because of the toxicological reasons, complexation of metal or rare earth ions to strong ligands is necessary before one can consider utilizing these paramagnetic pharmaceutical for MRI was Mn-EDTA (Mendonca-Dias et. al., 1982) followed by Cr-EDTA (Runge et. al., 1983a,b). Both these metal complexes have less proton relaxation enhancement characteristics compared to the parent cations. Nevertheless, significant relaxation rate enhancement was present in these two metal complexes.

We have studied 27 metal complexes representative of the transition metal and rare earth series (Wesbey et. al., 1983b). The parent cations included: Fe^{+3}, VO^{+2}, Mn^{+2}, Cu^{+2}, Cr^{+2}, Gd^{+3}, Ho^{+3}, Dy^{+3}, Eu^{+3}. These 9 cations were complexed to the following 3 ligands: DTPA (diethylene-triaminepentacetic acid), a well known metal chelator of the polycarboxcylic acid group; desferrioxamine mesylate, a hydroxyamate siderophore which is the drug of choice in iron chelation therapy in human pharmacology; and glucoheptonate, from the group of sugar acids. These 27 metal complexes were evaluated in the 15 MHz small animal MRI system and in a 100 MHz NMR spectrometer, under standard aqueous conditions (pH 7.3, 0.35 normal Hepes buffer, 23° C), and in concentrations ranging from 0.01 to 10 millimolar. The results of the study indicated that the complexes of manganese and gadolinium, six complexes in all, had the most superior relaxation enhancement characteristics. Chromium-DF and chromium-DTPA were also promising as was iron desferrioxamine (ferrioxamine B). This study demonstrated that complexation of potentially toxic metal or rare earth ions to known strong ligands far from eliminated paramagnetic proton relaxation enhancement properties. Although relaxation rates in the metal complexes were lower than the relaxation rates in the parent cations, potentially clinically useful relaxation rates were observed nonetheless. Urographic enhancement of rat renal parenchyma and urinary collecting structures in vivo has been demonstrated with several of these complexes (Huberty et. al., 1983).

One promising paramagnetic metal complex agent is ferrioxamine B (Huberty et. al., 1983). Of the paramagnetic intravenous MRI contrast agents proposed to date, only ferrioxamine B brings a prior background of safe, albeit indirect, human clinical pharmacological experience. This pharmaceutical is a stable ferric iron complex of desferrioxamine mesylate, a hydroxamate siderophore that is the drug of choice for iron chelation therapy. The association constant, Ka, of this metal complex has a log Ka of 31, an indication of high stability (Catsch et al., 1979; Martel, Smith, 1974-6). Ferrioxamine B is rapidly excreted into the urine. We have performed in vivo MRI experiments of the urographic system of normal and abnormal rats, as well as imaging of canine and rat models of cerebritis. With ferrioxamine B, contrast enhancement of the renal pelvis and parenchyma occurred at doses as low as 1 micromole/kg, considerably lower than the known toxic levels in animals. In mice, an LD50 of 500 micromoles/kg (IP) has been cited (Pfister et al., 1976).

In animal models of cerebritis, identification of focal blood-brain-barrier defects was facilitated by ferrioxamine B, producing T2 (Figure 7) shortening in the lesion, causing decreased MRI spin-echo signal intensity. In a rat with a right sided hydronephrosis, intravenous injection of ferrioxamine B provided direct functional assessment of the hydronephrotic right kidney, indicating good excretory function despite the presence of unilateral hydronephrosis.

Of the several paramagnetic pharmaceuticals studied to date, it is our opinion that gadolinium-DTPA (Gd-DTPA) affords the best combination of in vivo lesion relaxation rate enhancement with favorable toxicological and pharmacokinetic behavior (Weinmann et. al., 1983; Weinmann et. al., 1984; Brasch et. al., 1984). Clinical trials have already begun, making this agent the first intravenous paramagnetic pharmaceutical for human MRI (Carr et. al., 1985). DTPA (diethylenetriaminepentacetic acid) was chosen as the ligand for chelation of gadolinium, because of the various aminocarboxylic acids, DTPA has among the highest association constants, log Ka=23 (Martell, Smith, 1974-6). Of all the paramagnetic cations in the atomic table, Gd^{+3} has the strongest relaxation rate enhancement properties. Gd^{+3} contains 7 unpaired electrons. In addition, an important feature in relaxation rate enhancement by Gd^{+3} is the presence of a relatively long electron spin relaxation time ($\gamma_s = 10^{-10}$ sec) (Dwek, 1973). Pharmacokinetic studies of Gd-DTPA indicate that after injection of 0.5 mmoles/kg dose of Gd-DTPA, a blood half-life of 20

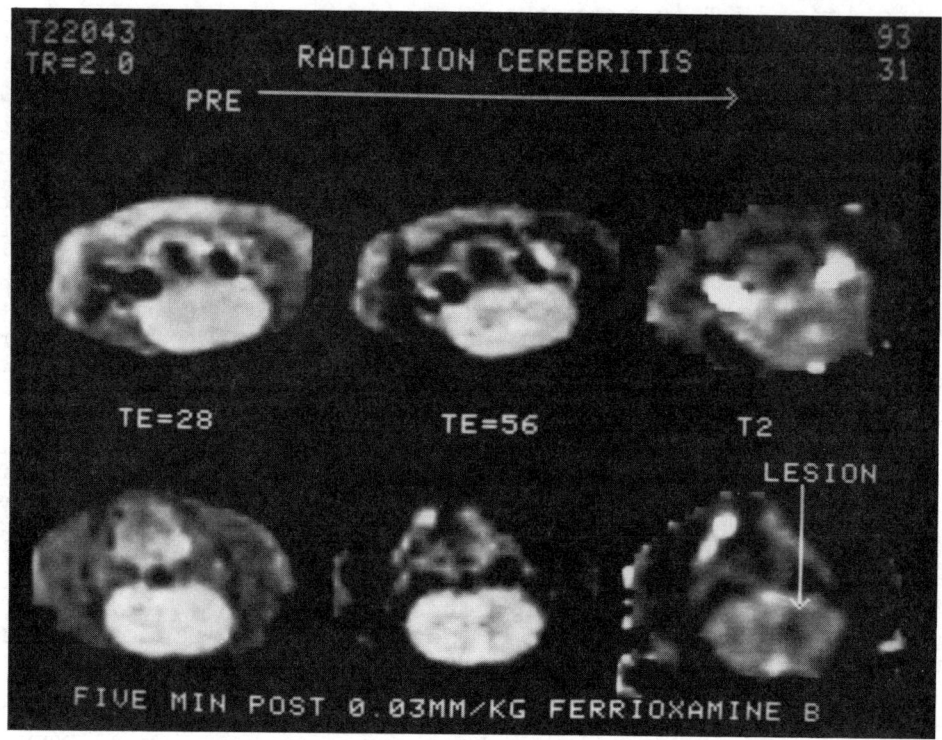

Figure 7. Transaxial MR images before and after intravenous administration of ferrioxamine B to a supine rat which was one week post-3000 rad exposure of heavy ion beam irradiation to the left cerebral hemisphere. Notice that the left hemisphere lesion is not appreciable on the pre-contrast MR images (upper row). Ferrioxamine B identifies the focal breakdown in the blood brain barrier as a region of low signal intensity on the TE = 56 msec image, due to T2 shortening as reflected in the calculated T2 image. (Courtesy of T. Richards, Ph.D., and T. Budinger, M.D., Ph.D.)

minutes is observed (Weinmann et. al., 1984). At three hours post-injection, 80% of the dose is excreted in the urine. At 7 days post-injection, 90% of the dose is recovered in the urine, 7% in the feces, and .4% is recoverable in the remainder of body tissues and fluids. An LD50 of 10 mmoles/kg is found in rats. This compares favorably with the LD50 for meglumine diatrizoate the well known iodinated radiographic contrast media which has an LD50 in rats of 18 mmoles/kg. The LD50 for gadolinium chloride for comparison is 0.4 mmoles/kg, far more toxic than that of the complexed Gd-DTPA. Surprisingly, Gd-EDTA has an LD50 of 0.3 mmoles/kg, even worse than that of the Gd^{+3} aquoion. This is observed despite the fact that Gd-EDTA has a relatively high in-vitro association constant of (log K = 17). Cardiovascular effects of Gd-DTPA have been studied by Fobben and Wolf (1983). At doses of 1 and 3 mmoles/kg, no arterial blood pressure or electrocardiographic changes were noted. At a dose of 10 mmoles/kg, minimal hypotension was noted.

MRI urographic imaging experiments with the dimeglumine salt of Gd-DTPA (Schering AG, Berlin) indicate rapid, easily observable increases in renal parenchymal and renal pelvis signal intensity after intravenous injection of doses as low as .01 mmoles/kg (Figure 8) (Brasch et al., 1984). After injection of 1 mmoles/kg, decrease in signal intensity in the renal parenchyma and urinary pelvis is noted, due to the predominant T2 shortening of paramagnetic Gd-DTPA at this concentration in the kidney (Figure 9). A wide variety of pathological lesions have been studied with the use of intravenous Gd-DTPA. Dramatic contrast enhancement of rat models of a sterile abscess has been observed (Figure 10). Similarly, identification of a focal breakdown in the blood-brain barrier with 0.5 mmole/Kg Gd-DTPA in a canine model of radiation cerebritis is appreciable (Figure 11).

In a study of the use of GD-DTPA in acute canine myocardial infarction, (Wesbey et. al., 1984b) 5 dogs with 24 hour old myocardial infarctions underwent cardiectomy 5 minutes after injection of 0.35 mmoles/Kg of Gd-DTPA. Three dogs underwent cardiectomy at 90 seconds post-injection. In dogs not given paramagnetic Gd-DTPA, T1 and T2 were longer in the infarct compared to normal myocardium. After injection of Gd-DTPA, conspicuous relaxation rate enhancement was noted in both the normal and infarcted myocardium. Greater relaxation rate enhancement in the normal myocardium was seen in the 90 second group, compatible with a perfusion phase. Greater infarct relaxation rate enhancement was seen in

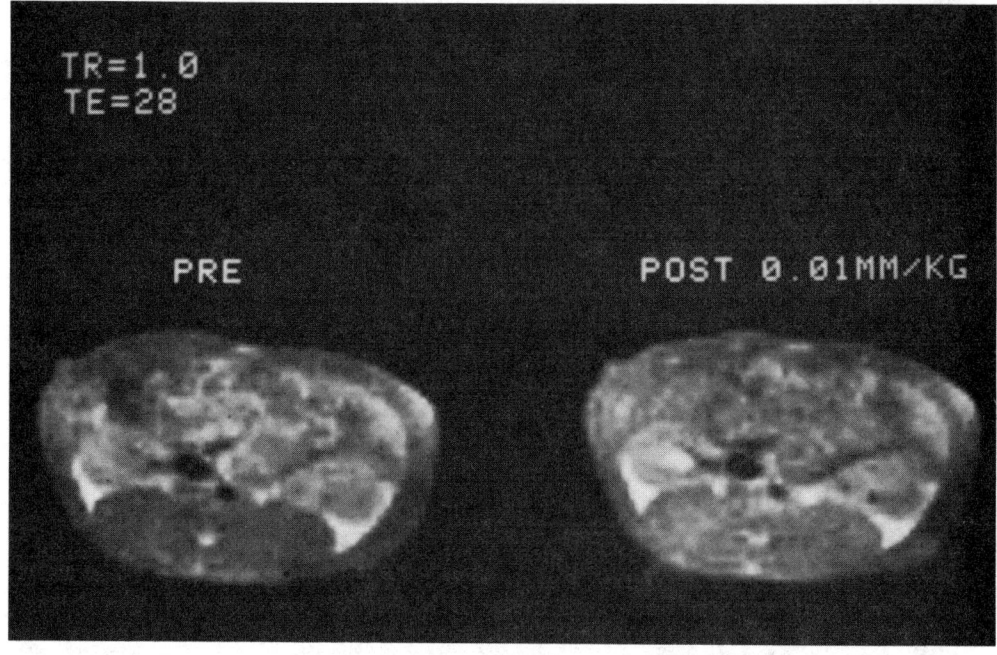

Figure 8. MR images in a supine rat through the level of the kidneys before and after intravenous administration of gadolinium-DTPA. Notice the conspicuous high signal intensity in the urine in the right renal pelvis on the post-contrast image, due to paramagnetic T1 shortening of water protons. (Reprinted with permission from Brasch RC, Weinmann HJ, Wesbey GE. AJR 142:625-630, 1984.)

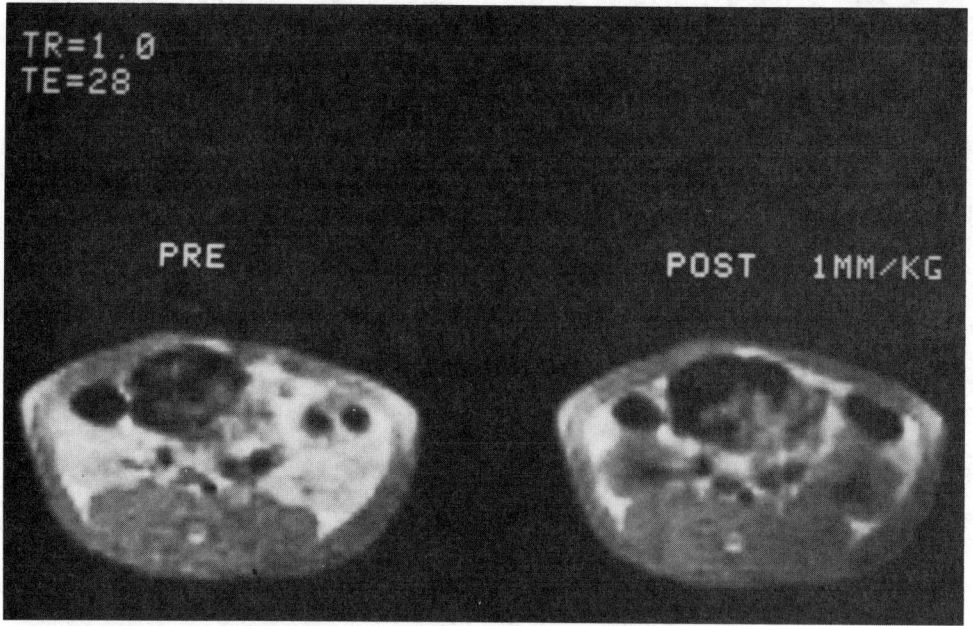

Figure 9. With a hundred-fold greater dose of intravenous gadolinium-DTPA, the urine in both renal pelves turns black, due to T2 shortening of water protons with the high concentration of paramagnetic excreted in the urine. (Reprinted with permission from Brasch RC, Weinmann HJ, Wesbey GE. AJR 142:625-630, 1984.)

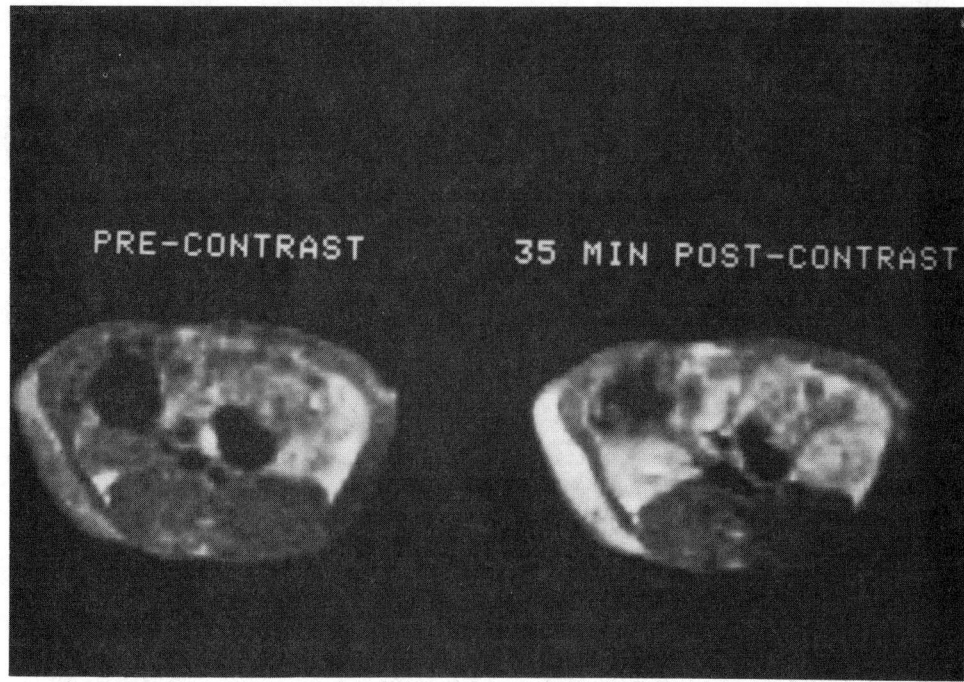

Figure 10. MR images in a supine rat before and after 0.1 mmol/kg intravenous gadolinium-DTPA. Contrast-enhancement of a sterile right flank abscess, as well as enhancement of both renal parenchyma and pelves is seen with Gd-DTPA. (Reprinted with permission from Brasch RC, Weinmann HJ, Wesbey GE. <u>AJR</u> 142:625-630, 1984.)

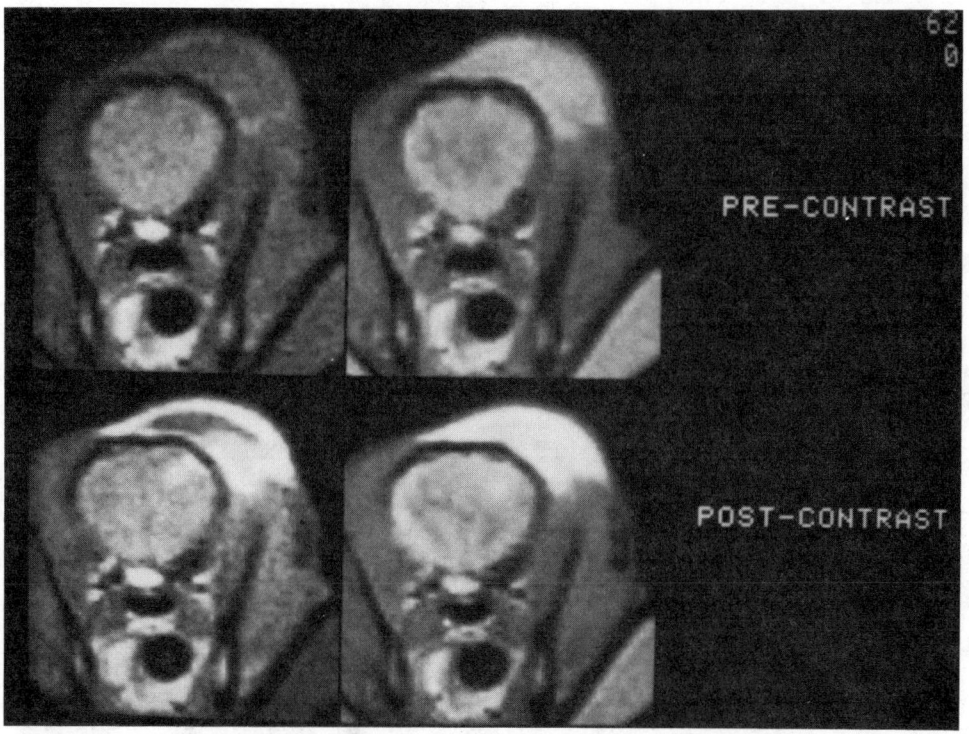

Figure 11. Coronal brain MR images with TR = 0.5 sec (right images) and TR = 1.5 sec (left images) (TE = 28 msec) in a prone dog which had received focal right hemisphere irradiation (1500 rads) by an implanted ^{125}I seed one week earlier. The lesion is barely discernible on the pre-contrast TR = 0.5 sec image as a region of low intensity, with adjacent scalp edema apparent. After intravenous administration of 0.5 mmol/kg of Gd-DTPA, dramatic contrast-enhancement of the focal defect in the blood-brain-barrier, as well as the scalp edema, is seen. (Reprinted with permission from Brasch RC, Weinmann HJ, Wesbey GE. <u>AJR</u> 142:625-630, 1984.)

the 5 minute group (Figure 12). This distribution of an extracellular pharmaceutical to regions of acute canine myocardial infarction 5 minutes post injection has also been noted with iodinated contrast media in x-ray computed tomography studies (Gerber et. al., 1983). The "wash in"and "wash-out" of Gd-DTPA from the normal myocardium, in assessing relative myocardial perfusion, may be of future clinical utility. Paramagnetics are not needed to discriminate acutely infarcted from normal canine myocardium with in vivo MRI (Wesbey et. al., 1984c).

In a subsequent study of canine myocardial ischemia with only sixty seconds of LAD coronary artery occlusion, McNamara et. al., (1984b) found significant relaxation rate enhancement in normal myocardium (compared to ischemic myocardium) one minute after injection of 0.5 mM/Kg Gd-DTPA. Thus, the potential exists for paramagnetic-enhanced MRI to challenge ^{201}Thallium myocardial perfusion scintigraphy in the identification of reversibly ischemic myocardium.

Human clinical trials with Gd-DTPA have been reported in forty patients with intracranial and abdominal tumors (Carr, 1985). Using a dose of 0.1 mM/Kg, contrast enhancement of cerebral lesions was seen in 18/20 patients. The Gd-DTPA-enhanced image showed better tumor margin definition in 13/20 patients in comparison with the iodinated contrast media-enhanced CT scan. In 2/20 cases, the contrast-enhanced CT study better imaged tumor margins. There were no changes in renal function or electrolytes; no change in blood counts or coagulation parameters; no change in liver function tests or urinalysis. However, a transient, reversible elevation in serum iron levels has been noted in a few patients.

Reticuloendothelial pharmaceuticals using a paramagnetic selectively distributed to the reticuloendothelial cells in the liver and spleen may be achieved by injection of collodial suspensions (Huberty et. al., 1983). In vivo imaging studies performed in our laboratory with the use of gadolinium-hydroxycolloid at a dose of 34 micromoles/kg demonstrates significant T2 shortening (from 40 msec to 24 msec) in the liver 10 minutes after injection. This T2 shortening results in easily observable reduction of MRI signal intensity in the liver (Figure 13). The clinical utility of this pharmaceutical could be that of providing assessment of normally functioning Kupffer cells. High intensity zones of liver parenchyma would represent abnormal liver

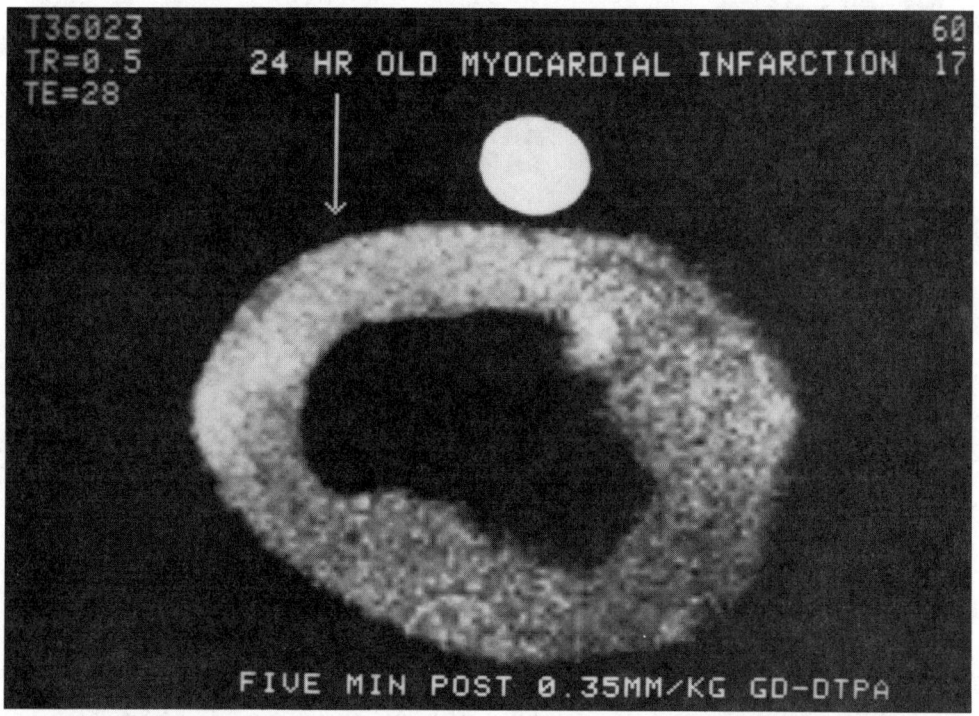

Figure 12. Transaxial MR image of an infarcted dog heart excised 5 minutes after intravenous administration of Gd-DTPA. The Gd-DTPA caused Tl relaxation enhancement in the anterior wall myocardial infarction, increasing the signal intensity in the infarct.

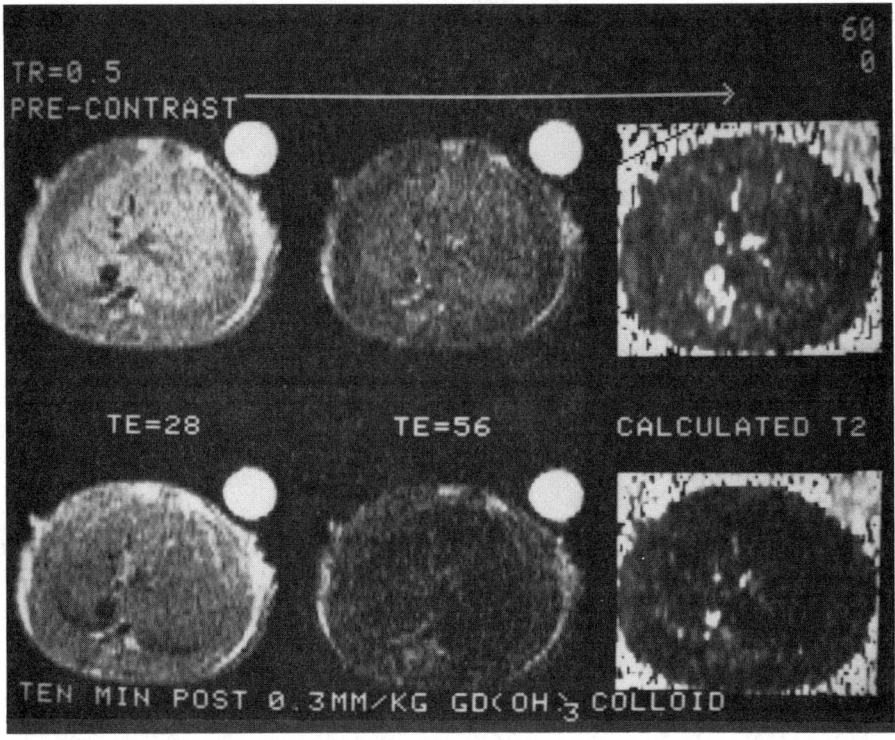

Figure 13. A) Transaxial MR images of a supine rat through the level of the liver before and after intravenous administration of a liver-spleen paramagnetic agent, gadolinium hydroxy-colloid. Notice on the pre-contrast images, the liver is brighter than surrounding skeletal muscle. Post-contrast images show the liver to be on the same intensity as muscle, due to selective T2 shortening in the liver.

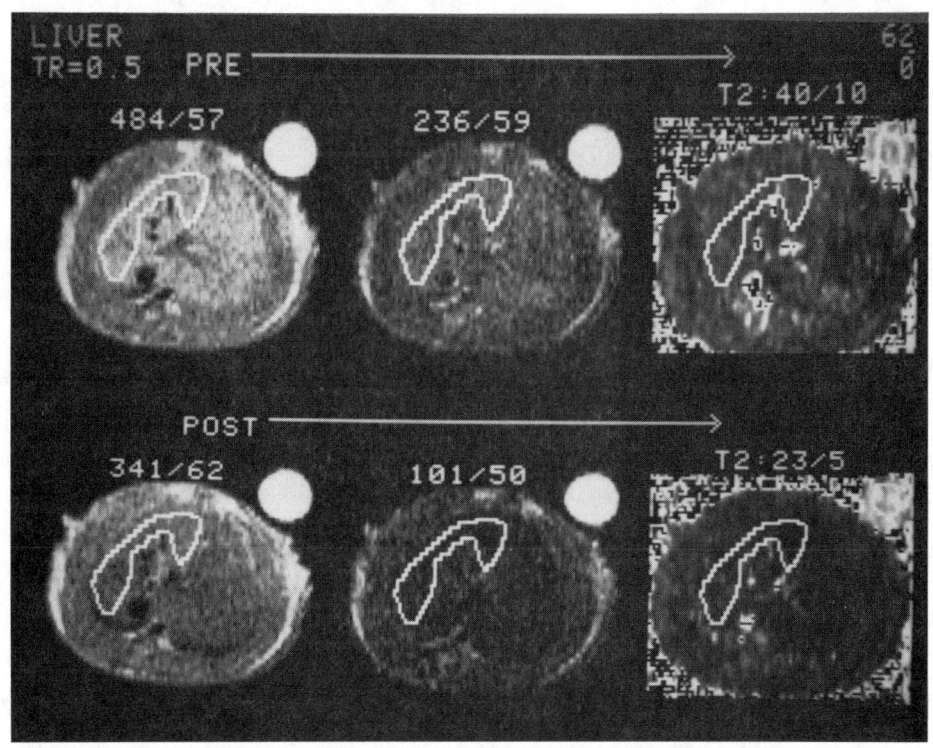

Figure 13. B) A 110 pixel region-of-interest drawn in the liver shows the mean/standard deviation of the liver intensity values and T2.

parenchyma, cast in a background of low signal intensity of normally functioning liver parenchyma.

Other investigators have reported promising results with paramagnetic metal complexes. Brady et. al. (1983) opened an exciting avenue in paramagnetic pharmaceutical research with the introduction of manganese-DTPA antimyosin monoclonal antibody complex. In two dogs given intracoronary injections of this agent at manganese doses of 1 micromole/kg, dramatic infarct T1 relaxation rate enhancement was seen in the excised heart. This antimyosin monoclonal antibody pharmaceutical has been bound to technetium in nuclear medicine studies. This agent binds specifically to irreversibly damaged myocardium, and thus has potential promise in the MRI discrimination of ischemic from infarcted myocardium. In addition, introduction of this agent opens the doors for paramagnetic immuno-imaging in neoplastic conditions, potentially providing the diagnostic specificity that proton MRI currently lacks.

Runge and others (1983b) have demonstrated urographic enhancement and lesion enhancement with the paramagnetic metal complex chromium-EDTA. A wide variety of lesions has been studied and contrast-enhanced by this agent.

Inhalation Paramagnetic Agents (Gases)

The third category of paramagnetics are gases, most notably molecular oxygen, which has potential use in both proton and fluorine-19 MRI.

Three well known noble gases have paramagnetic properties. These are nitric oxide, nitrogen dioxide, and molecular oxygen. The first two gases have little promise for human applications because of adverse limiting side effects. However, the obvious safety of inhaled 100% molecular oxygen is extremely appealing for potential clinical human use. Molecular oxygen has a magnetic moment of 2.8 Bohr Magnetons, and its concentration as dissolved oxygen in the blood is approximately 4 parts per million at 100 mm of mercury arterial oxygen saturation (Gore, 1981). It is estimated that the normal paramagnetic oxygen contribution to tissue proton relaxation rates is approximately only 1 to 2%. Two groups of investigators have found proton MRI relaxation rate enhancement after inhalation of 100% oxygen by human volunteers. Investigators at the Hammersmith (Gore, 1981) and Cleveland Case Western Reserve (Alfidi et. al., 1982) found intensification of the blood and myocardium in humans in nongated cardiac images. This was ascribed to paramagnetic T1 relaxation rate enhancement. However, problems with applications with molecular oxygen for human use can be raised. First, cardiovascular changes associated with inhalation of 100% molecular oxygen for 10 minutes, including changes in cardiac output and blood flow velocity, could be alternative explanations for the observed signal intensity changes in the blood in the nongated images of the heart previously mentioned. In addition, directed delivery of an inhaled paramagnetic gas to a specific biological tissue or organ would be extremely difficult. Finally, oxygen is not strongly paramagnetic and does not exhibit strong proton relaxation enhancement in water and blood (Runge, et. al., 1983a). T1 relaxation rate enhancement in blood after in vitro exposure to 100% oxygen at 700 millimeters mercury of arterial oxygen pressure, produces only a 2 or 3 fold increase in the T1 relaxation rate of blood. A greater enhancement of T1 relaxation rates is achievable in-vitro with use of stronger paramagnetics such as gadolinium, manganese, or iron complexes.

Paramagnetic molecular oxygen has potential biomedical applications in Flourine-19 MRI also. Two groups of investigators have proposed that Flourine-19 T1 measurements in injected oxygenated perfluorocarbon emulsion pharmaceuticals may be a sensitive parameter for the in vivo measurement of oxygen tension in blood vessels perfused with perfluorochemical blood substitutes (Lai et. al., 1983; Clark et. al., 1983).

CONCLUSION

Diagnostic pharmaceuticals offer promise in extending the diagnostic utility of MRI. The three most promising areas of potential clinical application of diagnostic pharmaceuticals are 1) the tissue, organ, or lesion specific pharmaceuticals, using well known nuclear medicine carrier biomolecules or monoclonal antibodies; 2) functional assessment of tissue perfusion at the capillary level; 3) assessment of organ function, such as renal excretion or Kupffer cell function in the reticuloendothelial system. Positive or negative labels of the gastrointestinal tract in MRI must continue to be developed, because identification of gut without use of bowel labeling agents is difficult, similar to the situation in abdominal CT. It is quite likely that safe positive or negative gastrointestinal agents will be developed and rapidly utilized for human clinical MRI. Very promising research has been conducted with intravenous metal complexes and nitroxide spin labels. However, development of intravenous paramagnetic pharmaceuticals for widespread human clinical trials still awaits important toxicity and kinetic research. Nitroxide spin-labels must be designed that are resistant to in vivo bioreduction; metal complexes must be proven not to undergo in vivo dissociation to the parent ion.

The field of paramagnetic pharmaceutical development for NMR imaging has progressed at rapid rates. The first animal experiments using Gd-DTPA began in 1981; human clinical trials were already underway in Europe by the fall of 1983. Clinical trials in the U.S. began in January, 1985. The intravenous injection of one gram (0.1 mM/Kg in a 70 kg man) of chelated gadolinium, a totally nonbiological lanthanide, without significant untoward effects is an unprecedented accomplishment in human pharmacology. Although Gd-DTPA is far from ideal in the specificity of its lesion enhancement, it stands out as a relatively safe "building block" upon which to design more tissue-specific paramagnetic pharmaceuticals, as well as even safer/more-effective nonspecific image enhancing agents.

REFERENCES

Afzal V, Brasch RC, Wolff S, Nitecki D. (1984). *Investigative Radiology* 19:549-552.

Aflidi RJ, Haaga JR, El Yousef SJ, et. al. (1982) *Radiology* 143; 175-182.

Baker CE (ed.) (1982) *Physicians' Desk Reference*. 36th Edition. Medical Economics Company, Inc., Oradell, New Jersey.

Beall PT. (1984). Physiological Chemistry and Physics and Medical NMR. 16:129-136.

Bloch F, Hansen WW, Packard M. (1946). *Physical Review* 70:474.

Brady TJ, Goldman MR, Hinshaw WS, Pykett IL, Buonano FS, Newhouse JH, Kistler JP, Levine FH, Pohost GM. (1982). *Radiology* 144:343-347.

Brady TJ, Rosen BR, Gold HK, Khaw BA, Fallon JT, Goldman MR, Ter Penning BJ, Yasuda T, Baber E. (1983). In: Works In Progress, Book of Abstracts, p10. The Society of Magnetic Resonance in Medicine. 2nd Annual Meeting. San Francisco, CA.

Brasch RC, Nitecki DE, Brant-Zawadzki MN, Enzmann DR, Wesbey GE, Tozer TN, Tuck LD, Cann CE, Fike JR, Sheldon P. (1983b). *AJR* 141:1019-1024.

Brasch RC, London DA, Wesbey GE, et. al. (1983a). *Radiology* 147:773-780.

Brasch RC, Weinmann HJ, Wesbey GE. (1984) *AJR* 142:625-630.

Brittenham GM, Farrepll DE, Harris JW, et. al. (1982). *N Engl J Medicine* 307:1671-1675.

Brown MA, (1985). *Magnetic Resonance Imaging* 3:3-9.

Caille JM, Lemanceau P, Bonnemain B. (1982) XII Symposium Neuroradiologicum, Washington D.C., October 10-16, 1982.

Carr DH. (1985). *Magnetic Resonance Imaging* 3:17-25.

Catsch A, Harmoth-Hoene AE. (1979) Pharmacology and Therapeutic Applications of Agents Used in Heavy Metal Poisoning. IN: The Chelation of Heavy Metals. Levine WG, ed. Pergammon Press, Oxford.

Christensen HE (ed). (1972). Toxic Substances List. U.S. Dept. of Health, Education and Welfare; National Institute for Occupational Safety and Health. Rockville, MD.

Clanton JA, Runge V, Lukehart CM, Partain CL, James AE. (1983). In: Works in Progress Book of Abstracts, Society of Magnetic Resonance in Medicine, p.13. 2nd Annual Meeting. San Francisco, CA.

Clark LC, Ackerman JL, Thomas SR, Millard RW. (1983) In: Book of Abstracts, Society of Magnetic Resonance in Medicine. pp.95-96. 2nd Annual Meeting, San Francisco, CA.

Couet W, Eriksson U, Tozer TN, et. al. (1984). Pharmaceutical Research 1:203-209.

Couet WR, Brasch RC, Sosnovsky G, et. al. (1985). Magnetic Resonance Imaging 3:83-88.

Crooks LE, Hoenninger JC, Arakawa M, Kaufman L, McRee R, Watts J, Singer JH. (1980). Radiology 136:701-706.

Crooks LE, Arakawa M, Hoenninger JC, et. al. (1982). Radiology 143:169-174.

Dornbluth NC, Potter JL, Fullerton GD. (1982). In: Scientific Program Book, Radiological Society of North America, 68th Annual Meeting, November 30, 1982. p.134. (Abstract).

Dwek RA, (1973). Nuclear Magnetic Resonance (NMR) in Biochemistry. Clarendon Press Oxford.

Ehman RL, Wesbey GE, Moon KL, et. al. (1985). Magnetic Resonance 3:89-97.

Engelstad BL, Wesbey GE, (1983). In: Book of Abstracts, pp.120-121. Society of Magnetic Resonance in Medicine, 2nd Annual Meeting, San Francisco, CA.

Fobben E, Wolf FL. (1983). Investigative Radiology 18:55. (Abstract).

Fukushima E, Roeder E. (1981). Experimental Pulse NMR. Addison Publishing Company, Inc. Reading, Massachusetts.

Gerber KH, Higgins CE. (1983). Investigative Radiology 18:238-244.

Gore JC. (1981). Proceedings of the Symposium on Nuclear Magnetic Resonance Imaging, Bowman Gray School of Medicine, Wake Forest University, Winston-Salem, NC, pp.15-23. Witcofski RL, Karstaedt N, Partain CL, eds.

Griffeth LK, Rosen GM, Rauckman EJ, Drayer BP. (1984). Investigative Radiology 19:553-562.

Grodd W, Paajanen H, Erikkson U, et. al. (1985). Proceedings of the Association of University Radiologists, 33rd Annual Meeting, Vanderbilt University, Nashville, Tennessee, April, 1985.

Herfkens R, Davis P, Crooks LE et al. (1981). Radiology 141:211-218.

Hollis DP, Bulkey BE, Nunnally RL, Jacobus WE, Weisfeldt MI. (1978). Clinical Research P. 240.

Huberty JP, Engelstad BL, Wesbey GE, et. al. (1983) In: Book of Abstracts. pp.175-176. The Society of Magnetic Resonance in Medicine, 2nd Annual Meeting. San Francisco, CA.

Hutchison JMS, Smith FW. (1983). In: Partain CL, James AE, Rollo FD, Price RR, Nuclear Magnetic Resonance (NMR) Imaging. W.B. Saunders Co., Philadelphia. Chapter 17.

Kyker GC, Anderson EB. (1956) United States Atomic Energy Commission. Rare Earths in Biochemical and Medical Research. Conference. Oakridge, Tennessee, Institute of Nuclear Studies.

Lai CS, Stair SJ, Miziorko H, Hyde JS (1983). In: Works in Progress Book of Abstracts, Society of Magnetic Resonance in Medicine, p.12. 2nd Annual Meeting, San Francisco, CA.

Lauterbur PC, Mendonca-Dias MH, Rudin AM. (1978). In Frontiers in Biological Energetics. ed PL Dutton. Academic Press. New York.

Martell AE, Smith RM. (1974-1976). Critical Stability Constants (Volumes 1-4). Plenum Press, New York.

McNamara MT, Wesbey GE, Higgins CB, et. al. (1985). Investigative Radiology 20:591-595.

McNamara MT, Higgins CB, Ehman RL, et. al. (1984b). Radiology 153:157-162.

McNamara MT, Ehman RL, Couet W, et. al. (1984a). *Investigative Radiology* 19(5):S-20.

Mendonca-Dias HM, Lauterbur H. (1982). In: Book of Abstracts. pp.105-106. The Society of Magnetic Resonance in Medicine. First Annual Meeting. Boston, MA.

Newhouse JE, Pykett IL, Brady TJ et. al. (1981). Prooceedings of the Symposium on Nuclear Magnetic Resonance Imaging, Bowman Gray School of Medicine, Wake Forest University, Winston-Salem, NC, 1981, 121-124. Witeciski RL, Karstadt N, Partain CL, eds.

Pauling LC. (1960). The nature of the chemical bond and the structure of molecules and crystals; An introduction to modern structural chemistry. Cornell University Press, Ithaca, NY.

Pfister G, Catch A, Nigrovic V. (1967). Argneim Forsch 22:748-751, 1967.

Poole CP, Farach HA. (1971). Relaxation in magnetic resonance. Academic Press, New York.

Pople JA, Schneider WG, Bernstein HJ. (1959). High-resolution nuclear magnetic resonance. McGraw-Hill Book Co., Inc. New York

Rauckman EJ, Rosen Gm, Lefowitz RJ (1976). *J Med Chem* 19:1254

Runge VM, Stewart RG, Clanton JA, James Ae, Partain CL. (1983a). *Radiology* 147:789-791.

Runge VM, Foster MA, Jones MN, James AE. (1983b). In: Book of Abstracts. pp.312-313. The Society of Magnetic Resonance in Medicine. 2nd Annual Meeting. San Francisco, CA.

Spector WS (ed). (1956). Handbook of Toxicology. W.B. Saunders, Philadelphia. pp.140-141.

Swartz HM (1982) ESR: Principles and applications. (abstract). Society of Magnetic Resonance in Medicine, First Annual Meeting, Boston, MA.

Weast RC, Astle MJ. (1981). CRC Handbook of Chemistry and Physics. CRC Press, Inc., Boca Raton, Florida.

Wehrli FW, MacFall JR, Grigsby N, Haughton V, Johansen J (1983). In: Book of Abstracts, pp.368-369. Society of

Magnetic Resonance in Medicine. 2nd Annual Meeting. San Francisco, CA.

Weinmann HJ, Brasch RC, Press WR, Wesbey GE. (1984). AJR 142:619.

Weinmann HJ, Gries H. (1983). In: Book of Abstracts. pp.370-371. The Society of Magnetic Resonance in Medicine. 2nd Annual Meeting. San Francisco, CA.

Wesbey GE, Moseley ML, Ehman RL. (1984a). Investigative Radiology 19:484-498.

Wesbey GE, Engelstad BL, Huberty JP, et. al. (1983b). In: Scientific Program Book (Scientific Sessions), Radiological Society of North America, 69th Annual Meeting, November, 1983.

Wesbey GE, Brasch RC, Engelstad BL, Moss AA, Crooks LE, Brito AC. (1983a). Radiology 149:175-180.

Wesbey GE, Higgins CB, Lipton MJ, et. al. (1984b). Radiology 153:165-170.

Wesbey Ge, Higgins CB, Lipton ML, et. al. (1984c). Circulation 69(1):125-130, 1984.

Wesbey GE, Brasch RC, Goldberg HI, et. al. (1985). Magnetic Resonance Imaging 3:57-64.

Wolf G., Baum L, (1983). AJR 141:193-197.

Young IR, Clarke GJ, Bailes DR, et. al. (1981). CT, 5:534-547.

ACKNOWLEDGEMENTS

The author wishes to thank Todd Richards, Ph.D, and Thomas Budinger, M.D., Ph.D., for preparation of the rat model of radiation cerebritis. We also wish to thank John Fike, Ph.D., and Christopher Cann, Ph.D. for preparation of the canine model of radiation cerebritis. We thank Helen Griffin, for preparation of this manuscript.

FLOW EFFECTS IN MAGNETIC RESONANCE IMAGING

Leon Axel, Ph.D., M.D.
Daniel Morton, M.S.E.E.
Department of Radiology, Hospital of the University of Pennsylvania
Philadelphia, Pa. 19104

ABSTRACT

A review of the effects of flowing blood on magnetic resonance images is presented. A summary is given of early investigations that noted flow effects in nonimaging techniques; attempts to measure flow in these experiments are also mentioned. Flow effects in magnetic resonance images are described in detail, as well as flow-related artifacts in spin warp imaging. Finally, a summary is presented of recent imaging techniques designed to measure blood flow by utilizing the various flow effects.

INTRODUCTION

In this paper, the effects of blood flow on magnetic resonance images (MRI) are examined. Several methods have been proposed for the utilization of these effects in order to quantitatively assess blood flow; a number of these methods are also presented here.

This discussion will be confined to flow effects originating in the larger vessels (veins and arteries, as opposed to the capillaries) because it is here that the most pronounced effects are evident. Indeed, it has not been established that tissue perfusion produces detectable effects in MRI. Flow in the larger vessels is highly directional, whereas flow in tissue is diffuse. Also, MRI flow effects are related to velocity, and perfusion occurs at lower velocities than that found within vessels. Furthermore, blood in tissue comprises only a small portion of the tissue volume, having much less influence on net signal than blood within a large vessel. The combination of these factors accounts for the difficulty in detecting flow effects in tissue. For that reason, these effects will not be considered here.

Motion effects due to blood flow in magnetic resonance imaging arise principally from three different sources: 1) The inflow of spins (magnetically resonant nuclei) into an imaging region, with a degree of saturation that differs from that of the displaced spins; 2) the outflow of excited spins from the imaging region; and 3) the shift in phase of excited spins due to motion along field gradients. The first two effects are generally grouped together as "washout" or "time of flight" effects.

Flow effects in magnetic resonance have been reported well before the advent of MRI. Suryan[1] discovered washout effects in his study of fluid flowing through a coil; with increasing flow rates, the signal first increased and then decreased. At slow flow rates, spins which were partially saturated (due to incomplete relaxation from previous excitation) were replaced by upstream spins that were fully magnetized; these spins contributed more signal, accounting for the initial increase. At rapid rates, the upstream spins did not have sufficient time in the magnet to be magnetized fully and hence contributed less signal. Hahn[2] noted the loss of spin echo signal resulting from motion through inhomogeneous magnetic fields, which results in incomplete refocusing of excited spins. Carr and Purcell[3] examined the relationship between motion along field gradients and spin echo formation. They found that spins that have lost phase coherence due to motion can regain phase coherence for even-numbered echoes. Early investigators attempted to exploit motion effects in nonimaging experiments which were designed to measure the velocity of moving fluid. Some of the earliest work in blood flow measurement using nonimaging MR was done by Singer[4], using separate excitation and detection coils to detect the time of flight of a bolus of partially saturated spins. Hahn[5] suggested employing a pulsed bipolar gradient to induce a phase shift in the spin echoes of moving fluid, which could be detected by beating the resultant signal against a reference signal from identical apparatus where the fluid velocity was zero; the amount of phase shift would be proportional to velocity.

Motion effects have also been observed in MR images where blood is flowing[6-12]; these effects are due to the sources noted above. The way in which flowing blood influences MRI depends not only on the nature of the flow, but also on the particular pulse sequence used. The de facto standard for MRI pulse sequences has come to be the so called "spin warp" pulse sequence[13-14], a conventional form

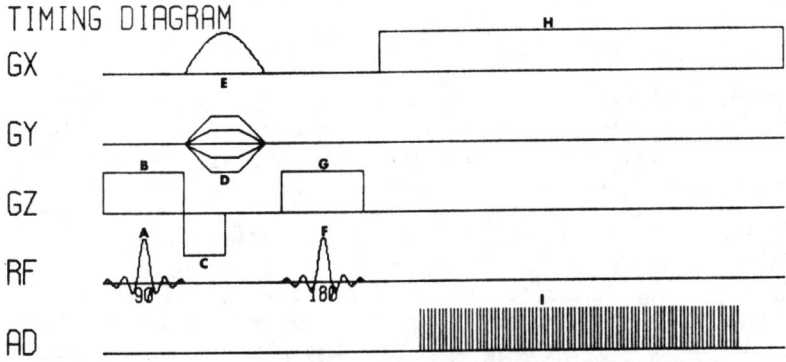

Fig. 1. Conventional spin warp pulse sequence. 90° RF excitation pulse is slice selective in Z due to presence of gradient (B). Rephasing gradient (C) rephases excited spins dephased during excitation. Phase-encoding gradient (D) varies for each excitation-detection cycle. Dephasing gradient (E) provides initial dephasing prior to rephasing that occurs during readout. Selective 180° RF pulse (F,G) produces spin echo which is then frequency encoded by the readout gradient (H) and sampled by the A/D converter (I).

of which is shown schematically in Fig. 1. Most imaging sequences form at least one spin echo through the use of 180° RF refocusing pulses. When a refocusing pulse is combined with a plane selection gradient, as is shown in Fig. 1, then only spins within the excited slice are affected by the refocusing pulse. In imaging where nonselective 180° refocusing pulses are used, spins outside of the excited slice are also affected. The choice of selective or nonselective refocusing pulses has implications for flow, as will be seen. Most of the flow effects mentioned in this review, as well as the techniques mentioned here to quantify flow, are discussed in the context of the spin warp imaging approach.

SOURCES OF FLOW EFFECTS IN MAGNETIC RESONANCE IMAGING

In spin warp imaging, the excitation-detection process is repeated (at least once) for each row of data in the two dimensional Fourier transform array. The repetition time is designated as TR; within each excitation-detection cycle, the time between excitation (the 90° RF pulse) and detection (of the spin echo) is designated as TE. Taking relaxation factors into account, the signal intensity is then

$$I \propto N(H)(1 - 2e^{-(TR-TE/2)/T1} + e^{-TR/T1})e^{-TE/T2} \qquad (1)$$

where $N(H)$ is proton density. TR is generally $\gg$ TE, in order to permit sufficient restoration of longitudinal magnetization. Given this premise, the expression for signal intensity is often simplified to

$$I \propto N(H)(1 - e^{-TR/T1})e^{-TE/T2} \qquad (2)$$

which is assumed valid for the purposes of this discussion.

This expression does, however, neglect the effects of moving spins. Consider a spin warp pulse sequence with a selective 180° refocusing pulse, such as that shown in Fig. 1. In a typical spin warp imaging sequence, TR is chosen to permit a substantial restoration of longitudinal magnetization before reexcitation; this is balanced against the need for rapid data acquisition. If TR is sufficiently long (compared to the time for excited spins to wash out of the slice, but shorter than or on the order of T1), then regions of the excited plane experiencing flow will have spins that are partially saturated (not fully relaxed) replaced with fully magnetized spins from upstream of the excited plane. If a slice thickness of L is assumed, then for a given element of the slice containing spins with a flow velocity of v, a fraction of partially saturated spins vTR/L within the element will be replaced with fully magnetized spins. Under conditions of relatively slow flow, the signal arising from this element following excitation will be approximately

$$I \propto N(H)\{vTR/L + (1 - vTR/L)(1 - e^{-TR/T1})\}e^{-TE/T2} \qquad (3)$$

(This neglects the loss of excited spins prior to refocusing, a phenomenon that has little effect with slow flow but has dominant effects with rapid flow.) This expression illustrates the so called "paradoxical" or flow-related enhancement, because the magnitude of the magnetization vector for the slice element has been increased by the influx of fully magnetized spins. When $vTR \geq L$, all the partially saturated spins have been replaced, and the signal is at a maximum. For more rapid flow, the loss of excited spins from the slice element becomes an overriding factor. For a time $TE/2$, the time between the excitation and refocusing pulses, excited spins which would otherwise contribute to signal if refocused are washed out of the slice element. They are replaced by fully magnetized spins which, when inverted by the 180° refocusing pulse, contribute nothing to the signal. The correction factor to (3) for this effect is $(1-vTE/2L)$. If intensity for the slice element is plotted as a function of velocity (Fig. 2), an initial increase is expected due

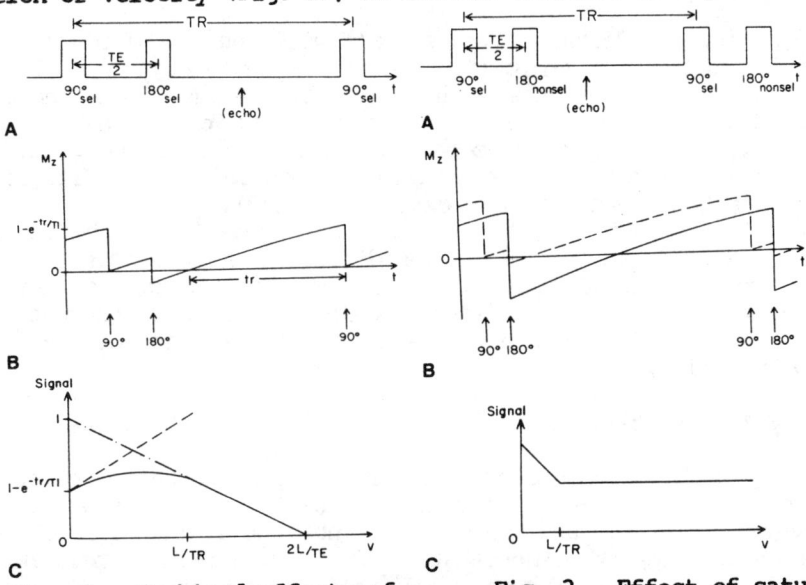

Fig. 2. Combined effects of saturated and excited spin washout. A, RF pulse sequence with selective 180° refocusing pulse. B, effect on longitudinal magnetization for spins remaining in the slice. C, signal intensity as a function of velocity. Reprinted courtesy of AJR[15].

Fig. 3. Effect of saturated spin washout. A, RF pulse sequence with nonselective 180° refocusing pulse. B, effect on longitudinal magnetization for in-slice spins (broken line) and out-of-slice spins (solid line). C, signal intensity. Reprinted courtesy of AJR[15].

to the influx of fully magnetized spins, and then a steady decrease due to the washout of excited spins, until the limit $vTE/2 \geq L$ is reached, when all excited spins have been removed from the slice element before they can be refocused, and any signal contribution to the spin echo has been eliminated.

For spin warp pulse sequences where nonselective 180° refocusing pulses are used, the washout of excited spins is not of significance since spins washed out of the plane of excitation are still refocused downstream, and contribute to the signal. However, while excited spins are refocused by the nonselective 180° pulse, fully magnetized spins upstream of the plane of excitation are inverted. If they are not reinverted by a second refocusing pulse (in a multiecho imaging sequence, where many such pairs may occur), then instead of partially saturated spins being replaced by fully magnetized spins before the next excitation pulse, they will be replaced by even more saturated spins. This leads to the expression

$$I \propto N(H)\{vTR(1 - e^{-TR/T1})/[L(1 + e^{-TR/T1})] + (1 - vTR/L)(1 - e^{-TR/T1})\}e^{-TE/T2} \qquad (4)$$

Thus a steady decrease in signal will occur with increasing velocity, until the limit $vTR \geq L$ is reached (Fig. 3). Then all partially saturated spins within the slice element will have been replaced by even more saturated spins, and the signal from the element will no longer decrease. For paired refocusing pulses, the upstream longitudinal magnetization is restored to near its initial state, and the signal is that expressed in (3).

The third flow effect, that of accumulated phase shifts in the presence of field gradients, is different in character from the first two effects of washout, and is not limited to flow normal to the excited plane. The explanation for the shift in phase of spins along the direction of the gradient is found in the integral of the Larmor equation,

$$\Delta\phi = \int_0^T \gamma G(t)x(t)\,dt = \int_0^T \gamma G(t)x_0\,dt + \int_0^T \gamma G(t)vt\,dt \qquad (5)$$

where $\Delta\phi$ is the accumulated phase shift, $G(t)$ is the magnetic field gradient and T is its duration, x_0 is the initial position of a spin and v is its (constant) velocity. Thus the first integral on the right hand side represents the phase increment experienced by excited spins as a function of their position, and the second integral represents the phase increment they experience as a function of their velocity. For a gradient of constant magnitude G and finite duration T, the net increase in phase will be

$$\Delta\phi = \gamma G x_0 T + \gamma G v T^2/2 \qquad (6)$$

By an appropriate choice of a bipolar gradient, where the magnitude and duration of each lobe can be different, it is possible to cancel the phase component due to either position or velocity[16]. If a balanced bipolar gradient is applied (where the duration of each lobe is the time T, and the magnitude of each lobe is equal but opposite), the first (position dependent) term on the right hand side of (6) will be eliminated. However, there will be a net shift in phase due to velocity,

$$\Delta\phi_1 = \int_0^T -\gamma Gvt\, dt + \int_T^{2T} \gamma Gvt\, dt = \gamma GvT^2 \qquad (7)$$

(Such a phase shift for moving spins will be produced, for example, by the bipolar gradient which is coupled with the 90° RF slice selection pulse in Fig. 1. This gradient is bipolar in order to rephase stationary spins within the slice that have become dephased by the slice selection gradient.) This phase shift due to velocity can be "undone" by the subsequent application of another balanced bipolar gradient, similar in form to the one that induced the shift, but where the polarities of the lobes are reversed. For example, suppose the second bipolar gradient starts at 3T; then

$$\Delta\phi_2 = \int_{3T}^{4T} \gamma Gvt\, dt + \int_{4T}^{5T} -\gamma Gvt\, dt = -\gamma GvT^2 \qquad (8)$$

and thus the sum total of acquired phase, $\Delta\phi_1 + \Delta\phi_2$, will be zero.

In the above example, if the magnitude of each gradient pulse is maintained at G for a duration of 2T, the same phase effect can be achieved by supplying a 180° RF pulse midway through each gradient pulse. In spin warp imaging where selective 180° refocusing pulses are employed, such as is shown in Fig. 4, the refocusing pulses are paired with constant gradient pulses. The result is a reduction in the range of spin phases for even echoes.

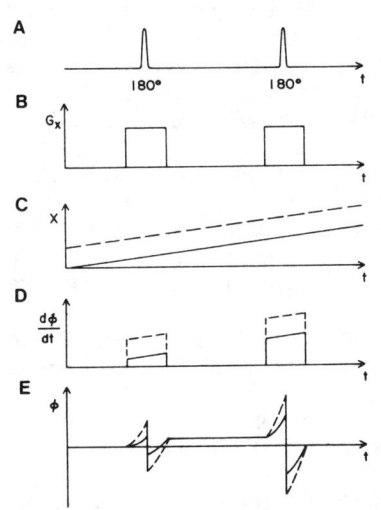

Fig. 4. Effect of constant velocity on phase of excited spins. A, RF pulse sequence. B, Corresponding gradient. C, position as function of time for spins with two different initial positions. D, rate of change of phase. E, net accumulated phase. Reprinted courtesy of AJR[15].

Another example from spin warp imaging is the use of a dephasing gradient prior to the 180° refocusing pulse (Fig. 1); coupled with the readout gradient during the spin echo, these gradients can be considered as an effective bipolar gradient.

In the blood vessels, flow is not constant across the lumen of the vessel[17]. The velocity profile of blood in a large, unbranched and relatively straight vessel (far from the norm, to be sure) is approximately parabolic. Thus, although blood velocity is relatively low near the perimeter of the vessel, the velocity gradient there is quite large. This means that within finite elements of the excited slice located near the perimeter of vessels, it is possible for spins to possess a wide range of velocities, and hence acquire a wide range of phase during the application of gradients such as those used in spin warp imaging. This will lead to a loss of coherence within the element and concomitant loss of signal. As Carr and Purcell first demonstrated[3], and as was detailed above, it is possible to reverse the dephasing effects of certain balanced gradients for even echoes, resulting in higher signal during these echoes. Whether or not such an increase will be observed in multiecho spin warp imaging depends on what pulse sequence is used and on what cumulative dephasing effects other gradients may have. For example, the gradient employed for the phase-encoding of spin position is generally not a balanced bipolar gradient, nor does it occur more than once in an excitation-detection cycle; therefore, it will tend to dephase moving spins, independent of whatever efforts may be made with other gradients to rephase them.

Finally, consideration must be given to the effects of pulsatile blood flow. If blood velocity varies from one excitation-detection cycle to the next, as is the case with MRI unsynchronized with the cardiac cycle, then the effects on acquired data of spin washout and phase shifts will also vary. When these effects are not consistent, they cause the reconstruction algorithm to distribute across the reconstructed image the signal that originated from regions of flow. The distribution will occur in the spin warp phase-encoding direction, appearing as streak or "ghost" artifacts across the image. Gating the pulse sequence to the same point in the cardiac cycle will alleviate the artifact, provided the cardiac pulse is not too erratic; if it is, then TR will vary significantly, as will the extent of spin relaxation, and the same type of artifact will be manifested.

In the next section, methods which attempt to exploit flow-related effects in MRI for the measurement of blood flow are examined.

TECHNIQUES FOR THE INVESTIGATION OF BLOOD FLOW

Singer and Crooks[18] have investigated blood flow using MRI, employing a partial saturation washout scheme; in Fig. 5 the pulse sequence is shown. Modifications to the conventional sequence include an initial saturation pulse, followed by a delay TD coupled with a homospoil gradient to disperse transverse magnetization. The method is one dominated by the first flow effect, that of the replacement of partially saturated spins with fully magnetized spins. In this technique, images are made for a number of values for TD. This permits varying degrees of spin replacement, with attendant increase in signal, up to the point where all partially saturated spins are replaced with fully magnetized ones. Since velocities will vary across the lumen of the vessel, the TD which will permit full replacement for a given element of the resulting image will depend on the location of the pixel within the vessel.

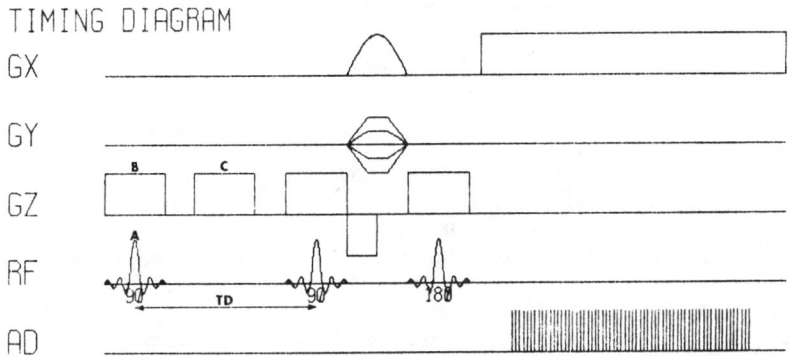

Fig. 5. Saturated spin washout technique. Differences from standard spin warp technique include selective saturation pulse (A,B) with delay TD, and homospoil pulse (C).

Given the thickness of the slice, the area of the lumen and the TD's which produce maximum signal for pixels within the lumen, an average velocity and volume flow rate can be established for the vessel. Disadvantages of this approach include the dependence of signal strength on T1 as well as on flow, and the need for the acquisition of a large number of images in order to accurately determine washout times. In addition, the loss of excited spins after excitation but prior to refocusing, since selective 180° refocusing pulses are used, is not taken into account. As with other velocity measurement techniques, gated data acquisition would be necessary to measure pulsatile flow.

Another technique devised by Feinberg[19] relies in part on the second flow effect, that of excited spin washout. The method is employed to evaluate (pulsatile) flow in arteries. The pulse sequence is basically that of Fig. 1, except that the RF is modulated in the presence of a plane selection gradient in order to select refocusing planes downstream of the excitation plane in a multiecho sequence. The timing of the echoes and the spacing of the planes is chosen in the expectation of a particular velocity range. The first refocusing plane overlaps the excitation plane slightly, so that the image produced from this echo provides an anatomical reference as well as displays the location of vessels with moving blood, since spins within the lumen experience dephasing and produce relatively dark pixels in the resulting image. The second downstream refocusing plane will yield an image of only excited spins that have washed out of the excitation plane into the refocusing plane, outlining the location of the vessels. The intensity of a given pixel within the vessel will be a measure of flow velocity; its value will be determined by the product of the shape of the moving excited spin bolus with the shapes of the refocusing "planes". The position and shape of the bolus will vary depending upon where in the cardiac cycle the pulse sequence is gated, demonstrating the pulsatile character of flow in the vessel.

The chief limitation of this technique is the lack of a precise measure of blood flow in the resulting image. In order to overcome this limitation, it would be necessary to obtain a number of images with different echo delays or refocusing plane displacements, and then deconvolve the selective "plane" profile from the resulting intensity data set.

A second technique has been implemented by Axel[20] for the direct visualization of excited spin washout. In this approach, the selective refocusing plane is orthogonal to the selective excitation plane (Fig. 6), along the direction of flow; the readout gradient is along the direction of flow as well. In the absence of flow, this yields a straight line of refocused, excited spins. Flow will cause the excited spins to move from the excited plane, and the orthogonal refocusing plane will yield a "snapshot" of the velocity profile of these spins. The degree of displacement is proportional to velocity. The principal advantage of this technique is that it provides in one image a direct measure of velocity. A relative disadvantage of this approach is that like many others, it is limited to measuring flow velocities at right angles to the plane of excitation.

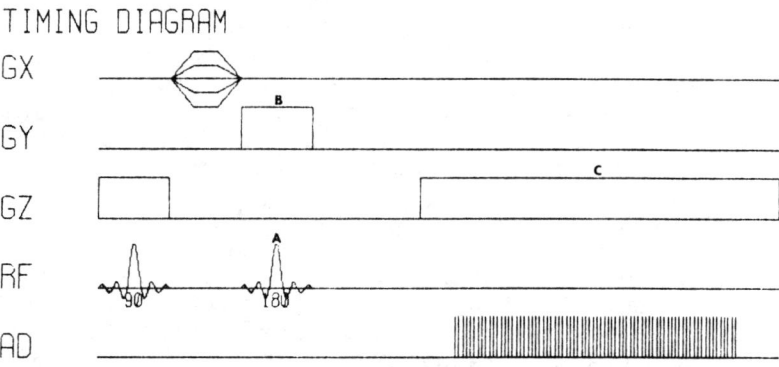

Fig. 6. Excited spin washout technique. Selective refocusing pulse (A,B) selects refocusing plane orthogonal to excitation plane. Readout gradient (C) is along the direction of flow.

A number of techniques have been devised to characterize flow by the introduction of balanced, bipolar gradients to produce a phase shift in moving spins, without influencing stationary spins. Moran[21] proposed the superposition of such a phase shifting gradient upon the gradient whose direction corresponds to the desired imaging direction for flow, as exemplified in Fig. 7. The resulting phase differences between images with and without this phase-encoding gradient provide a measure of flow. Furthermore, the magnitude of the velocity phase shifting gradient can be varied from image to image, much as the positional phase-encoding gradient is varied from iteration to iteration in conventional spin warp imaging. Thus a third dimension has been added, that of image number. If the ensemble of images so produced is then Fourier transformed in this dimension, the resulting images will correspond to particular ranges of phase shift, with the median image corresponding to unshifted, stationary spins. The amount of displacement for moving spins along this dimension will be proportional to their shift in phase, which in turn is proportional to their velocity. The chief disadvantage of this approach is that a large amount of time must be spent making a sufficient number of images that will permit the resolution of different velocities.

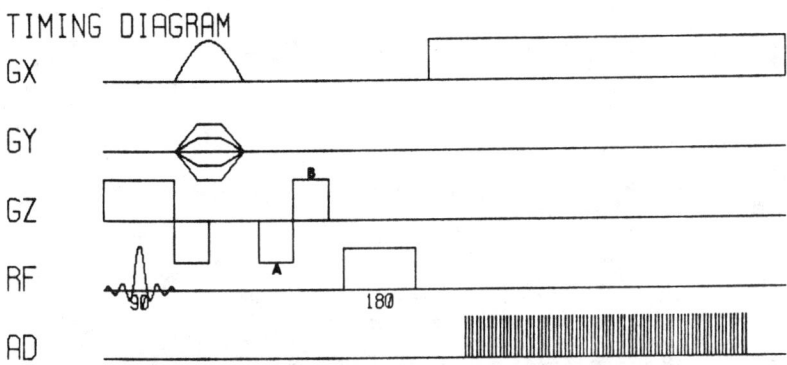

Fig. 7. Phase shift technique. Balanced bipolar gradient (A,B) produces a phase shift for moving spins without affecting stationary spins. The magnitude of (A,B) can be varied from image to image to produce an ensemble of phase shift images.

Alternatively, the velocity component of (6) can be rewritten to yield

$$v = 2\Delta\phi/\gamma GT^2 \qquad (9)$$

so that a more direct measure of velocity for a given pixel can be obtained by evaluating the amount of phase accumulated for the duration of the gradient. However, since the range of velocities within a vessel with approximately parabolic flow can be quite large, this approach suffers from one of two problems: 1) the gradient chosen to affect relatively slow moving spins is so large that fast moving spins "wrap around" in phase, and cannot be discriminated from slower spins, or 2) the gradient chosen to prevent aliasing of fast spins is so low that it produces very small phase changes in slower spins, and the effect cannot be discriminated from that due to noise. O'Donnell[22] has proposed a pulse sequence (Fig. 8) which can potentially surmount this obstacle. In this method, the flow phase-encoding gradient is chosen small enough to prevent aliasing for the first echo in a multiecho imaging sequence. After each refocusing pulse, and before each echo, the same bipolar gradient is applied, except that the sign of each lobe alternates from echo to echo. Consequently, flow-induced phase accumulates with each echo. This improves the signal to noise ratio for slow spins; although the accumulated phase for fast spins may still "wrap around" for later echoes in the sequence, it can be "unwrapped" since no aliasing will be produced on the first echo. For a given pixel, the set of unwrapped phases from all the echoes can be plotted as a function of the echo number; the slope of the line fit to these points will yield the velocity.

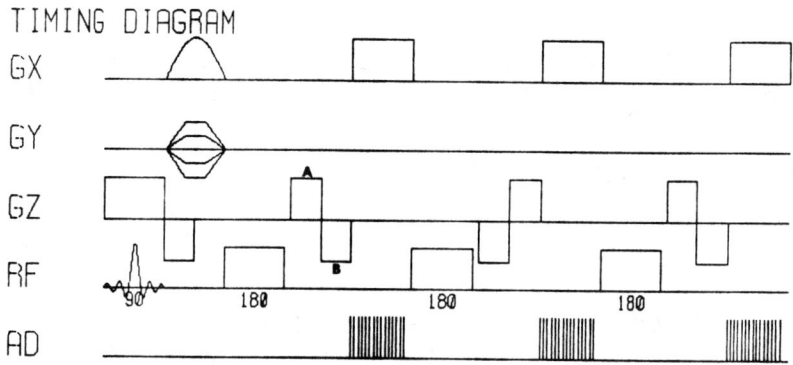

Fig. 8. Phase shift technique. The balanced bipolar gradient (A,B) induces a phase shift in moving spins, as does each successive bipolar gradient, for a cumulative phase shift effect.

SUMMARY

The sources of flow effects in magnetic resonance imaging have been discussed, namely: 1) the inflow of spins with a different saturation level than that of displaced spins; 2) the loss of excited spins during refocusing, and 3) the accumulation of phase shifts by excited spins due to motion along field gradients. Washout effects can either increase or decrease the magnitude of the net magnetization vector within an element of the excited plane, causing a corresponding change in the signal arising from that element. Phase shift effects can cause coherence loss among excited spins within an element of the excited plane, resulting in a net decrease in signal intensity for that element. Deleterious streaking artifacts can result from the failure to synchronize the excitation-detection cycle with the cardiac cycle, due to these flow effects.

Several modifications to the conventional spin warp imaging pulse sequence have been proposed that would utilize flow-induced MRI effects to provide measures of blood flow. All of these approaches enjoy some success when applied to phantom studies; however, it remains to be proven that these methods are efficacious in clinical settings.

ACKNOWLEDGEMENTS

Leon Axel is an Established Investigator of the American Heart Association, and is supported in part by funds from the Southeast Pennsylvania chapter. This work was supported in part by NIH grant R01 HL33236.

REFERENCES

1. G. Suryan: Proc Indian Acad Sci [A] 33, 107 (1951).

2. E.L. Hahn: Phys Rev 80, 580 (1950).

3. H.Y. Carr, E.M. Purcell: Phys Rev 94, 630 (1954).

4. J.R. Singer: Science 130, 1652 (1959).

5. E.L. Hahn: J Geophys Res 65, 776 (1960).

6. W.S. Hinshaw, P.A. Bottomley, G.N. Holland: Nature (London) 270, 722 (1977).

7. I.R. Young, M. Burl, G.J. Clarke, et al: AJR 137, 895 (1981).

8. L. Crooks, P. Sheldon, L. Kaufman, W. Rowan, T. Miller: IEEE Trans Nuc Sci NS-29, 1181 (1982).

9. L. Kaufman, L.E. Crooks, P.E. Sheldon, W. Rowan, T. Miller: Invest Radiol 17, 554 (1982).

10. L.E. Crooks, J.C. Hoenninger, M. Arakawa: (In) Nuclear Magnetic Resonance and Correlative Imaging Modalities, p. 69. C.L. Partain, ed. New York: Society of Nuclear Medicine (1984).

11. J.P. Grant, C. Back: Med Phys 9, 188 (1982).

12. F.W. Wehrli, J.R. MacFall, L. Axel, D. Shutts, G.H. Glover, J.R. Herfkens: Noninv Med Imag 1, 127 (1984).

13. A. Kumar, D. Welti, R. Ernst: J Mag Res 18, 69 (1975).

14. W.A. Edelstein, J.M.S. Hutchison, G. Johnson, T. Redpath: Phys in Med and Bio 25, 751 (1980).

15. L. Axel: AJR 143, 1157 (1984).

16. A. Constantinesco, J.J. Mallet, A. Bonmartin, C. Lallot, A. Briguet: Nuc Med Comm 5, 671 (1984).

17. C.G. Caro, T.J. Pedley, R.C. Schroter, W.A. Seed: The mechanics of the circulation. New York: Oxford University Press (1978).

18. J.R. Singer, L.E. Crooks: Science **221**, 654 (1983).

19. D.A. Feinberg, L. Crooks, J. Hoenninger, M. Arakawa, J. Watts: Radiology **153**, 177 (1984).

20. L. Axel, A. Shimakawa, J. MacFall: A time-of-flight method of measuring flow velocity by magnetic resonance imaging. Presented at the 70th Scientific Assembly of the RSNA, Nov. 25-30, 1984.

21. P.R. Moran: Mag Res Imag **1**, 197 (1982).

22. M. O'Donnell: Med Phys **12**, 59 (1985).

CLINICAL APPLICATIONS: CARDIAC

Ronald M. Peshock
University of Texas Health Science Center at Dallas
Dallas, Texas 75235

ABSTRACT

Nuclear magnetic resonance imaging is particularly well suited to the evaluation of the heart and vascular system. However, cardiac motion introduces a number of technical problems and potential artifacts which must be addressed. Major areas of application at present include the the evaluation of disease of the great vessels, ischemic heart disease, and congenital heart disease. Although clinical experience is limited as compared with that in the evaluation of the central nervous system, initial experience suggests that nuclear magnetic resonance imaging will play an important role in cardiac diagnosis and management.

INTRODUCTION

Cardiovascular disease is one of the leading causes of morbidity and mortality in this country. A variety of imaging techniques including contrast angiography, echocardiography, and radionuclide ventriculography have been utilized in an effort to deal with this clinical problem. Recently, nuclear magnetic resonance imaging (MRI) has been applied to the evaluation of the cardiovascular system and the potential of MRI in cardiology has been the subject of a number of recent reviews[1,2,3,4]. In many ways MRI is well suited to the evaluation of the heart. Advantages of MRI include high inherent contrast between rapidly flowing blood and chamber or vessel wall, good spatial resolution, relative ease of gating to the cardiac cycle and the ability to obtain images in three orthogonal planes. In addition, the fact that ionizing radiation and iodinated contrast material are not necessary allows serial studies to be performed with relatively little risk. Disadvantages of MRI in cardiac evaluation include its rather long imaging time (typically in the range of 6-8 minutes for each imaging sequence), artifacts related to arrhythmias and respiration, significant partial volume effects, and complex alterations of signal intensity in regions of relatively slow blood flow. The goals of this section are (1) an examination of the technical considerations which are relatively unique to cardiac imaging and cardiac patients, (2) an introduction to the clinical aspects of flow effects, (3) a presentation of some examples of the use of this tool in clinical practice, (4) a discussion of artifacts encountered in cardiac imaging, and (5) a brief overview of recent technical developments in this area.

TECHNICAL CONSIDERATIONS

In imaging the heart one has to deal with the fundamental problem that the heart is constantly in motion. In imaging techniques such as cineangiography or echocardiography one is able to acquire images rapidly enough to minimize blurring of the image with cardiac motion. Unfortunately, most methods for acquiring magnetic resonance images require minutes to carry out the number of phase encoding steps necessary for imaging of an acceptable resolution. Ungated MRI has been performed in the past and, in general, has been of poor quality except in relatively specialized circumstances[5]. To obtain good structural resolution in the majority of subjects it is necessary to synchronize or gate the data acquisition to the cardiac cycle[6].

In comparison to gated computed tomography, gated MRI is quite straight forward. A physiologic marker, such as the QRS complex on ECG, is used to indicate to the control computer when to begin the pulse sequence. Initially there were concerns regarding the use of ECG leads within the imager, and attempts were made to use peripheral pulses to control data acquisition[6]. However, these efforts were limited by the variability of the time delay between cardiac contraction and the transmission of the pulse to the periphery. With use of short ECG leads, ECG preamplifiers without ferromagnetic components, and transmission of the ECG signal to the control computer via telemetry or fiber optic cable, it is possible to use the ECG as the physiologic trigger in most presently available imaging systems.

It is important to realize that the imager causes two "artifacts" to appear on the ECG. First, since blood is a conductor which is moving in the presence of a magnetic field, it generates a current which is superimposed on the patient's ECG. Due to the pulsatile nature of blood flow, this effect is maximum during systole when the velocity of the blood being ejected is greatest. Hence, the current generated is maximized in the ST segment and T wave of the electrocardiogram. This is a magnetohydrodynamic effect which has been previously described in animal studies and appears to have no physiologic significance[7]. In particular, it does not appear to induce arrhythmias or alter thresholds for electrical instability in the heart. The changes in the electrocardiogram resolve when the patient is removed from the magnetic field. However, these changes mean that this portion of the ECG is of limited use for monitoring the patient during imaging. Second, the switching of gradients during multislice imaging induces currents in the ECG leads which are also superimposed on the patient's ECG. This can lead to autogating and makes it essentially impossible to evaluate the ECG during the portion of the cardiac cycle during which the gradients are being switched. In some systems this is handled by disabling the ECG from the control computer for the required period of time following the detection of a physiologic trigger.

The motion of the heart has important implications for multislice imaging. Multislice is a very efficient technique for obtaining images with a relatively long pulse repetition interval. However, in imaging the heart the use of multislice means that each slice is acquired at a different point in the cardiac cycle. It appears that the interpretation of images obtained in this way is not a major problem when one is dealing with strictly structural abnormalities of the heart or vascular system, but it is a significant problem in the evaluation of chamber size, wall thickness and wall motion, all of which vary during the cardiac cycle.

The fact that the pulsing is controlled by the ECG has several additional implications for image interpretation. First, the repetition time or TR is controlled by the patient's heart rate. Since the heart rate in different patients typically varies from 40-120 beats per minute, repetition intervals correspondingly vary from 1500 to 500 milliseconds. Depending upon the type of imaging sequence being used, this means that images from different patients may have considerably different amounts of relative T_1 weighting present in the image. Second, there is intrinsic variability in the heart rate of most people. In a young, normal volunteer it is not unusual for the heart rate to vary by 10-20 percent during the period of signal acquisition. Hence, almost all gated cardiac MRI includes effects due to a varying TR during acquisition. By imaging every second or third heart beat and forcing a long repetition interval, it is possible to minimize the effect of variable repetition times. However, this is at the expense of an increase in the total amount of time required to carry out the necessary number of phase encoding steps.

Variations in heart rate can also lead to problems in images obtained late in the cardiac cycle. The timing of mechanical events early in the cardiac cycle are relatively unaffected by small changes in heart rate. However, following end systole or completion of the contraction of the heart, events are more dependent on the heart rate. Hence, images obtained early in diastole, typically more than 400 msec after the QRS, may suffer significant degradation in image quality due to variability in heart position, particularly at high heart rates.

An additional consideration is that of temporal resolution or the effect of motion during the acquisition of each imaging sequence. If a spin echo sequence is being used, the signal obtained depends on the position of the heart at the time of the 90 degree pulse and the position of the heart at the time of the 180 degree pulse. Hence, the image represents a composite of the heart position at those two times. Typically, in the case of a single spin echo image, the interval between these two times is approximately 14 msec which is short relative to the mechanical events. However, this is considerably longer than the time interval represented in a frame from a cineangiogram or a line in an M-mode echocardiogram. In the case of later spin echoes this problem becomes more severe, and in the case of double spin echo images the interpretation of what the image actually represents becomes even more complex in terms of the mixture of effects from the two 180 degree pulses.

SPECIAL CONSIDERATIONS IN CARDIAC PATIENTS

Patients with cardiac disease undergo a variety of surgical interventions. The insertion of coronary artery bypass grafts, prosthetic heart valves, and cardiac pacemakers are frequent treatments and need to be considered as potential sources of problems in magnetic resonance imaging of these patients.

Interestingly, the wire sternal sutures and vascular clips used in cardiac surgery do not appear to be a significant problem in terms of image degradation or patient safety. This may relate in part to the fibrosis that occurs following surgery. The thought that fibrosis may be important in fixing a clip would make one hesitant to study patients very early after surgery prior to significant fibrosis, although this has not been tested.

Recently, the force generated on various prosthetic heart valves has been evaluated at a number of fields[8]. These studies indicate that the force generated on these valves at relatively low magnetic fields (0.35 T) should not pose a hazard to imaging these patients for the valves studied as long as the valve is sutured securely in position. However, at higher fields these forces may be significant. Surprisingly, the imaging artifacts related to these valves at low field appear to be minimal. Patients with prosthetic valves have been imaged at a number of centers without difficulty. However, it has been suggested that prior to imaging that the force exerted on that particular type of valve be evaluated and that it be establish that the patient's valve is securely sutured in place.

A major point of concern has been the effect of MRI on patients with cardiac pacemakers. Several theoretical concerns exist. First, pacemakers contain a magnetic reed switch which is used to convert the pacemaker from a demand mode (in which the pacemaker fires only when no intrinsic cardiac activity is present above a certain rate) to an asynchronous mode (in which it fires at a preset rate independent of cardiac activity). In a study by Pavlicek[9] the switch was closed at a field of 17 gauss in the most sensitive pacemaker. However, it appears that the field strength required to close this switch is quite variable and is quite dependent on the orientation of the pacemaker with respect to the field. In the majority of patients switching to the asynchronous mode would not be expected to cause a problem, although there is a very small but finite probability that going into this mode could induce a significant arrhythmia in a patient. Second, the RF pulses or gradient pulses could induce currents in the pacemaker lead which could directly pace the heart or effect the pacemaker in a manner that would suppress its output. Experimental studies suggest that the former effect is unlikely, whereas the latter may be possible. Pacemakers are generally designed to reject such electromagnetic interference but one can propose the situation in which the output of the pacemaker is supressed in a pacemaker in which the magnetic reed switch is not operating, thus leaving the patient with no pacemaker activity. Third, the electrical components in the pacemaker could be directly effected by the RF and gradient pulses.

Lastly, the body of the pacemaker might experience sufficient force that it would move in the chest wall. An additional related concern is that the presence of a pacemaker lead in the right ventricle could significantly degrade the image quality of the heart, particularly if the lead contained ferromagnetic material. Hence, at present there are many unanswered questions regarding the safety of imaging patients with cardiac pacemakers and the presence of a cardiac pacemaker must be considered a contraindication to MRI.

BLOOD FLOW

Blood flow plays a particularly important role in the interpretation of cardiovascular magnetic resonance images. The effects of flow on the NMR experiment have been extensively studied by Singer[10] and others. The manifestations of these effects on spin echo magnetic resonance imaging have been the subject of several recent excellent reviews[11,12]. From a clinical perspective these effects have been grouped under three main headings: (1) high velocity signal loss, (2) flow related enhancement, and (3) even echo rephasing. Briefly, high velocity signal loss relates to the fact that rapidly flowing blood moves out of the excited slice prior to refocusing and, hence, yields no signal. Flow related enhancement involves the movement of unsaturated spins into the imaging slice so that moving blood yields more signal than stationary blood. Even echo rephasing describes the fact that spins moving with respect to a magnetic field gradient are more completely rephased on even spin echoes than on odd spin echoes. Each of these effects is seen frequently in clinical images and can be extremely helpful in the evaluation of pathologic states. Unfortunately, they can also lead to significant problems in interpretation because the flow profiles and velocity distributions in normal and abnormal vessels in the body can be quite complex. In particular, these effects can be affected by the direction of the vessel with respect to the slice, the degree of turbulent flow present, the exact position of the slice in the imaging sequence, the exact timing of the slice with respect to the cardiac cycle, and a host of other factors. It is hoped that some of these problems can be addressed through the use of imaging techniques purposely designed to encode flow velocities[13].

CLINICAL RESULTS

The first area in which magnetic resonance imaging has emerged as an important clinical tool in the evaluation of the cardiovascular system is in the diagnosis and management of great vessel disease. In conditions such as aortic dissection, aortic aneurysm, and disease involving the superior and inferior vena cava, the clinician is interested in the structural abnormality present but also in the blood flow in the abnormality, i.e. is there rapid or slow flow in the region and clotted blood present? MRI has been shown to correlate well with the standard techniques such as computed tomography and angiography in these patients with these problems[14,15,16]. Typical images from a patient with a markedly dilated aortic root is shown in figure 1. The

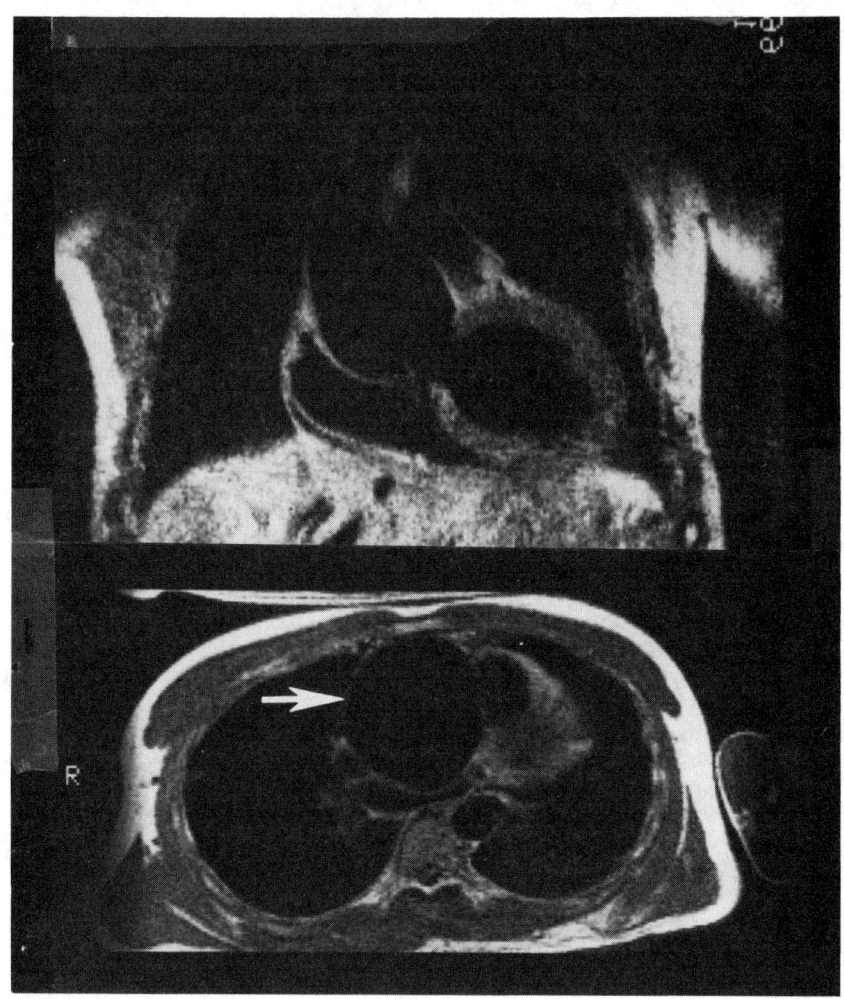

Figure 1. Coronal and transaxial images from a patient with aortic insufficiency. A markedly dilated aortic root is indicated by the arrow. (Reproduced with permission from reference 31).

primary advantages of MRI in these patients are that ionizing radiation and iodinated contrast material are not required. The primary disadvantages are the time required for a complete study using MRI and concerns regarding placing critically ill patients in the confines of the magnet where they may be difficult to monitor. In addition, there is, as in all methods, the potential for false positives. These relate not only to anatomic considerations but also to variability in the flow profile in major vessels in patients without great vessel pathology. The variability of normal blood flow has not really been open to study in the past and, hence, our knowledge in this area is limited. With greater experience and with MRI methods that specifically encode flow, it may be possible to deal with these problem cases.

A second major area of interest has been in the use of MRI in patients with ischemic heart disease. Efforts in this area have involved the study of chronic ischemic heart disease, acute myocardial infarction, assessments of myocardial perfusion, and the possibility of evaluating the patency of coronary arteries. Several investigators have demonstrated that remote from the time of infaction MRI shows thinning of the wall of the heart corresponding to the scar that forms following damage to the heart muscle[6]. A typical image from a patient with a remote infarction is shown in figure 2. More interesting are studies indicating that MRI can detect regions of acute myocardial damage due to alterations in tissue relaxation times. Studies performed by Williams[17] demonstrated that tissue proton T1 increased in regions of myocardial infarction correlating with changes in tissue water content. Subsequently, excised heart and then _in vivo_ studies have indicated that changes in T1 and T2 can be detected in magnetic resonance images[18,19,20] both in animals and in man. However, significant concerns exist regarding the sensitivity and specificity of these findings. Different pathologic conditions such as cardiomyopathy have been shown to lead to lengthening of relaxation times similar to those seen in ischemia[21]. A more fundamental concern involves the fact that the determination of whether infarction is present or not rests on the degree of signal heterogeneity present. Although variations in signal intensity may be due to infarction or another pathologic process, there are many other sources of heterogeneity in signal intensity including poor signal to noise, phase encoding artifacts related to incomplete gating, and B_1 field in homogeneity.

Questions regarding sensitivity and specificity, as well as interest in the assessment of myocardial perfusion, have lead investigators to examine the use of paramagnetic contrast agents in the heart. Work by Wesby[22], McNamara[23] and others[24] in animal models suggests that agents such as Gadolinium diethylene triamine pentaacetic acid can serve as markers of perfusion. However, the rapid redistribution of this agent compared to the time required to obtain magnetic resonance images limits its use in this regard. It is likely that new agents or more rapid imaging will become available that will allow one to better address questions of myocardial perfusion.

Coronary arteries, particularly the right coronary artery, are frequently seen on routine magnetic resonance images. MRI is the

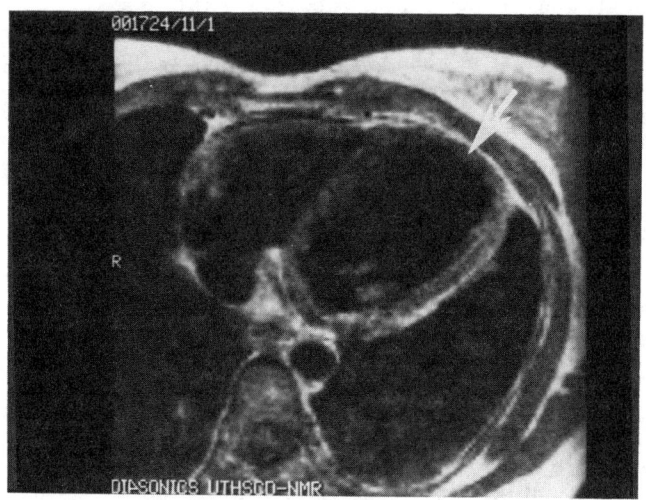

Figure 2. A transaxial image from a patient with an old anterior myocardial infarction. Thinning of the wall is indicated by the arrow.

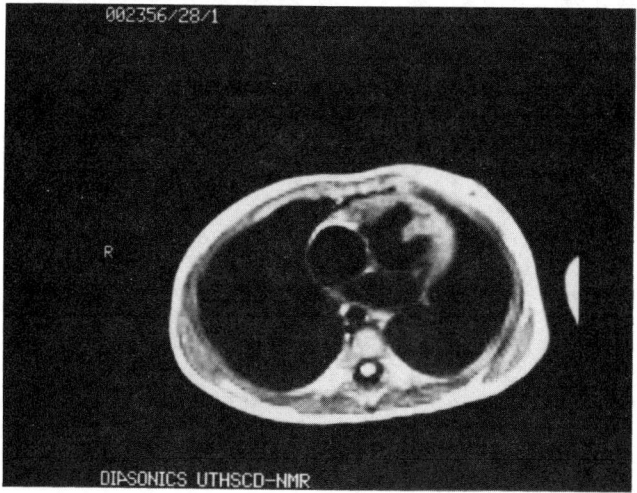

Figure 3. A transaxial image from a 20 month old infant with a ventricular septal defect.

first non-invasive imaging technique that has demonstrated coronary arteries with such frequency and ease. Hence, it shows promise as a means of assessing the coronary arteries. However, phantom studies suggest that to deal with real clinical situations improvements in resolution will need to occur.

A third major area of utilization of MRI in cardiology has been in the evaluation of congenital heart disease. A typical image from a child with congenital heart disease is seen in figure 3. The ability of MRI to examine the thoracic contents completely in a single study in multiple planes has made it useful in the evaluation of complex congenital heart disease[25]. In addition, the fact that ionizing radiation and contrast material are not used in MRI studies makes this technique attractive in examining infants who may need repeated evaluation.

MRI can be used to examine a wide variety of other cardiac conditions including pericardial disease, cardiomyopathy, and possibly valvular heart disease. However, at present the exact role of MRI in the evaluation of these conditions is unclear.

ARTIFACTS

Another area of importance in image interpretation is the recognition of potential artifacts. A major source of artifacts is inconsistent gating or ungated motion. Motion in the phase encoding direction which is not correctly encoded due to inaccurate gating is misplaced in the image and appears as ghosting in the phase encoding direction[26]. Motion in the frequency encoding direction which is inadequately gated may be manifest as blurring. Ghosting can be a significant problem in patients with arrhythmias as it leads to heterogeneity in signal intensity which may appear to be localized depending upon the rate and direction of motion of a particular structure. Not surprisingly, this may be more of a problem in patients whose hearts are moving well and may be less of a problem in hearts which are contracting poorly as less motion occurs. A second source of ungated motion relates to the fact that respiratory gating is rarely used. In the majority of patients respiratory gating is not necessary to obtain satisfactory images; however, in a small number of ill patients it appears that respiratory gating might be helpful. Unfortunately, at the present time most devices for respiratory gating appear to be unreliable and poorly tolerated by many patients. In addition, respiratory gating at least doubles imaging time which makes it very unattractive in terms of patient throughput.

RECENT DEVELOPMENTS

Until recently, MRI of the cardiovascular system has concentrated on the structural aspects of cardiac disease. However, for MRI to assume a major role in cardiovascular diagnosis it is important that it yield more functional information. Several recent advances have occurred which should allow one to obtain more information regarding cardiac function. First, by altering the gradients, it is possible to obtain oblique slices through the body. This is important because the position and orientation of the heart in the chest is variable and assessments of functional status require the heart to be viewed in a standard position. Present coronal, sagittal and transaxial images obtained with respect to the fixed external reference frame do not show the heart in these standard positions. Second, to acquire functional information requires that all of the heart be imaged at several points in time. Gate multislice imaging yields different slices at different points in the cardiac cycle which is unacceptable. Several methods might be used to overcome these problems[27].

First, true 3D volume signal acquisition might be used at several points during the cardiac cycle. Unfortunately, the heart rate sets a limit on how rapidly the pulsing can be done making this approach relatively time inefficient. Another approach is to carry out multislice imaging and altering the order in which the multislice images are obtained. It is then possible to construct a matrix of images which shows each slice through the heart at multiple points during the cardiac cycle. This allows one to obtain information regarding both the global and segmental function of the heart. This still requires a significant amount of time in that many images are required; however, it appears to be more time efficient than present 3D techniques. Clearly, if more rapid imaging schemes such as echo planar[28] or hybrid imaging[29] schemes can be implemented over the volume of the adult thorax, it may be possible to obtain this functional information in much less time.

An interesting and more efficient means of obtaining information regarding wall motion may involve the use of pulsing schemes to encode wall motion in the image, similar, in a sense, to the phase images employed in nuclear medicine. This type of approach has been demonstrated by Van Dijk[30] and others. However, the clinical utility of this technique has not been demonstrated.

CONCLUSION

Magnetic resonance imaging is rapidly emerging as an important tool in the evaluation of cardiac disease. With technical developments to add functional information to the structural information presently available, it is anticipated that the role of magnetic resonance imaging in clinical diagnosis and management will continue to grow.

REFERENCES

1. Adda, G: Br Heart J 50:197-201, 1983.
2. Steiner RE, Bydder GM, Selwyn A, et al: Br Heart J 50:202-208, 1983.
3. Kaufman L, Crooks L, Sheldon P, et al: Circulation 67:251-257, 1983.
4. Pohost GM and Ratner AV: JAMA 251:1304-1309, 1984.
5. Choyke PL, Kressel HY, Reichek N, et al: Am J Rad 143:1143-1150, 1984.
6. Herfkins RJ, Higgins CB, Hricak H, et al: Radiology 147: 749, 1983.
7. Budinger TF and Cullander C: Biophysical phenomena and health

hazards of in vivo magnetic resonance. (In) Clinical Magnetic Resonance Imaging. San Francisco, Radiology Research and Education Foundation, 1983.
8. Soulen RL, Budinger TF, and Higgins CB: Radiology 154:705, 1985.
9. Pavlicek W, Gessinger M, Castle L, et al: Radiology 147:149-153, 1983.
10. Singer JR: J Phys E: 11:281-291, 1978.
11. Bradley WG, Waluch V, Lai A, et al: Am J Rad 143:1167-1174, 1984.
12. Axel, L: Am J Rad 143:1157-1166, 1984.
13. Singer JR and Crooks LE: Science 221:654, 1983.
14. Amparo EG, Higgins CB, Hricak H, et al: Radiology 155:399-406, 1985.
15. Gesinger MA, Risins B, O'Donnel JA, et al: Radiology 155:407-412, 1985.
16. Peshock RM, Weinreb J, Cohen JC, et al: (submitted).
17. Williams ES, Kaplan JI, Thatcher F, et al: J Nucl Med 21:449-453, 1980.
18. Wesby GE, Higgins CB, Lanzer P, et al: Circulation 69:125-130, 1984.
19. McNamara MT, Higgins CB, et al: Circulation 71:717-724, 1985.
20. Peshock RP, Filipchuk NG, Malloy CR, et al: J Am Coll Cardiology 5:435, 1985.
21. Ratner AV and Pohost GM: Presented at the Society for Magnetic Resonance in Medicine meeting, San Francisco, 1983.
22. Wesbey GE, Higgins CB, McNamara MT, et al: Radiology 153:165-169, 1984.
23. McNamara MT, Higgins CB, Ehman RL, et al: Radiology 153:157-163, 1984.
24. Brady TJ, Goldman MR, Pykett IL, et al: Radiology 144:343-347, 1982.
25. Fletcher BD, Jacobson MD, Nelson AD, et al: Radiology 150:137-140, 1984.
26. Schultz CL, Alfidi RJ, Nelson AD, et al: Radiology 152:117-121, 1984.
27. Crooks LE, Barker B, Chang H, et al: Radiology 153:459-465, 1984.
28. Mansfield P, Ordidge RJ, Redzian RR, et al: J Mag Res Med.
29. Twieg DB: Med Phys 10(5): 610-621, 1983.
30. Van Dijk P: JCAT 8:429, 1984. 31. Rehr RB, Filipchuk NG, Malloy CR, et al: Am J Cardiology 55: 1243-1244, 1984.

MAGNETIC RESONANCE IMAGING OF THE ABDOMEN AND PELVIS
Nolan Karstaedt
Department of Radiology
Bowman Gray School of Medicine
Winston-Salem, NC 27103

ABSTRACT

This paper reviews many of the common diseases of the abdomen and pelvis that have been studied with magnetic resonance imaging (MRI). The disease appearance with regard to T1 and T2 has been described in order to de-emphasize equipment-specific differences.

The problems induced by multiple tissue contrast in the abdomen are discussed. Present approaches to MRI have resulted in disease-sensitive rather than disease-specific images. In view of the high capital cost of equipment, further improvements in pulse sequence selection, contrast agents, and reduction of motion artifacts will be required to assure a major clinical role for MRI.

INTRODUCTION

Remarkable progress has been made in MRI of the abdomen and pelvis in the past 4 years. However, the difficulties in imaging this anatomical area have not been fully overcome. I will discuss the major organs in the abdomen and pelvis separately and also review the physiological information that can be learned from MRI. Pulse sequences and imaging planes will also be discussed.

PULSE SEQUENCES

For convenience, pulse sequences can be grouped according to their tendency to produce either T1 contrast, T2 contrast, or a reflection of proton density. Using the inversion-recovery (IR) pulse sequence, image contrast is produced by the differing T1 relaxation times of tissue. The time of inversion (TI) is set to an average value for the tissues being examined. A typical TI is 400 msec. The repetition time (TR) is usually set at a multiple of the average T1 of the tissue to allow T1 relaxation to occur. A typical TR is 1000-3000 msec. Spin-echo (SE) pulse sequences can also demonstrate T1 contrast in the image if a short time-to-echo (TE) 12-30 msec and a short TR 150-500 msec are chosen. The TE time is set short with respect to the T2 of the tissue to minimize T2 effects. The TR is set short with respect to the T1 of the tissue. It is important to understand that T1 time increases with increasing field strength and that identical pulse sequences may not produce identical contrast if the main magnet field strength differs.

Spin-echo pulse sequences are also used to produce images dependent on T2 contrast. In this case, the longest possible TE is chosen to maximize T2 contrast, bearing in mind that the longer the TE the noisier the final image. A long TR is also chosen to allow

T1 relaxation processes to occur and therefore to contribute little to image contrast. It should be remembered that increasing the TR increases the total imaging time. Typically the TE time will be 60-120 msec and the TR time will be 1000-3000 msec.

Proton density images will be produced when the TE and TR times are in the intermediate range, TE 30-50 msec and TR 500-1000 msec. These images are usually high in signal and produce "pretty" images with good anatomical outlines. However, with the exception of fat, the proton density of abdominal tissues varies little and overall contrast in these images is low.

It is important to realize that the above statements are convenient clinical simplifications. The pixel signal intensity of every image is composed of contributions from all the parameters, but by selecting pulse times as described above, the contrast from one parameter can be made to dominate the image. It is also important to understand that the pulse sequence descriptions apply only to the radiofrequency pulses, yet the application of the slice select and phase encoding gradients can affect the image, particularly in relation to the production of artifact and the appearance of flow and motion in the image(1).

PHYSIOLOGY

The promised capability of MRI to demonstrate physiologic phenomena in vivo has been studied in few cases because the emphasis placed on obtaining acceptable anatomic delineation mandates pulse sequences yielding a high signal-to-noise ratio. The pixel signal intensities resulting from the commonly used pulse sequences reflect a complex mixture of T1 and T2 relaxation times which may obscure physiologic information while providing good anatomic detail.

The major physiologic phenomenon demonstrated on all MRI scans is flow in the major blood vessels(1,2,3,4). Depending on the pulse sequence used, flow will manifest either as high signal or, more often, as no signal in the vessel. The latter case is referred to as the flow void. It should be noted that flow is not quantitated by the standard imaging sequences. Techniques devised to quantitate flow in the image have not yet proven to be clinically useful because of their sensitivity to patient motion as well as blood flow. An important secondary effect of flow is the production of a motion artifact on two dimensional Fourier transform images resulting in a stream of artifacts arising from the vessel and extending on either side of it in the phase encoding direction. The blood vessels are major landmarks in the abdomen and pelvis and are sometimes involved by disease processes arising in adjacent organs. Therefore the flow signal (or lack thereof) providing very high contrast between the blood vessels and surrounding tissues has been one of the major advantages of the MR image.

Two other physiologic phenomena have been described by MRI. The state of hydration of the kidney can be crudely assessed by the degree of difference in the T1 contrast between the renal cortex and medulla. The more hydrated the kidneys, the greater the differential on Tl contrast scans(5). With MRI, gallbladder bile can be differentiated from hepatic bile(6). On Tl contrast scans, bile which has been stored in the gallbladder for some time has a bright signal thought to be due to the resorption of water by the gallbladder, producing a highly concentrated bile with a short Tl. Bile recently entering the gallbladder from the liver, as when a patient has just eaten or a cholecystagogue has been administered, has a low signal reflecting a long Tl presumably due to its higher water content. A layering effect of liver bile over the higher specific gravity gallbladder bile may be seen in the gallbladder.

PATHOLOGY

I will now discuss the contributions MRI has made in evaluating the diseases that affect individual organs and regions of the abdomen and pelvis.

LIVER

The liver is subject to a wide variety of diseases that are classified most conveniently as focal or diffuse.

FOCAL LIVER DISEASE

Our experience and the reports of others suggest that MRI is a highly sensitive technique for identifying focal liver disease(7,8,9). Focal lesions appear as low intensity areas on scans demonstrating Tl contrast and as high intensity areas on T2 contrast scans (Fig. 1). The proton density technique has been abandoned for evaluation of focal liver disease since lesions are often invisible.

Differentiation by MRI between benign and malignant focal lesions has been poor. No difference in signal intensity has been reported for metastatic disease to the liver irrespective of the primary tumors(7,8). Benign cystic lesions have demonstrated very long Tl times and in general, long T2 times. This, coupled with the typical smooth, round cyst morphology, has allowed most of these lesions to be diagnosed(7,8).

Hepatomas have also been identified as focal or infiltrating lesions, but with signal intensities too similar to those of metastatic tumors to allow differentiation.

Cavernous hemangioma, the most common benign tumor of the liver, has shown a unique pattern which may allow differentiation from other tumors of the liver. Although cavernous hemangiomas appear dark on Tl contrast scans as do many other tumors, they have demonstrated increasing signal intensity on spin-echo scans as the TE and TR are lengthened. Too few cases have been evaluated to determine the reliability of this appearance.

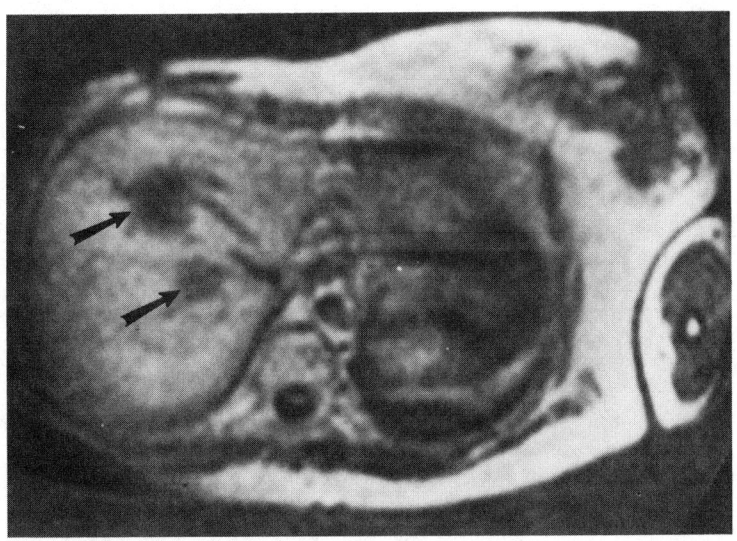

Fig. 1-(A) Transverse IR 400/1750 scan through the liver. Two rounded, irregular, low intensity lesions are seen (arrows) representing metastases from breast cancer.

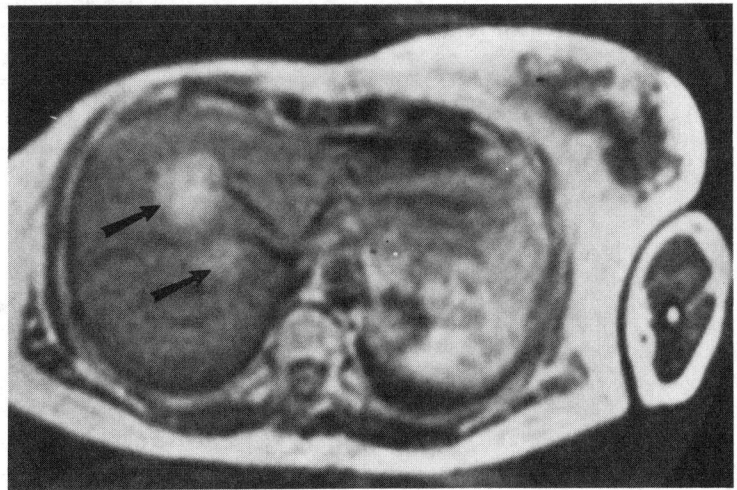

Fig. 1-(B) Transverse SE 60/2000 scan through the liver of the patient in Fig. 1(A). The metastases are now seen as high signal lesions (arrows).

A few comparisons of the sensitivity, specificity and accuracy of MRI with those of other modalities in detecting focal liver disease have been published(7,10). We have found MRI to be a sensitive but not specific test for focal liver disease. One disadvantage is its inability to detect calcification of a lesion, a capability that improves specificity with computed tomography.

DIFFUSE DISEASE OF THE LIVER

MRI has not been useful in detecting diffuse malignant disease of the liver. Investigation of a typical infiltrative malignant disease, lymphoma, has been disappointing although the total number of cases is small(11).

Results in detecting diffuse benign diseases of the liver such as cirrhosis, fatty infiltration, hemochromatosis and Wilson's disease have been mixed. Fatty liver, unless marked, is not identifiable on scans performed with standard pulse sequences. Using pulse sequences that allow imaging of the chemical shift caused by fat, MRI is very sensitive to the presence of fat(12). The clinical problem is that unless these pulse sequences are used routinely, fatty infiltration may be missed, but the utility of the chemical shift sequence in other diseases of the liver has not been established. Hemochromatosis and Wilson's disease result in liver deposition of iron and copper, respectively. Since these are paramagnetic, they should be detectable with MRI. Lengthening of the T1 of the liver has been noted in patients with hemochromatosis, and results in a lower signal intensity than in normal liver(7,9,13,14). However most reported cases of Wilson's disease had normal T1 times for the imagers used(15).

Hepatitis also results in lengthening of the T1 and T2 values of the liver. Stark et al., in a rat model, quantified the T1, T2 and pixel signal intensity with respect to duration of disease and found that MRI was sensitive to increased liver hydration, primarily manifesting as increased T2 values, and to cell necrosis manifesting as a lengthening of T1 values(16). In clinical studies, active liver inflammation appears to be detectable as an increased signal on T2 contrast scans and as a low signal on T1 contrast scans; however, the clinical manifestations vary with the nature of the pathology and timing of the scan. We have scanned a single case of granulomatous hepatitis (presumed sarcoid) in which the abnormality was not detected.

Cirrhosis of the liver produces morphological changes, decrease in size of the right lobe with relative sparing of the left and caudate lobes, which are visible on MRI. The situation with respect to the relaxation times is somewhat more complex. Several authors have shown that the T1 time in cirrhotic livers is increased resulting in a darkening of the liver(7,9) while Goldberg et al. have shown in rats that pure collagen deposition in the liver does not significantly change either of the relaxation times(17). The discrepancy between experimental and clinical findings has not been explained. The signal change in the clinical setting may be due to the inflammation rather than the collagen deposition seen in the disease.

PANCREAS

MRI of the pancreas has generally been disappointing. Because the splenic and superior mesenteric vessels are well seen, the posterior margins of the pancreas are well delineated on MRI but the close association of the anterior margins of the gland with the posterior stomach and medial duodenum causes problems. The bowel commonly is dark on T1 contrast scans and bright on T2 contrast scans reflecting the fluid nature of its contents. Both inflammatory and malignant diseases of the pancreas produce signal changes resulting in lengthened T1 and T2 of the tissue and a loss of contrast between the abnormal pancreas and the normal bowel (Fig. 2).

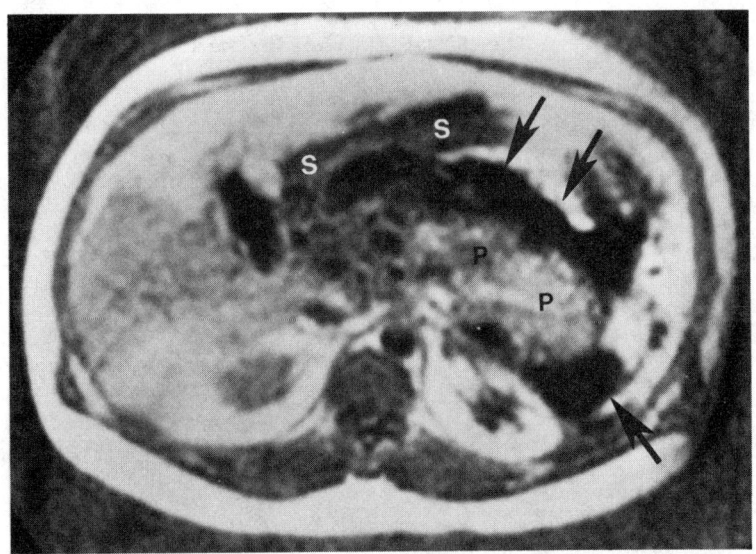

Fig. 2 Transverse IR 400/1750 scan through the pancreas (P) which is markedly swollen. The pancreas is surrounded by low signal material (arrows) representing peripancreatic fluid in this patient with pancreatitis. The stomach (S) is distinguishable from the fluid because it is empty.

MRI fails to detect two other important indicators of pancreatic disease, calcification and pancreatic duct dilatation. Increased spatial resolution may solve the latter problem but detection of small calcifications may always be difficult because of the lack of signal from calcium. Many authors have published reports demonstrating pancreatitis, its complications, and pancreatic neoplasms on MRI but the consensus is that until the problems are solved, computed tomography will remain the preferred imaging technique(18,19,20).

KIDNEYS

Renal imaging presents two sets of problems, those encountered in imaging surgical renal disease (evaluation of a renal mass) and those encountered in medical renal disease. The essential task in imaging a renal mass is to differentiate benign from malignant disease. The imaging method must be able to separate the solid from the cystic mass and to stage renal malignancy. MRI seems very promising in this regard. Several reports agree on the ability of MRI to distinguish solid masses from benign simple and hemorrhagic cysts(21,22,23), and recent experience suggests that accurate staging of renal tumors is possible(24).

A renal cyst on MRI appears as a smooth, round lesion with uniform signal intensity and is very dark on T1 contrast scans reflecting a long T1. The T2 of the lesion also tends to be long producing a high signal on T2 contrast scans. Hemorrhagic cysts have a short T1 and a prolonged T2 and therefore appear bright on T1 and T2 contrast scans. One author has suggested that the age of the hemorrhagic cyst may be estimated by MRI since fresh hemorrhage has a higher signal intensity than does older hemorrhage on T1 contrast scans(25).

Renal cell carcinoma, in contrast, presents as a contour-deforming renal mass with a variable T1 and on T1 contrast scans the lesion may appear brighter than, darker than, or the same as renal parenchyma (Fig. 3).

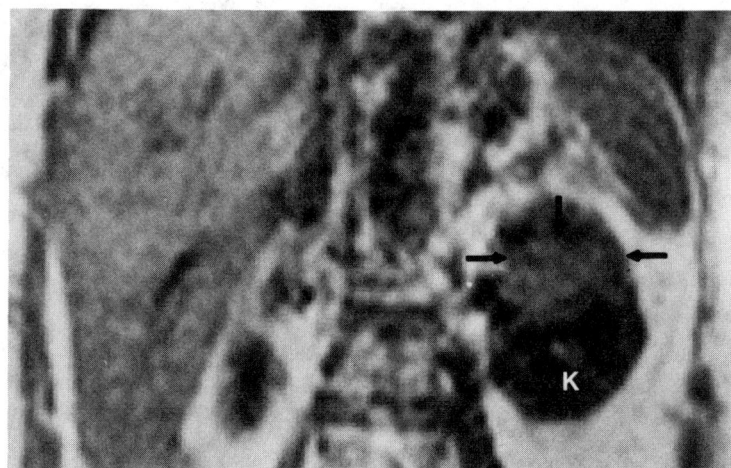

Fig. 3 Coronal IR 400/1750 scan through the left kidney. A tumor (arrows) with brighter signal than normal kidney (K) is seen.

A tumor that has a shorter T1 than its host tissue is somewhat unusual on MRI. This appearance has been attributed to the fat content of the clear cells typical of renal carcinoma(23). The T2 of renal tumors is generally longer than that of renal tissue and the lesions therefore appear bright on T2 contrast scans. The lateral margins of the tumor may be difficult to delineate on T2 contrast scans as the signal intensity of the tumor approaches that of perirenal fat. The morphology of the renal tumor also allows differentiation from renal cyst; tumors are more irregular, may have varied internal signal intensity and may demonstrate a pseudocapsule, seen as a thin dark line surrounding the tumor on either T1 or T2 contrast scans.

The secondary effects of renal tumors are seen well on MRI. The dilated collecting system in hydronephrosis can be easily defined by the long T1 of its contents. Metastatic lymph nodes appear as intermediate signal masses in the renal hilum and retroperitoneum. The most striking finding on MRI of the kidney is the ability to see tumor invasion of the renal vein and inferior vena cava. The tumor thrombus is easily identified as high signal soft tissue within the low signal lumen of the vessel. The craniad extent of the tumor thrombus is defined by the contrast between the bullet-shaped edge of the thrombus and the low signal flowing blood. In one series, a 96% accuracy rate was achieved in staging renal cell carcinoma with MRI(24).

The effectiveness of MRI in evaluation of medical renal disease is unproven since only a few results in each disease category have been reported(26). Certainly MRI can provide the basic information required for evaluatiion of renal failure. The renal size can be established and the presence or absence of hydronephrosis can be determined. It has been suggested that obstructive hydronephrosis can be differentiated from nonobstructive hydronephrosis by the fact that the corticomedullary junction definition is lost in obstructed kidneys(25). The accuracy of MRI in detecting an obstructing lesion is not known but it is unlikely that small calculi will be seen. In many of the glomerulonephritides and in renal artery thrombosis, definition of the corticomedullary junction, best seen on T1 contrast scans, is lost. Leung et al. and LiPuma have observed that in acute tubular necrosis in transplant kidneys, corticomedullary differentiation is preserved, with enlargement of the medulla, while it is lost in transplant rejection(25,26). These initial observations suggest that MRI will play a role in evaluating renal medical disease and especially in evaluation of the transplant kidney.

ADRENALS

The adrenal glands and their pathology can be identified with MRI. The adrenal cortex can be differentiated from the medulla since the cortex shows higher signal intensity on T2 contrast scans probably due to its higher lipid content. If this differentiation can be made reliably on MR images it would be unique among imaging techniques.

Adrenal disease can be identified by changes in the morphology of the glands, but no unique signal changes have been observed that allow specificity of diagnosis. Adrenal hyperplasia is diagnosed as increased thickness of the gland, while benign and malignant tumors are seen as masses of either uniform or variable signal intensity distorting the gland. Differentiation of benign from malignant tumors has not been possible(27).

RETROPERITONEUM

The aorta and inferior vena cava are well defined and coronal and sagittal scanning planes are well suited for the evaluation of the major vessels. Thrombus in the inferior vena cava is easily identified as discussed above and aortic aneurysms are accurately depicted(28,29).

Diseased lymph nodes are easily identified on T1 contrast MRI scans taken with short TE and TR because the resulting medium signal of the node contrasts well with the low signal vessels and the high signal fat(28,29). On T2 contrast scans the nodes yield high signal which may make them difficult to differentiate from retroperitoneal fat. The best plane for nodal imaging has yet to be determined. The longitudinal coronal and sagittal planes are attractive since the entire retroperitoneum can be imaged with a few slices, but the transaxial plane is best understood by radiologists because of their previous experience with computed tomography. As with all previously discussed areas, the MRI findings are nonspecific. The nodes show similar signal intensities irrespective of the disease process.

PELVIS

In contrast to the upper abdomen where motion artifact presents serious problems in MRI, the pelvic organs are relatively motionless enabling high quality images to be obtained despite long imaging times(30,31). The superior contrast resolution of MRI coupled with the ability to obtain scans in longitudinal axes make MRI a promising technique for evaluation of this area.

PROSTATE

On spin-echo images using a short TE/TR the normal prostate has a medium signal intensity that increases with longer TE and TR values. The gland is clearly distinguished from the lower intensity levator ani muscles and higher intensity fat as well as from the bladder base(32,33).

Despite early enthusiastic reports, differentiation of prostatic hyperplasia from carcinoma is not possible. Both have low signal intensity on T1 contrast scans and high signal intensity on T2 contrast scans and both may have an inhomogeneous appearance. It

is of interest that in one published series of seven patients with
benign prostatic hypertrophy and 25 with prostatic carcinoma, the
authors were unable to define nodular lesions of the prostate.
Despite the use of a wide variety of pulse sequences they were
unable to differentiate benign from malignant enlargements of the
prostate. Others have been able to define local inhomogeneous
signal in both prostatic hyperplasia and carcinoma(32). However it
appears that prostatic carcinoma can be staged with MR since tumor
extension into the adjacent fat, seminal vesicles, and local nodes
can be identified. The reliability of staging and detection of
prostatic carcinoma are unproven and false positive and false
negative diagnoses using MRI have been reported(35).

UTERUS

The most striking feature of MR scanning of the uterus is the
ability to differentiate normal endometrium from myometrium. This
cannot be done using any other imaging modality(30) (Fig. 4).

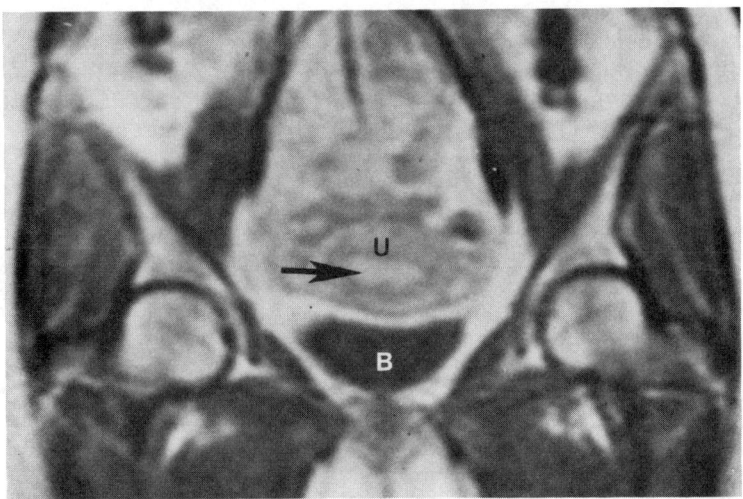

Fig. 4 Coronal SE 40/1400 scan through female pelvis. The high
signal area (arrow) in the center of the uterus (U)
represents endometrium. A thin, dark line surrounding the
endometrium and thought to represent the stratum basale is
visible. The partially filled bladder (B) is seen.

This distinction is most easily seen using sequences with a long TE
and TR. A thin, dark line separating endometrium from myometrium
and thought to represent the stratum basale has been noted. Hricak
and colleagues have described the normal premenarchal, menarchal and
post-menopausal uterus(30). The ability to define the normal
endometrium has led to the hope that staging of endometrial

carcinoma using MRI is possible but to date only anecdotal cases have been reported(31,35).

Benign uterine fibroleiomyomas (fibroids) have a T1 longer than myometrium, giving them a slightly lower signal intensity on short TE/TR scans. These masses show little T2 difference from the myometrium and are surrounded by a thin, low signal band thought to represent compressed muscle tissue(35).

The normal uterine cervix has been described by Hricak as having three zones; a high intensity central zone probably representing cervical mucus, a low intensity band external to the central zone which she felt represented glandular and stromal tissue of the endocervix, and an adjacent outer zone which increased in signal intensity with increasing TR(30). Results with MRI and CT in staging cervical carcinoma were comparable with a 64% accuracy of staging and a 75% accuracy in evaluating recurrent disease(37). These results are expected to improve with the use of higher resolution scanners.

OVARY

There have been several anecdotal reports on the use of MRI in evaluating ovarian cysts and tumors(30,36,38). Functional ovarian cysts have demonstrated an intermediate signal intensity slightly greater than the ovary itself on short TE/TR scans and the signal intensity has increased with increased TR. In a report of two serous cystadenomas, the signal intensities have differed. One had a short T1 and short T2, the other a long T1 and T2 which was more consistent with a watery fluid(36). The authors postulate that the difference is due to different protein or lipid contents within the cysts. The ovarian tumor with the most consistent MRI appearance has been the dermoid tumor. Most dermoid tumors have a very high signal intensity on both T1 and T2 contrast scans due to their high fat content(30,36,38). Dermoids with low fat content and atypical MRI appearance have been described(30). The endometriomas studied have had varying T1 relaxation times and therefore a variable appearance on T1 contrast scans(36).

BLADDER

The urine-filled bladder appears dark on T1 contrast scans and the contents increase in signal intensity as the TE and TR are increased. On the long TE/TR scans the bladder wall can be distinguished as a low intensity rim surrounding the high intensity urine(33). Good contrast between bladder tumors and urine is achieved on short TE/TR scans. Contrast between bladder tumors and the bladder wall is best on long TE/TR scans (Fig. 5).

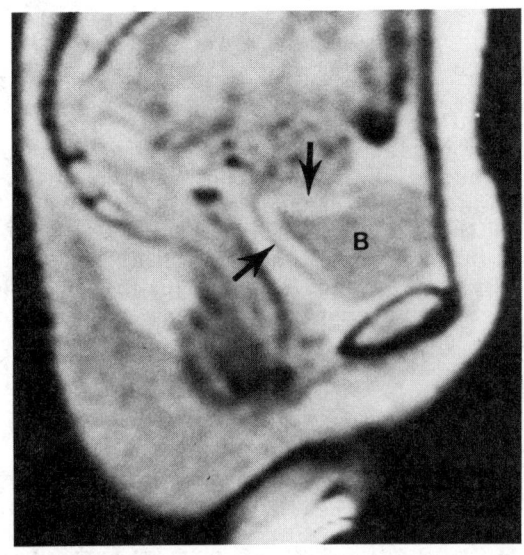

Fig. 5 Sagittal SE 60/2000 section through the mid-pelvis of a patient with prior resection of cancer of the uterine cervix. The bladder (B) is seen anteriorly. A v-shaped area of high signal intensity (arrows) identified on the posterior and superior aspect of the bladder represents bladder wall invasion by the cervical tumor.

Short TE/TR scans are preferred for demonstrating tumor infiltration in the perivesical fat so the tumor appears dark against the bright signal of the fat(33). The claim has been made that MRI is at least as accurate as CT in staging of bladder carcinomas(39).

BOWEL

Peristaltic motion and variable contents make the bowel a difficult organ to evaluate with MRI. Various authors have commented on the need for a bowel contrast agent, chiefly to enable separation of the bowel from other intra-abdominal organs but also to allow evaluation of the bowel itself. Geritol, which contains the paramagnetic ferrous ammonium citrate, has been used for this purpose but tends to dilute out in the distal small bowel and has not proved to be totally satisfactory. The only reported MR investigation of bowel disease is that of a rectal carcinoma which was seen on all three planes and could be seen to be invading the perirectal fat(39).

CONCLUSION

MRI has been very successful in the central nervous system where the organs to be imaged are relatively immobile and only three tissues, gray matter, white matter and cerebrospinal fluid need to be imaged. The pulse sequences needed to evaluate the limited number of tissue contrasts encountered in the central nervous system are few in contrast with MRI of the abdomen which presents the problems of motion and the necessity for evaluating a large range of tissue contrasts in a large anatomical area. Yet MRI already shows promise for evaluating several abdominal areas, the liver, kidney, male and female pelvic organs, and major blood vessels. Despite these successes, it is premature to speculate on the future role of MRI in evaluating the wide range of organs and diseases of this anatomical region.

REFERENCES

1. Moran P.R., Moran R.A., Karstaedt N.: Radiol. 154, 433 (1985).
2. Feinberg D.A., Crooks L., Hoenninger J., et al.: Radiol. 153, 177 (1984).
3. Bradley, Jr. W.G., Waluch V.: Radiol. 154, 443 (1985).
4. Singer J.R., Crooks L.E.: Science 221, 654 (1983).
5. Hricak H., Crooks L., Sheldon P., Kaufman L.: Radiol. 146, 425 (1983).
6. Hricak H., Filly R.A., Margulis A.R., et al.: Radiol. 147, 481 (1983).
7. Smith F.W., Mallard J.R.: Br. Med. Bull. 40, 194 (1984).
8. Moss A.A., Goldberg H.I., Stark D.B., et al.: Radiol. 150 141 (1984).
9. Doyle F.H., Pennock J.M., Banks L.M. et al.: AJR 138, 193 (1982).
10. Heiken J.P., Lee J.K.T., Ling D., Glazer H.S.: Radiol. 153(P), 265(A) (1984).
11. Weinreb J.C., Brateman L., Maravilla K.R.: AJR. 143, 1211 (1984).
12. Dixon W.T.: Radiol. 153, 189 (1984).
13. Stark D.D., Moseley M.E., Bacon B.R., et al.: Radiol. 154, 137 (1985).
14. Runge V.M., Clanton J.A., Smith F.W., et al.: AJR. 141, 943 (1983).
15. Aisen A.M., Martel W., Trygve O., et al.: Radiol. 153(P), 264(A) 1984.
16. Stark D.D., Bass N.M., Moss A.A., et al.: Radiol. 148, 743 (1983).
17. Goldberg H.I., Moss A.A., Stark D.D., et al.: Radiol. 153, 737 (1984).
18. Haaga J.R.: Radiol. Clin. North Am. 22, 869 (1984).
19. Stark D.D., Moss A.A., Goldberg H.I., et al.: Radiol. 150, 153 (1984).

20. Smith F.W., Reid A., Hutchinson J.M.S., et al.: Radiol. 142, 667 (1982).
21. Smith F.W., Hutchinson J.M.S., Mallard J.R., et al.: Diagn. Imaging 50, 61 (1981).
22. Hricak H., Williams R.D., Moon, Jr. K.L., et al.: Radiol. 147, 765 (1983).
23. Choyke P.L., Kressel H.Y., Pollack H.M., et al.: Radiol. 152, 471 (1984).
24. Hricak H., Demas B.E., Williams R.D., et al. Radiol. 154, 709, (1985).
25. LiPuma J.P.: Radiol. Clin. North Am. 22, 925 (1984).
26. Leung A.W-L., Bydder G.M., Steiner R.E., et al.: AJR. 143, 1215 (1984).
27. Davis P.L., Hricak H., Bradley, Jr. W.G.: Radiol. Clin. North Am. 22, 891 (1984).
28. Lee J.K.T., Heiken J.P., Ling D., et al.: Radiol. 153, 181 (1984).
29. Dooms G.C., Hricak H., Crooks L.E., Higgins C.B.: Radiol. 153, 719 (1984).
30. Hricak H., Alpers C., Crooks L.E., Sheldon P.E.: AJR. 141, 1119 (1983).
31. Bryan P.J., Butler H.E., LiPuma J.P. et al.: AJR. 141, 1111 (1983).
32. Buonocore E., Hesemann C., Pavlicek W., Montie J.E.: AJR 143, 1267 (1984).
33. Hricak H., Williams R.D., Spring D.B., et al.: AJR. 141, 1101 (1983).
34. Poon P.Y., McCallum R.W., Henkelman M.M., et al.: Radiol. 154, 143 (1985).
35. Steyn J.H., Smith F.W.: Br. J. Urol. 54, 726 (1982).
36. Butler H., Bryan P.J., LiPuma J.P., et al.: AJR. 143, 1259 (1984).
37. Bies J.R., Ellis J.H., Kopecky K.H., et al.: AJR 143, 1249 (1984).
38. Thickman D., Kressel H., Gussman D., et al.: Am. J. Obstet. Gynecol. 149, 835 (1984).
39. Bryan P.J., Butler H.E., LiPuma J.P.: Radiol. Clin. North Am. 22, 897 (1984).

MAGNETIC RESONANCE IMAGING:
CLINICAL RESULTS IN THE CHEST AND BREAST

C. Leon Partain, M.D., Ph.D.
Madan V. Kulkarni, M.D.
Martin P. Sandler, M.D.
James A. Patton, Ph.D.
Ronald R. Price, Ph.D.
Vanderbilt University Medical Center, Nashville, TN 37232

ABSTRACT

A review of current clinical results in MRI evaluation of the chest and breast is presented. This summary discusses the current role and future potential of MRI in the diagnosis of diseases of the thorax. Unique capability together with limitations of MRI are presented. Illustrative examples demonstrate results in imaging using the Vanderbilt University 0.5 Tesla superconducting MRI system.

INTRODUCTION

Magnetic resonance imaging of the chest and of the breast are active areas of investigation at numerous medical centers. The diagnostic capability of MR scanning in the chest is being widely recognized as a strongly compatititve modality in the evaluation of soft tissue masses of the thorax and mediastinum. Progress has been somewhat more difficult in the evaluation of parenchymal diseases of the lungs. In addition, a specialized study of the breast using total body and surface coil techniques is being actively pursued at several medical centers. While there is great potential for improved breast imaging, the results to date have failed to demonstrate significantly improved specificity in distinguishing malignancy from benign lesions of the breast.

This report will summarize and illustrate the clinical results and potential of chest and breast magnetic resonance imaging in 1985.

CHEST

The evaluation of soft tissue masses of the thorax and mediastinum by magnetic resonance imaging is usually superior to other imaging modalities (1,2). This is the result of increased soft tissue contrast resolution (3,4) and the power of thoracic imaging with either cardiac gating alone or with combined cardiac and respiratory gating (5,6).

On the other hand, current difficulties in thoracic imaging include evaluations of the anatomy and function of the intracardiac valves, coronary arteries, and lung parenchyma. Additional safety limitations, of course, apply to all patients with cardiac pacemakers and cerebral aneurysm clips.

Recent results are illustrated by several cases as follows: Hodgkin's disease (Figure 1); chest wall mass (Figure 2); coarctation of the aorta (Figure 3); and pericardial cyst (Figure 4).

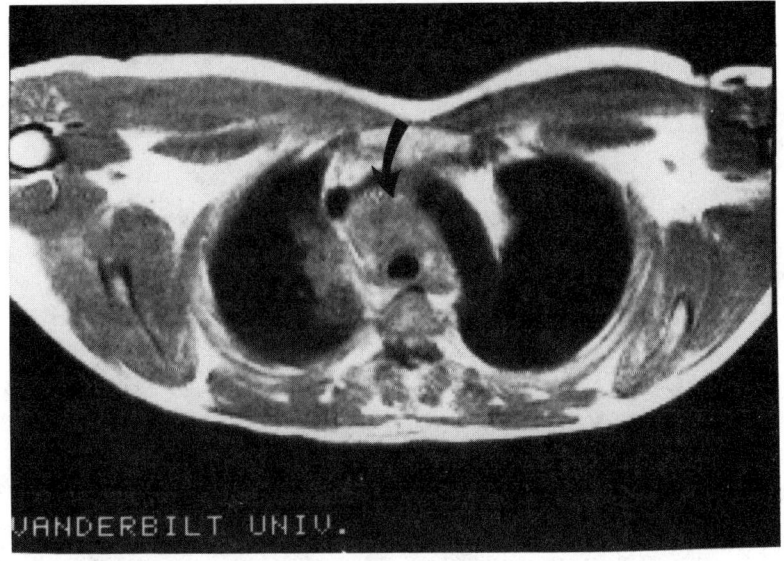

Fig. 1.   Transverse MRI view of mediastinum mass (arrow) in Hodgkin's disease.

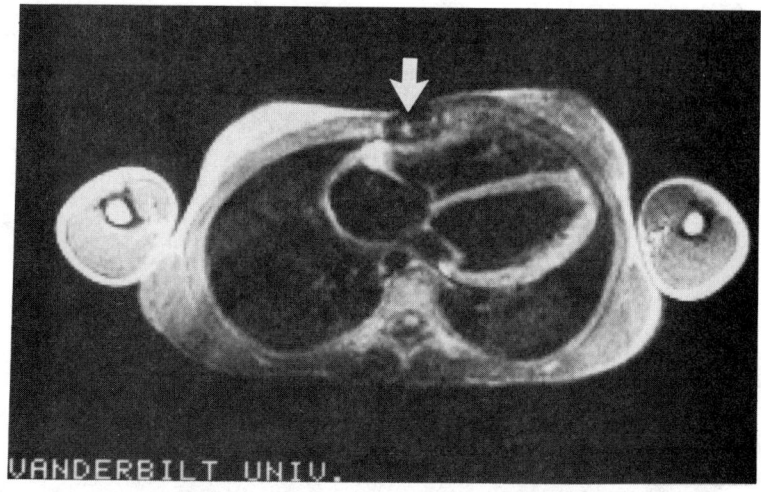

Fig. 2. Chest wall abscess (arrow) in gated cardiac MRI image.

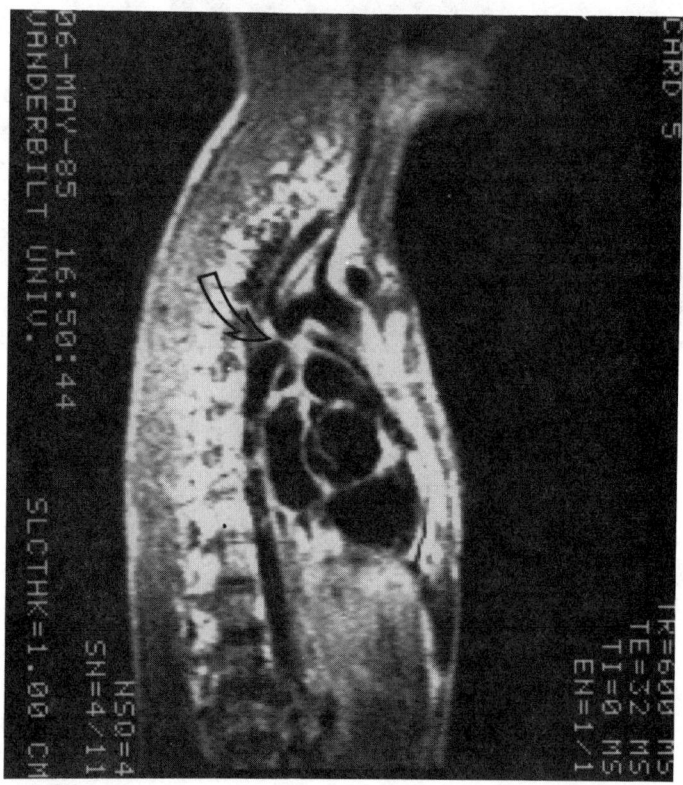

Fig. 3. Gated sagittal MR image of coarctation (arrow) of aorta.

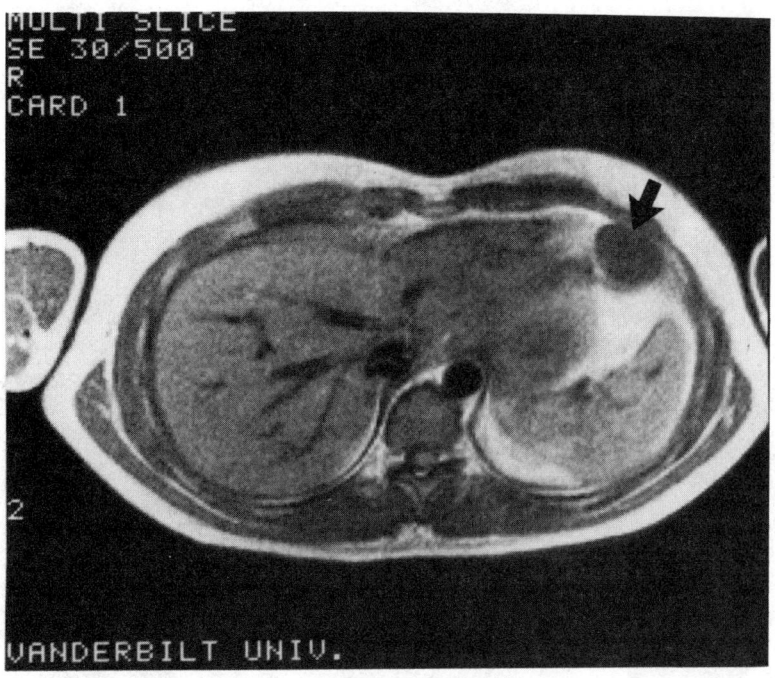

Fig. 4. Gated MR image of upper abdomen in patient with pericardial cyst.

BREAST

Breast imaging body coil results have been complemented and extended by surface coil imaging. The majority of our specialized breast coil images utilize a circular cylinder 16 cm wide by 8 cm deep. The surface coil is installed as a routine modification of the patient cot and fits easily into the gantry of the total body imaging device. Our experience extends over approximately 50 cases, and the results are very similar to those at other medical centers (7,8). Basically, MRI of the breast yields thin section tomographic images at any angle and utilizing any available pulse sequence. If a breast mass exists in the background of fat, there is at least equal soft tissue contrast sensitivity compared to x-ray mammography. However, in a background of fibrocystic disease and other dense breast tissue, several cases have demonstrated inferior soft tissue contrast sensitivity when compared to x-ray mammography. With regard to specificity, calculated T1 and T2 images together with spin echo and inversion recovery pulse sequence techniques seem to have significant clinical potential for characterizing breast lesions. However, once again it appears to be most applicable, in the initial stages, in cases of breast masses in a fatty background. Significant overlap of NMR parameters (T1, T2, and spin density) in breast masses which exist in a breast stroma of fibrocystic disease cause considerable difficulty in identifying abnormal breast masses.

Illustrative examples of breast magnetic resonance images include a normal, transverse, spin echo 30/500 image (Figure 5); adenoma (Figure 6); carcinoma using spin echo 30/500 (Figure 7); and carcinoma using calculated T1 image (Figure 8).

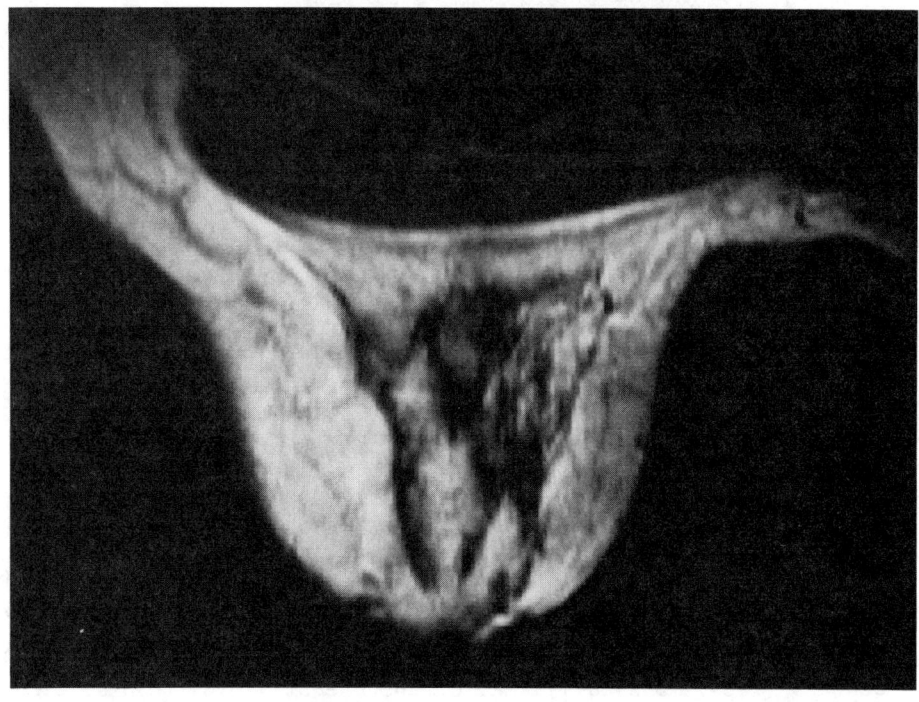

Fig. 5. Transverse MRI, normal breast.

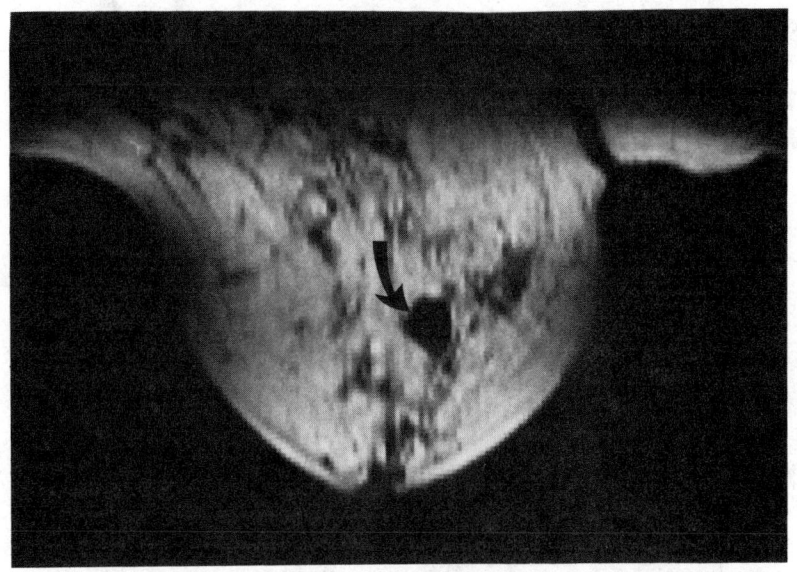

Fig. 6. Transverse MRI, adenoma (arrow), of the breast.

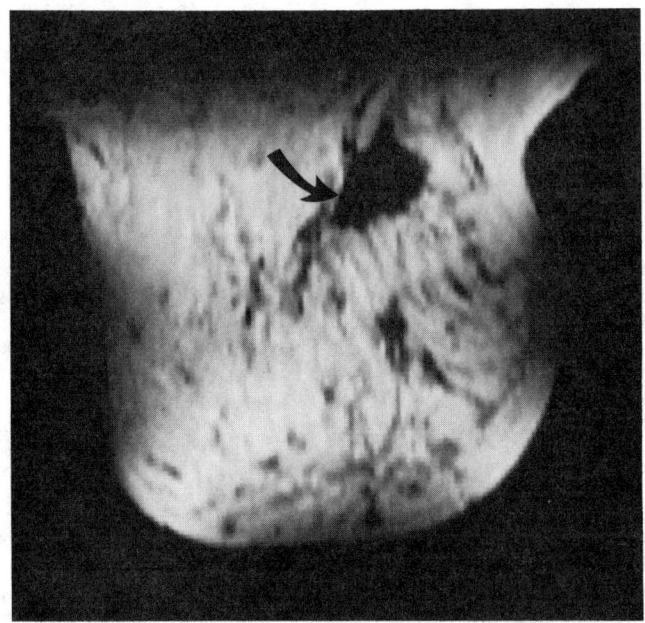

Fig. 7. Transverse MRI, carcinoma (arrow) of the breast, SE 30/500.

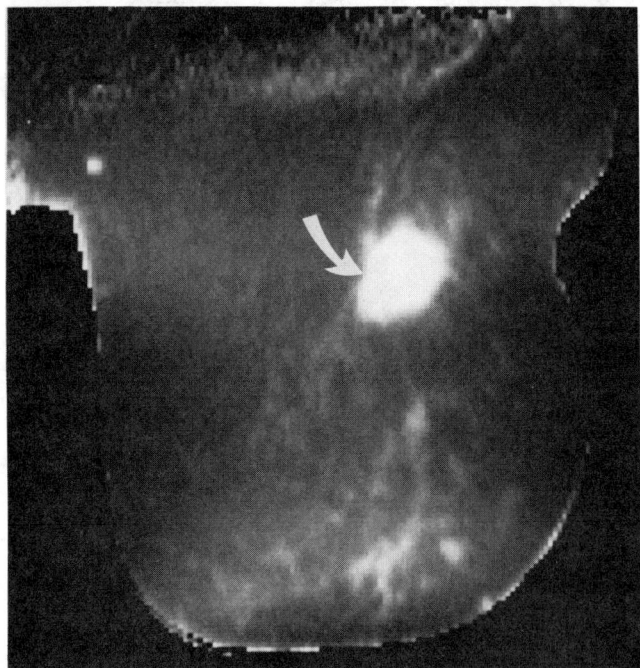

Fig. 8. Transverse MRI, carcinoma (arrow), calculated T1 image of the breast.

CONCLUSION

In order to realize the full potential of magnetic resonance imaging in the chest and breast, additional work is needed in pulse sequence optimization, surface coil techniques, MRI contrast agent development and evaluation, and possibly correlation with other functional imaging modalities. The potential of the technique, as with other anatomical and functional studies, lies with the power of magnetic resonance to provide thin section, tomographic, functional images at any angle, in some cases with superior anatomical resolution and, in most cases, with superior contrast resolution to any alternative modality.

REFERENCES

1. Webb WR, Jensen GB, Gamsu G, Sollitto R, Moore EH: Coronal magnetic resonance imaging of the chest: normal and abnormal. Radiology, 153:729-736 (1984).

2. Cohen AM, Creviston S, LiPuma JP, et al: Nuclear magnetic resonance imaging of the mediastinum and hili: early impressions of its efficacy. AJR 141:1163-1169 (1983).

3. Gore JC: The meaning and significance of relaxation in NMR. In Witcofski RL, Karstaedt N, Partain CL: NMR Imaging. Winston-Salem, Bowman Gray School of Medicine (1982).

4. Mitchell MR, Conturo TE, Gurber TJ, Jones JP: Two computer models for selection of optimal magnetic resonance imaging (MRI) pulse sequence timing. Invest Rad 19(5):350-360 (1984).

5. Herfkens RJ, Higgins CB, Hricak H, et al: Nuclear magnetic resonance imaging of the cardiovascular system: normal and pathological findings. Radiology 147:749-759 (1983).

6. Runge VM, Clanton JA, Partain CL, James AE: Respiratory gating in magnetic resonance imaging at 0.5 tesla. Radiology 151(2):521-523 (1984).

7. El Yousef SJ, Duchesneau RH, Alfidi RJ et al: Magnetic resonance imaging of the breast. Radiology 150:761 (1984).

8. Partain CL, Kulkarni MV, Cook LT, et al: Nuclear magnetic resonance imaging of the breast: Functional T1 and three dimensional imaging. In D Adams (ed), Nuclear Magnetic Resonance Imaging: A Special Issue, Cardiovascular and Interventional Radiology, Vol 8 (1985).

CLINICAL APPLICATIONS OF CORRELATIVE IMAGING: MRI/NM/US/CT

C. Leon Partain, M.D., Ph.D.
Madan V. Kulkarni, M.D.
Martin P. Sandler, M.D.

Vanderbilt University Medical Center, Nashville, TN 37232

ABSTRACT

The clinical correlation of multiple imaging modalities is increasingly important because of the accelerating complexity of instrumentation and because of the growing pressures of government control which demand optimal use of high technology based medical diagnostic equipment. This presentation reviews the current clinical utilization of major tomographic imaging modalities including magnetic resonance imaging, nuclear medicine, single photon emission tomography, positron emission tomography, ultrasound, and x-ray computed tomography.

INTRODUCTION

Today's imaging instrumentation allows the generation and presentation of diagnostic images based upon information not previously available by alternative techniques and with less risk to the patient. These images tend to be quantitative, tomographic, thin section and, sometimes, dynamic, high-resolution magnification images without ionizing radiation or any known adverse biological effect. In addition, there is an unprecedented explosion of multiformatted digital images which must be displayed, reviewed, and appropriately archived and retrieved.

Many pressures come to bear in the proper application of computer based, complex, and expensive medical imaging instrumentation. There is the need to appropriately distribute this equipment in ways that are medically, economically, socially, and politically feasible. Beyond that, there is the need for continuing research and development, in spite of significant limitations to funding bases for these investigations. It is also abundantly clear that cooperative teams of physicists, engineers, computer scientists, physiologists, biochemists, and physicians are and will be required to realize the full potential of the newer metabolic functional imaging modalities including, in particular, magnetic resonance imaging, single photon emission computed tomography, and positron emission tomography.

Below are example cases illustrating correlative principles of magnetic resonance imaging in relationship to other imaging modalities.

Nuclear Medicine

An intriguing comparison exists between conventional radioisotope imaging and the newer radioisotope techniques of SPECT and PET in comparison with MRI because each involves quantitative functional imaging using isotopes: unstable isotopes in the first case and stable isotopes in the second case. In particular, there is a special opportunity to compare and correlate the pathophysiological significance and metabolic/biochemical basis for imaging in magnetic resonance imaging and positron emission tomography. These two modalities are described by some as the only true physiologically based imaging modalities and are already generating significant new data providing fresh insights into disease processes and response to therapeutic modalities (1,2).

One disease process in which conventional nuclear medicine and magnetic resonance imaging have teamed together in a study of relative sensitivity and specificity is the orthopedic problem of avascular necrosis of the femoral head. Multiple centers are evaluating the relative role of these modalities in this entity. There is continuing debate about whether MRI or nuclear medicine is more sensitive for the diagnosis of AVN. Most investigators claim that MRI is more sensitive. In our experience, nuclear medicine has been more sensitive in two cases out of ten. Figure 1 illustrates an abnormal coronal magnetic resonance imaging view through the femoral heads in a patient with avascular necrosis in this region. The bone scan was also abnormal in this region. An example of the correlation of nuclear medicine and MRI in the evaluation of the single "cold" palpable nodule is shown in Figure 2.

Ultrasound

The absence of ionizing radiation and ease of utilization make both ultrasound and magnetic resonance imaging attractive modalities from the viewpoint of patient safety. Clinical areas of potential correlative imaging include the evaluation of cystic structures and the evaluation of intrauterine pregnancy. One clinical area where MRI appears possibly more sensitive than ultrasound is in the detection of placenta abruptio illustrated in Figure 3. Ultrasound and MRI comparative studies of breast disease are in progress in multiple centers (3,4). An example case of a cyst and tumor in the same breast are illustrated in Figures 4A and 4B. A coronal MRI of third trimester intrauterine pregnancy is shown in Figure 5.

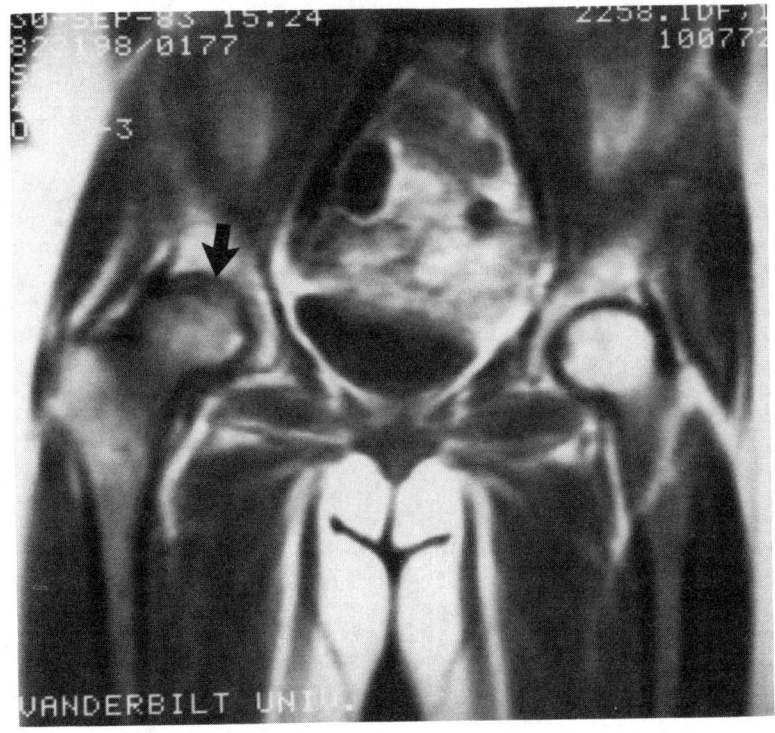

Figure 1. Avascular necrosis, right femoral head (arrow), coronal MRI view, SE 30/500 pulse sequence.

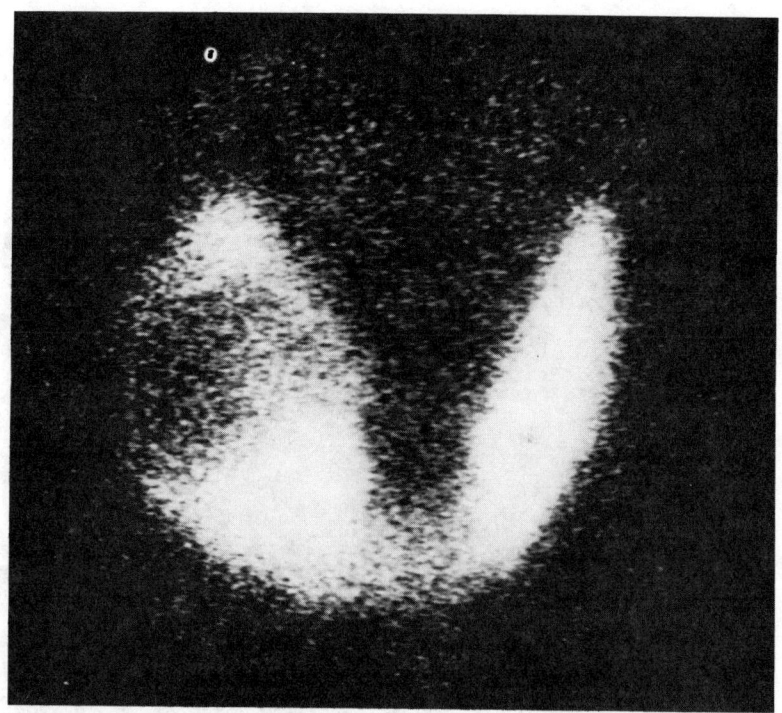

Figure 2. Papillary carcinoma, right lobe thyroid.
A. Technetium-99m pertechnetate scan.

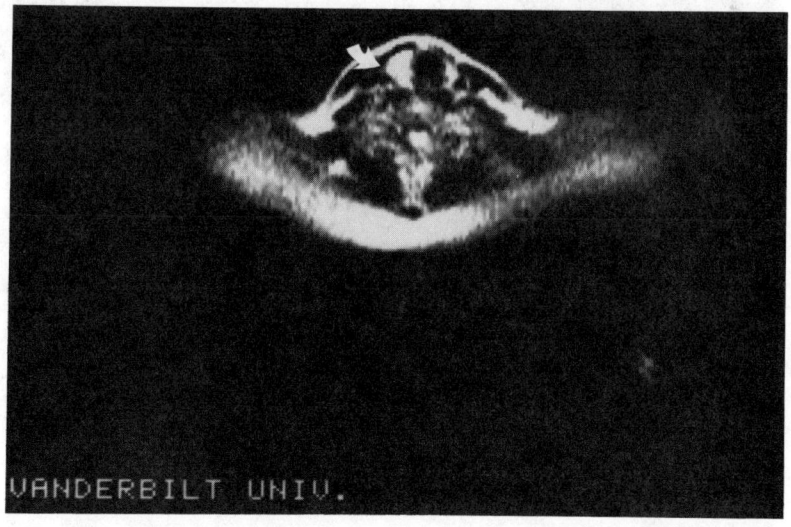

B. Transverse MRI, SE 120/2000, (arrow at mass).

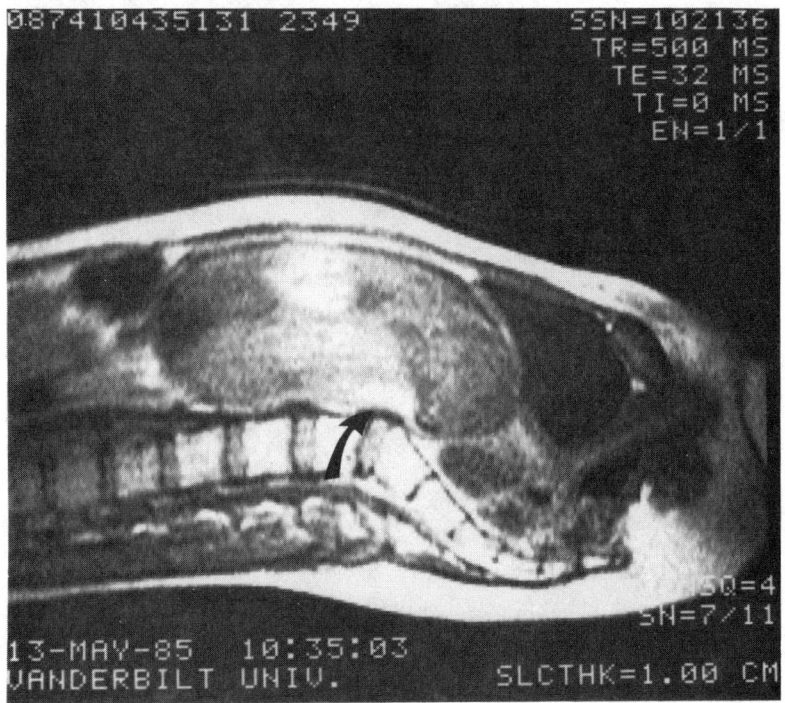

Figure 3. Placenta abruptio, SE 32/500, hematoma between placenta and uterus (arrow).

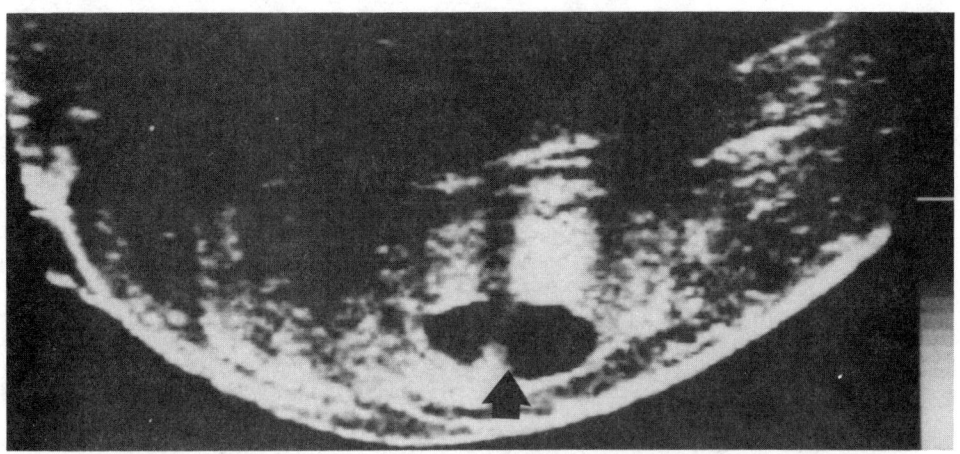

Figure 4. Breast cyst and mass. A. Ultrasound, arrow at cyst.

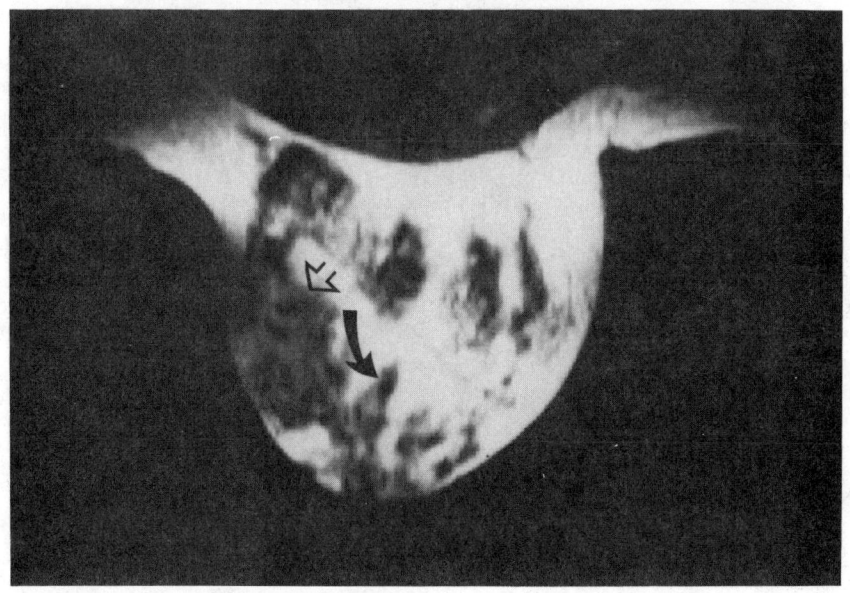

B. MRI, SE 30/500, closed arrow at cyst, open arrow at mass.

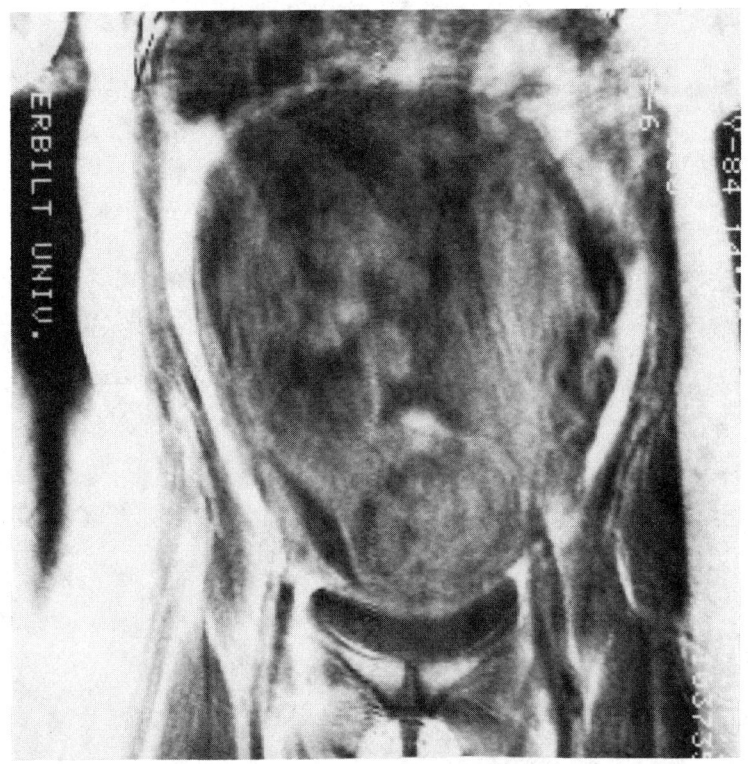

Figure 5. Third trimester normal intrauterine pregnancy.

Computed Tomography

The tomographic imaging capability in the transverse plane of computed tomography has been equalled in most parts of the body, except the mesentery and bowel, using magnetic resonance imaging. This position is likely to be solidified with the recent developments in MRI of contiguous thin-slice, multislice, multiecho imaging where slice thickness now approaches 1 mm. This presumes that there are no contraindications for magnetic resonance study where obviously CT would be required; these contraindications include cardiac pacemaker and aneurysm clip.

The continuing evolution of relative roles of CT and MRI is actively under investigation at multiple centers (5,6). It is our view that most moderate sized community hospitals and, certainly, medical centers need x-ray computed tomography as the first tomographic imaging modality with high anatomical resolution. Beyond that, the second tomographic unit probably should be magnetic resonance imaging because of the metabolic and biochemical basis for imaging which is possible with this technique.

A comparison of MRI and CT in metastatic disease to the liver is shown in Figure 6. Metastatic disease to the L-4 vertebral body is shown in midline sagittal section in Figure 7; this finding correlated well with plain radiography. Midline sagittal imaging in a child with meningomyelocele and a multicompartmental syringomyelia is shown in Figure 8. A myelogram was not needed in this case.

CONCLUSION

Tomographic, thin-section, quantitative, dynamic medical imaging is extending once again the diagnostic capabilities of the physician. Magnetic resonance imaging is evolving as a powerful tool which is the first line of defense for patients who can tolerate an imaging procedure taking several minutes in the evaluation of such diseases as intracranial mass and spinal cord abnormality. Tomographic viewing at multiple angles allowed by MRI lends itself very well to correlative imaging wih other modalities including functional nuclear medicine and anatomic images from CT and ultrasound.

Acknowledgment is made of the editorial assistance and photographic assistance of Margaret Moore and John Bobbitt, respectively.

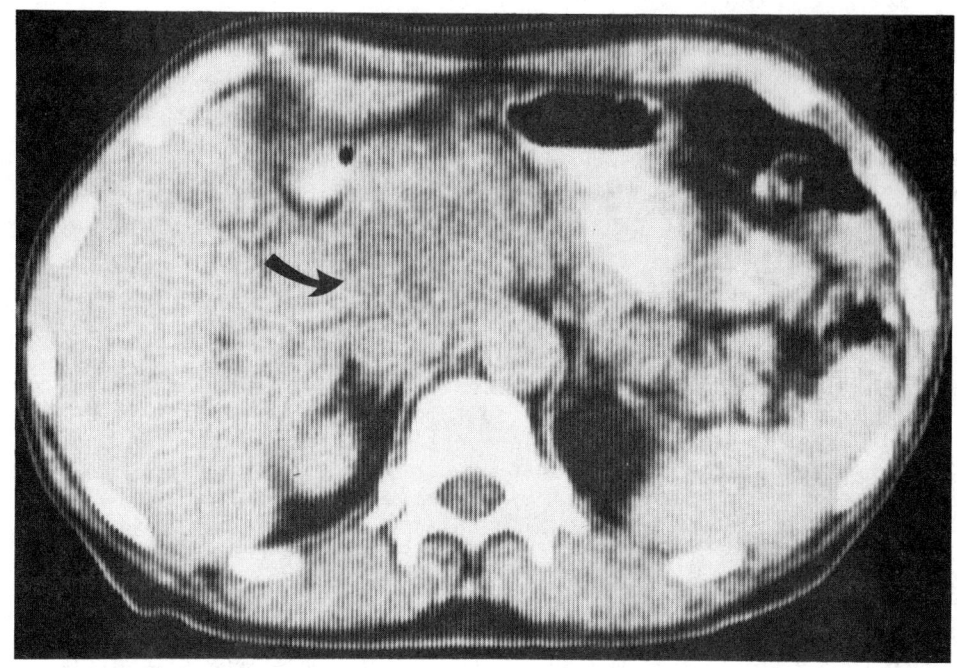

Figure 6. Metastatic disease to liver. A. CT, arrow at mass.

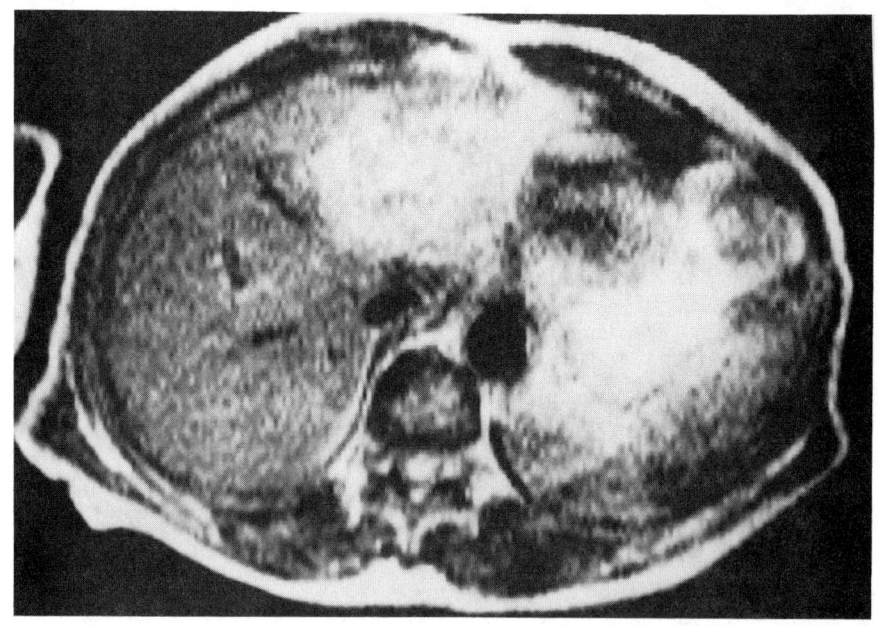

B. MRI, SE 90/1000

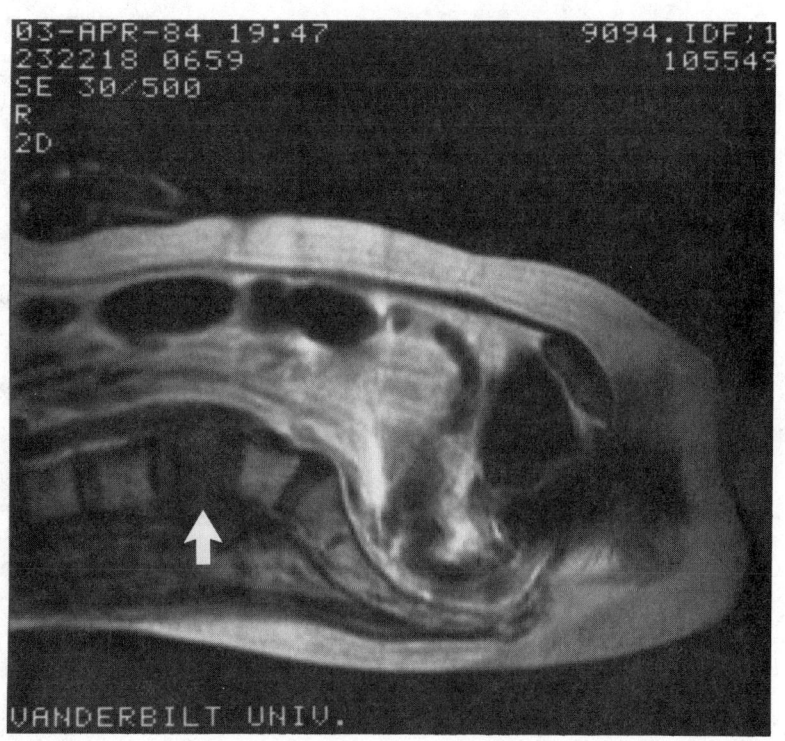

Figure 7. Metastatic disease to L-4 vertebral body.
A. MRI, SE 30/500.

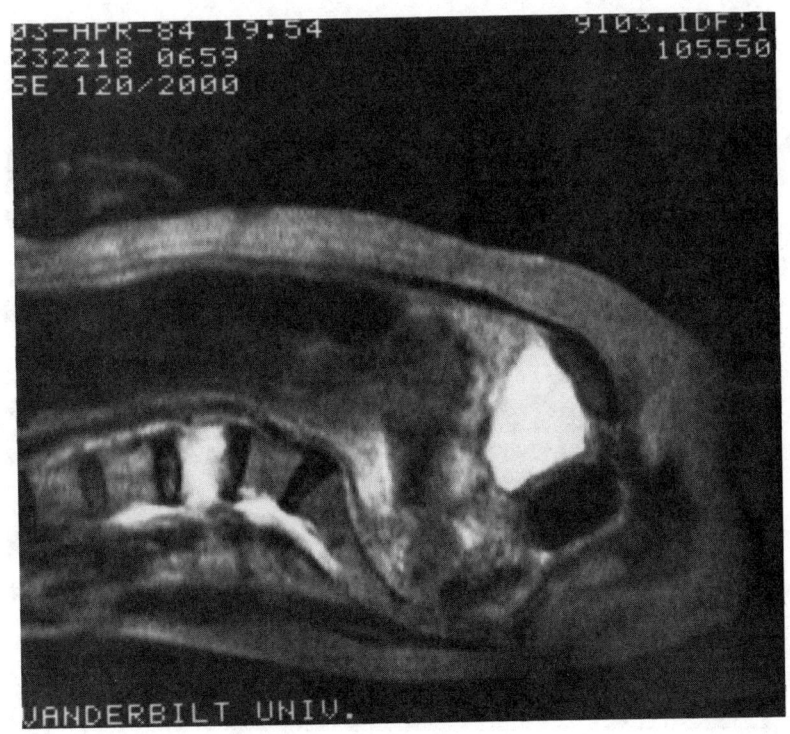

B. MRI, SE 120/2000.

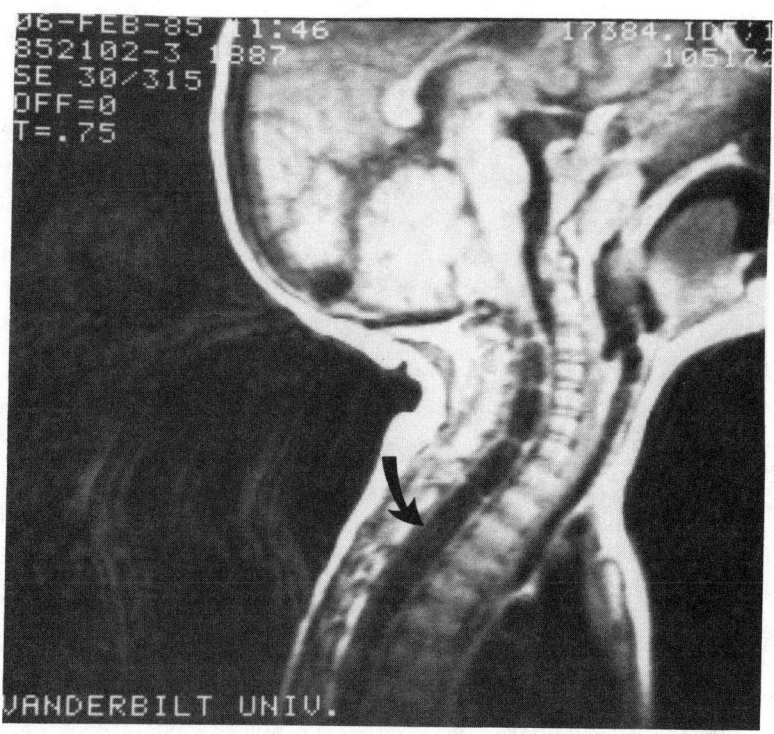

Figure 8. Meningomyelocele and multicompartmental syringomyelia (see arrows). A. Cervical spine, MRI, SE 30/315.

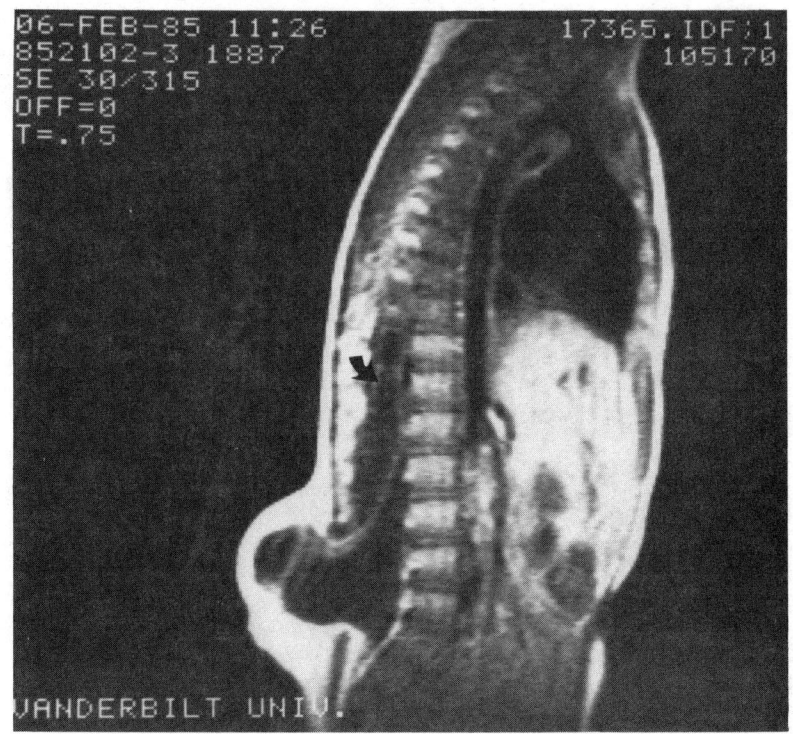

B. Lumbar spine, MRI, SE 30/315.

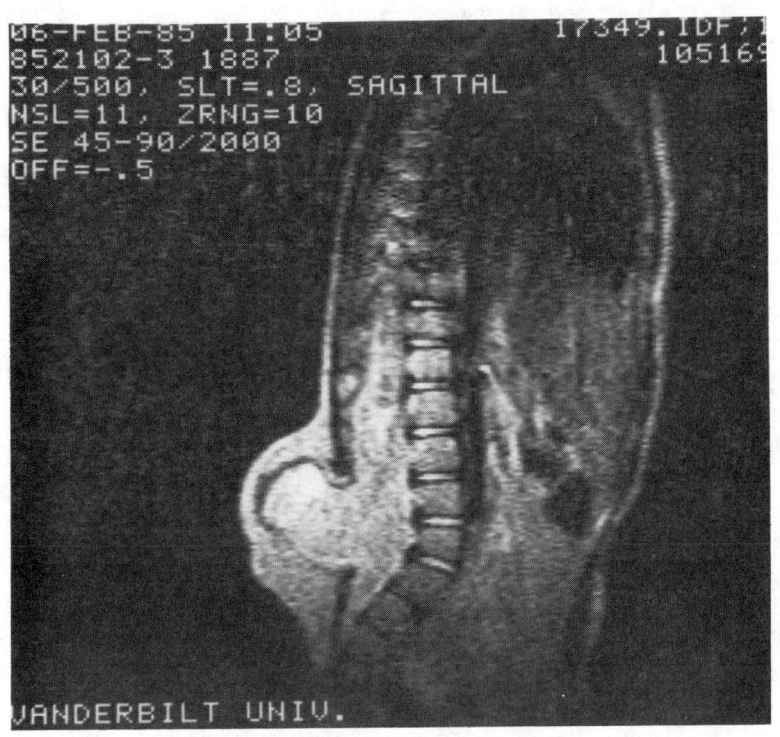

C. Lumbar spine, MRI, SE 90/2000.

REFERENCES

1. Brownell GL, Budinger TF, Lauterbur PC, McGeer PL: Positron tomography and nuclear magnetic resonance. Science 215, 4533:619-626 (1982).

2. Kulkarni MV, Sandler MP, Shaff MI, Jones JP, Patton JA, Partain CL, James AE: Clinical magnetic resonance imaging with nuclear medicine correlation. J Nucl Med 26(8) (1985).

3. Cole-Benglet C, Soriano R, Pasto M et al: Solid breast mass lesions: Can ultrasound differentiate benign & malignant? In Jellins J and Kobayashi T (eds): Ultrasonic Examination of the Breast. New York, John Wiley & Sons (1984).

4. Partain CL, Kulkarni MV, Cook LT et al: Nuclear magnetic resonance imaging of the breast: Functional T1 and three dimensional imaging. In Adams D (ed): Nuclear Magnetic Resonance Imaging: A Special Issue, Cardiovascular and Interventional Radiology, Vol. 8 (1985).

5. Stark DD, Moss AA, Goldberg HI, et al: Magnetic resonance and CT of the normal and diseased pancreas: A comparative study. Radiology 150(1):153-162 (1984).

6. Dooms GC, Hricak H, Crooks LE et al: Magnetic resonance imaging of the lymph nodes: Comparison with CT. Radiology 153(3):719-728 (1984).

SITE PLANNING FOR MAGNETIC RESONANCE IMAGING

P. L. Carson, S. R. Thomas*, M. Koskinen**, M. Lassen[+]
W. Pavlicek[++], R. R. Price[+++], M. J. Bronskill[++++]

Department of Radiology
University of Michigan Medical Center
Ann Arbor, MI 48109

ABSTRACT

The data and material presented in this paper have been extracted from a more extensive interim report document entitled "Site Planning for Whole Body Magnetic Resonance Systems." This report was prepared by Task Group #2 on Site Planning and Preparation for NMR Installations. Members and others participating in the writing of the document include: Paul L. Carson (Chairman), Elizabeth Amari, Michael J. Bronskill, Stephen Einstein, Jon Erickson, Michael Koskinen, Margit Lassen, Seong Ki Mun, William Pavlicek, Ronald R. Price, and Ann Wright. Task Group #2 is part of the AAPM Committee on Nuclear Magnetic Resonance, Stephen R. Thomas, Chairman. The full interim report is available upon request for review and comment from the New York AAPM office. Subjects discussed in this larger document of which the following paper represents a subset include: I. Introduction and NMR systems description; II. Facility layout including structural and utility requirements; III. Health and safety including forces on ferromagnetic objects; IV. Effects of metals on image quality; V. Effects of magnetic fields on other equipment; VI. Status of magnetic shielding; VII. RF interference and shielding; VIII. Checklist; and IX. Bibliography.

INTRODUCTION

The planning of magnetic resonance imaging facilities still offers challenging opportunities for creativity and courage, as siting practice is changing rapidly with systems changes and with accumulation of more experience and understanding. It is clear that many relatively recent siting decisions have been overly costly or have produced unnecessary inconvenience in patient management. There is, however, a growing consensus on the range of practical methods for meeting the many requirements with the foremost of these being related to magnetic field containment and RF shielding.

*Department of Radiology, University of Cincinnati, Cincinnati, OH.
**Joint Center for MRI, Harvard Medical School, Boston, MA.
[+]Department of Radiology, Thomas Jefferson University, Philadelphia, PA.
[++]Department of Radiology, Cleveland Clinic, Cleveland, OH.
[+++]Department of Radiology, Vanderbilt University, Nashville, TN.
[++++]Ontario Cancer Institute, Toronto, ON.

Site selection and preparation for a clinical Nuclear Magnetic Resonance (NMR) installation requires special considerations that have not been encountered previously. The items which must be considered before locating an NMR unit in a diagnostic facility are more numerous than for radiological imaging equipment. In addition to the usual requirements for appropriate structural foundation one must now examine the effect of the surroundings on magnetic field uniformity within the magnet core and the effect of the magnet's fringe fields on other devices. Interference is also possible by the radio-frequency (RF) signals from the NMR installation on equipment in adjacent facilities and on electronic devices worn by patients in the NMR facility or nearby areas. Other considerations involve interference, this time from RF radiation in the environment, on the operation of the machine. There may also be consequences of locating another NMR machine in the same vicinity as well as emergencies such as quenching during patient examination, that have not previously been encountered in the medical facility. Present knowledge in these areas is both limited and dispersed especially with regard to whole-body imaging machines.

Suppliers of NMR systems have gained considerable expertise in many aspects of site planning and installation. However, the medical physicist can contribute significantly to a successful NMR operation by drawing on in-depth knowledge of physics phenomena. The physicist's involvement can often save the hospital a considerable amount of money, prevent irreversible mistakes and promote maximum flexibility in the clinical operation of the machine. By being involved in the early planning stages, the physicist can direct the decision process effectively and help evaluate potential machines and sites as well as architectural firms, before any commitments are made.

Task Group #2 under the Nuclear Magnetic Resonance Committee of the American Association of Physicists in Medicine was formed with the charge to assemble information currently available, follow technical developments, gather results and experiences from new installations and suggest areas for further research. The Task Group intends to make this information available to the medical and manufacturing communities in the form of a manual. The plan is to have the manual updated and expanded as more knowledge and experience are gained.

SYSTEMS SPECIFICATIONS

The block diagram in Figure 1 shows an NMR Imaging system as presented in Reference 1. Key Parameters impacting on system performance are presented in Table 1. A detailed list of systems specifications has been compiled by Task Group #6 on NMR Systems Specifications and Acceptance Testing Protocols and is included elsewhere in this Proceedings.

Table 1:   General Components of an NMR Imaging System.

I. Static Magnet System
    A. Magnet Siting and Access control/restriction
    B. Types of Magnets--Special Considerations
       - Superconducting Electromagnets
         Cryogen consumption, Gas recovery and refrigeration system, Extent of Fringe Fields
       - Resistive Electromagnets
         Power and Cooling Requirements
       - Permanent Magnets
         Floor Loading
       - Hybrid Magnet Systems
    C. Patient Access
    D. Magnet Stability/Homogeneity
       - Type of Shim Coils required: Active/Passive control

II. Gradient system
    A. Field Characteristics
       - Maximum Gradient Strength for each axis
       - Linearity and Stability of gradients
    B. Electrical and Operational Characteristics
       - Power consumption and cooling requirements
       - Maximum switching speed
       - Audio Noise Levels

III. RF System
    A. Spectrometer Components
       - Synthesizer
         Frequency Range, Stability, Multi-nuclear capability
       - Transmitter--Peak power output, bandwidth, and stability
       - Receiver--input impedance, noise figure, tuning requirements, total available gain
    B. Tuning/Coil Components
       - Remote/Local Tuning
       - Types of Head, Body and Surface Coils available with some figure of merit

IV. Data Acquisition System
    A. Available Techniques
       - 2DFT, 2DPR, 3DFT, 3DPR, echo planar, FLASH, etc.
    B. Electrical Specification
       - # of bits/data point, sampling speed and jitter
    C. Performance Specifications
       - Slice profile, continuity, interleaving, gaps, etc.

V. Computer/Image Processing System
    A. Capacity
       - Operating system--single or multi-user
       - Memory, Disk, Tape, etc.
    B. Performance
       - Array Processor, matrix size, reconstruction time.

Table 1 (Continued): General Components of an NMR Imaging System.

VI. Patient Handling System
    A. Operational Specifications
       - Clearance within Magnet/RF Coils
       - Maximum Patient Weight
       - Position Indicators/accuracy
    B. Convenience/Comfort Features
       - Automatic/Manual Positioning
       - Illumination/Ventilation inside Magnet Bore
       - Patient Alarm/Panic Button

Table 2: Typical Magnetic Field Strengths

	Tesla (T)
Air Core Resistive-Large Bore Imaging	0.02– 0.2
Air Core Resistive-Spectrometer	0.04– 1.45
Superconducting-Large Bore Imaging	0.15– 2.0
Superconducting-Spectrometer	1.5 –15
Superconducting-Medium Bore	2.0 – 4.9
Imaging/Research Spectrometer	1.9 – 4.2
Permanent	0.35
Hybrid (combination of permanent and resistive)	0.35– 1.0

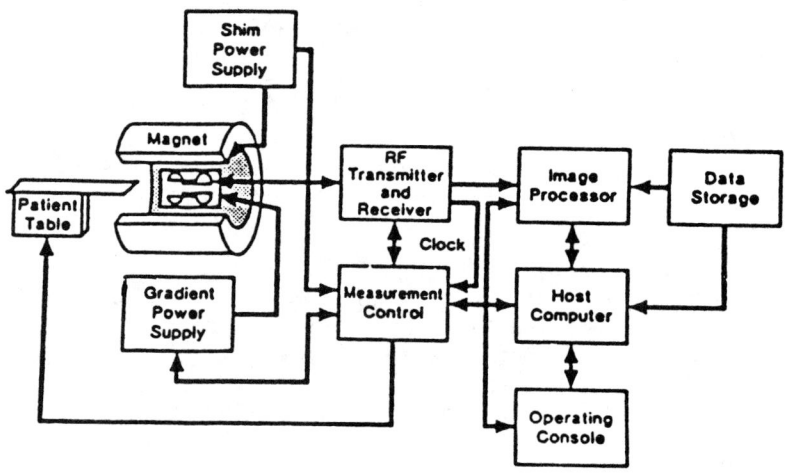

Figure 1. Block diagram of an NMR imaging system (1).

At the present time there is a wide range of magnetic field strengths available; with advancing technology, this range is likely to continue to expand. Table 2 shows some typical magnetic field strengths available commercially ranging from 0.02T to approximately 15T. Physical specifications for the different imaging systems can be obtained from individual manufacturers. Typical examples of system specifications are listed in Table 3.

Table 3: Examples of Typical Installation Specifications for NMR Imaging Systems.

	Superconducting	Resistive	Permanent
Minimum Magnet Room Area (ft^2)	450-800	250-500	250
Minimum Imager Area (ft^2)	850-1600	~1200	225-360
Volume of 5G field without shielding			
height (ft)	35	30	8
width (ft)	35	30	10
length (ft)	50	40	6
Air Conditioning (x1000 BTU/h)	50-101	12-80	0-80
Chilled Water (gal/min)	10-30	15-30	0
Total Electrical Requirements (KVa)	30-110	18-100	3.3-20
Total weight (tons)	7-10	1.5-8.8	7-100

I. Magnet Systems:

In some instances, manufacturers have established boundary conditions by defining zones within which the primary magnet system is contained. Table 4 specifies zone dimensions for superconducting air core units of 0.5, 0.6 and 1.5T (5). Typical floor plans for these systems are shown in Figure 2.

Multiple System Facilities

Magnets now can be shimmed for operation in close proximity to one another (6). Even without magnetic shielding, it is feasible to place 1.5T magnets as little as thirty feet apart. However, such close placement is generally undesirable since removing the field from one magnet, or adjusting it significantly, will necessitate reshimming of the second magnet. It may be possible to have fixed locations for metal shim pieces or fixed settings for shim coils, for the cases in which the adjacent magnet(s) are and are not energized.

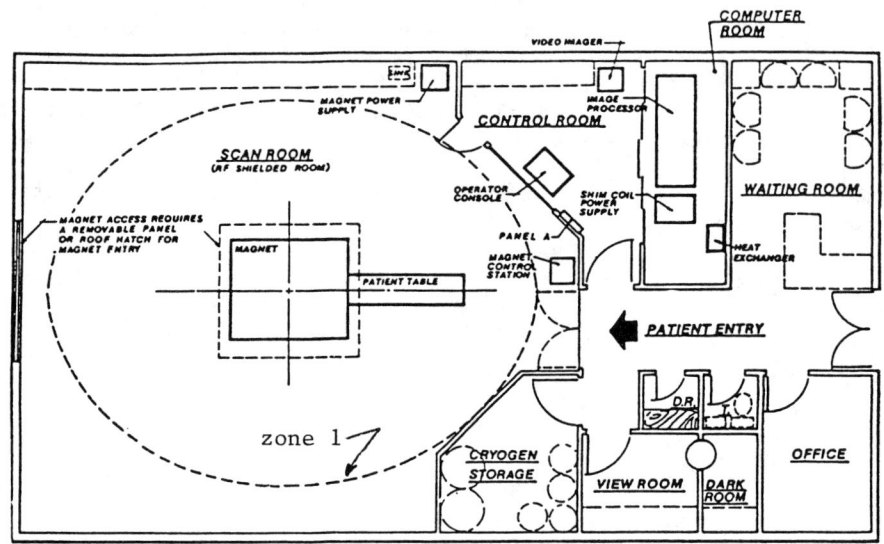
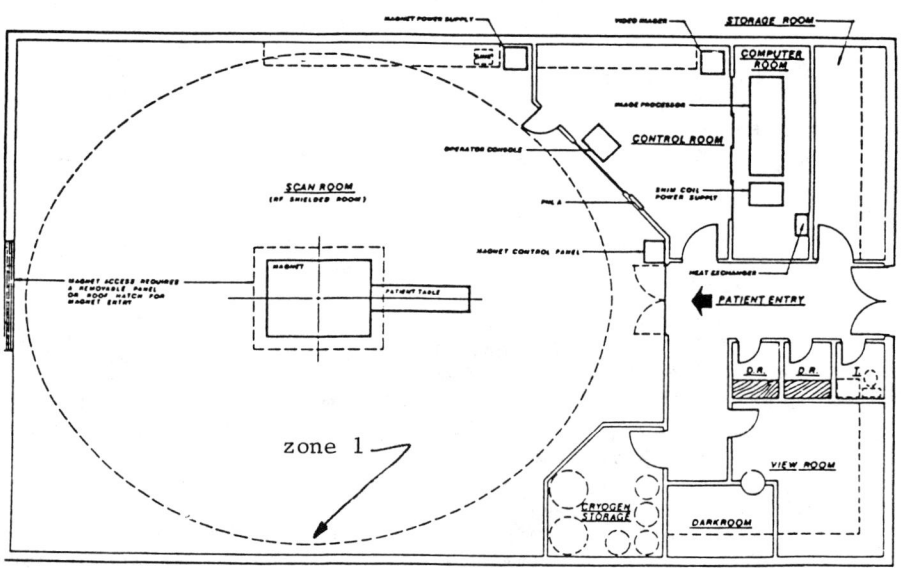

Figure 2. Typical installation floor plans indicating the zone boundaries (5). (a) 0.5 and 0.6 T. (b) 1.5 T.

Table 4: Examples of zone dimensions which might be established to contain the primary magnet system and the 15 G field lines for superconductive units of 0.5, 0.6 and 1.5T (5).

	ZONE DIMENSIONS (In Feet)					
	0.50 Tesla		0.60 Tesla		1.5 Tesla	
	Bore	Side	Bore	Side	Bore	Side
Zone 1	18	14	19	15	25	21
	(In Meters)					
	Bore	Side	Bore	Side	Bore	Side
Zone 1	5.49	4.27	5.80	4.58	7.62	6.40

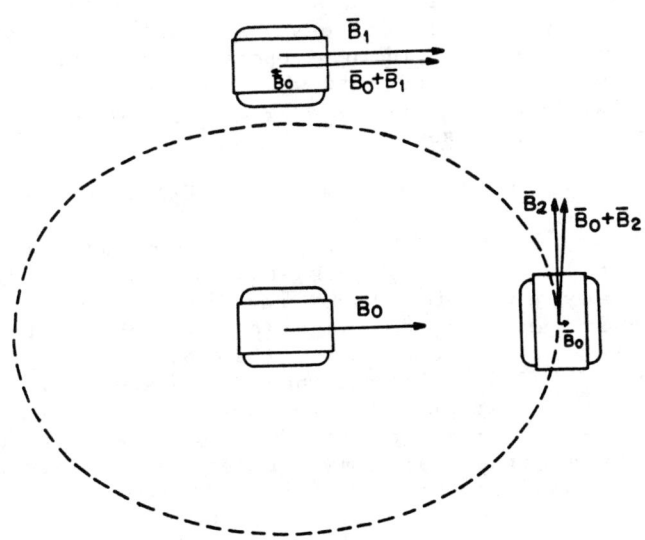

Figure 3. Inhomegeneity considerations for two-magnet facilities (6).

A wide variety of magnet orientations is now possible. If the magnet axes are perpendicular to each other, as shown in Figure 3, the inhomogeneity induced in one magnet by the other is actually reduced compared with the case in which the two magnet axes are parallel. This is true even though the absolute field in one of the magnets is greater for the perpendicular case than for the parallel case at the same center to center distance. The inhomogeneity of concern for imaging and spectroscopy is primarily the inhomogeneity of the B_0 field in the Z direction within the imaging volume. When the two magnets' axes are parallel, the fringe field from system 1 lies in the Z direction for system 2 and vice versa. However, when the magnet axes are perpendicular, the fringe field from either magnet within the other is perpendicular to the Z direction and, therefore, does not contribute to B_0 within the other magnet.

However, shimming can now be performed relatively easily and a more significant constraint is the force between the magnet coils and the torques on the coils. Placement of two systems in symmetric parallel and antiparallel orientations results in zero torque, with the distance between magnets being set by the maximum allowed force between the coils.

The difference between the various magnet orientations and separation distances are slight. It is probably now possible to design relative magnet locations to optimize operational efficiency and flexibility, within constraints of magnetic field containment for public safety guidelines and trouble free operation of magnetically susceptible devices. An optimal design for a two facility system probably includes operation and image interpretation areas between the two scanners which are relatively spacious to minimize down-time for shimming a second system if the first must be shut down for other reasons.

HEALTH AND SAFETY CONSIDERATIONS

A unique feature of MR is the presence of the high magnetic fields produced by the large magnets. With such large magnets a major safety consideration is simply the development of administrative and physical barriers to prohibit the accidental introduction of ferrous materials into the magnet room (7). Conventional I-V fluid poles and wheelchairs are easily pulled into a magnet. Large ferrous objects such as oxygen tanks and floor buffers may be attracted to the magnet with such force that they cannot be restrained, and smaller ferrous objects could become projectiles. Image distortions will result from ferrous objects on patients or from those pulled into the magnet and accidentally secured to the inside bore of the magnet. Superconducting and permanent magnets in particular should be secured against unauthorized entry at all times. At reasonable distances from the magnet, the field falls off according to the dipole approximation at approximately $1/r^3$. Large distances are necessary to reach background levels.

At fields greater than 15G, warnings may be posted with signs reading "CAUTION-HIGH MAGNETIC FIELD" (a corollary to the "CAUTION-HIGH RADIATION AREA" signs that are found within radiology departments). At greater than 15G, pacemakers may not operate properly and health and safety considerations must be addressed. Other guidelines recommend a 5G limit (9). A "CAUTION-MAGNETIC FIELD" warning (comparable to a "CAUTION-RADIATION AREA") can be specified for the area between 15 and 5G. Within this region, administrative controls for excluding patients with pacemakers can be applied. Further, the MR operators can control the movement of large ferrous objects and the entry of computer tapes, discs, and color television sets. Individuals wishing to enter the magnet room must pass through this administratively controlled area to ensure the removal of credit cards, watches, and loose ferrous objects. In areas having magnetic fields less than 5G, no administrative controls may be necessary since little or no possibility exists for health and safety problems or effects on the magnetic field due to the environment.

Fringe fields can be substantially decreased through the use of magnetic shielding. Shielding of magnets has the advantage of reducing the space requirements necessary for administrative control. Numerous electronic devices found in a hospital radiology department (i.e., x-ray tubes, CRT, scintillation cameras, and image intensifiers) may be affected by environmental levels on the order of 1 to 50 gauss. Siting an MR unit in an area in which fringe fields impact on these devices or on human safety will require shielding of the magnet, shielding or the removal of the devices and/or control of access in the fringe field area (7). Additional aspects of electromagnetic specifications related to patient safety are provided in Table 5 (10). Guidelines provided by British and American agencies are contained in references 11 and 12.

Table 5: Electromagnetic Specifications Related to Patient Safety (10).

FIELD PROPERTY	UNITS	0.35T SYSTEM (1983)	1.5T SYSTEM (1984)	DRH GUIDELINES (1982)	NRPB GUIDELINES (1980)
STATIC B FIELD	TESLA	0.35	1.5	2.0	2.5 (0.35 for protons)
RATE OF B FIELD CHANGE	T/S	1.0	12.4	3	20 (IF 10 ms)
RF DOSE	W/KG				
BODY AVERAGE		0.3	0.2	0.4	(1°C rise)
HEAD AVERAGE		0.13	0.2	0.4	(1°C rise)
PEAK		?	2.0	2.0	

Approximate calculations, using a dipole to simulate the fringe field of a magnet, can be helpful in understanding the magnet's pull on ferromagnetic objects. A typical 1.0T imaging magnet has a field of five Gauss at an axial distance of ten meters from the magnet center. This yields an equivalent dipole strength of 2.5×10^6 Amp-turn-meter^2 (1.989 Tesla-meter^3). The fringe field of such a dipole is shown in Figure 1. The outline of the magnet housing is shown to suggest the limits of validity of this approximation.

If a ferromagnetic object is allowed to rotate so that its induced dipole moment is parallel to the applied field, the attractive force, $\vec{F}$, is given by

$$\vec{F} = M \cdot \text{grad } B , \tag{1}$$

where M = magnitude of the induced dipole and
B = magnitude of the magnetic field.

The simplest case for computing the induced dipole moment is that of a long slender object, aligned with the field. Flux is concentrated in the object and the iron is saturated. This produces the maximum dipole moment and, therefore, the maximum force per unit mass of iron. The dipole moment per unit volume of saturated iron is approximately 20 kiloGauss (1.59×10^6 Amp-turn/meter). Introducing this, and the density of iron, into Eq. (1) yields surfaces of constant force per unit mass as shown in Figure 4. The variation of this force along the axis of the magnet is shown in Figure 5. It varies inversely with the fourth power of the distance. In the case of fixed magnet geometry, the force, at a fixed position, scales linearly with the strength of the central field of the magnet. Some objects may not fully saturate and the above calculation can, therefore, overestimate the actual force.

A solid sphere of iron has the smallest induced dipole moment and, therefore, the minimum force per unit mass of iron (assuming a freely rotatable object). Its dipole moment is

$$M = 3 \cdot \frac{B}{\mu_o} \cdot \frac{4\pi}{3} R^3 \cdot \left[\frac{\mu/\mu_o - 1}{\mu/\mu_o + 2} \right] , \tag{2}$$

where R = radius of sphere,
μ = permeability of iron, and
μ_o = permeability of free space.

Since μ is much greater than μ_o, the term in brackets is approximately equal to unity. Combining Eqs. (1) and (2) with the density of iron yields a lower limit on the force per unit mass of iron, which is shown in Figure 5. It varies inversely with the seventh power of distance. At a fixed position, it scales as the square of the magnet's central field.

Complex ferromagnetic objects will have their force versus position curves between the two extremes shown in Figure 5. At short distances and high fields, the gap between the two curves narrows as the sphere approaches saturation. In Figure 6, the gap between the two limiting cases is shown in three dimensional, cylinderical coordinates for a force equal to one tenth the weight of the iron.

Unless there is a strong reason to do otherwise, the fully saturated case, together with an appropriate value for the force, should probably be used to calculate safety limits.

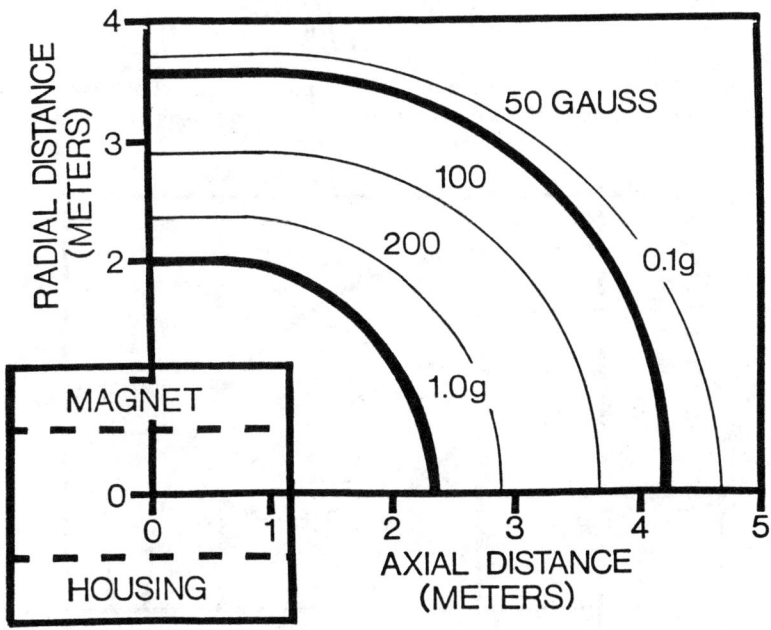

Figure 4: Lines of constant force per unit mass of magnetically saturated iron for the force equal to the weight of iron (1.0g) and one tenth the weight (0.1g). Based on a dipole simulation of a 1.0T imaging magnet. Lines of constant magnetic field strength are shown.

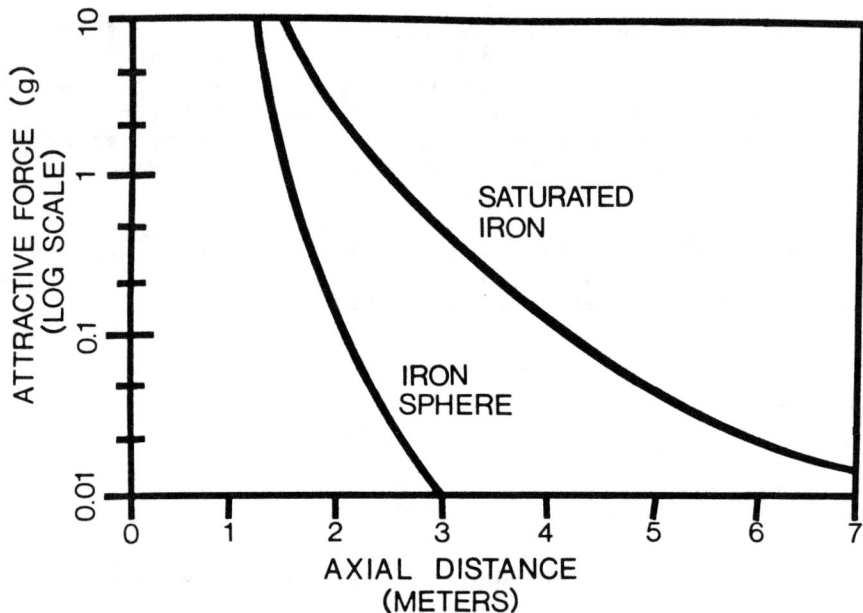

Figure 5: Force per unit mass of iron along the central axis for saturated iron and for an unsaturated iron sphere. Based on a dipole simulation of a 1.0T imaging magnet.

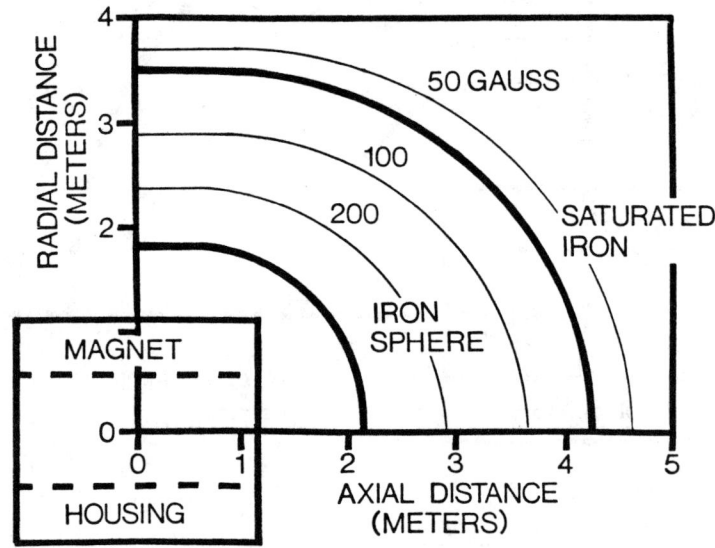

Figure 6: Lines of constant force per unit mass of iron equal to one tenth the weight of the iron (0.1g) for saturated iron and for an unsaturated iron sphere. Based on a dipole simulation of a 1.0T imaging magnet. Lines of constant magnetic field strength are shown.

EFFECTS OF MAGNETIC FIELDS ON OTHER HOSPITAL EQUIPMENT

Potentially adverse effects on the operation of many medical devices and a few more generally available consumer products are observed as the magnetic induction or "B" field is increased above a certain level dependent upon the particular device. For example, devices which depend on the precise positioning of a relatively slow-moving electron beam such as an image intensifier tube or a television monitor, may suffer noticeable effects at relatively low field strengths. Most medical and consumer devices function well in the earth's magnetic field, but documentation on the effects of stronger magnetic fields on various devices as a function of magnetic induction or field strength is quite limited. In available site planning guides, known or estimated magnetic field thresholds are often listed for potentially significant effects on various devices. Thresholds quoted in manfacturers' literature and other articles (3-5, 13-16) are summarized in Table 6 along with the current best threshold estimates. As can be seen, recommendations do not exist for many devices and there are considerable variations when thresholds are recommended. Little information is given on the severity of effects to aid decisions as to whether it might be possible to exceed the guidelines to reduce facility costs or increase operational efficiency. In relation to Table 1, it is worth noting that devices such as color and black and white TV systems and magnetic storage media and computer systems are particularly important because they are associated with the control of an NMR system and should be as close as possible to the magnet for efficient operation. TV monitors also are of concern because they are becoming so common in almost any room in a medical facility. Computer electronics are not affected by the lowest fields, but computer system locations are usually limited because of the accompanying magnetic storage media. To completely erase magnetic storage media such as that on credit cards requires a relatively high static field over a period of time. Thresholds as high as 200 gauss have been reported (17). However, fixed or changing magnetic fields or motion of the media within a static magnetic field at the levels quoted in Table 6 can increase the loss of marginally recorded information in a manner normally associated with aging.

Since the output of photomultiplier (PM) tubes is affected by the magnitude and orientation of magnetic fields, a device whose operation is extremely sensitive to PM tube gain (e.g. a scintillation camera (18) or a CT scanner which utilizes PM tubes) can be among the most sensitive to magnetic fields. The entire device or individual PM tubes can be magnetically shielded (19), but the large entrance window of a scintillation camera will make magnetic shielding difficult in most cases. It is not known to what extent magnetic shielding is already done by various manufacturers of existing equipment. Electroencephalographs and electrocardiographs may be relatively common in areas near prospective NMR sites, the former being extremely sensitive to oscillating magnetic fields and the latter being relatively insensitive. However, quantitative data is limited at this time.

Table 6: Maximum Magnetic Induction (B-field in Gauss) Expected For Acceptable Operation of Sensitive Devices

Device	Informational Source (See Reference List)								Recommended Maximum Field (Best Est.)
	#13	#4	#3	#14	#12	#15	#16	#5	
Scintillation Camera	1	1	1	1.5	-	1	0.5	2	1
Rotating ECAT	0.6	-	0.6	-	-	-	-	-	0.6
CT Scanner Utilizing PMTs	1-2	1	-	1.5		1	0.5	2	1
CT Scanner Non PMT	-	-	-	-	-	1	-	-	5
Shielded PMTs	10	10	-	-	-	-	-	-	10
Cyclotron	1	-	1	-	-	-	-	-	1
Image Intensifier	1	1	1	-	-	1	0.5	2	1
Electron Microscope	1	-	-	-	-	-	0.01	-	1
LINAC	-	-	-	-	-	-	-	1	1*
Ultrasound	3	-	-	-	-	-	-	-	3
Analytical Balance	-	-	-	-	-	-	-	-	2
Color TV	1.5	-	-	-	-	-	-	-	1.5
EEG	-	-	-	-	-	-	-	-	1
Mass Spect	1	-	-	-	-	-	-	-	1
Video Camera Unshielded	3	10	10	2	-	10	-	5	3
Video Camera Steel Case	10	10	-	-	-	-	-	-	10
B&W Monitor Non-critical	10-20	-	-	-	-	-	-	-	15

*More sensitive to changing field (gradient fields) than B_o.

Table 6 (Continued): Maximum Magnetic Induction (B-field in Gauss) Expected For Acceptable Operation of Sensitive Devices

Device	Informational Source (See Reference List)								Recommended Maximum Field (Best Est.)
	#13	#4	#3	#14	#12	#15	#16	#5	
Cardiac Pacemaker	5-15	5	3	10	5	5	5	15	5-15
ECG	-	-	-	-	-	-	-	-	-*
Neuro-Stimulator	-	-	-	-	-	-	-	-	5*
Mechanical Watches	10	-	-	10	-	30	-	15	10
High Density Magnetic Storage	1-10	10	10	5	-	10	5	15	5
Magnetic Credit Cards	10-200	20	-	10	-	30	-	15	20
Disc & Tape Drives	-	-	-	-	-	10	-	15	10
Computers	1-10	-	-	5	-	10	-	-	10
X-ray Tube	10	-	-	-	-	-	-	-	10
Operator Console	-	-	-	<50	-	-	-	-	15
MRI Power Supplies, etc	-	-	-	-	-	-	-	-	-
Rescussitation Equipment	-	-	-	-	-	-	-	-	-
Hearing Aids	-	-	-	10	-	-	-	-	10
Electric Motors	-	-	-	10	-	30	-	-	20
Photographic Equipment	-	-	-	-	-	30	-	-	30
Metal Detector	-	-	-	-	-	-	-	-	-

*More sensitive to changing field (gradient fields) than B_o.

STATUS OF MAGNETIC SHIELDING

The field outside the magnet bore may extend over an extremely large area. This area extends in all directions and frequently goes beyond the boundary of the NMR imaging suite. The area beyond the imaging suite is referred to as the fringe field region and in the absence of magnetic shielding is proportional to the strength of the magnet. Table 7 illustrates the approximate maximum field extent of the 5 gauss fringe field of magnets of different strengths.

Table 7: Maximum Distance From Magnet Center Yielding 5 Gauss Field

		MAGNETIC FIELD STRENGTH			
		0.15	0.30T	0.50T	1.50T
Distance in:	meters	6.1	7.6	9.0	12.8
	feet	20	25	29	42

An extended fringe field region is undesirable in a hospital environment because of the influence and interference it may have on other hospital activities. The most serious of these are the interference with cardiac pacemakers, interference with electron beam devices, influence on small iron objects and on magnetically stored information. Consequently, a detailed knowledge of a magnet's fringe field and its relationship to surrounding activities is an essential part of any site planning and installation program.

The most common method employed to date to limit the extent of the fringe field is the use of high flux return paths with sheets of ferrous alloys to confine or alter the shape of the field lines-of-force. This solution is not without complications since the use of large amounts of iron for shielding establishes forces on the magnet coil and also affects the uniformity of the field within the bore of the magnet. In addition, in some partially shielded configurations, edge effects along the periphery of the shield may result in field strengths in excess of those present without shielding. Iron in the fringe field will become magnetized, causing the main magnet to see other magnets in the surrounding area with a resulting distortion in the imaging volume and a distortion of isointensity contours in the vicinity of the iron.

At least three possible approaches to the magnetic field screening can be identified (20).
1. Closed-flux path screens with iron alloys.
2. Partial screening with iron alloys.
3. Active shields using equivalent current shells.

One example of an active shield at the entrance to an MRI room is presented in reference 21. Active shields have not been used extensively to date and will not be discussed further.

Choice Of Magnet Screens

When the zone has been identified in which the fringe field is unacceptably high, one may choose from various forms of passive shielding methods:

1. A screen which shields the local zone by enclosing the zone itself in a closed-flux path, e.g., an iron box around the computer.

2. A closed-flux path screen around the magnet which can be either within the magnet housing (so-called self-shielding magnets) or around the magnet so that most of the magnetic field energy is diverted from the outside boundary of the box.

3. Partial or discontinuous high-flux screens which are positioned to cause local distortions of the field sufficient to accommodate the need of specific local zones, e.g., a distortion just large enough to accommodate a CT scanner.

Generally, a closed-flux path shield will be more efficient at screening than partial screening, such as a single iron sheet placed between the magnet and the zone to be shielded. With proper design, the closed shield can save cost and space by serving as an RF shield (22). The general criterion for shielding is to use as little iron as possible because of cost, weight, and effect on magnet homogeneity.

Rules-of-thumb For Closed-flux Shields

For local shielding under the assumption of a spherical screen (rather than a box), the following equation can be used to relate the (source) field outside the screen H_{out} to the field inside the screen H_{in}:

$$H_{in} = (2d/\mu t) H_{out}$$

where the screen thickness is t and diameter is d. The permeability of the screen material is assumed to be independent of H (20). In most shielding the iron is partially saturated, so that these equations overestimate the field reduction.

For more extensive shielding, it is generally better to consider shielding the entire magnet. The rule-of-thumb estimate for the thickness of the iron (d2-d1) needed to reduce the field by a factor of f can be obtained from the following equation:

$$f = \{1 + 2/9 \, (1-(d1/d2)^3) \, (\mu-1) \, [1-1/\mu)]\}$$

Where d1 and d2 are the average inner and outer diameter of the screen and μ is the permeability (Ref. 1).

Such rule-of-thumb equations are generally not adequate for specific installations which must include both screening and structural iron and their effects on homogeneity. It is also true with closed-flux path shields, that the mass of the screen remains approximately constant for a given field reduction and magnet strength regardless of the shields average distance from the magnet. In addition, the effects of partial screens are not easily calculated. For partial screening situations a handbook giving screening values for various isolated, finite plates of different thickness and locations relative to the magnet center ray are used (20). Even though high-permeability materials are very efficient shields, in many cases the real concern is the maximum flux density obtained in a material. In many cases, steel may satisfy the requirements thus minimizing cost.

Configurations Used In Existing Sites

Magnetic field shielding and site planning is becoming more complex as magnet field strengths increase. In many sites, installation of magnets greater than 0.5T would be impossible without some sort of shielding.

Self-shielding Designs

The Siemens Corporation and Oxford Magnet Technology offer self-shielding options which are installed as part of the magnet housing. The Siemens option offers the field reduction factors shown in Table 8 (23).

Table 8: Self-shielding Field Reduction Factors (23)

Field Strength	Field Reduction Factor	Weight of Shield
0.5T	5	21,000 kg
1.0T	4.5	21,000 kg
1.5T	2.8	21,000 kg
1.5T	7.5	31,000 kg

Discrete Steel Plate Shielding

Opposed pairs of steel plates have been used in the walls surrounding the system by the Philips Corporation and others to substantially reduce the fields outside the magnet room. The increased steel thickness will reduce the magnitude of the fringe field lines (4). The use of such steel plates will disrupt the homogeneity of the central imaging volume. However, by using opposing plates the effects on the homogeneity is significantly reduced (24, 25).

A variation on the use of large discrete plates has also been proposed. This variation is referred to as the "bird cage" shield or as a magnetic dome (4). In this method a dome is constructed from relatively small modular sheets. This may reduce construction costs and is quite aesthetically pleasing.

Closed-flux Shield

Several installations have been completed which use closed-flux path shielding (26). The Diasonics approach of an enclosed steel box resting on a copper floor to accomplish RF as well as fringe field shielding seems particularly cost effective, as only the inside layer of steel requires welding or other electrical connection for the RF shielding. An interesting variation between the discrete plate geometry and the closed-flux shield design has recently been installed at the Henry Ford Hospital in Detroit, Michigan. In their installation they used a continuous steel cylinder to enclose the magnet (25).

Magnetic Shielding Software

Most manufacturers now possess special purpose software packages which can analyze fringe fields in three dimensions and can custom design both closed-flux path shields and discrete plate shields to meet the varying requirements of individual customers. A complete 3D field calculation program may be obtained at considerable expense (27).

For geometries which can be simulated adequately by a 2-dimensional arrangement, a Fortran code is available in the public domain which uses the Poisson group of codes (28).

RADIOFREQUENCY SHIELDING

Various interference coupling pathways are present between potential sources of noise and the MR detection coil. These include: (1) radiative noise from fluorescent lights, capacitors and power supplies; (2) conductive current or voltage elements which establish linking magnetic fields; (3) the presence of conduits which couple noise generated externally into the magnet room; and (4) lines connected directly to the magnet from the computer, the RF power supply, and the gradient power supply. It is generally agreed that this last point represents the dominant noise pathway for MRI systems. The proton frequencies associated with NMR cover a relatively wide frequency range from 4.26 MHz at 0.1T to 85.1 MHz at 2T. Although this portion of the electromagnetic spectrum is very heavily populated, the MR unit can be adjusted easily to avoid a specific RF frequency. Manufacturers specifications for shielded rooms vary from 60 dB isolation to 120 dB, the latter being for spectroscopic applications. Since it is relatively easy to attain

80 to 100 dB isolation without significantly increased cost over lower isolation, most manufacturers specify 80 to 100 dB isolation (29). Siemens Corporation specifies for their 21 MHz (0.5T) system--80 dB isolation at 2 MHz, 100 dB at 5 MHz and 110 dB from 30-100 MHz (30). Shielding requirements do depend on the ambient electromagnetic noise in the area and a few MR system suppliers specify ambient electric and magnetic field strengths which will allow prior system operation with the specified RF shielding or system properties alone. One company has established quantitative electrical field specifications of 100 mV/m for acceptable ambient RF prior to RF shielding for their 1.5T system.

One hundred dB is difficult to achieve in practice without a Faraday cage since any construction other than a solid shield allows for RF leakage. RF shielded enclosures are sold by numerous companies specializing in this field. The information on various manufacturers of shielded enclosures may be obtained from an MR Site Planning Consultant or from manufacturers of MR systems. A typical rectangular shielded enclosure costs $50,000 to $110,000 installed. A physicist or other hospital representative should verify performance of the RF enclosure with the supplier after the enclosure is installed.

All users and vendors of MR imaging systems agree that radiofrequency shielding is necessary. However, disagreement exists as to the type and extent of RF protection required. Radiative interference from ambient RF is thought to be of minimal concern in comparison to the noise conducted by the lines leading into the MR unit. Thus some vendors feel that magnets could be shielded at the magnet through the use of zinc (or other mterial) coating the inside of the fiberglass housing. The opening of the magnet bore provides a waveguide effect for incident RF. The effectiveness of the bore opening as an attenuator decreases as the magnetic field size increases since shorter wavelengths easily pass through to the RF coil. Magnets operating at 0.15T have much less signal than magnets operating at 1.0T and greater. Thus noise reductions will result in improvements more readily with lower field magnets.

SITE PLANNING CHECKLIST AND PLANNING FORM

The following list identifies most topics to be considered in designing an MRI facility.

I. <u>Functional Areas</u>   Sq. Ft.

The first group is normally required for an MRI facility:

```
Scan Room                                      _____
Control Room                                   _____
Computer Equipment Room (include rf
  equipment and power supplies)                _____
Reading Rm. (include physician's console)      _____
Cryogen Storage                                _____
```

The second group is required adjacent to the MRI facility but some areas can be shared with other imaging services when necessary or when spaces can be designed properly.

```
Film Processing                                _____
Quality Control and Service                    _____
Patient Preparation Recovery, and
  Emergency Procedures area                    _____
Patient Reception and Waiting                  _____
Stretcher Holding Area                         _____
Storage (supplies, magtapes, films, etc.)      _____
Washrooms                                      _____
Soiled Utility                                 _____
Clean Utility                                  _____
```

The third group lists additional functions, likely to be required, but which can be both remote from the MRI unit and shared with other services in extenuating circumstances.

```
Secretarial and Transcription Services         _____
Conference Area                                _____
Additional Storage (e.g. film library,
  magtapes)                                    _____
Offices                                        _____
```

II. Construction and Access Considerations   Comments

    Equipment transportion, unloading and installation access
    Floor loading (including access routes)
    Floor levelness
    Ceiling heights (especially magnet room and access console)
    Access for cryogens
    Cryogen venting (normal and quench)
    Controlled access to facility and well-controlled access to magnet room

III. Protecting Magnetic Field Homogeneity   Possible problems

    Structural iron and steel (include reinforcing rod in concrete)
    Other large ferrous structures or objects
    Symmetrical location of ferrous structures
    Moving ferrous objects (vehicles, lift trucks, elevators, carts, etc.)

IV. Protecting Surrounding Environment from Magnetic Fields

    A three-dimensional survey of magnetically sensitive devices and equipment should be undertaken. Actual distance from the center of the magnet will depend on magnet field strength and design. Use the field strengths in Table 6 as a conservative guide or the current best estimates.

DEVICE	MAGNETIC FIELD LINES (GAUSS)	AXIAL DISTANCE (feet)	TRANSVERSE DISTANCE (feet)
A. Color TV monitors			

B. B&W monitors
   1. Precise spatial measurements
   2. Unacceptable for visual use			

C. Magnetic storage media			
D. Scintillation			
E. Emission tomography scintillation cameras			
F. CAT scanners			
G. Image intensifier systems			
H. Computer systems			
I. Electroencephalographs (sensitive to oscillating fields from gradients)			
J. EKG			
K. Electron microscopy			
L. Mass spectroscopy			
M. Other systems with low potential electron beams or sensitive electronics in the 10 Hz to 3 KHz frequency range of gradient fields			

V. **Radiofrequency Shielding**

   Complete rf shield enclosing magnet and patient table (to manufacturer's specifications and site survey).

   Avoid light dimmers, fluorescent lighting ballasts near scan room.
   Check for:
A. Paging system, nearby
    radio stations and
    citizens band transmitters

B. Electrocartery devices

C. Diathermy equipment

D. Site survey necessary ?

VI. **Facility Environment**

   Electrical supplies--voltages, current, and phases

   Air conditioning--general
                   --computer room (temperature, humidity, and
                                    filtration)
   Water supply and floor drains (include sink for phantom
                                  filling)
   Chilled water supply--temperature, flow rate and tolerable
                         temperature fluctuation
   Personnel protection--pacemaker, credit card and watch limits
                        --metal detection
   Fire Detection and Safety--no sprinklers; non-ferrous
                              extinguishers
   Telephone Service--separate lines for operator, physician and
                      service personnel (near computer)
   Housekeeping--no carpet, no ferrous cleaning tools or supplies

References:

1. Faul DD. An Overview of Magnetic Resonance System Design. Technology of Nuclear Magnetic Resonance. (PD Esser and PE Johnston, editors.) Society of Nuclear Medicine Inc., New York, NY, 1984. p. 3-14.

2. Holland GN. Systems Engineering of a Whole-Body Proton Magnetic Resonance Imaging System. In Nuclear Magnetic Resonance (NMR) Imaging. (CL Partain, EE James, FD Rollo, et. al. editors.) WB Saunders Co., Philadelphia. 1983 p. 128-151.

3. Magnetic Resonance Site Planning Considerations. General Electric Company. 1982 and 1984.

4. NMR Site Planning Considerations. Philips Medical Systems. 1982 and 1983.

5. NMR Imaging Superconductive Magnet Systems Site Planning Guide. Technicare Corporation, 1983.

6. Patz S and Moore WS. The placing of many large superconducting magnets in a limited space. Magnetic Resonance in Medicine $\underline{2}$:262-274, 1985.

7. Pavlicek W, MacIntyre W, Go R, et. al. Special Architectural Considerations in Designing a Magnetic Resonance Facility. Technology of Nuclear Magnetic Resonance. (PD Esser and PE Johnston, editors.) Society of Nuclear Medicine Inc., New York, NY, 1984.

8. Pavlicek W and Meaney TF. The Special Environmental Needs of Medical Magnetic Resonance. Applied Radiology $\underline{13}$:23-33, 1984.

9. Pavlicek W, Geisinger M, Castle L, et. al. The Effect of Nuclear Magnetic Resonance on Patients with Cardiac Pacemakers. Radiology $\underline{147}$:149-153, 1983.

10. Saunders RD and Orr JS. Biological Effects of NMR. in Nuclear Magnetic Resonance Imaging. (L. Partain, AE James, FD Rollo, et. al. editors.) Saunders, Philadelphia, 1983.

11. Revised Guidance on Acceptable Limits of Exposure During Nuclear Magnetic Resonance Clinical Imaging. National Radiological Protection Board. BJR $\underline{56}$:974-977, 1983.

12. Gundaker WE. Guidelines for Evaluating Electromagnetic Risk for Trials of Clinical NMR Systems. Letter of Dec. 28, 1982. Office of Radiological Health, National Center for Devices and Radiological Health.

13. Carson PL, Martel W, Gabrielsen TO, et. al. Facility Planning for Magnetic Resonance Imaging. (Abstract) Radiological Society of North America. Annual Meeting, 1982 (RSNA Program p. 193).

14. Preliminary Site Planning Guide--Diasonics NMR Scanner. Diasonics NMR Division, South San Francisco, CA, May 1983.

15. Morneburg H. Factors in Site Determinations and Planning for a Magnetom. Electrtometica 51:65-72, 1983.

16. NMR Selection Guidelines--Resistive and Superconducting Systems. Picker Internatonal, Solon, OH. July 1983.

17. Shaw D. Oxford Research Systems, Oxford England. Private Communication.

18. Thomas SR, Ackerman JL, and Kereiakes JG. Practical Aspects Involved in The Design and Set Up of a 0.15T, 6-Coil Resistive Magnet, Whole Body NMR Imaging Facility. Magnetic Resonance Imaging 2:341-348, 1984.

19. Ross RJ, Thompson JS, Kim K, et. al. Site Location and Requirements for the Installation of a Nuclear Magnetic Resonance Scanning Unit. Magnetic Resonance Imaging 1:29-33, 1982.

20. Magnets in Clinical Use--Site Planning Guide. Oxford Magnet Technolgoy Ltd., Oxford, England, 1983.

21. Den Boer JA. Hybrid Shielding of the Static Magnetic Stray Field Generated by a 0.5 tesla Whole Body NMR System. (Abstract) Society of Magnetic Resonance in Medicine 3rd Annual Meeting. New York, New York. August 13-17, 1984. 188-190.

22. Ries G and Frese G. Magnetic Shielding of Whole Body MR Magnets. (Abstract) Society of Magnetic Resonance in Medicine 3rd Annual Meeting. New York, New York. August 13-17, 1984. 625-627.

23. Magnetom^{tm} Magnetic Self-shielding, Siemens Corporation, Erlangen, Federal Republic of Germany (in the U.S., Siemens Medical Systems, Iselin, NJ), 1985.

24. Einstein SG. Siting and Shielding. (Abstract) Society of Magnetic Resonance in Medicine 3rd Annual Meeting. New York, New York. August 13-17, 1984. 212-215.

25. Flynn MJ, Vavrek RM, Ewing MJ, et. al. Magnetic Fields from MR Imaging Magnets with Axially Symmetric Iron Shields. Radiology 153(p):304, 1984.

26. Ewing JR, Timms W, Helpern J, et. al. Magnetic Shielding and Site Planning for a Large Bore, High Field Magnet. Society of Magnetic Resonance in Medicine 3rd Annual Meeting. New York, New York. August 13-17, 1984. 224.

27. TOSCA 3D Magnetic Field Calculation Program. Available from Infolytica Corporation; Suite 430, 1500 Stanley Street, Montreal, Canada H3A LR3.

28. Two-D Field Calculation Program. Contact John L. Warren, Group AT-6, Los Alamos Scientific Laboratories, Los Alamos, NM.

29. RF Shielding for NMR Imagers. RNM Images 1983. The Keene Corporation, Ray Proof Division, 50 Keeler Avenue, Norwalk, CT 06856.

30. MR Imaging Site Planning, 0.5T Unistat Superconducting Magnet. Siemens Corporation, Erlangen, West Germany. November 1984.

CONCEPTS OF QUALITY ASSURANCE AND PHANTOM DESIGN FOR NMR SYSTEMS

R.R. Price, J.A. Patton, J.J. Erickson
D.R. Pickens, C.L. Partain, A.E. James
Department of Radiology and Radiological Sciences
Vanderbilt University Medical Center, Nashville, TN   37232

ABSTRACT

This document attempts to explore test methods which can be used on a routine basis to assure the quality of performance of NMR imaging systems. These tests are to be distinguished from acceptance tests which are used to determine whether or not an instrument meets the manufacturer's specifications at the time of purchase and which are specifically designed to test the limits of a system's performance. Potential NMR phantom materials are categorized as either proton rich materials or as paramagnetic metal ions. Imaging parameters which are suggested to be monitored on a routine basis are categorized as either geometric parameters or signal intensity parameters. Several specific phantoms which could be included as part of a quality assurance program are described along with required measurements, calculations, and suggested interpretation.

INTRODUCTION

The goal of a quality assurance program is to provide a set of tests which when performed on a regular basis can be used to determine if the system is performing in a reproducible and predictable manner. Unfortunately, at the present time clinical NMR imaging does not enjoy the benefit of a large body of knowledge from which one can design definitive procedures and protocols for routine system performance testing. On the other hand, NMR is fortunate in that it shares many common features with multiplane transmission and emission computed tomography systems and for those features can draw from those modalities. Many of the test procedures and phantom designs presented in this document have in part been borrowed from protocols now being used in the evaluation of CT and nuclear medicine systems.

The goals of a quality assurance program should be differentiated from the goals of an acceptance testing protocol. In an acceptance testing protocol one attempts to measure quantifiable system parameters which are then compared to the manufacturer's specifications. Acceptance tests should be designed to be instrument independent and should produce absolute parameters which can be compared between various manufacturers' equipment. Quality assurance tests, on the other hand, are most useful for an individual user for assessing relative changes in the system performance, the distinction being primarily the difference between absolute and relative measurements.

NMR presents numerous special problems not encountered in other imaging modalities. These problems result from the fact that NMR systems are "tuned" systems and for optimized performance must be tuned to the object being imaged. The logical extension of this line of reasoning would be to conclude that phantoms could not be used in determining how an NMR system would perform when imaging a patient. Fortunately, this conclusion is not correct and the fact that phantoms are useful tools has already been established in several laboratories[1-3]. However, the problem of tuning which includes coil loading or filling factor, remains an exceedingly important factor in quality assurance measurements. Because of these unique problems NMR phantom design and the interpretation of their results probably requires a more detailed understanding of the instrumentation and their underlying physical principles than is required for any other imaging modality.

Another complexity not encountered in other imaging modalities is the phenomenon that the subject contrast (as well as image contrast) may vary from instrument to instrument. This is due to the fact that the T_1 and T_2 relaxation times of the subject are field dependent and will thus depend upon the operating field strength of the imaging system. This fact also leads to images of the same subject with different signal-to-noise levels.

Further, additional complexities are introduced by the infinity of different pulse sequences, receiver coil geometries and image processing steps which may be used to create an image. All of these factors must be specified and kept constant for comparison measurement to be meaningful.

NMR PHANTOM MATERIALS

A variety of different agents and compounds have been proposed as potential standard materials for NMR phantoms. These can be roughly divided into two categories; (1) proton rich materials (mineral oil, various vegetable oils, vaseline, ethylene glycol, propylene glycol, other like compounds) and (2) paramagnetic metal ions (Cr^{3+}, Mn^{2+}, Fe^{3+}, Cu^{2+}, Eu^{3+}, Gd^{3+}, and others).

Some proton rich compounds are water soluable and can be easily diluted to yield T_1 and T_2 values that are in the range of normal tissue. Table 1 includes the results of a set of T_1 and T_2 measurements made in our 0.5 T (20 MHz) imager, on various mixtures of 1,2 propanediol and distilled water. The T_1 values were estimated using a two pulse sequence technique produced by the manufacturer and the T_2 values were determined from a single exponential fit to a series of 8 echoes from a spin-echo pulse sequence. It should be noted that both T_1 and T_2 increase with increasing water content. T_2 values in particular tend to be shorter when measured in an imaging system relative to a spectrometer. This effect is presumed to be due to gradient effects. The values presented in Table 1 are presented for comparison only and can not be guaranteed to be accurate.

Phantom material derived from various concentrations of D_2O/H_2O has also been proposed[4]. Since the deuterium yields no NMR signal the detected signal is linearly related to the water concentration (proton density) while both T_1 and T_2 remain constant.

A problem that has been noted with proton rich materials in regard to phantom design is that since they are generally non-conductive, coil-loading may not be representative of tissue loading.

TABLE 1
1,2 Propanediol
(20 MHz)

% Propanediol and distilled water	T_1 (m sec)	T_2 (m sec)
0	2134	485
10	1808	313
20	1068	185
40	754	118
60	503	112
80	328	99
100	217	72

Transition elements and rare-earth elements constitute a group of paramagnetic substances which are now widely used as NMR contrast agents. Unlike the proton rich agents, the paramagnetic ions are added to water to shorten the effective T_1 and T_2 of the mixture and thereby increase the detected signal relative to unmodified water protons. The relative influence of the various ions on the proton spin-lattice relaxation time is roughly proportional to the ions magnetic moment (Table 2)[5].

As seen in Table 2, the ion of gadolinium (Gd^{3+}) which has seven unpaired electrons has an unusually strong hydrogen proton spin-lattice relaxation effect. For this reason it is this ion in its chelated form (Gd-DTPA) which is being suggested as a likely in vivo contrast agent.

TABLE 2

Atomic Number	Ion	Unpaired Electrons	Magnetic moment (Bohr magnetons)
24	Cr^{3+}	3	3.8
25	Mn^{2+}	5	5.9
26	Fe^{3+}	5	5.9
29	Cu^{2+}	1	1.7-2.2
64	Gd^{3+}	7	7.9

TABLE 3*
(20 MHz)

$MnCl_2$ Concentration (mM)	T_1 (m sec)
0.0	3269
0.01	2660
0.05	1475
0.10	982
0.25	518
0.40	316
0.50	262
0.80	164
1.00	132
5.00	27

*Beale P.T., Amtey S.R., Kasturi S.R.: <u>NMR Data Handbook for Biomedical Applications</u>. Pergamon Press, New York (1984)

TABLE 4
(12.5 mHz)

$CuSO_4$ Concentration (mM)	T_1 (m sec)
6.2	225
12.5	101
25.0	47
50.0	28
100.0	15

TABLE 5
(6.25 MHz)*

Ni(NO$_3$)$_2$ concentration (mM)	T$_1$ (m sec)	T$_2$ (m sec)
1.0	–	283
2.5	274	–
5.0	193	151
10	112	57
20	60	–
40	32	–

*Coffey, C., Smith, S., Wang, P., Bellis, G., Hines, H.: Early generation phantoms and test objects for quality control in NMR. AAPM handout (1984).

$CuSO_4$, $MnCl_2$, $Ni(NO_3)_2$, and $CrCl_3$ are all compounds that have found frequent use as NMR phantom materials[6]. The general behavior of aqueous solutions of all of these agents is to decrease both T_1 and T_2 of the solution with increasing concentrations of the paramagnetic ion.

Several investigations have recognized the problem in the use of paramagnetic ion solutions in that one is unable to vary the magnitude of one relaxation time without changing the other. These investigators have generally sought to use combinations of metal ions and agar gels. Their work has shown that the T_2 values of the solutions are dependent on the gel concentrations while the T_1 values are primarily dependent upon the metal ion concentration[7-9]. An important need for phantom construction is the availability of materials with standard traceable T_1 and T_2 values.

NMR IMAGE PARAMETERS

NMR imaging parameters can be subdivided into geometric parameters, signal intensity parameters and general system parameters. In the category of geometric parameters we have included spatial resolution, slice geometry, sensitive volume and spatial linearity. Included in slice geometry is slice location, multi-slice adjacency, slice alignment, and slice thickness. In the category of signal intensity parameters included are noise, signal-to-noise, contrast-to-noise, signal linearity, T_1 and T_2 accuracy, and signal response uniformity. In the category of general system parameters is 90° and 180° tip-angle accuracy, RF field uniformity, resonance frequency stability, video display parameters, and light localizer accuracy.

The next section will be devoted to the description of a number of specific phantom designs, the associated measurements and calculations, and suggested results interpretation. The content of this section is not intended to be a recommendation of any specific phantom, but is intended rather to illustrate the range of phantom designs which are currently being proposed. There are surely many acceptable phantom designs and test procedures which could be used for assessing any individual image parameter. With more experience, it is hoped that the AAPM, or some other like organization, will be able to identify those methods which have been found to provide adequate and useful quality assurance test measurements.

SPATIAL RESOLUTION

Unlike other imaging modalities, the intrinsic spatial resolution of most NMR systems currently on the market is limited by the image acquisition matrix size. Consequently, many manufacturers quote the spatial resolution in terms of the pixel size rather than perceived or measured resolution. This specification of resolution is inappropriate since it not only assumes optimal instrument operation including display as well as image processing, but also will likely be voided by the availability of increased matrix sizes.

A number of different resolution phantom designs familiar to us from use with other imaging modalities are also applicable to NMR imaging.

Phantom designs:
- ° Parallel-line bar phantoms
- ° Star design bar phantoms
- ° Hole phantoms (hot or cold)
- ° Edge-response phantoms

These phantoms are usually made by forming grooves or drilling holes in an acrylic block and then filling the holes with a high signal producing material (Fig. 1). An alternate design uses acrylic rods suspended in a signal producing medium to produce a "cold" hole image. The result for each design is a high contrast phantom since acrylic produces no signal in imaging systems (Fig. 2).

The purpose of the spatial resolution measurement is to determine the size of the smallest high contrast object, which when placed with separations equal to the width of the objects, that can be distinguished as individual objects. The classical approach to this has been to determine the MTF from either an edge-response or line response function (10, 11). However, for practical reasons, the use of images of line-pair phantoms (bar and hole arrays) with varying spatial frequency is generally accepted as the preferred method for routine assessment of spatial resolution. MTF values may be calculated for specific line pair groups by using intensity profiles to determine the modulation decrease as a function of line pair spatial frequency relative to a reference frequency.

Since the spatial resolution may be positron dependent, resolution measurements are generally made at the slice center and at the slice periphery at the position of the four compass points.

In systems that use the 2-DFT imaging technique, it is frequently found that the spatial resolution will be different along the frequency encoding and phase encoding directions. Most systems keep the sampling in the frequency encoding direction fixed while allowing the user the option of changing the number of gradient steps to vary the resolution in the phase encoding direction (Fig. 3A and 3B).

Resolution estimates are also made using phantoms of isolated holes of different sizes (Fig. 4). The resolution is estimated as the hole size at which the measured intensity drops to 50% of its maximum value (Fig. 5).

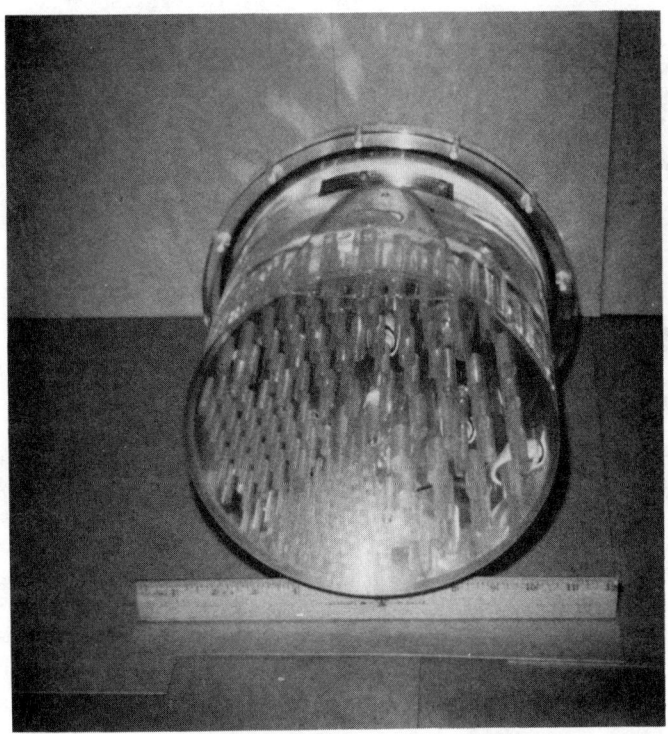

Fig. 1 Photograph of a commercially available "hot" hole phantom used originally for emission computed tomography.

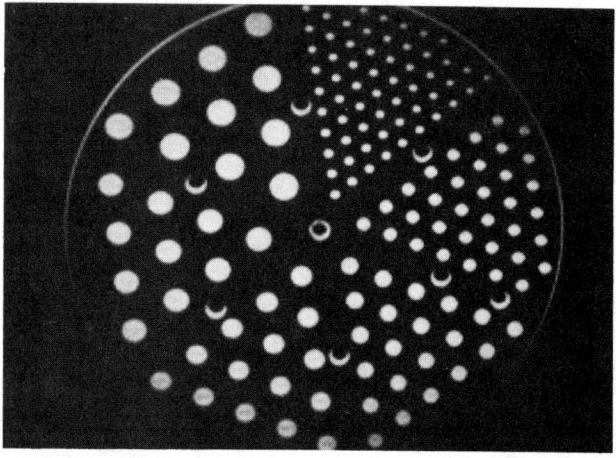

Fig. 2 NMR scan of "hot" hole phantom. Minimum hole separation 3 mm.

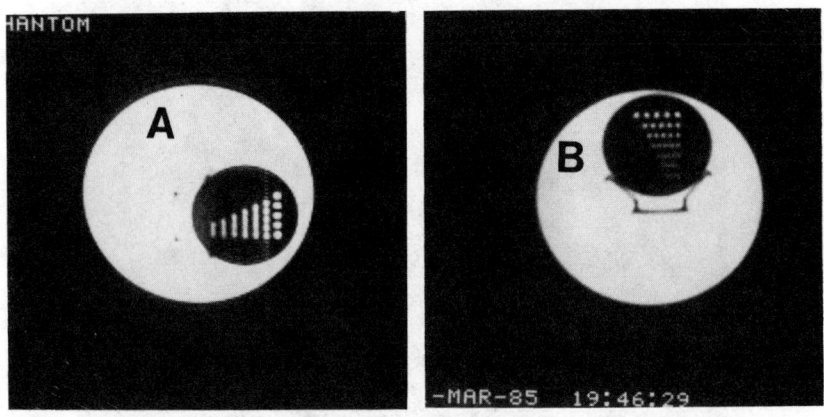

Fig. 3 (A) Resolution hole phantom scanned with orientation along the phase encoding direction using only 128 phase encoding gradient steps. Acrylic insert with 7 sets of 5 holes (2.5, 2.0, 1.75, 1.5, 1.25, 1.0, and 0.75 mm square) spaced longitudinally on 5 mm centers and vertically on centers equal to twice the side of the square (2 mm/pixel).
(B) Hole phantom scan with orientation along the frequency encoding direction with 256 samples (1 mm/pixel).

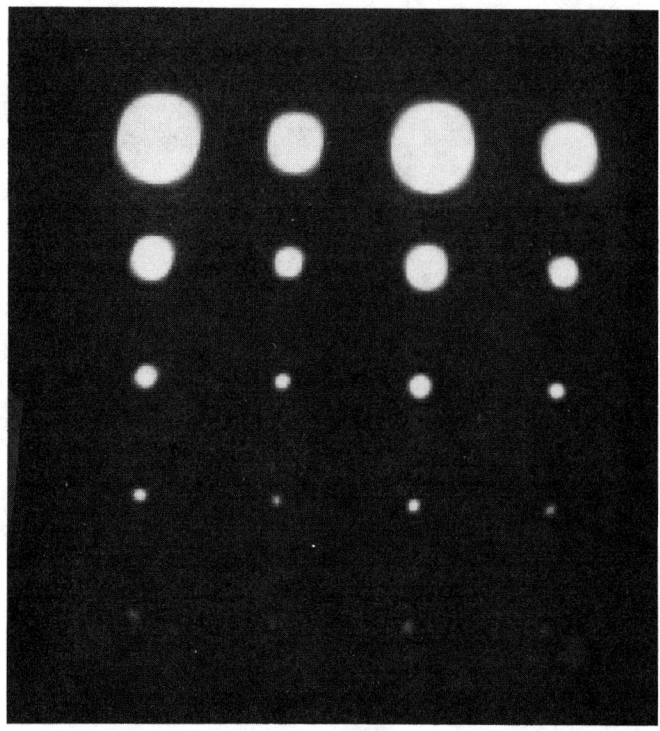

Fig. 4 Discrete hot-hole phantom. Hole sizes 19, 13, 10, 6, 5, 3.2, 2.4, 1.6, 1.2, and 0.8 mm.

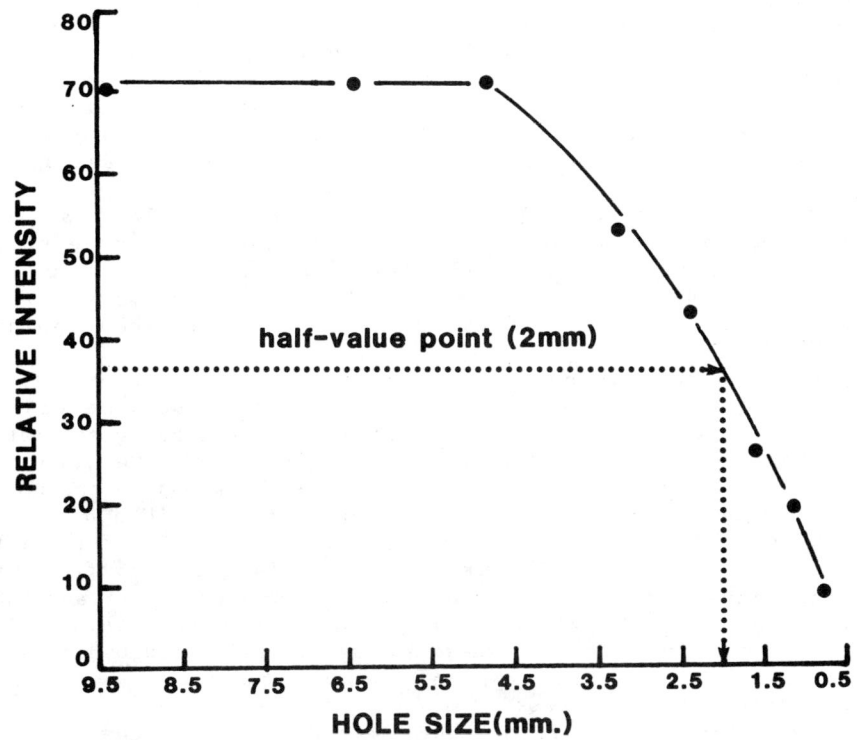

Fig. 5 Plot of intensity over center of each hole versus hole size. Resolution defined as hole size where intensity drops to 50%.

SLICE GEOMETRY

The most common slice geometry parameters are slice thickness, multi-slice position accuracy, and slice alignment.
        Slice thickness phantoms:
         ° Inclined ramps
         ° Continuous wedge (either hot or cold)
         ° Discrete stepwedge
         ° Double or single signal producing helix

The most commonly used phantom for slice thickness determination is an inclined signal producing ramp whose thickness is small with respect to the slice thickness. If the ramp is inclined at 45° relative to the slice plane, then the intensity profile will be equal to the slice sensitivity profile and can be used directly to estimate slice thickness by the FWHM. Problems associated with this phantom design result from low signal strength and noisy profiles requiring either long scan times with multiple averages or the averaging of many scan lines to reduce the noise.

A modification of this design is the continuous wedge (Fig. 6). The wedge, because of the integrating effect of including more signal producing material as the slice progresses up the ramp, yields a less noisy image. This advantage, however, is traded for the disadvantage of requiring a more detailed analysis. Since the profile is now an integral response, the true slice profile is estimated by differentiation. Figure 7A shows the integral response function of a 45° wedge and the estimated slice response function using first differences of adjacent points (Fig. 7B).

A discrete stepwedge can also be used to estimate slice thickness (Fig. 8). The stepwedge is analyzed in the same way as the continuous ramp with the integral response being generated from regions of interest measurements from each step plotted against position (Fig. 9). Total slice thickness to the noise level can be estimated by counting the number of visible discrete steps and then multiplying by the step thickness. The full width at half-max thickness is determined by plotting the differences of the signal value of the steps versus the step number and then assessing the distance between the two half-max points. The accuracy of the slice thickness estimates is limited by the step thickness with the accuracy being equal to approximately $\pm$ one-half the step thickness.

A modification of the wedge method has led to the use of a phantom consisting of signal producing helical tubes. The helical phantom has generally found less use than the wedge design for slice thickness measurements. The helical phantom design, however, has found considerable acceptance for determining slice location and adjacency in multi-slice techniques. Helical phantoms have been constructed from blown glass tubing but suffer from being too fragile. A more rugged design is to machine spiral grooves on the surface of an acrylic cylinder and then to place plastic tubing (usually 1 mm) filled with signal producing material in the groove. A somewhat less costly design can be made by placing plastic tubing formed in the shape of a double helix on the surface of an 18 cm high cardboard cylinder (Fig. 10). The phantom is designed so that the tube rotates through exactly 180° over the 18 cm height of the cylinder. Tubes placed on opposite sides of the cylinder parallel to the long axis are used for orientation and reference. Thus for each displacement of 1 cm along the axis of the cylinder, the tubes move through 10° of arc. Slice position is then determined by making multiple planar images through the axis of the phantom and measuring the relative rotation in degrees of the position of the image of the tubing (Fig. 11). The actual rotation is 10°/cm.

A phantom for determining slice orthogonality and alignment can be easily constructed. The phantom consists of a planar rectangle formed from plastic tubing filled with signal producing material. An improved version of the phantom consists of multiple rectangles of different sizes in slightly different planes separated approximately by the slice thickness. The largest rectangle should be as large as the receiver coil will accommodate. Deviation of the plane of the slice from the plane of the rectangle can easily be identified by a decreased signal in the portion of the rectangle outside of the image plane.

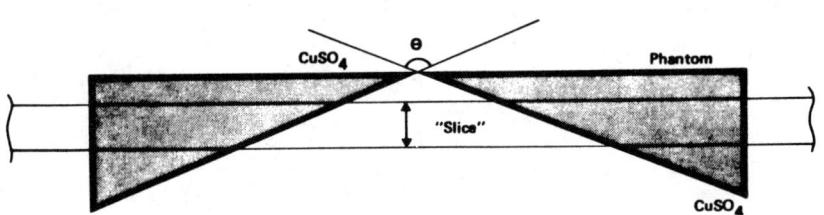

Fig. 6 Continuous signal producing wedge used for slice thickness determination.

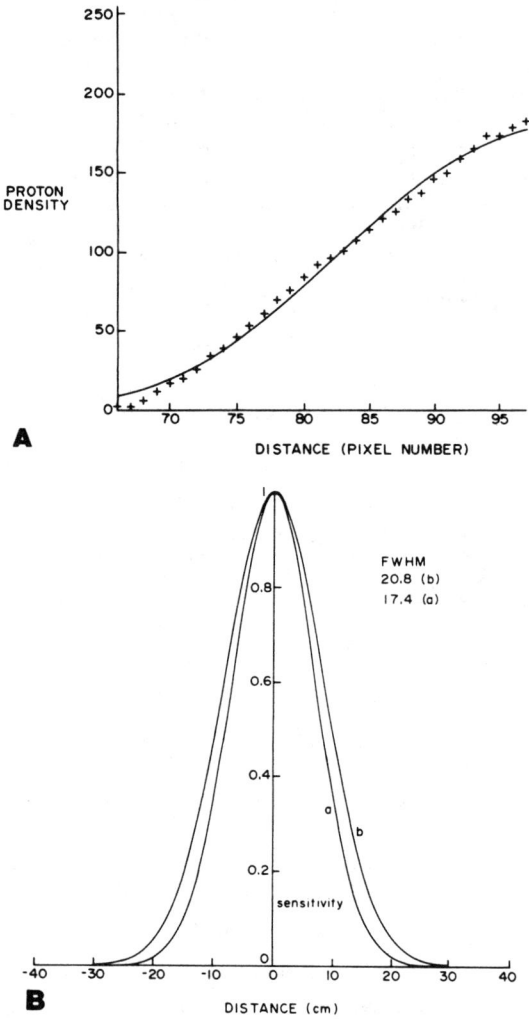

Fig. 7 (A) Plot of signal intensity versus position expressed in pixel numbers for a continuous wedge filled with $CuSO_4$.
(B) First difference of adjacent pixels to estimate true slice sensitivity response. Slice thickness estimated by FWHM response.

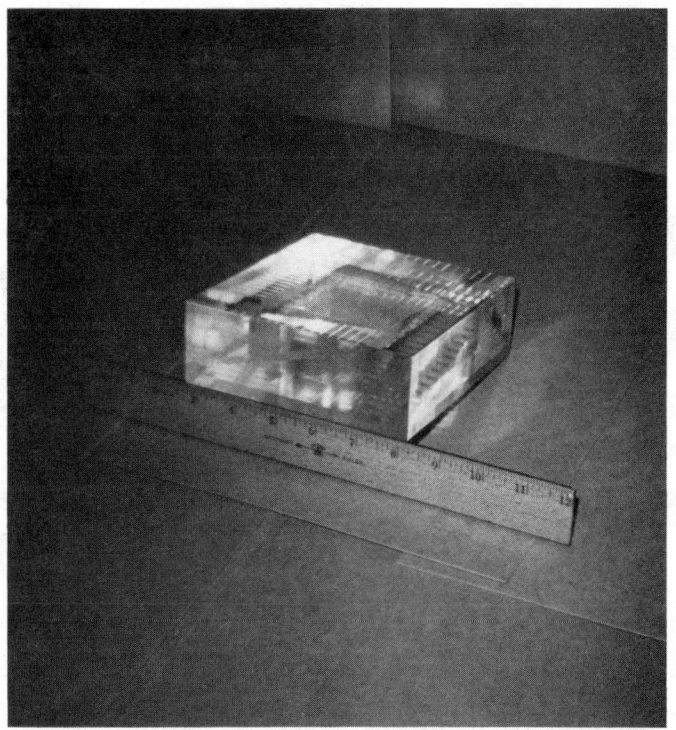

Fig. 8 Photograph of discrete step-wedge phantom. Phantom design includes four orthogonal signal producing wedges with 2 mm step thickness.

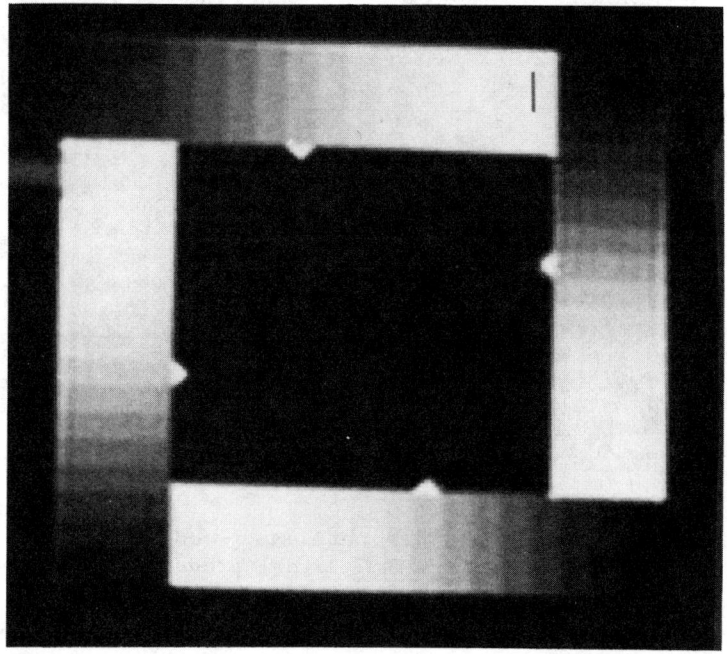

Fig. 9 Scan of discrete step-wedge phantom used for slice thickness determinations. Bright tabs are used to determine orthogonality of slice relative to wedge axis.

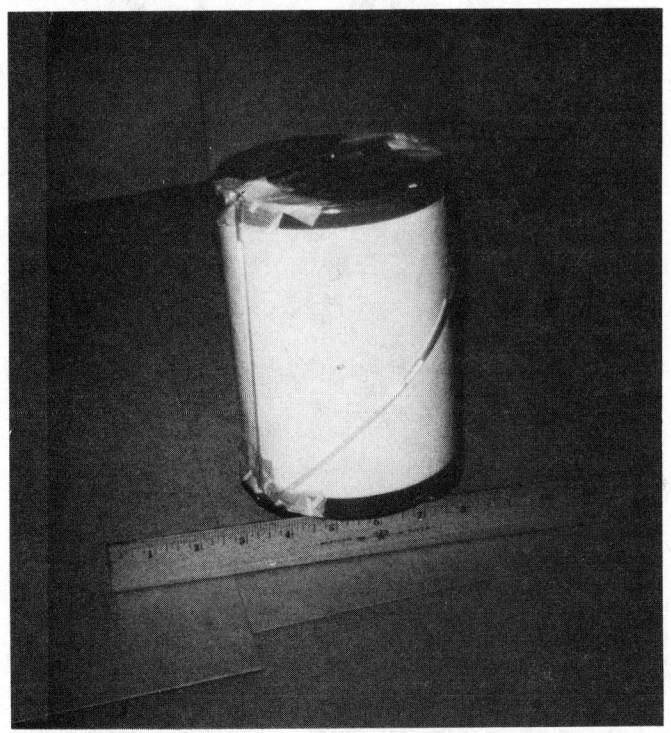

Fig. 10 Photograph of a double helix phantom used for slice position accuracy in a multi-slice sequence. Tubing is 1 mm in diameter and is filled with 1,2 propanediol.

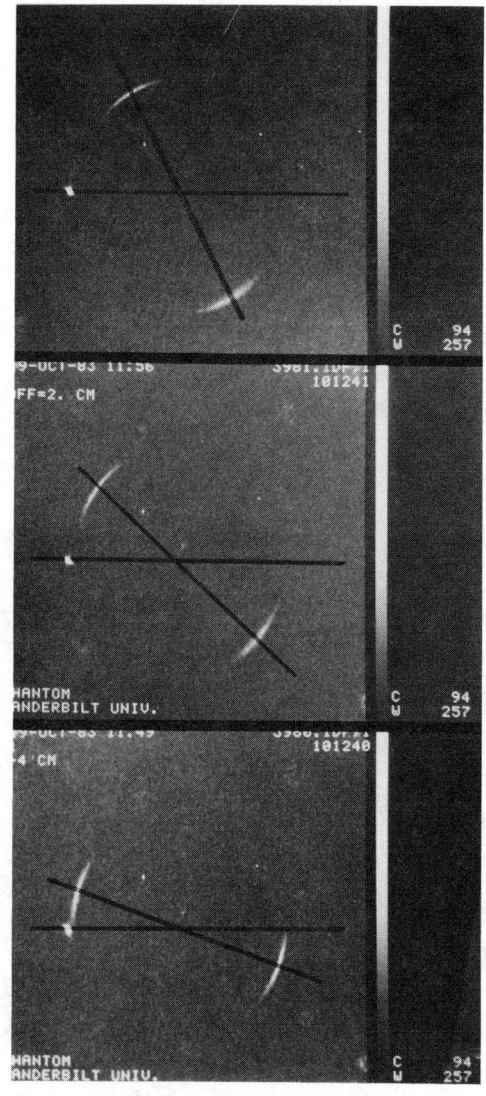

Fig. 11 Scans of double helix phantom. Requested scan separation was 2 cm. (Top) Angle relative to reference line = 60°. (Middle) Angle relative to reference = 40°. (Bottom) Angle relative to reference = 20°. Helix pitch = 1 cm/10°. Slice separation equals angular separation x 1 cm/10°= 2 cm.

SPATIAL LINEARITY

Spatial linearity refers to the ability of the imaging system to accurately reproduce the spatial features of an object without distortion. Since NMR images can be produced as either planar or volumetric, 3-dimensional distortions should be assessed.

Spatial linearity phantoms:
° Orthogonal hole
° Parallel line (grid)
° 3-D parallel grid

The approach to assessing spatial linearity is to image a regular array of objects with known array dimensions and to determine variations or distortions in the imaged distribution from the known distribution. This is usually done by measuring the differential linearity and the overall or integral linearity of the image. Differential linearity is measured in terms of pixels/cm between the centroids of adjacent array elements. Integral linearity is measured in terms of the average pixels/cm over the entire field-of-view in both vertical and horizontal directions. Linearity measurements also produce an assessment of spatial distance calibration.

The orthogonal hole phantom consisting of a rectangular array of "hot" holes drilled in an acrylic block is the most common phantom employed for spatial linearity measurements (Fig. 12). The hole diameters should be larger than the spatial resolution of the system. The separation of the hole is not critical but should be small enough to be able to assess linearity over relatively small areas (1-2 cm separation is common). A variation on this design is a rectangular array of small vials filled with signal producing material (Fig. 13). Images of each of these phantoms are evaluated in much the same way. Rapid evaluations are done visually by assessing the straightness of the image rows and columns and their orthogonality (Fig. 14).

A similar linearity phantom has been constructed by sawing an orthogonal groove pattern in a block of lucite and filling the grooves with signal producing material. In this design the coordinates of intersection points are used to measure differential linearity (Fig. 15).

The ideas of linearity can be extended to 3-dimensions by creating a 3-D array of intersecting tubes. With this geometry volumetric linearity can be evaluated.

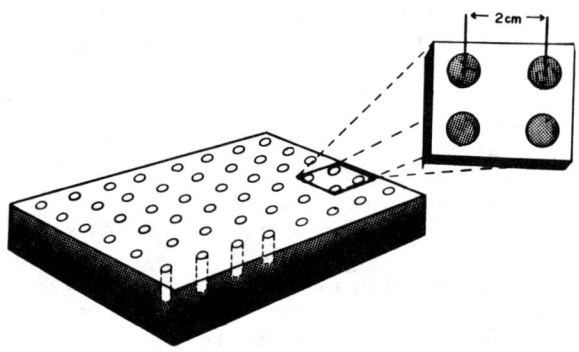

Fig. 12 Orthogonal-hole phantom. Filled with signal producing material, scans are used to assess presence of spatial distortions.

435

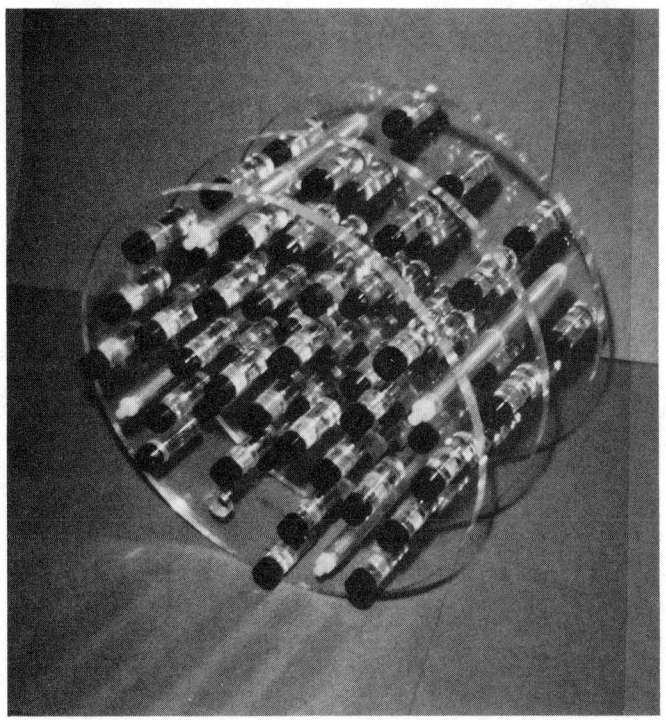

Fig. 13 Photograph of phantom used to assess spatial linearity and spatial distortions. Vials are 1 cm in diameter and separated by 2 cm in one direction and 4 cm in the orthogonal direction. Three parallel planes of vials allow volumetric assessment.

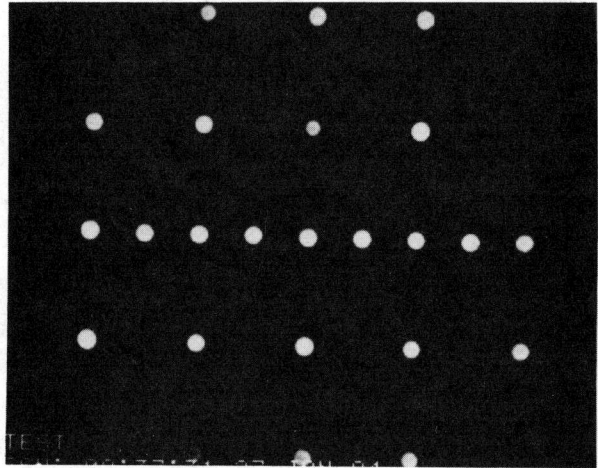

Fig. 14 Scan of phantom shown in Fig. 13. Size calibration in terms of cm/pixel is determined by measuring actual distance between vial centroids and then dividing by pixel distance.

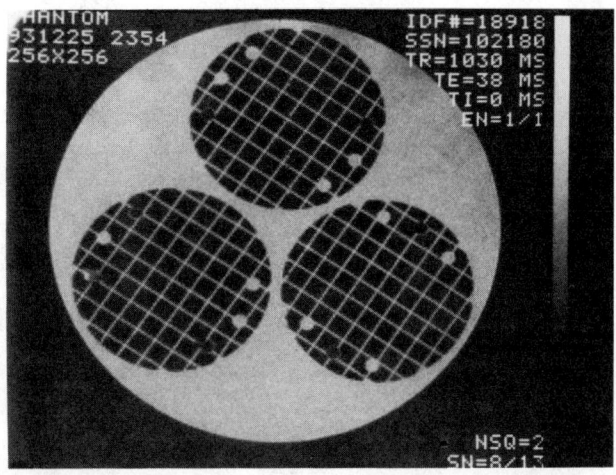

Fig. 15 Orthogonal line phantom constructed from grooves sawed into lucite blocks. Multiple inserts approximately 10 cm in diameter allow linearity to be evaluated on a regional basis.

SPATIAL UNIFORMITY

Spatial uniformity refers to the ability of the imaging instrument to reproduce the same signal response throughout the image volume. Spatial uniformity can also be assessed using the phantoms described previously for spatial linearity. The analysis differs in that the variations in the signal intensity are calculated rather than the variations in spatial location. An alternate and probably more common phantom used for spatial signal uniformity is the homogenous so-called flat-field flood phantom. The phantom simply consists of a large signal producing volume (much thicker than the slice thickness). The volume is scanned and the variations in signal intensity are measured throughout the slice and quoted in terms of the deviation from the mean intensity.

The image shown in Figure 16 is a scan of a 25 cm diameter, 10 cm thick cylinder, filled with a uniform mixture of 1, 2 propanediol. Intensity measurements taken from a vertical and horizontal line across the phantom are plotted in Figure 17. The intensity plots reveal that the center is less sensitive than the peripheral portion and differs on the average of about $\pm$ 5%.

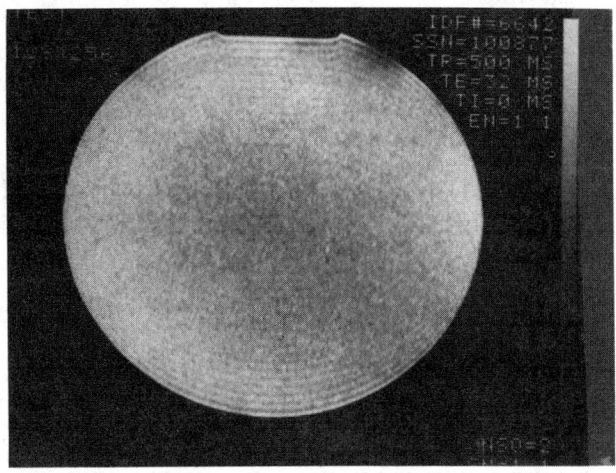

Fig. 16 Scan of a flat-field phantom. Phantom is 25 cm in diameter and 10 cm in thickness, filled with 1,2, propanediol. Display window settings have been narrowed to illustrate the degree of non-uniformity of response.

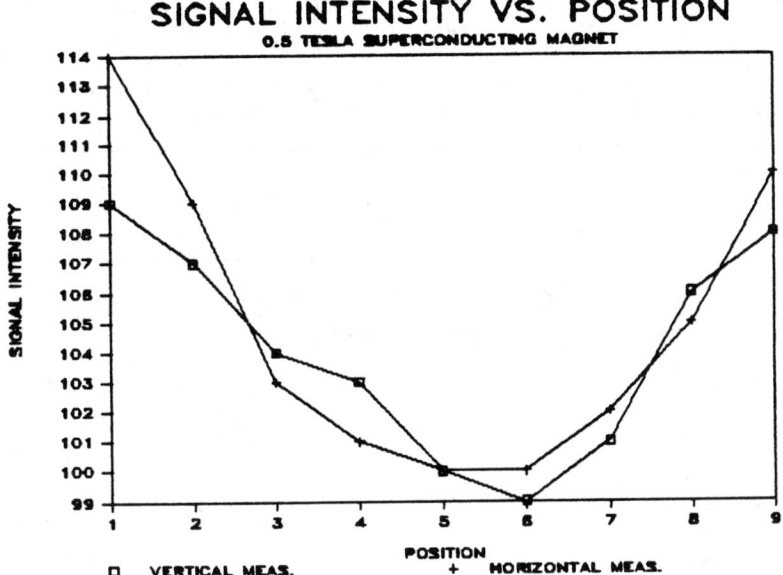

Fig. 17 Vertical and horizontal profiles taken from phantom scan shown in Fig. 16. Profiles demonstrate non-uniformities characterized by a cold center and hot rim. Relative to the mean value the non-uniformity is equal to approximately ± 5%.

SIGNAL-TO-NOISE

Signal-to-noise can be assessed by a number of different phantoms[12]. The signal uniformity phantom described in the previous section is commonly used for this measurement. It is also possible to measure signal-to-noise for a variety of different signal strengths. This is accomplished by using a phantom which contains components with different concentrations of contrast agents.

The signal (S) is usually defined as the difference in the signal mean from a region selected over a signal producing area (Sp) and the signal mean from a background region containing no signal producing material (Sb). The noise is defined to be equal to the standard deviation in the measurements from the background area (S.D.). Thus:

$$S/N = \frac{S_p - S_b}{S.D.}$$

A plot of S/N for two different NMR imaging systems is shown in Figure 18. The phantom used consisted of vials of different concentrations of D_2O/H_2O and therefore should produce a linear response in signal strength. The signal will increase with higher field strengths and larger pixels or slice thicknesses. Noise will generally decrease with larger pixels or greater slice thicknesses and with increased signal averaging.

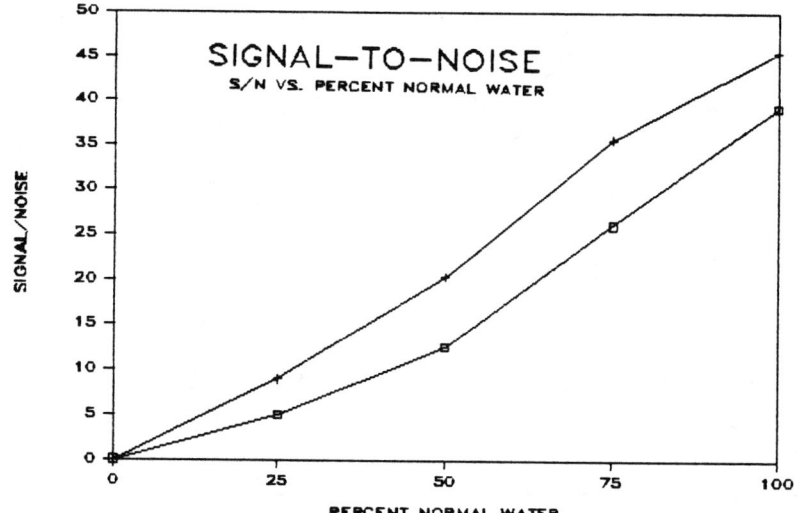

Fig. 18 Plots of signal-to-noise ratios versus concentration of D^2O/H^2O. The two plots correspond to measurements taken from two different NMR imaging systems.

SIGNAL LINEARITY

Signal linearity refers to the ability of the system to respond linearly to linear increases in material proton density (P), T_1 or T_2. Since detected signal strength depends greatly on the timing parameters of the pulse sequence used and the fact that it is presently very difficult to make materials with linear variations in either P, T_1 or T_2 independent of the other two consequently, signal linearity is not easily measureable for all three parameters. As mentioned earlier, this may soon change as combination gel/metal ion phantoms become available. At the present time however, signal linearity is usually measured only for proton density using D_2O/H_2O mixtures which have been doped with paramagnetic ions to produce proton density changes while maintaining constant T_1 and T_2 values.

Figure 19 shows the results of a signal linearity check on two different systems with signal strength plotted against H_2O concentration. The linearity is assessed by a least square fit to a straight line. Since these data are presented as a percent of the maximum H_2O signal, the slope of the line should be unity. Until the problem of contrast standardization is solved, low contrast detectability using different contrast agents may remain difficult to address. The technique of partial volume averaging used in CT may be an approach which also could be adopted for NMR imaging. In this approach a single contrast agent is placed in holes of different depths so that the image slice intersects progressively smaller portions of signal producing material (averaging larger portion of non-signal producing material) to produce a low-contrast image.

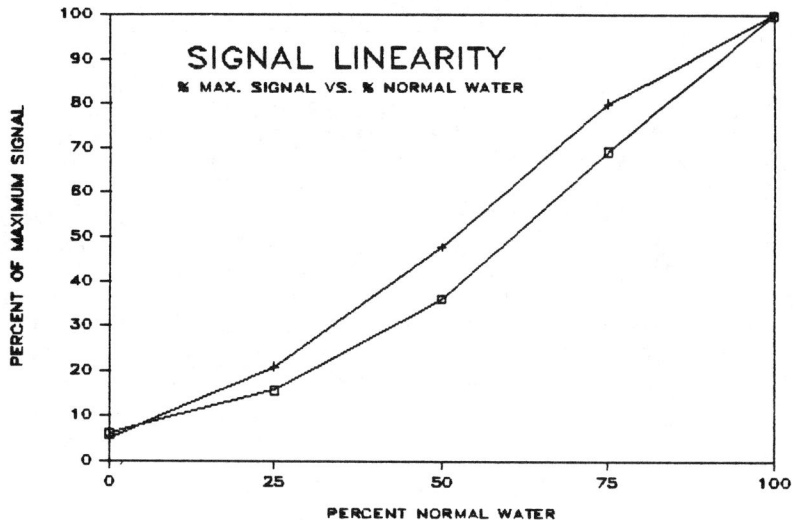

Fig. 19 Assessment of signal linearity using D_2O/H_2O to vary proton density. Plots correspond to measurements made on two different NMR imaging systems. Ideal response would be a straight line with slope equal to unity.

T_1 and T_2 CALIBRATION

Quantitative T_1 and T_2 images or point measurements have been actively pursued goals of most of the manufacturers of NMR imaging equipment. At the present time, however, since there are many different operating field strengths, T_1 and T_2 standards must generally be produced locally with available NMR spectrometer operating at the appropriate field strength.

It is predicted that standard materials which are temperature stable and with T_1 and T_2 values within the clinically important range (T_1 200-1600 m sec, T_2 50-1600 m sec) will soon be available.

GENERAL SYSTEM PARAMETERS

The assessment of general system parameters is frequently very machine dependent and can not be described in a generic manner. It is therefore necessary for each user to work with the manufacturer's representative to establish an appropriate procedure for monitoring those parameters. Among these parameters are the resonance frequency check, 90° and 180° tip angle checks and display intensity and spatial linearity checks. The RF checks are generally best performed using the field-uniformity phantom; however, any strong signal producing phantom would probably be adequate. For resistive systems both the field strength and RF pulse freqency can be changed in an effort to seek the maximum response. In superconducting systems, only the RF is changed.

Tip-angle optimization programs are usually available as part of the manufacturer set-up procedures. These consists of varying the 90° pulse width and intensity until maximum response is obtained. Similarly, the 180° pulse is found by looking for a null signal.

Display monitor linearity checks are performed using computer generated grids and intensity step wedges. Display quality assurance protocols are available from the Center for Medical Devices and Radiation Health.[13]

ROUTINE QUALITY ASSURANCE PROGRAMS

The specification of exactly which Q.A. tests should be performed and their frequency must wait until more experience is gained. Early experience however, seems to indicate that a frequent check (probably daily) of field uniformity and noise may be necessary. Other checks can probably be performed on a less frequent basis (possibly weekly or monthly).

CONCLUSION

In conclusion, it can be said that there already exists numerous NMR phantoms and proposed quality assurance tests which can be incorporated into an adequate quality assurance program. At the present time however, it must be the responsibility of each individual installation to choose which test procedures best suit their need and then to determine the frequency at which they are to be performed. An essential part of any Q.A. program which must not be overlooked is the maintenance of proper records of the test results including a careful review of trends on a regular basis.

It is hoped that a document will soon be available from AAPM which lists those Q.A. protocols for each image parameter which are considered to be adequate tests and which will yield reliable results. This document will hopefully also contain a recommendation as to which parameters are to be monitored and the frequency at which these measurements should be made.

REFERENCES

1. Schneider, N.J., Bryan, R.N., Willcott, M.R.: Nuclear Magnetic Resonance Imaging: Partain, James, Rollo and Price, editors. W.B. Saunders, 436-445 (1983).

2. Redpath, T.W.: Phys. Med. Biol. 27, 1057-1065 (1982).

3. Runge, V.M., Johnson, C.T., Smith, F.W., Erickson, J.J., Price, R.R., Partain, C.L., James, A.E.: Noninvas. Med. Imag. Vol. 1 No 1: 49-60 (1984).

4. Leiski, R.A., Stroughan, K., Orr, J.S.: Phys. Med. Biol. 29, (3) 271-276 (1984).

5. Weinmann, H.J., Brasch R.C., Press W.R., Wesbey G.E.: A.J.R. 142, 619-625 (1984).

6. Morgan, L.O., Nollo, A.W.: J. Chem. Phys. 31, 365-368 (1959).

7. Mitchell, M.D., Axel, L., Kundel, H.L.: Mag. Res. Med. 1, 207 (1984) Abstract.

8. Mathur-DeVre, R., Gruner, R., Parmentier, F., Binet, J.: Mag. Res. Med. 2,, 176-179 (1985).

9. Madsen, E.L., Fullerton, G.D.: Mag. Res. Imag. 1, 135-141 (1982).

10. AAPM 1, Phantoms for Performance evaluation and quality assurance of CT Scanners (1977).

11. Rossman, K.: Image Quality, Proc. AAPM Summer School, San Antonio, Texas. D.J. Wright, editor. (LHEW Publication [FDA], Rockville, MD.) 220-281 (1971).

12. Ortendahl D.A., Hylton N.M., Kaufman L., Crooks L.E.: Mag. Res. in Med. 1. 316-338 (1984).

13. Goldstein, A.: "Hardcopy Care", section 4,5 Quality Assurance in Diagnostic Ultrasound. HHS Publication. FDA 81-8139, 11-15 (1980).

14. Mitchell M.D., Axal L., Kundel H.L.: Mag. Res. Med. 1, 206 (1984) Abstract.

Systems Specifications and Acceptance Testing[*]

Charles W. Coffey, II
University of Kentucky Medical Center, Lexington, KY   40536

Ronald T. Droege
Mt. Sinai Medical Center, Cleveland, OH   44106

Kenneth E. Ekstrand
Bowman Gray School of Medicine, Winston-Salem, NC   27103

ABSTRACT

This presentation is intended to assist in the selection of an NMR imaging system and the formulation of an appropriate purchase contract. System components listed in the appendix are identified to provide a basis by which NMR systems may be compared. Quantitative comparisons are preferred, and require that performance specifications be obtained from the vendor. Such specifications should be used for purchase deliberations and should be incorporated into the final purchase agreement. Since there are no AAPM-approved NMR performance testing protocols, this presentation can only suggest image parameters and associated variables to be evaluated and test methods to be followed. To avoid any misunderstandings, prior to purchase, the consumer and vendor should identify and agree on the test phantom(s) and evaluation method(s) to be employed. A thorough, well-defined purchase agreement is a guarantee that the selected vendor will deliver and install the system he has described.

INTRODUCTION

In response to the introduction of Nuclear Magnetic Resonance (NMR) Imaging to clinical radiology in the United States, the AAPM Board of Directors, following the recommendation of the Science Council, voted to form the NMR committee. The general goals of this committee include: education, patient safety, site planning, system specifications, the development of imaging techniques and patient protocols, and the standardization of test phantoms and procedures for NMR image analysis. A number of individual task groups were created to accomplish these goals. Task Group #6 was formed to assist in the planning and writing of purchase specification documents and to recommend protocols for the acceptance testing of purchased NMR imaging equipment.

The task group membership was constituted in December, 1982. Task group members were chosen because of interest and experience with NMR installations at their respective institutions. Task group members, NMR manufacturers, and physicists with NMR experience were asked to assist in the preparation of a document

[*]Partial Report of Task Group #6 of the AAPM Nuclear Magnetic Resonance Committee

which would address the issues of specifications and acceptance testing. A consensus document was adopted by the task group and circulated to the total NMR Committee of the AAPM. Following adoption by the NMR Committee, the document was given to members of the AAPM Science Council for review. The completed, approved document was printed in the January/April Newsletter of the AAPM (1). The document represents input from scientists, consumers, and manufacturers; it is intended to assist in the selection of an NMR imaging system and the formulation of an appropriate purchase contract. This presentation is an elaboration upon the content and rationale of the task group report.

THE DOCUMENT

The document in its entirety is included as an appendix to this presentation. It consists of thirteen major categories which are listed in Table I. We will take a focused look at Sections I and XIII, Magnet Specifications and Administrative Considerations, as examples of the document's specific contents.

Table I. NMR System Components

Category	System
I	Magnet Specification
II	Imaging Gradients Systems
III	RF Transmitter/Receiver
IV	Computer Specifications
V	Console Specifications
VI	Multiformat Camera
VII	Patient Couch Specifications
VIII	Image Acquisition
IX	Image Processing Specifications
X	Image Quality Performance
XI	Spectroscopy
XII	Safety
XIII	Administrative Considerations

Magnet Specifications

The chief component of an NMR Imaging unit is, of course, the magnet. The physical size, type of construction, and strength of the magnetic field depends critically on the anticipated uses of the machine (2). We suggest one should consider the fourteen parameters suggested in Table II.

Table II. Magnet System Components

Design
Physical Dimensions
Weight and Maximum Floor Loading
Field Strength: Range and Typical Operation
Fringe Field Maps
Field Direction Relative to Patient Axis
Shim Coils
Uniformity
Stability
Power Consumption
Electrical Requirements
Power Dissipation/Cooling System
Shut-down Capability
Magnet Protection System

Following decisions on anticipated uses of the unit (3), e.g. proton imaging, multi-nuclei imaging, and/or spectroscopy, the consumer must determine a magnetic field strength range and typical-operation field strengths. Next, the design of the anticipated unit will have to be investigated. Will the unit be a permanent, resistive, superconducting, or hybrid magnet system? Along with the decisions on design and aperature size are the constraints of physical size and weight requirements. Size, weight, and floor loading must be carefully considered in siting discussions and planning (4). Concomitant with high strength magnets produced by electromagnet systems are other site planning issues: fringe fields, significant electrical and power dissipation requirements, and cooling systems. However, after site installation, the major concerns are that the magnet, with shim coils operational, produce a uniform and stable magnetic field. A final important concern is one of safety after installation. Does the unit have emergency shutdown capability for the safety of patients and staff? In the event of an emergency, will the expensive magnet system be protected? These safety issues must be addressed during the planning stages of installation.

Administrative Considerations

NMR imagers must become cost-effective for institutional administrators, or their future in clinical radiology will be short-lived. We suggest that in addition to medical and scientific deliberations, administrative consultation must be sought before an NMR purchase agreement is written. Pertinent administrative considerations are listed in Table III. Of course, the major concern to administrators will be the cost of the installed system including site preparation and site surveys (5). Associated with costs may be the issue of Certificate of Need (CON) approval by the appropriate health systems regulation agency (6,7). Further, for some facilities, delivery time and installation time become important factors.

Table III. Administrative Considerations

Cost of Installed System
Estimated Cost of Site Preparation and Site Surveys
Dates of Delivery and Completed Installation
"Normal" Patient Throughput
Estimated Operating Cost
Service Contract and/or Warranty Agreement
Upgrade Options
Downtime
QA Phantoms and Protocols
Listing of Operational Clinical Sites
Pre-Market Approval (PMA) Status

After installation the most common concern will probably be that of patient throughput. Patient throughput and operating costs will determine the amortization schedule (8,9) and consequently, the cost of the procedure to the individual patient.

A further administrative concern is the loss of patient-generated revenues by down-time interruptions. Thus, service contracts, warranty agreements, engineering support, and staff training are essential elements of any contract to insure the maximum machine uptime. Another concern is the availability of system upgrade options. Administrators would probably be hesitant to purchase an expensive system having no alternatives for upgrade with the exception to buy the "newer-improved" model. A present concern is the Pre-Market Approval (PMA) status of the manufacturer with the Federal Food and Drug Administration (FDA) (11). Finally, there are medical-legal issues (11,12) that must be addressed by in-house investigational review boards including: patient safety and comfort during normal operation and during an emergency, and the exclusion of patients who are at risk from high magnetic field strengths.

Quantitative Specifications

The document in its present form does not provide quantitative recommendations for any system specifications. This was not an oversight. The task group did not desire to recommend quantitative specifications which might be outdated very quickly.

HOW TO USE THE DOCUMENT

Formation of Imager Selection Committee

Each institution considering purchase of an NMR imager should form an "in-house" selection committee consisting of, but not limited to, the following: basic NMR scientists, clinical physicians, medical physicists, physical plant engineers, and administrators. Important to any decision making is the consensus of the committee members concerning the needs, goals, and important concerns for the particular institutional site. Basic questions of siting and safety must be addressed. Other questions will have to be answered. Will the unit be used clinically and/or for research? Will the unit be capable of imaging and spectroscopy? Members of the selection committee must reach some agreement on what capabilities the NMR imager unit will be expected to demonstrate.

NMR Components List

We suggest that a representative of the institution's selection committee (i.e. the clinical physicist) prepare a list of the needs and wants expressed by the various committee members. This list may be very similar to the task group report (1). In addition to the Task Group #6 document, meetings with manufacturer representatives, equipment shows and exhibits, manufacturer brochures, and visits to other operational clinical sites can help establish a list of wants/needs.

Specifications Chart

After preparation of a list that most completely meets the anticipated needs, one should further prepare a chart including system components with the addition of quantitative specifications and proposed methods of testing. An example of a specifications chart is presented in Table IV. The testing may involve specific test procedures, visual inspection, and/or passive testing. Passive testing may be defined as the acceptance of a subsystem by inference from the acceptable test results of the major component. An example of passive testing would be that the shim coils are assumed to be correctly operational if the magnetic field uniformity was demonstrated to have met specification values. Where applicable, the designation of factory tested and/or site tested should be indicated.

Table IV. Specifications Chart: Numbers and Evaluation Methods

System Specifications	Factory Tested Y/N	Site Tested Y/N	Method of Evaluation (describe) A. Specific Test Procedures B. Visual Inspection C. Passive (Inference)	Instrumentation and/or Phantom(s) (describe)

The next phase of the purchase agreement is communication with the manufacturers. Meetings should be arranged with all institutional members and manufacturer representatives present. Manufacturer plant visits and visits to operational clinical sites can be scheduled. Each manufacturer asked should respond to the information requested in the chart of specifications and testing methods. Vendors should provide specifications and describe testing procedures for each component identified. The vendor should also distinguish between prototypes and production model capabilities.

Imager Selection

After collection of all the data from the vendors, the "in-house" committee should meet again for the final consideration. Since no one imager is likely to satisfy all the specifications as initially discussed, compromises will invariably be required. The "in-house" committee must make the final decision on the vendor and the unit which is most suitable to the overall goals of the institution.

Writing the Purchase Contract

Once the vendor selection has been made, representatives from the "in-house" committee and the manufacturer should meet and reach agreement upon each individual system component including quantitative specifications, evaluation methods, and test equipment. The agreements reached in these discussions should be incorporated into the purchase contract. For example, factory testing versus on site demonstration and testing should be indicated. In addition, details as to site preparation, installation, and specification testing should be included. Specifications testing should be completed before the imager is released to the purchasing institution.

Clauses concerning non-compliance and resultant penalties must be included. Administrative concerns involving installation scheduling, payment, training, and warranty must, of course, be written into the purchase contract agreement. Remember, this purchase agreement is the single guarantee that the manufacturer will install the unit that he and your institution agreed upon.

SPECIFICATIONS TESTING OF MAJOR SYSTEM COMPONENTS

Pre-Testing Considerations

Prior to imager installation, representatives of the institution may arrange for a factory site visit to observe the various stages of imager assembly. Also, the representatives may observe a number of factory tests including results and methods of testing performed on similiar units. These observable results can serve only as representative values and are not necessarily indicative of the imager assembled for your institution. However, a detailed factory test check list of your purchased unit should be made available upon customer request. We further suggest that an individual be assigned to monitor carefully the on-site installation proceedings. This has a two-fold purpose: first, to observe the installation techniques and on site pre-specifications testing; secondly, to provide an interface for any questions that may arise between installers and on-site personnel. A smooth interface between installers and on-site engineers and physical plant personnel can only make the installation shorter and more correct.

Testing Considerations

The following discussion includes suggested testing of specific components of an NMR imager unit. The suggestions are personal preferences and do not reflect testing procedures approved by the AAPM. (To date, there are no AAPM approved specifications testing procedures).

Magnet System.

Particular to the magnet system is the specification of uniformity over the imaging volume after installation and with shim coils operational (13,14). The manufacturer representative should demonstrate the procedures for and the experimental data obtained from the mapping of the magnetic field with the manufacturer-provided magnetometer. Important parameters include the ppm and the size and shape of the resulting test volume. (The demonstrated procedure should be that agreed upon in the agreement purchase contract). Both short-term and long-term magnetic stability can be demonstrated by the use of a magnetometer, or by monitoring change in resonance frequency. Fringe field maps can be verified after installation by the use of a moderately priced gauss meter. Other magnet system components, the cooling system, shutdown capability, and protection system can be evaluated by the visual demonstration and passive inspection of normal and emergency operating conditions.

Gradients and RF Transmitter/Receiver Systems.

The subcomponents of both the imaging gradients system (15,16) and the RF transmitter/receiver (17) can be demonstrated via electronics testing techniques using a high frequency oscilloscope and other commonly available electronics test meters (18). In addition, the gradient field strength and linearity may be passively demonstrated by the formal evaluation of the slice sensitivity profile parameters. Of important concern to patient comfort is the audio noise produced by the gradient system during the scan procedure. An acoustic powermeter free of magnetic field interference should be available for on-site testing. The audio levels will be dependent on the pulse sequence and data acquisition scheme (single slice, multi-slice, and/or volume imaging). In this test one should be careful to select the machine data aquisition parameters that yield a maximum dB level. Other components of the RF system can be visually demonstrated/tested, i.e. coil dimensions can be measured and the time required for coil tuning and coil changing can be observed.

Computer System.

Most computer system components can be visually and/or passively evaluated. Individual computer components including the printer can be demonstrated and the computer manufacturer's specifications reviewed. Overall system performance (image quality and scan time) infer the correctness and efficiency of each working subcomponent. The interface capability of the computer hardware and software with other imaging and recording systems should be demonstrated and the format documentation released to the purchaser. Further, software capabilities and functions should be individually demonstrated and verified, i.e., Region of Interest (ROI) statistics, distance measurement, line plot function and etc.

Console and Multiformat Camera Specifications.

The console component specifications can be evaluated by simple demonstration, visual inspection, and/or passive testing. Of primary importance is the number of grey levels displayed, the image monitor resolution, and the reconstruction matrix size versus the display matrix size. The multiformat camera can be visually inspected for film sizes, formats, film loading type, and computer control. The image quality of the multiformat camera can be actively evaluated by the SMPTE video test pattern (19).

Patient Couch Specifications.

Patient couch positioning performance can be visually demonstrated and measured for accuracy and range of motion. The accuracy of positioning indicators and patient localizers with respect to the center of the imaging volume should be carefully established. Availability and demonstration of a two-way patient communication system and a patient-activated alarm should be recorded. Finally, emergency procedures for patient removal should be demonstrated.

SPECIFICATIONS TESTING OF IMAGE QUALITY

Image Quality Parameters

The true test of image acquisition and image processing is the image quality. In Table V is listed those image quality parameters of importance in any tomographic imaging modality. At the time of this report image quality parameters specific to NMR have not been comprehensively identified and defined. Furthermore, there is little agreement in methods to measure such parameters. Therefore, the parameters listed in Table V are offered as a guide for NMR applications.

Table V. Image Quality Parameters

Spatial Resolution
Signal-To-Noise
Image Uniformity
Spatial Linearity
Signal Linearity
Slice Sensitivity Profile (Slice Thickness)
Slice Position Accuracy
Slice Angulation Accuracy

To date, it is left to the purchaser and manufacturer to agree on definitions and measurement methods. (Image quality definition and phantoms for test measurements are the task of TG#1 of the NMR Committee. Task Group #1 (20) has presented a report earlier in this Conference).

Image Quality Factors

As a result of the many factors (21,22) involved in NMR image acquisition and processing, each image parameter must be investigated under a variety of conditions. The specific factors to be investigated are included in Table VI.

Table VI. Image Quality Factors

Pulse Sequence
RF Coil
Image Plane
Location Along the Coil Axis
Radial Dependence Within the Field of View
Orientation Within the Field of View
Number of Acquisitions
Dynamic Range
Type of Image Acquisition

Pulse Sequence.

There are potentially a number of clinical images obtained by varying the pulse sequence and pulse parameters. Image parameters should be minimally evaluated for the major pulse sequences - Spin Echo and Inversion Recovery. Probably, for minor changes within the major pulse sequences (small changes in TR and TE), few image quality parameters will have to be re-evaluated.

RF Coil.

Individual image parameters must be investigated for the available RF imaging coils. For some units this may be a head coil and body coil; for others this may include breast coils and surface coils. Further, it may be important to investigate a number of the image parameters as a function of RF coil loading (17,23).

Image Plane.

Since NMR is a three-dimensional imaging modality, it is important to evaluate the image parameters in each of the three major planes - transverse, sagittal, and coronal. A potential problem existing between image planes is the change in the magnitude and linearity of the gradients along the X,Y, and Z axes. A poor slice sensitivity profile test result may be indicative of misaligned or miscalibrated gradients.

Location Along the Coil Axis.

Due to spatial variations in RF power, magnetic field uniformity, and gradient linearity, image quality should be investigated as a function of distance from the central axis of the coil. One should also investigate the dependence of various image parameters on the alignment or misalignment of the RF coil with the center of the magnet.

Radial Dependence Within the Field of View (FOV).

Likewise, image quality may vary between locations within the field of view. It has been suggested that image parameter analysis should be evaluated for five locations: central axis, and the four points of the compass at approximately 80% of the maximum or specified field of view (24).

Orientation.

Image resolution may differ in the X and Y directions of a 2DFT image. This is especially evident if the number of samples per view differs from the number of independent acquisitions. Thus, the orientation or alignment of the test phantom object with respect to the raster lines of the video display can have a significant effect even if the video display system has raster-blend or raster-erase features (19).

Number of Acquisitions.

Increasing the number of acquisitions will generally improve resolution but signal-to-noise will generally decrease and the scan time will increase. Duplication of acquisition (i.e. signal averaging) will increase signal-to-noise.

Dynamic Range.

Much investigation (25) has been done on the dependence of NMR relaxation times with tissue type and NMR frequency. Since the dynamic ranges for Spin Density (N), T1, and T2 will be large for the tissues imaged, it may be important to evaluate the image parameters over the full range of these parameters. It has been suggested (24) that the image parameter test materials be evaluated over the following ranges: T1 (150-1600 msec), T2 (25-1600 msec), and N (50-100% water).

Type of Image Acquisition.

Image resolution, signal-to-noise, and slice sensitivity profile parameters should be investigated as a function of the type of image acquisition (single slice, multi-slice, and/or volume imaging).

Which Factors to Investigate?

For the eight image quality parameters listed and the nine factors quoted, the resulting combinations and permutations are astronomical! It is not practical to test all parameters under all conditions. However, one must perform a sufficient number of evaluations to be confident about the overall machine performance.

Parameter Calculations: N, T1, T2, and Flow

Another important consideration in specifications testing is the accuracy of N, T1, T2, and flow measurements (26,27,28). It is important to evaluate the measurable range, the accuracy of the measurements, and the measurement reproducibility for each. The reproducibility should be investigated for scan to scan variation and for day to day variation. Accuracy measurements for N, T1, and T2 depend on the availability of stable, inert standards. Presently the AAPM NMR committee is addressing this issue (29).

Demonstration of Artifacts

In addition to specifications testing, artifacts should be investigated. Artifacts may be caused by ferromagnetic materials within the scanning volume (30), motion (31), partial volume effects, and chemical shift misregistration (32). Artifact demonstration enables "abnormal scans" to be more readily categorized as normal, abnormal, or artifact.

Decisions Concerning Measured Specification Values

The "in-house" committee should review all acceptance testing results and decide upon the acceptance or rejection of the imager. The decision should be made promptly and delivered in writing to the manufacturer since most contracts provide a time limit beyond which the imager is deemed to be accepted by default.

GENERAL SUGGESTIONS FOR SPECIFICATIONS TESTING

Test Method Selection

Presently there are no AAPM endorsed methods for specifications testing of any image quality parameters. The NMR committee of the AAPM hopes to identify phantoms and test methods for NMR image parameter analysis. Until that time, we can only suggest that each NMR parameter test method be chosen from analogous methods shown to be effective for tomographic imagers.

Summary of the Process

After selection of the test phantom and evaluation method for each image parameter, we presently suggest the following three step specifications testing process:

1. In agreement with the manufacturer, write into the purchase contract the test phantom(s) and evaluation method(s) to be followed to test the specifications numbers.
2. With the "agreed-upon" phantom(s) and testing method(s), evaluate an existing state-of-the-art clinical imager at a manufacturer-designated site.
3. Write into the purchase contract that your purchased, installed, and clinically operational unit shall meet or exceed the specifications so tested (#1) on the unit evaluated and located off-site (#2).

Following this three-part process should eliminate any confusion as to phantom design(s), test method(s), and/or interpretation of results.

CONCLUSION

Specifications testing is the guaranteed insurance for the consumer against the manufacturer. Specifications not met or out of "agreed-upon" tolerances can lead to penalties or even removal and exclusion of the machine and vendor from the institution. A manufacturer which produces a specific imager that does not meet specifications must remain liable for that non-compliance, not the purchasing institution.

The task group report in its present form is limited to a listing of the components of an NMR imager. This presentation has only made suggestions concerning procedures, purchase contract agreements, and specifications test methods. Individual task groups of the NMR Committee of the AAPM are actively working toward approval of a set of test phantoms and evaluation methods for acceptance testing that are both efficient and theoretically accurate. Hopefully, these phantoms and evaluation methods will become the industry's standards.

REFERENCES

1. Droege, R.T., Ekstrand, K.E. and Coffey, C.W.: Systems Components for Consideration in Purchasing an NMR Imager. In: AAPM Newsletter and Bulletin. American Association of Physicist in Medicine. January/April p. 4-8 (1985).

2. Gordoen, R.E. and Timms, W.E.: Comput. Radiol. **8**, 245 (1984).

3. Bradley, W.G.: J. Comput. Assist. Tomogr. **9**, 220 (1985).

4. Carson, P.L.: Site Planning Considerations for NMR Installations. In: NMR in Medicine: The Instrumentation and Clinical Applications. Proceedings of AAPM Summer School, Portland, Oregon, August 1985.

5. Bradley, W.G., Opel, W., and Kassabian, J.P.: Radiol. **151**, 719 (1984).

6. Lille, K.J.: RNM Images - Technology Management J., June, 22 (1983).

7. AHA Hospital Technology Series Guideline Report: Nuclear Magnetic Resonance. American Hospital Association. Chicago, Illinois. 66 p. (1983).

8. Frankel, A.N.: Applied Radiol. **13(4)**, 55 (1984).

9. Stephens, W.H., James, A.E., Winfred, A.C. and Pendergrass, H.P.: Financial Implication of NMR Imaging. In: Nuclear Magnetic Resonance Imaging. Philadelphia, W.B. Saunders Co., (1983).

10. Freedman, G.S., Stephens, W.H., and Fisher, B.: Applied Radiol. **13(3)**, 55 (1984).

11. Gray, J.E., Phillips, R.A., Schenck, J., and Wagner, L.K.: Task Group #4 Report: A Tour Through the FDA, NCDRH, IDE, PMA, and IRB Maze vis-a-vis Nuclear Magnetic Resonance Equipment. AAPM Newsletter and Bulletin. American Association of Physicists in Medicine. April/May (1984).

12. James, A.E., Partain, C.L., Rollo, F.D., Bundy, A.L. et al.: Nuclear Magnetic Resonance: Certain Legal and Proprietary Questions. In: Nuclear Magnetic Resonance and Correlative Image Modalities. New York, Society of Nuclear Medicine Publishers, (1983).

13. Roos, C.E., Coffey, H.T., and Efferson, K.R.: Superconducting Magnets. In: Nuclear Magnetic Resonance Imaging. Philadelphia, W.B. Saunders Co., (1983).

14. Pykett, I.L.: Seminars Nuc. Med. **13**, 319 (1983).

15. Kaufman, L. and Crooks, L.E.: Hardware for NMR Imaging. In: Nuclear Magnetic Resonance Imaging Medicine. New York, Igaku-Shoin, Medical Publishers, (1982).

16. Thomas, S.R. and Ackerman, J.L.: The Instrumentation of Nuclear Magnetic Resonance Imaging. In: Proceedings 5th Annual Conference IEEE Engineering in Medicine and Biology Society. Columbus, Ohio, September (1983).

17. Mansfield, P. and Morris, P.G.: Some Hardware Considerations. In: NMR Imaging in Biomedicine, Supplement 2, Advances in Magnetic Resonance. New York, Academic Press, (1982).

18. Holland, G.N.: Systems Engineering of a Whole-body Proton Magnetic Resonance Imaging System. In: Nuclear Magnetic Resonance Imaging. Philadelphia, W.B. Saunders Co., (1983).

19. Gray, J.E., Lisk, K.G., Haddick, D.H., Harshbarger, J.H., et al.: Radiol. 154, 519 (1985).

20. Price R.R.: Concepts of Quality Assurance and Phantom Design for NMR Systems. In: NMR in Medicine: The Instrumentation and Clinical Applications. Proceeding of AAPM Summer School, Portland, Oregon, August (1985).

21. Pykett, I.L., Newhouse, J.H., Buonanno, F.S., Brady, T.J., et al.: Radiol. 143, 157 (1982).

22. Young, I.R., Bailes, D.R., Burl, M., Collins, A.G., et al.: J. Comput. Assist. Tomogr. 6, 1 (1982).

23. Edelstein, W.A., Bottomley, P.A., and Pfeifer, L.M.: Med. Phys. 11, 180 (1984).

24. Morgan, T.J.: Private Communication.

25. Bottomly, P.A., Foster, T.H., Argersinger, R.E., and Pfeifer, L.M.: Med. Phys. 11, 425 (1984).

26. Feinberg, D.A., Crooks, L., Hoenninger, J., et al: Radiol. 153, 177 (1984).

27. George, C.R., Jacobs, G., MacIntyre, W.J., et al: Radiol. 151, 421 (1984).

28. Moran, P.R., Moran, R.A., and Karstaedt, N.: Radiol. 154, 433 (1985).

29. Thomas, S.R.: Private Communication.

30. New, P.F.J., Rosen, B.R., Buonanno, F.S.: Radiol. 147, 139 (1983).

31. Schultz, C.L., Alfidi, R.J., Nelson, A.D., et al: Radiol. 152, 117 (1984).

32. Soila, K.P., Viamonte, M., and Starewicz, P.M.: Radiol. 153, 819, (1984).

APPENDIX

SYSTEMS COMPONENTS FOR CONSIDERATION IN PURCHASING AN NMR IMAGER

COMPILED BY

TASK GROUP #6: NMR SYSTEMS SPECIFICATIONS AND ACCEPTANCE TESTING PROTOCOLS

Ronald T. Droege
Kenneth E. Ekstrand
Charles W. Coffey, II, Chairman

The TASK GROUP is part of the AAPM Nuclear Magnetic Resonance Committee. Stephen R. Thomas, Chairman

INTRODUCTION

This document is intended to assist in the selection of an NMR imaging system and the formulation of an appropriate purchase contract. System components are identified to provide a basis by which NMR systems may be compared. Quantitative comparisons are preferred, and require that performance specifications be obtained from the vendor. Such specifications should be used for purchase deliberations and should be incorporated into the final purchase agreement.

A three part evaluation is suggested before purchasing an NMR imaging system:

1. Identify All Important Performance Characteristics - Reveiw this document and select those items judged to be relevant to the intended use of the equipment. The vendor should be requested to provide quantitative descriptions of these items (when possible) so that individual imagers may be objectively compared. In these responses, the vendor should distinguish between prototype and production model capabilities.

2. Review Vendor Response - A systematic review of component specifications should give special weight to those items uniquely important to the buyer's particular needs (e.g. a difficult site environment may require careful consideration of field uniformity and site preparation expenses). If appropriate, the buyer may request a vendor to update his information if it is insufficient or non-competitive.

3. Write A Purchase Contract - Finally, the collected specifications should be incorporated into the purchase agreement contract so that the selected vendor is obligated to deliver the system he has described. The specifications identified in the contract form the basis by which the installed system can be tested for acceptance. The contract should identify those components to be factory and/or site tested by the vendor. Where relevant, the contract should also identify the test equipment and testing procedures so the buyer can perform acceptance tests in a manner agreed upon by the vendor.

The performance required of any NMR imaging system will depend on the intended use of the buyer. It is inappropriate for this task group to speculate on the potential applications of NMR systems, so it is left to the individual buyers to select from the enclosed list those items deemed to be relevant to the intended applications.

NMR SYSTEM COMPONENTS

I. <u>Magnet Specification</u>

   A. Design

      1. Type

         a. Resistive
         b. Superconducting
         c. Permanent
         d. Hybrid systems

      2. Manufacturer

   B. Dimensions (m)

      1. Individual components
      2. Totally assembled
      3. Bore size and shape

   C. Weight and Maximum Floor Loading (kg, kg/m^2)

      1. Individual components
      2. Totally assembled

   D. Field Strength: Range and Typical Operation (T)

   E. Fringe Field Maps (down to 0.1 mT)

      1. Without magnetic shielding
      2. With magnetic shielding, specific to site

   F. Field Direction Relative to Patient Axis: parallel/transverse

   G. Shim Coils (yes/no)

      1. Routine mechanical re-alignment necessary (yes/no)
      2. Frequency (times per year)

   H. Uniformity (ppm) Over The Imaging Volume After Installation With Shim Coils Operational

      1. Shape of test volume
      2. Volume (cm^3)
      3. Protocol for measuring uniformity (describe)

I. Stability

   1. Long term: ppm per hour
   2. Short term: ppm per min

J. Power Consumption (kW)

K. Electrical Requirements (V, kVA)

L. Power Dissipation/Cooling System (BTU/hr)

   1. Heat exchanger

      a. dimensions (m)
      b. electrical requirements (V, kVA)
      c. coolant system: closed loop, open loop or both (describe)
      d. coolant flow (l/min)
      e. coolant water storage requirements (l)
      f. temperature and flow monitoring (yes/no)

   2. Dewars, vacuum pump, replenishment system

      a. dimensions (m)
      b. cryogen(s) reservoir size (l)
      c. cryogen(s) consumption (l/week)
      d. cyrogen(s) recovery system (yes/no)
      e. rapid exhaust of cryogen vapors if quench occurs (specify)
      f. precautions if uncontrolled quench raises room "air" pressure (yes/no)
      g. cryogen(s) consumption during controlled quench (l)
      h. cryogen(s) level monitoring (describe)

   3. Room environment

      a. temperature requirements
      b. humidity requirements
      c. monitoring (describe)

M. Shutdown Capability

   1. Emergency shutdown controls readily accessible at magnet and console (yes/no)

   2. Time (min) required to complete emergency, controlled, or normal shutdown

   3. Time (hrs) required to resume imaging after emergency, controlled, or normal shutdown

N. Magnet Protection System (yes/no, describe)

II. **Imaging Gradients Systems**

   A. Gradient Field Strength for X,Y, and Z axes (mT/m)

      1. Maximum achievable
      2. Typical operation

   B. Coil Configuration (describe)

   C. Rise Time (msec from 10% to 90%)

   D. Linearity (over the imaging volume)

   E. Stability (%)

   F. Audio Noise Levels (dB) (describe measurement method)

   G. Electrical Requirements (V, kVA)

   H. Heat Exchanger

      1. Power dissipation (BTU/hr)
      2. Dimensions (m)

   I. Gradient Power Supply Protection System (yes/no, describe)

III. **RF Transmitter/Receiver**

   A. Maximum Power to Transmitter Coil (W)

   B. Average Power Limits to Transmitter Coil (Duty Cycle)

   C. Frequency Range (MHz)

   D. Phase Shift Control (yes/no)

   E. Programmable Pulse Shaping (yes/no)

   F. Rise Time (msec from 10% to 90%)

G. Coil Configuration

1. Separate transmitter/receiver coils

   a. body (yes/no)
   b. head (yes/no)
   c. breast (yes/no)
   d. surface (yes/no)
   e. other (yes/no: describe)

2. Coil dimensions (cm) and configuration for each of the above

3. Time (mins) required to change from one coil to another and to resume imaging

4. Tuning procedure required for each patient (yes/no)

5. Time (sec) required to tune (describe procedure)

H. Type of Detection

1. Single phase
2. Quadrature

IV. Computer Specifications

A. Manufacturer and Model

B. Electrical Requirements (V, kVA)

C. Dimensions (m)

D. Word Size

E. Memory Size (M byte)

F. Array Processor (yes/no)

G. Interface Capability (yes/no)

1. Compliance with ACR/NEMA interface standards (yes/no)
2. RS232 port availability (yes/no)
3. Software and documentation for data transmission (yes/no)
4. Image and header format documentation if not ACR/NEMA interfaced

H. Disk

1. Storage capacity (M Byte)
2. Removable (yes/no)
3. Floppy (yes/no)
4. Optional added storage (M Byte)

I. Tape Drive

   1. Speed (ips)
   2. Density (bpi)

J. Software/Hardware Capabilities (yes/no)

   1. Cursor with joystick, trackball, or mouse

   2. Region of Interest (ROI): shape and size variable, with means and standards deviations computed, and histograms displayed

   3. Convenient grey scale adjustment (mean and window), color

   4. Annotation at any location

   5. Distance and angle measurements, reference grid

   6. Profile plot

   7. Reformat images (e.g. transverse to sagittal)

   8. Magnification of selected region (without resolution improvement) specify 2x, 4x, 6x, etc.

   9. Time to display image

      a. time to "paint the screen" for a single image (specify matrix size)
      b. time to display multi slice images (number per minute)

   10. Simultaneous display of multiple images (number displayed)

   11. Scout view can be used to select location of image

      a. sagittal, coronal, transverse views
      b. time (sec)
      c. slice thickness: thin and thick (specify)

   12. Labeling of images (patient ID, date, left/right, sequence parameters, slice thickness, slice location, etc.)

   13. Image processing: addition, subtraction, filtering, other (describe)

   14. Capability to display MR side by side with CT images from same manufacturer, other manufacturers

K. Printer (yes/no)

   1. Characters per second
   2. Column width

L. Heat Dissipation/Cooling Requirements (BTU/hr)

M. Thermal Alarm System (yes/no)

V. Console Specifications

A. Electrical Requirements (V, kVA)

B. Dimensions (m)

C. Scan Control Capabilities

   1. Separate console (yes/no)
   2. Screen size (cm)

D. Image View Capabilities

   1. Separate console (yes/no)
   2. Screen size (cm)
   3. Image display functions and photography are independent of scan control functions (yes/no)

E. Number of Grey Levels Displayed (i.e. bit depth of image display)

F. Image Monitor Resolution (i.e. 512, 1024, etc)

G. Reconstruction Matrix Size Versus Display Matrix Size

H. Heat Dissipation/Cooling Requirements (BTU/hr)

I. Patient Observation

   1. Ability of operator to view patient handling area and room accesses when seated at console (yes/no)
   2. Ability of operator to view patient during scan (i.e. remote TV) (yes/no)
   3. Diagnostic (not blanked) ECG (yes/no)

J. Video Signal: Standard RS170 (yes/no)

VI. Hard Copy Device

    A. Dimensions (m)

    B. Separate TV Monitor with Same Display as Operator's Console (yes/no)

    C. Expose and Film Advancement Under Computer Control (yes/no)

    D. Specify Cassette, Roll-Film, or Magazine Loading (films/load)

    E. Film Sizes (cmxcm)

    F. Formats

        1. Images per film, variable, (identify)
        2. Capability for 35 mm slides (yes/no)

    G. Image Quality During Scanner Operation Documented (e.g. SMPTE test pattern) (yes/no)

VII. Patient Couch Specifications

    A. X,Y,Z Positioning

        1. Ranges (cm)
        2. Controls at couch and console (yes/no)

    B. X,Y,Z Positioning Indicators

        1. Indicators at couch and console (yes/no)
        2. Accuracy (mm)
        3. Relative to center of imaging volume (yes/no)

    C. Patient Localizer (e.g. laser to indicate slice position)

        1. Accuracy (mm)
        2. Localization for X,Y,Z axes (yes/no)

    F. Dimensions (m): Extension from Gantry

    G. Alarm: Patient Activated (yes/no)

    H. Minimum Time Required to Remove Patient in Emergency (sec)

    I. Communication: Audio and Visual Links to Patient (yes/no)

    J. Maximum Couch Load (kg)

    K. Head Holder Permits Angular Adjustment (yes/no)

VIII. Image Acquisition

Note: Separate specifications for the various sequences, imaging modes, or coils may be required (e.g. head versus body modes, body versus surface coils). In particular, single versus multiple image acquisitions can be expected to differ in their specifications.

A. Single Image

1. Number of identical acquisitions NSA, i.e. signal averaging (specify possible NSA values)

2. Slice thickness

   a. slice sensitivity profile provided (yes/no)
   b. full width half maximum (FWHM) available (specify thickness)

3. Slice orientations

   a. transverse, sagittal, coronal
   b. others (specify)

4. Shift of image plane other than mechanical (e.g. frequency offset)

   a. range of shift (cm)
   b. shift increments (mm)

5. Spin echo

   a. TR/TE Combinations (msec)
   b. Multiple echoes (number)
   c. Carr-Purcell-Meiboom-Gill (CPMG) echoes (yes/no)

6. Inversion recovery: TR/TI: TE combinations (msec)

7. Other sequences (yes/no)

   a. rapid "scout view" for selection of image slice locations (yes/no), time (sec)
   b. saturation recovery
   c. echo planar or alternate "fast" scan
   d. chemical shift imaging
   e. other sequences provided by manufacturer (specify)
   f. effort and expertise required by operator to design pulse sequences (describe)

B. Multiple Simultaneous Images: Multi-Slice and/or Volume Imaging Acquisition

1. Number of identical acquisitions NSA (specify possible NSA values)

2. Slice thickness

   a. slice sensitivity profile provided (yes/no)
   b. full width half maximum (FWHM) available (specify thickness)

3. Slice orientations

   a. transverse, sagittal, coronal
   b. others (specify)

4. Shift of image planes other than by mechanical means (e.g. frequency offset)

   a. range of shift for the entire set of images (cm)
   b. shift increments for the entire set of images (mm)
   c. spacing between images of a set (mm), variable (yes/no)

5. Spin echo

   a. TR/TE combinations (msec)
   b. Multiple echoes (number)
   c. Carr-Purcell-Meiboom-Gill (CPMG) echoes (yes/no)

6. Inversion Recovery: TR/TI: TE combinations (msec)

7. Other sequences

   a. rapid "scout view" for selection of image slice locations (yes/no), time (sec)
   b. saturation recovery
   c. echo planar or alternate "fast" scan
   d. chemical shift imaging
   e. other sequences provided by manufacturer (specify)
   f. effort and expertise required by operator to design pulse sequences (describe)

C. A/D Conversion

1. Digitization depth (bits)
2. Conversion rate (kHz)

D. Time (min)

1. Time to acquire representative images, Time=PxNSAxTR where P is the number of projections (i.e. different acquisitions)
2. Time to measure T1, T2, or spin density (N) (specify pulse sequences)

E. Acquisition Geometry

1. Useable imaging volume: sphere or ellipsoid dimensions (cm)
2. Reconstruction region

   a. standard head and body diameters (cm)
   b. maximum and minimum diameters (cm)
   c. variable field of view (FOV) (describe)

3. Patient access limitations for head and body (cm)

F. Gating

1. Cardiac and/or respiratory (yes/no)
2. Single slice (yes/no)

   a. single phase
   b. multiple phase simultaneously acquired

3. Multi images simultaneously acquired (yes/no)

   a. different locations have different phases: time to acquire (min)
   b. different locations have same phase: time to acquire (min)

4. Operator selectable phase (yes/no), accuracy (msec)

IX. Image Processing Specifications

A. Parameter Calculations: Spin Density (N), T1, T2 and Flow (yes/no)

1. Range measurable
2. Accuracy of measurements (%)
3. Reproducibility (%)
   a. scan to scan
   b. day to day
4. Absolute calibration
   a. standards available (yes/no)
   b. accuracy of standards (%)
5. Entire image or selected region
6. Method of calculation documented (yes/no)

B. Image Reconstruction

  1. Type

      a. filtered back projection (yes/no)
      b. 2DFT (yes/no)
      c. 3DFT (yes/no)
      d. phase information retained (i.e. negative pixel values are possible)

  2. Time (sec) for the available matrix size

      a. single slice time (sec): end collection to end display
      b. multi slice time (sec, sec/image): end collection to end of all images displayed

  3. Variable field of view (FOV) (describe)

  4. Reconstruction filters, variable (identify)

  5. Raw data storage such that different reconstructions of a given image are possible (yes/no)

  6. Pixel depth (bits)

X. Imaging Quality Performance

  Note: At the time of this report image quality parameters specific to NMR have not been comprehensively identified and defined. Furthermore, there is little agreement in methods to measure such parameters. Therefore, the following parameters are offered as a guide. It is left to the purchaser and manufacturer to agree on definitions and measurement methods.

  A. Spatial Resolution

  B. Signal-to-Noise

  C. Image Uniformity

  D. Spatial Linearity

  E. Signal Linearity

  F. Slice Sensitivity Profile (Slice Thickness)

  G. Slice Position Accuracy

  H. Slice Angulation Accuracy

XI. Spectroscopy (yes/no)

   A. Magnetic Field Uniformity (ppm): specified for the maximum and minimum selected volumes

   B. Volume Sample Selection

      1. Shapes of selection volumes (eg. spheres, ellipsoids, etc.)
      2. Maximum to minimum selection volumes (cm^3)
      3. Accuracy of selected volumes (%)
      4. Location accuracy of selected volumes (mm)

   C. Resolution: NMR linewidth (FWHM in ppm)/chemical shift (δ) (ppm), for specified nuclei

   D. Time Required for Change-over (min)

      1. From one nuclei to another (specify via example)
      2. From spectroscopy to imaging mode and vice versa (specify via example)

XII. Safety (see BRH Guidelines)

   Note: The factors which affect patient safety are still being debated. Listed below are four items of concern. It is left to the purchaser (institution) and manufacturer to consider these factors, establish limits, and agree upon methods of acceptance testing. Single slice, multi-slice, multi-echoes, etc. should be considered in assessing maximum risk.

   A. Magnetic Flux Density (Fringe Plots) (T)

   B. Maximum Rate of Change of the Magnetic Field (T/sec)

   C. Maximum RF Absorption in tissue (W/Kg)

      1. Single slice
      2. Multi slice
      3. Multi echo

   D. Metal (ferromagnetic) Detector(s) at Entrance(s) to Magnet Room (yes/no)

XIII. Administrative Considerations

　　A. Cost of Installed System Exclusive of Site Preparation and Site Surveys

　　B. Estimated Cost of Site Preparation and Site Surveys

　　C. Dates for Delivery and Completed Installation

　　D. "Normal" Patient Throughput: Typical Scan Times/Patient (This could be indicated by patient numbers, types of exams, average scans per patient from other clinical sites with similar imaging units).

　　E. Estimated Operating Cost

　　　　1. Electrical
　　　　2. H_2O and/or cryogen(s)

　　F. Service Contract and/or Warranty Agreement

　　　　1. Technical/engineer support

　　　　　　a. normal maintenance (hours/week)
　　　　　　b. emergency response time (hours)
　　　　　　c. cost for the above

　　　　2. Provide operating manuals, service manuals, and schematics (yes/no)

　　　　3. Provide training for staff technologists, radiologists, and physicists (yes/no)

　　G. Upgrade Options

　　　　1. Magnet (field strength)
　　　　2. Computer and software (describe)
　　　　3. Spectroscopy (describe)
　　　　4. RF system (describe)

　　H. Downtime (%) (Maximum per year, per month)

　　I. QA Phantom and Protocols, provided by Manufacturer (yes/no) (describe in detail)

　　J. Provide List of Operational Clinical Sites

　　K. Specify Pre-Market Approval (PMA) Status

ECONOMIC CONSIDERATIONS IN MAGNETIC RESONANCE

William Pavlicek, M.S., Meredith A. Weinstein, M.D.
Thomas F. Meaney, M.D., Paul Intihar, M.S.
The Cleveland Clinic Foundation, Cleveland, Ohio 44106

ABSTRACT

Magnetic resonance imaging programs range from a mobile resistive system to a 2.0 Tesla superconductive unit placed in an existing Radiology Department. This presents an equally broad spectrum of economic considerations and financial importance. Clearly, the single most important decision to be made in lowering the break even cost for an MR exam is the initial decision; selecting the magnet type and its location of operation. Due to relatively minor variable costs associated with the procedure (i.e. film, forms and magnetic tape), the cost incremental increase for doing additional patients is essentially inconsequential. The responsibility for an MR program to develop a positive return on investment lies in these critical decisions. The role of the medical physicist is instrumental in the architectural designs of siting magnets since health and safety considerations determine to a large extent whether or not a magnet can be safely sited or whether compromises in image quality would occur. Additionally, since many medical physicists are hospital based, the challenge exists for these individuals to demonstrate economic savings to the hospital in the area of customized ferrous shielding and factors affecting patient throughput such as development of patient protocols.

INTRODUCTION

Any analysis of MR, including an economical one, must recognize that it is making a statement that is valid for a certain period of time. Changes occur in technical development which affect clinical utility and in turn, the economic soundness of this new imaging modality (1,2). With these requisite statements made, one can make certain assumptions which simplify the economic analysis. The most important factors in the economic analysis are which magnet system is purchased, where it is to be located, and what are the number of patients per day that can be examined. The reasons for this are that the variable costs of performing an examination are generally quite small in comparison to the purchase price and facility modification or construction necessary to provide the service. Summarized in Table I are the various magnet types which are found in use today. Each magnet type has advantages and disadvantages. A resistive magnet is the type most conveniently installed in an existing facility since minimum restrictions for modification are required. Permanent magnets have siting needs which include a consideration for structural support while superconducting magnets cannot be broken down into small components which can fit in conventional hospital elevators or doorways.

TABLE I: MAGNET TYPES AND THEIR CHARACTERISTICS

Characteristic	Permanent	Resistive	Superconductive
Source of field	Permanent magnetization of magnetic domains in ferromagnetic material	Current circulating in solenoidal coil	Current circulating in solenoidal coil
Configuration	Frame/Air Gap	Solenoid	Solenoid
Determinants of homogeneity	Geometry/Finish of pole pieces, metallurgy, temperature	Winding accuracy, current regulation	Winding accuracy, current rgulation
Operating costs	Special air conditioning system	High power consumption to maintain field*	Replenishment of cryogenic gases
Siting needs	Inherently shielded to conserve flux, site must stand high weight	Water to remove generated heat	Requires large areas because of extensive fields. Magnetic shielding will decrease room size.**

* Besides power for magnet, power is needed for chiller to remove heat

** Besides costs of shielding material, added costs are incurred for structural support

Typical purchase price of MR magnet systems are shown in Table II. The cost of the additional capital for going to the highest available field strength is not insignificant, since the higher field strengths markedly increased site preparation costs (3).

TABLE II: COSTS OF MR IMAGING SYSTEM

Magnet Technology	Field	Cost List
Persistive	.15 T	$1,000,000
Permanent	.3 T	$1,600,000
Superconductive	.6 T	$1,500,000
Superconductive	1.5 T	$2,000,000

Site preparation costs differ markedly depending upon whether a new free-standing facility is to be constructed or whether renovation is to be performed. Additionally, substantial differences occur in whether hospital code construction is required for the MR facility or whether outpatient medical facility construction is specified. While the area requirements for the ancillary equipment (console, power supplies, computer room) are relatively constant regardless of which magnet type is selected (typically 300 to 400 square feet), the scan room varies depending upon the field strength of the selected magnet. Typical ancillary and scan room areas for several magnet types are given as Table III.

TABLE III: MR MAGNET AREA REQUIREMENTS

Field Strength	Ancillaries*	Scan Room	Total
.15 T	330	560	890
.3 T Perm. **	375	625	1000
.3 T	330	750	1080
.5 T	330	1020	1350
.6 T	330	1150	1480
1.5 T	330	2100	2430

* Includes control room, computer room and storage

** Requires special reinforcement to handle weight and special temperature control

Table IV gives typical cost per square foot and cost for a 3,000 square foot facility. Note that renovation of a hospital site to accommodate an MR system is quite high. The total square feet required for a 1.5 Tesla system can be reduced if magnetic shielding is employed. However, this adds to the renovation cost due to the cost of the shielding and the need for added structural support to carry the weight of the shielding.

TABLE IV: MR CONSTRUCTION COSTS

Construction Type	Cost per Square Foot	Cost for 3000 Ft Facility
New freestanding		
- Bare	$85	$255,000
- Furnished	$112	$336,000
- Hospital grade bare	$120 - $170	$360,000 - $510,000
Renovation		
- Hospital grade	$180 - $255	$540,000 - $765,000

The key point to observe is that the selection of the magnet and its location of operation will be shown as the single most important consideration from an economical viewpoint.

MR COST ANALYSIS

Fixed Costs

Fixed costs can be separated into the areas of capital related costs, operating costs, and overhead. Capital related costs include the equipment financing cost and interest to be paid on the loan as well as the facility rental or amortization. As mentioned earlier, it will be shown that the selection of the magnet and its physical location are the major determinants of the MR program cost.

The fixed operating costs include personnel, utilities (power, cryogens, water, etc.) and maintenance (both MR system and facility).

Overhead costs include insurance on the MR facility and service as well as other administrative accounting and legal fees.

In Table V, typical capital expenditures for MR systems are given for the magnet types shown. Integrated RF shielding is being provided in a new facility construction of minimal square feet for the magnet type given. Construction quality is of hospital grade. The total capital expenditures cover a two-fold range of between 1.3 and 2.7 million dollars.

TABLE V: MR CAPITAL EXPENDITURES

	Resistive .15 T	Permanent .3 T	Superconductive .6 T	Superconductive 1.5 T
Capital Expenditures:				
Imaging System	$1,000,000	$1,600,000	$1,500,000	$2,000,000
Radiofrequency Shielding	$ 75,000*	$ 75,000	$ 75,000	$ 75,000
Facility Construction	$ 226,950	$ 285,000	$ 377,400	$ 619,650
TOTAL	$1,301,950	$1,960,000	$1,952,400	$2,694,650

* Free standing RF shielding is not recommended by all vendors

The more expensive approach would be to site a 1.5 or 2 Tesla magnet in an existing Radiology Department by employing the use of magnetic shielding. The use of magnetic shielding can markedly decrease the total square feet requirement necessary for the imaging room. Additionally, the siting of the magnet in an existing Radiology Department permits the use of existing reception areas and waiting rooms as well as possibly increase the efficiencies of the existing medical staff.

Free standing RF shielding is not a requisite by all vendors of resistive units. Also note that if existing facility chillers cannot handle heat removal, a capital purchase (approximately $30,000 - $40,000) must be made.

Flynn, et al (4) have shown the costs associated with shielding a magnet "in house" to be $227,000. An analysis of this amount of space saved by the use of shielding coupled with improved patient flow and non-duplication of ancillary services must be made. In departments where space is at a premium, shieldings may become the norm.

In figure 1, the effect of interest rates upon the annual capital cost for 5 year financing is given for various magnet types. A 15% interest rate is assumed for this analysis.

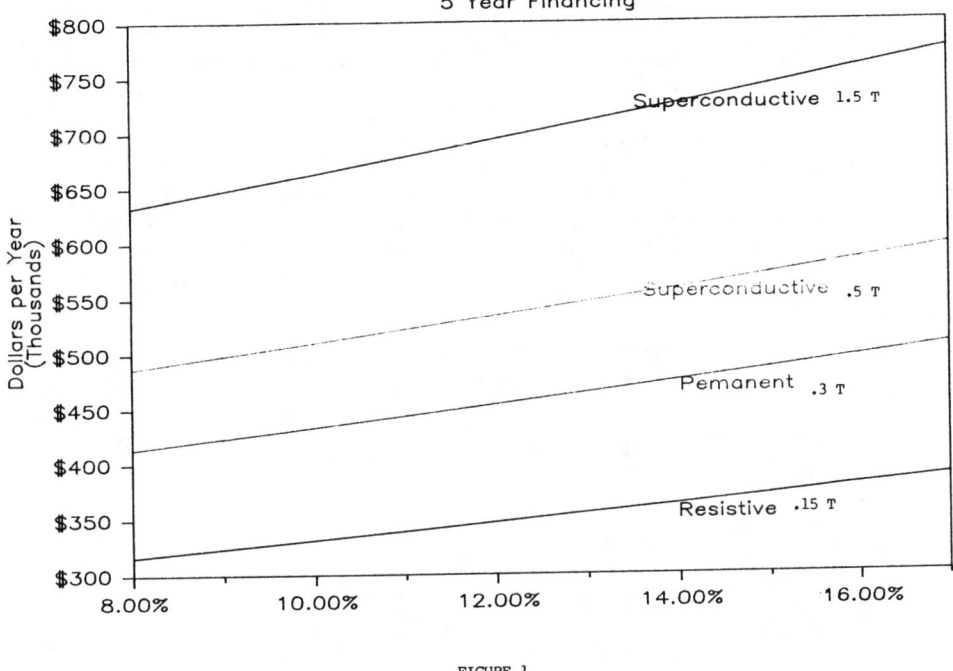

FIGURE 1

Personnel costs are calculated assuming that two technologists, a clerk or patient coordinator work 5 days a week, 8 hours a day providing a 10 to 12 hour MR service. A physicist is not assumed to be a part of the MR service while the personnel costs related to equipment service are covered by the maintenance contract with the MR vendor.

Fixed operating costs related to utilities are driven by the cost of electrical power. For these calculations, it is assumed that 24 kilowatts at 10 cents per kilowatt hour are typical values for the air conditioning and MR system needs. This calculates to approximately $6,000 per year.

Cryogen costs are assumed to be $36,000 per year based upon a cost of 50 cents a litre for nitrogen and $5 a litre for helium. Boil-off rates on the order of .2 to .3 litres per hour of helium and 1.0 to 1.5 litres per hour of nitrogen are assumed. The initial fill of cryogens is included in the purchase cost of the MR system.

Variable Costs

The estimated costs per procedure which are variable and depend upon the number of examinations performed are given in Table VI. The costs per procedure for CT and conventional and digital angiography are also included. MR costs are primarily related to filming the examination while the other modalities have expensive replacement parts or disposable items. The key point to gain from this data is that variable costs associated with MR are quite small in comparison to the fixed operating costs. Conversely and even more importantly, the costs associated in doing additional patients during a work day are minimal. Consequently, patient throughput is a dominant factor in MR economic liability (5,6).

TABLE VI: COST PER PROCEDURE FOR MR AS COMPARED WITH CT AND ANGIOGRAPHY

Variable Cost	MR	CT	Angio-Film	Angio-Dig
Film	10	10	50	5
Magnetic Tape	5	5		5
Forms	5	5	5	5
Tube Wear		20	20	20
Contrast		6	6	6
Disposables			70	20
TOTAL	$20	$46	$151	$61

In Table VII, a summary of the data presented here is shown with the total first year costs associated with various magnet types. It is assumed for these calculations that 10 patients per day (1 patient per hour) for a total of 2,500 patients are performed annually. Again, a factor of 2 is noticed between the total annual costs associated with the highest to lowest magnetic field strength.

TABLE VII: TYPICAL TOTAL SYSTEM COSTS BY MAGNET TYPE

Fixed Operating Cost	Resistive .15 T	Permanent .3 T	Superconductive .6 T	Superconductive 1.5 T
Capital Related:				
Financing cost per year, 15% interest, 5 year term	$390,806	$588,333	$586,052	$ 808,853
Floorspace	$ 22,250	$25,000	$ 33,750	$ 60,750
Operating:				
Personnel 2 technicians, 1 clerk	$ 80,000	$ 80,000	$ 80,000	$ 80,000
Utilities Power	$ 41,000	$ 12,500	$ 6,000	$ 6,000
Cryogens			$ 36,000	$ 36,000
Maintenance Facility	$ 6,000	$ 6,000	$ 6,000	$ 6,000
Equipment @ 7% of capital (not incurred until second year)	$ 70,000	$112,000	$105,000	$ 140,000
Overhead:				
Insurance	$ 10,000	$ 16,000	$ 15,000	$ 20,000
Other	$ 60,000	$ 60,000	$ 60,000	$ 60,000
TOTAL FIXED COST	$610,056	$787,833	$822,802	$1,077,603
Variable cost Supplies $20/study	$ 50,000	$ 50,000	$ 50,000	$ 50,000
TOTAL COST	$660,056	$837,833	$872,802	$1,127,603

Break Even Charge per Procedure

Using the data given in the above section, it is possible to determine the costs associated for a procedure for several magnet types in comparison with CT. This is given as figure 2 and it is noted that in all cases MR is more expensive than CT.

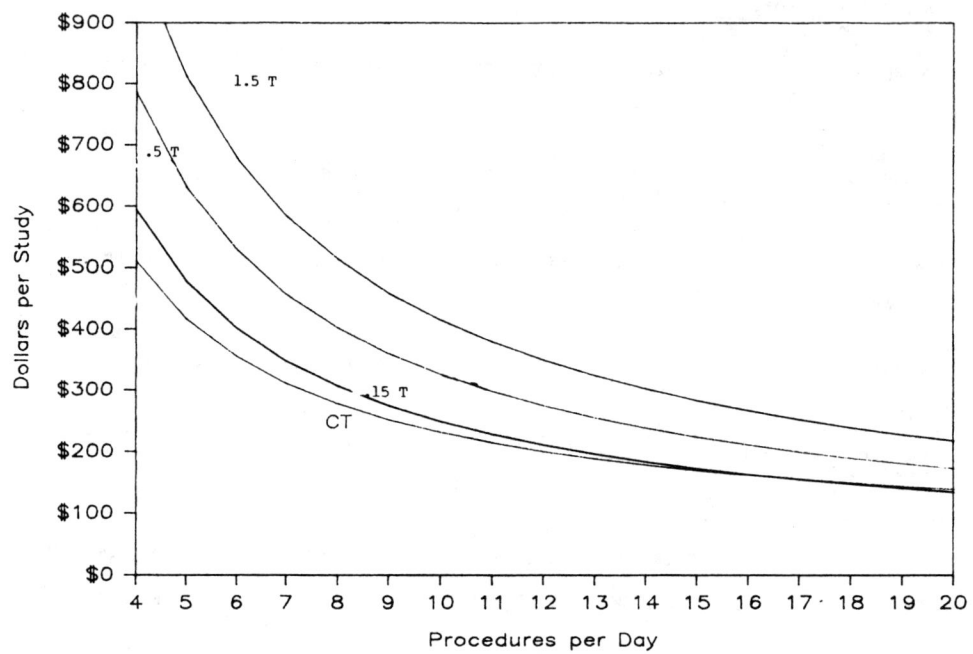

FIGURE 2

Additionally, it is noted that the break even cost per procedure markedly decreases until approximately 10 to 12 patients are examined daily. The data indicates that importance must be placed upon the facility construction to maximize patient throughput not unlike the same efforts typically made with CT facilities.

In a typical MR imaging cycle, patient preparation requires 4 to 5 minutes during which the patient is placed upon the table and given instructions for the examination. A localization scan, if required, can require 2 minutes for proper identification of anatomical site to be examined. Setting up an MR protocol with the proper pulse sequences can be minimized if clinical interaction is given prior to patients being situated on the table. Data acquisition for most MR systems is limited by the number of slices necessary to cover the anatomical area of interest since 2DFT imaging is normally selected. This means that the examination runs approximately 20 to 40 minutes. Completing the reconstruction and removing the patient may take 4 to 5 more minutes. Because of the large number of optional approaches to an MR study (projection, T1, T2, or spin density weighting), clinical monitoring is essential to high throughput.

MR INCOME

It is in the area of MR reimbursement that major uncertainties exist (7). The rapidity with which MR is expanded into the community service depends upon major decisions made by third party reimbursors. Medicare Part A (hospital based) has embarked upon the program of diagnostic related gorups (DRG's). This method of payment fixes the costs associated with standard clinical conditions and does not reimburse based upon fee for service. As a consequence, an expensive technology such as MR within a hospital must demonstrate to be an improved modality over conventional imaging tests or it must be of equal value but of less expense. In one analysis (8), a comparison was made of MR for the indications of multiple sclerosis, syringomyelia, normal pressure hydrocephalus and vertebrobasilar infarction. Based upon the technical charges associated with the conventional workup of these patients, including hospital stay, the technical charges associated with MR at the Huntington Medical Research Institutes MR Facility (Table VIII) shows that MR can result in considerable savings for these examinations. With the case of MS, the savings is $1,244 per patient for patients with myelopathic findings and $268 for patients not having myelopathic findings. The savings per patient for syringomyelia are $976 while a savings of $700 is possible in the workup for normal pressure hydrocephalus and acoustic neuromas. Vertebrobasilar infarction examinations with MR can result in a savings of $1,318 per patient.

TABLE VIII: MR TECHNICAL CHARGES

	Acquisition Time (Min)	Charge	Patients*
Head	0 - 17	$379	114
	18 - 34	$515	173
	35+	$606	49
	AVERAGE	$482	TOTAL: 336
Body	0 - 17	$422	6
	18 - 34	$574	48
	35 - 51	$675	22
	51+	$774	6
	AVERAGE	$605	TOTAL: 82

* October 1 - November 15, 1984

Data courtesy of W. Bradley, M.D., Ph.D.
Pasadena, California

This analysis ignores other than economic affects upon the patients and obviously the elimination of intravenous contrast or lumbar puncture is of improved care with respect to risk and pain.

Medicare Part B (outpatient based) reimbursement, is not currently under the directives to reimburse using DRG's. Reimbursement is dependent upon local state policies and practices. Likewise, Blue Cross and Blue Shield reimbursement is dependent upon local decisions but in general, has not approved MR as a reimbursable service. Blue Cross and Blue Shield plans apply a criterion of "usual, customary and reasonable" fees and do not reimburse for a research investigational device.

Clinical examinations are being performed full time (10 hours/day) on a 0.6 T magnet since August, 1983 and 2.5 days/week on a 1.5 T system since April, 1984 at the Cleveland Clinic Foundation. Although close to 5,000 patients have been examined to date, differentiation between inpatients/outpatients and billing startd in August, 1984.

Outpatient reimbursement is of paramount importance for MR. In Table IX, the computerized data for the last 1,500 patients at the Cleveland Clinic Foundation shows 60% outpatients. More importantly, 75% of billings are outpatients. In Table X, billings by clinical distribution are given. Note that neurological exams account for 80+%.

TABLE IX: INPATIENT VS OUTPATIENT MR EXAMS

	Patient Count		**Percent**	
	Inpatient	Outpatient	Inpatient	Outpatient
1984 August	79	103	43.4%	56.6%
September	73	75	49.3%	50.7%
October	94	77	55.0%	45.0%
November	67	110	37.9%	62.1%
December	52	84	38.2%	61.8%
1985 January	89	98	47.6%	52.4%
February	66	80	45.2%	54.8%
March	69	127	35.2%	64.8%
April	57	113	33.5%	66.5%
TOTAL	646	867	42.6%	57.3%

Data courtesty Cleveland Clinic Foundation

TABLE X: DISTRIBUTION OF MR BILLINGS*

Cardiac	.7%
Brain	44.0%
Spine	38.4%
Chest	1.8%
Abdomen	3.0%
Pelvis	2.1%
Muscular/Skeletal	3.5%
Multiple Site	6.5%

* Billings after December 1, 1984

Data courtesy of Cleveland Clinic Foundation

Many commercial insurance companies are reimbursing for MR examinations. In an analysis of collection rate for an 8-month period in 1984, Bradley has found that collections are currently 78% of the billings for private patients including those with Medicare (6). While Medicare does not reimburse for MR, many patients have supplemental plans which cover non-Medicare expenses following a formal denial by Medicare. However, since insurance checks are usually sent directly to the patient, it is difficult to determine whether the collection rate (78%) is originating from third party carriers as opposed to those patients who are paying directly.

In Table VIII, it is noted that with a typical MR examination comprising 30 minutes, a technical fee of $515 is the fee for a head exam (9). Since this facility operates at almost 14 procedures per day, a break even charge of approximately $300 is expected (using figure 2). The difference ($215) represents the cost of doing those patients that are either research protocols or in-house investigations as well as non-collectibles including Medicaid. Additionally, in a capital intensive modality such as MR, a reasonable return on the investment is needed or capital will not be available (10). Considering that interest rates are in the neighborhood of 15%, a 20% return on investment is not unreasonable to attract capital necessary for MR purchase and subsequent update.

Mobile MR Systems

The surprising development in MR imaging is the observation that mobile MR is especially cost effective and avoids certain risks. When a major capital expenditure in MR is simply the renovation or construction of a facility, the value of mobile or placement of an MR system in a van becomes apparent. A mobile MR system can be sold if an MR service fails to materialize. The cost of the system as well as the facility then becomes less of a risk. Additionally, if patient referral patterns do not develop and/or a lower number of patient exams is performed, mobile MR becomes economically more advantageous. In figure 3, the cost sensitivity of mobile versus fixed 0.6 Tesla system is shown. For less than 5 to 6 patients per day, the return on an investment of a mobile system is markedly superior. For patient throughput at rates of 10 to 12 patients a day, fixed site facilities do not represent major savings over mobile units in terms of cost per procedure to break down.

The break even costs per procedure for a 0.6 T fixed unit are quite high for low patient volume. The data for the mobile unit are from a mobile service company, which can offer a low cost to a low volume hospital since multiple hospitals are being serviced.

Data courtesy Technicare Corporation

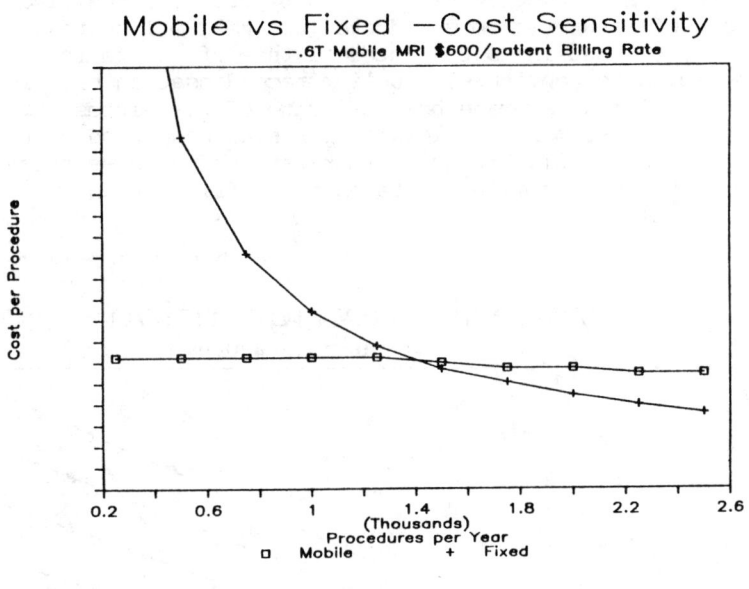

FIGURE 3

Beyond the cost of a van ($400,000) and siting at a hospital ($35,000 to $50,000), an additional cost incurred with mobile superconductive systems is the increased loss of liquid helium. The leads to the magnet are normally kept fixed so that the magnets can be ramped up and ramped down as sites are changed. This decreases the thermal separation and increases the boil off rate.

While refrigeration systems do not appear financially justifiable for fixed MR systems in the United States due to the low cost of liquid helium and nitrogen, low cryogen consumpton, and high cost of purchasing and operating the refrigeration system, they do appear justifiable for mobile systems. For example, assuming 2 ramp up and ramp down occurances per week and 20 litres of helium loss per occurance, as well as a boil off rate of 1 litre of helium per hour with leads in place, a boil off rate of at least 1.1 litres per hour is expected from a mobile system visiting 2 hospitals a week. As shown in figure 4, a positive internal rate of return is observed even for helium less than $4.00 per litre. Assuming a 20% internal rate of return for reasonable capital expenditure, a helium recondensation unit is favorable even with an average boil off rate of 0.8 litres per hour. This graph assumes 15 kilowatts per hour power consumption for an annual cost of $10,250 and a refrigerator purchase price of $130,000 with $3,000 for maintenance on the refrigeration unit.

Data courtesy Technicare Corporation

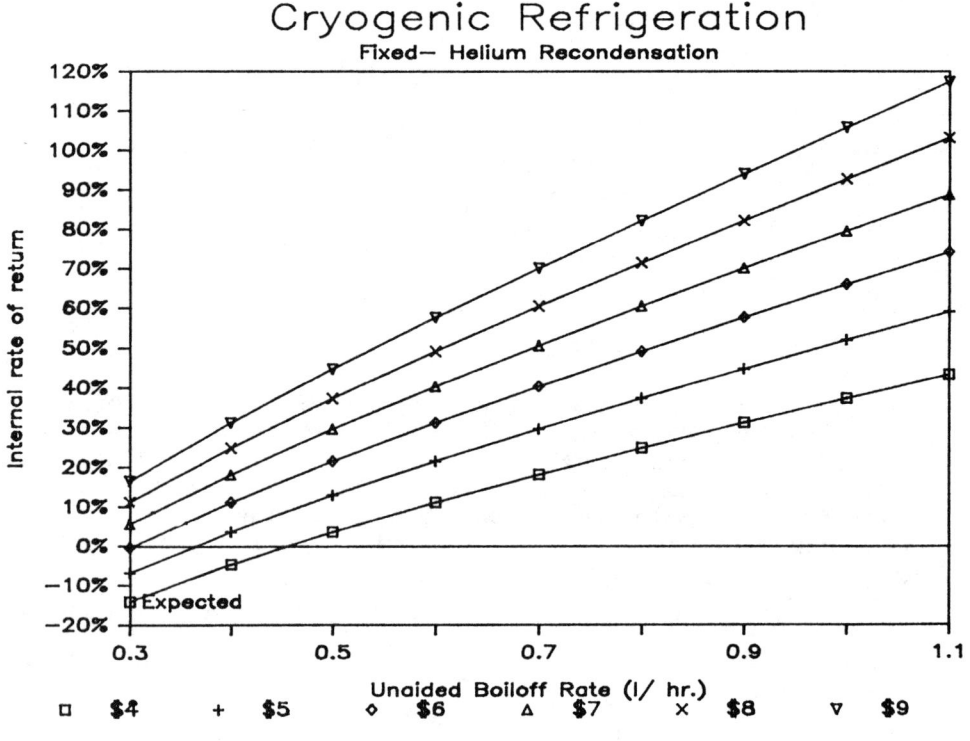

FIGURE 4

Note also that if a mobile system is to be sited at a single setting, the leads can be removed, the boil-off rate reduced to 0.31/hr, and cost of $9.00 per litre of helium is necessary for cryogenic refrigeration to be realistic.

CONCLUSION

The role of the medical physicist in magnetic resonance can have a major impact on the economic return of this modality. As observed in the discussion under fixed costs, the selection of the magnet and its site is of utmost importance in the fixed capital costs associated with an MR service. Whether an MR system should be incorporated into an existing facility with the use of magnetic shielding depends, among other things, upon the expected patient throughput advantage a site provides. Additionally, design of magnetic shielding and the specification of the 5 and 15 gauss lines around the MR system determine the controlled space requirements.

Acknowledgement

The authors are pleased to thank David J. Nuechterlein, Director of Corporate Planning, Technicare Corporation for his many contributions and Sharon McFadden for manuscript preparation.

REFERENCES

1. Steinberg EP, Cohen AB: Health technology case study 27: Nuclear magnetic resonance imaging technology. A clinical, industrial and policy analysis. Office of Technology Assessment, September, 1984. Published by Congress of United States.

2. DiMonda, R: Hospital technology series guideline report. NMR issues for 1985 and beyond. 4:3-4, 1985. Published by American Hospital Association.

3. Freeman GS, Stephens H, Fisher B: Economic considerations in MRI. Applied Radiology, May/June, 1984, p. 55.

4. Flynn MJ, Vavrek RM, Ewing JR, Froelich J, Issa J: Magnetic fields from MR imaging magnets with axially symmetric iron shields. Works in progress. Presented at RSNA, Washington, D.C., 1984. Abstract in Scientific Program, p. 304.

5. Meaney TF, Intihar P: Cost projections of NMR units. Proceedings of course "Basic MR Principles. A Clinical Program for Radiologists." Cleveland Clinic Foundation, Cleveland, Ohio, October 20, 1984.

6. Bradley W, Johnson KC: Hints for establishing a profitable MR practice. Diagnostic Imaging, March 1985, p. 39.

7. Osborn RR: Keeping your cool while medicare puts on the squeeze. Diagnostic Imaging, April, 1984, p. 46.

8. Bradley W, Stuart B, Kortman K: Magnetic resonance imaging in the cost sensitive environment of patient care. Presented at MRI: A National Conference on Clinical Application and Issues, sponsored by the Cleveland Clinic Foundation, San Diego, California, April 1-3, 1985.

9. Bradley W, Opel W, Kortman K, Kassabian J: MR installation: 18 Months clinical experience. Presented at RSNA, Washington, D.C., November 25, 1984. Abstract in Scientific Program, p. 39.

10. Shannon K, ed: Money woes cloud MRI's clinical success - Hospital physician venture cuts cost of MRI. Management Rounds of Hospitals, October, 1984, p. 60.

BIOLOGICAL EFFECTS AND PHYSICAL SAFETY ASPECTS OF
NMR IMAGING AND IN VIVO SPECTROSCOPY

T.S. Tenforde and T.F. Budinger
Division of Biology and Medicine, Lawrence Berkeley Laboratory,
University of California, Berkeley, California 94720

ABSTRACT

An assessment is made of the biological effects and physical hazards of static and time-varying fields associated with the NMR devices that are being used for clinical imaging and in vivo spectroscopy. A summary is given of the current state of knowledge concerning the mechanisms of interaction and the bioeffects of these fields. Additional topics that are discussed include: (1) physical effects on pacemakers and metallic implants such as aneurysm clips, (2) human health studies related to the effects of exposure to nonionizing electromagnetic radiation, and (3) extant guidelines for limiting exposure of patients and medical personnel to the fields produced by NMR devices. On the basis of information available at the present time, it is concluded that the fields associated with the current generation of NMR devices do not pose a significant health risk in themselves. However, rigorous guidelines must be followed to avoid the physical interaction of these fields with metallic implants and medical electronic devices.

INTRODUCTION

The primary objective of this chapter is to summarize the theoretical and experimental bases for judging the safety of human exposure to the static and time-varying fields associated with NMR imaging and in vivo spectroscopy. Unlike ionizing radiation, the interaction of these fields with living objects is generally subtle and frequently difficult to detect. A few exceptions include magnetically-induced potentials in the circulatory system, the induction of magnetophosphenes by extremely-low-frequency (ELF) magnetic fields, and tissue heating by radiofrequency (RF) fields with sufficiently high power densities. These phenomena, and the direct interaction of NMR fields with electronic devices and metallic implants, will be discussed within the context of established interaction mechanisms that can be characterized using elementary physical principles. A summary and critique will also be given of several human health studies that have been reported in the literature, with a particular emphasis on evaluating the soundness of the methodology used in these epidemiological surveys. Detailed discussions of these topics have also been given in several recent review articles and monographs.[1-16]

FIELDS ASSOCIATED WITH NMR DEVICES

The present generation of devices for NMR imaging and in vivo spectroscopy use static magnetic fields with flux densities less than 2.5 Tesla (1 T = 10^4 Gauss). Most of the existing machines for whole-body imaging contain large-volume superconducting magnets that produce highly stable, uniform fields of 0.6 T or less. Several of the newer whole-body imaging units use fields up to 2.0 T, and fields up to 2.5 T are currently used for in vivo spectroscopy. Higher field levels are being considered for future NMR units.

The magnetic field gradients that provide spatial information defining the location of magnetic nuclei are less than 10 mT/m, and generally lie in the range of 1-5 mT/m in the existing NMR devices. The rapid switching of gradient fields leads to a time variation of the magnetic flux density (dB/dt) which is less than 3 T/sec in the current imaging devices, with typical values in the range of 0.5-1.5 T/sec. Higher values of dB/dt are anticipated in future NMR units using faster rates of data projection.

The frequencies of the RF fields used in current NMR devices are a function of the static field strength and the Larmor frequencies of the magnetic nuclei being studied. For example, in a 1 T field the resonant frequencies of ^1H, ^{13}C, ^{23}Na, ^{31}P and ^{39}K are, respectively, 42.576, 10.705, 11.262, 17.235 and 1.987 MHz. Under the near-field imaging conditions used for in vivo NMR, the absorption of RF energy is primarily associated with the magnetic component of the field, which is typically on the order of 0.5 mT. As discussed in a later section of this chapter, the specific absorption rate of RF energy is a function of frequency, tissue conductivity and dielectric constant, geometric factors, and the NMR pulse characteristics used for imaging.

STATIC MAGNETIC FIELDS

Interaction Mechanisms

Although numerous mechanisms have been proposed through which static magnetic fields could potentially influence biological functions,[13] only three classes of physical interactions are well established on the basis of experimental data: (1) electrodynamic interactions with ionic conduction currents; (2) magnetomechanical effects, including the orientation of magnetically anisotropic structures in uniform fields and the translation of paramagnetic and ferromagnetic materials in magnetic field gradients; (3) effects on electronic spin states of the reaction intermediates in charge transfer processes. Each of these physical interaction mechanisms, along with relevant experimental data, will be described in this section.

Electrodynamic interactions. Ionic currents interact with static magnetic fields as a result of the Lorentz forces exerted on moving charge carriers. Under steady state conditions this electrodynamic interaction gives rise to a local electric field $\vec{E} = -\vec{v} \times \vec{B}$, where $\vec{v}$ is the velocity of current flow and $\vec{B}$ is the magnetic flux density. This phenomenon is the physical basis of the Hall effect in solid state materials, and it also occurs in several biological processes that involve the flow of electrolytes in an aqueous medium.

One example of electrodynamic interactions with weak magnetic fields is the electromagnetic guidance system of elasmobranch fish, a class of marine animals that includes sharks, skates and rays.[17-19] The heads of these fish contain long jelly-filled canals with a high electrical conductivity, known as the ampullae of Lorenzini. As an elasmobranch swims through the lines of flux of the geomagnetic field, small voltage gradients are induced in its ampullary canals. These induced electric fields can be detected at levels as low as 0.5 µV/m by the sensory epithelia that line the terminal ampullary region.[20] The polarity of the induced field in an ampullary canal depends upon the relative orientation of the geomagnetic field and the compass direction along which the fish is swimming. As a consequence, the $-\vec{v} \times \vec{B}$ fields induced in the ampullae of Lorenzini provide a sensitive directional cue for the elasmobranch fishes.

A second example of electrodynamic interactions is the electric field resulting from blood flow in the presence of a static magnetic field. It is a direct consequence of the Lorentz force exerted on moving ionic currents that blood flowing through a cylindrical vessel of diameter, d, will develop an electrical potential, ψ, given by the equation:[13]

$$\psi = |\vec{E}| d = |\vec{v}| |\vec{B}| d \sin \Theta \qquad (1)$$

where Θ is the angle between $\vec{B}$ and the axial velocity vector, $\vec{v}$. This equation, which was first derived by Kolin, describes the physical principle upon which the electromagnetic blood flowmeter operates.[21-23] The induced blood flow potentials within the central circulatory systems of several species of mammals exposed to large static magnetic fields have also been characterized from electrocardiogram (ECG) records obtained with surface electrodes.[24-30] As demonstrated by the data shown in Fig. 1 for a Macaca monkey exposed to static fields up to 1.5 T, the primary change in the ECG is an augmentation of the signal amplitude at the locus of the T-wave. Based on its temporal sequence in the ECG record, this change in T-wave amplitude has been attributed to the electrical potential that is induced within the aortic vessel during pulsatile blood flow in the presence of a magnetic field.[25-30] The opening and closing of the aortic heart value have been shown to correspond with the timing of the appearance and disappearance of the magnetically-induced potential at the locus of the T-wave.[31] In small animal species such as rats, the aortic blood flow potential can be detected in the ECG when the magnetic flux density exceeds 0.3 T.[29] For larger animal species such as dogs, monkeys and baboons, the threshold field level which induces a measurable potential is approximately 0.1 T.[27,30,31] For all of these animal species, the change in T-wave signal amplitude observed during magnetic field exposure has been shown to be completely reversible upon removal of the field. In addition, the linear dependence of ψ on magnetic field strength and its variation as a function of animal orientation within the field [see eqn. (1)] have been experimentally confirmed.[27,29-31]

The linear dependence of a magnetically-induced blood flow potential on vessel diameter, as shown in eqn. (1), leads to the prediction that these potentials should have greater magnitudes in humans than in the smaller animal species that have been studied in the laboratory. This prediction is supported by a calculation based

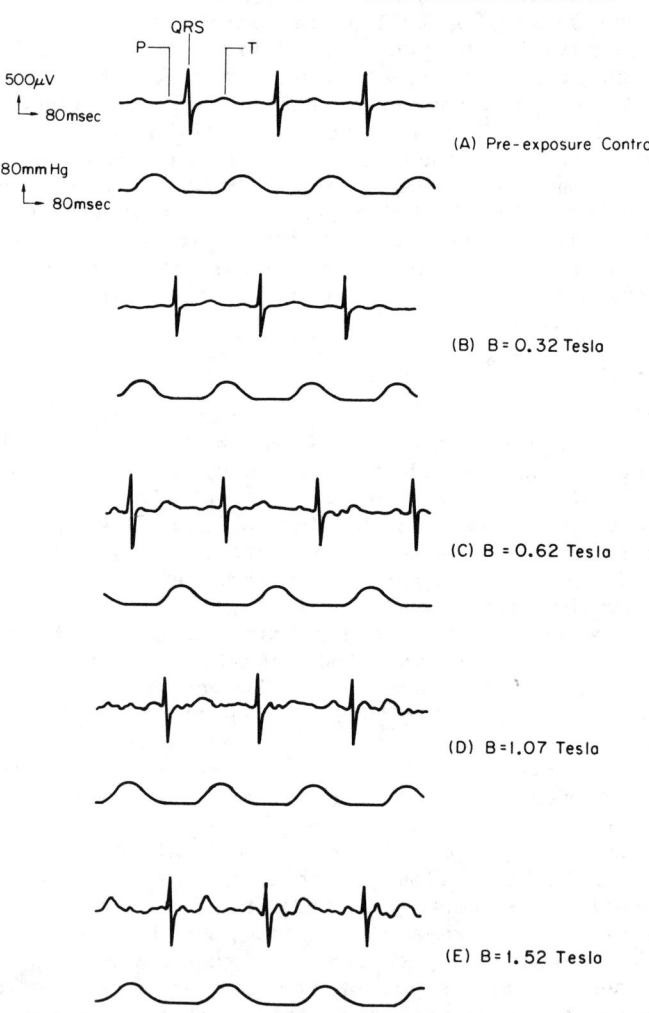

Fig. 1: Electrocardiogram and intraarterial blood pressure records are shown for a Macaca monkey exposed to uniform static magnetic fields up to 1.5 T. The ECG clearly demonstrates the increase in signal amplitude at the locus of the T-wave during magnetic field exposure. No measurable change occurred in the intraarterial blood pressure at field levels up to 1.5 T. [Adapted from Fig. 1 of ref. 30.]

on eqn. (1) that the maximum magnitudes of the induced aortic blood flow potentials in a rat and a man placed within a 2 T field should be 0.5 and 13.4 mV, respectively. An increase in the magnitude of magnetically-induced blood flow potentials as a function of animal size has also been demonstrated directly by experimental data obtained for rats, baboons, monkeys and dogs.[14,27-31]

The electrodynamic interaction between a static magnetic field and a flowing conductor such as blood also produces a net volume force within the fluid that is equal to $\vec{J} \times \vec{B}$, where $\vec{J}$ is the ionic conduction current. The hydrodynamic consequence of this electrical force is a reduction in the axial blood flow velocity. From magnetohydrodynamic theory the fractional reduction in blood flow rate can be predicted to a good approximation by the equation:[31]

$$\frac{v(B=0) - v(B)}{v(B=0)} = \frac{R^2 B^2 \sigma}{4\eta} \qquad (2)$$

where R is the vessel radius and σ and η are, respectively, the electrical conductivity and kinematic viscosity of blood. From eqn. (2) the estimated reduction in aortic blood flow rate for a man in static fields of 1 T and 5 T is about 1% and 7%, respectively. In accord with theoretical predictions, less than a 1% reduction in aortic blood flow rate was observed in direct laboratory measurements on 9 adult rats exposed to a 1.5 T field.[31] Also, as demonstrated by the intraarterial blood pressure measurements shown in Fig. 1, no hemodynamic alterations were observed during the exposure of three Macaca monkeys to a 1.5 T field.[30] Contrary to earlier speculations,[32-34] the extent to which magnetohydrodynamic interactions alter blood flow dynamics is therefore expected to be minimal even in relatively large magnetic fields.

Another important physiological process that is potentially sensitive to electrodynamic interactions with static magnetic fields is the conduction of nerve impulses. Simple theoretical calculations, however, demonstrate that the interaction of a magnetic field with the ionic currents in an axonal membrane is extremely weak.[35,36] For example, it has been estimated that a magnetic field in excess of 24 T would be required to produce a Lorentz force on nerve ionic currents equal to one tenth the force they experience from the electric field of the nerve membrane.[35] The absence of a measurable interaction of a 2 T static field with the ionic currents of an isolated sciatic nerve is demonstrated by the action potential recordings shown in Fig. 2. In other studies with isolated nerves, fields of 1.2-2.0 T applied in either a parallel or perpendicular configuration relative to the nerve axis have been found to have no influence on the amplitude or conduction velocity of evoked action potentials.[37-39] Static magnetic fields were also found to have no effect on other bioelectric properties of sciatic nerves, including the threshold for nerve excitation and the duration of the absolute and the relative refractory periods that follow the passage of an action potential.[39]

<u>Magnetomechanical effects</u>. Macromolecules with a high degree of magnetic anisotropy will rotate in a static magnetic field and reach an equilibrium orientation that represents a minimum energy state.

In general, these macromolecules have a rodlike shape and magneto-orientation occurs as a result of anisotropy of the magnetic susceptibility tensor along the different axes of symmetry. The total interaction energy with the field, U, is obtained by integrating the tensorial product of the magnetic flux density, B, and the magnetic moment per unit volume, M, over the molecular volume, V. The resulting expression for U is:[13]

$$U = - VB^2[\chi_z + (\chi_z - \chi_r)\cos^2\Theta]/2\mu_o \qquad (3)$$

where χ_z and χ_r are the axial and radial components of the magnetic susceptibility, Θ is the angle between the direction of the field and the z axis, μ_o is the magnetic permeability of free space ($\mu_o = 1$ in CGS units and $4\pi \times 10^{-7}$ N/A^2 in MKS units). Because the rodlike

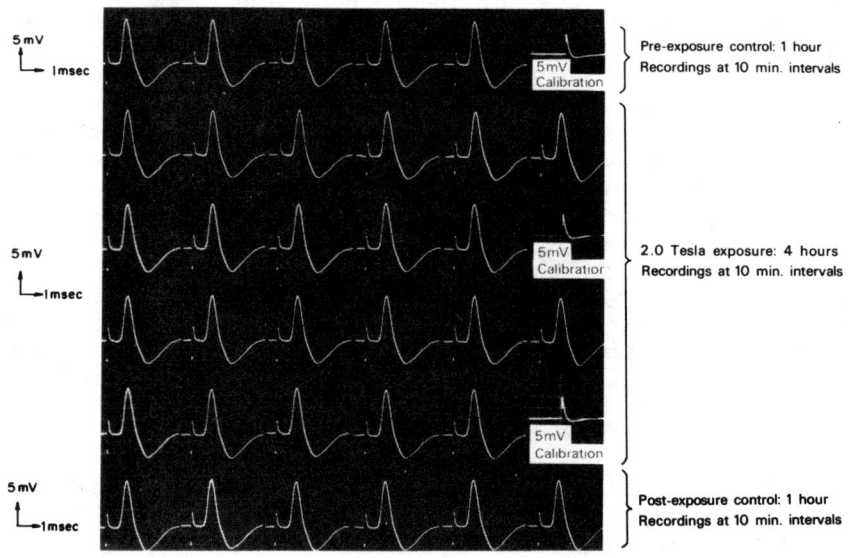

Fig. 2: Evoked action potentials in a frog sciatic nerve are shown before, during and after a 4-hr exposure to a uniform static 2.0-T field. The nerve axis was oriented parallel to the magnetic field lines, and there was no significant variation in the 20-mV amplitude of the maximal action potential during exposure to the field. [Adapted from Fig. 1 of ref. 39.]

molecules will rotate in the field to achieve a minimum energy, then the equilibrium orientation will be at $\Theta = 0$ or π if $\chi_z > \chi_r > 0$ (paramagnetic molecules) or $\chi_r < \chi_z < 0$ (diamagnetic molecules). The equilibrium orientation will be at $\Theta = \pi/2$ if $\chi_r > \chi_z > 0$ (paramagnetic) or $\chi_z < \chi_r < 0$ (diamagnetic).

For individual macromolecules of biological importance, the magnetic interaction energy given by eqn. (3) is small compared to the thermal energy, kT, where k is Boltzmann's constant and T is the absolute temperature. As a result, the extent of orientation of individual molecules in strong magnetic fields is very small. For example, optical birefringence measurements on calf thymus DNA in solution have demonstrated that a field of 13 T is required to produce orientation of 1% of the molecules.[40] In contrast, there are several examples of macromolecular assemblies that can be oriented in fields of 1 T or less. These assemblies behave as structurally coupled units in which the summed magnetic anisotropy is large, thus giving rise to a large magnetic interaction energy. Examples of molecular aggregates that orient in fields of 1 T or less include retinal rod outer segments,[41-47] muscle fibers,[48] photosynthetic systems (chloroplast grana, photosynthetic bacteria and Chlorella cells),[49-53] and purple membranes of Halobacteria.[54] Although the magneto-orientation of biologically important structures such as retinal rods can be demonstrated by optical techniques when these units are suspended in an aqueous medium, the implications of this effect for visual functions in vivo is unclear. As discussed in a later section of this chapter, there is no experimental evidence that the visual apparatus of mammals is influenced by static fields up to 2 T. It is likely that a magnetic orientational torque has little influence on the strong structural matrix in which retinal rods are embedded within the intact retina.

There are also biological examples of cellular structures with permanent magnetic moments in which significant magnetic orientational effects occur. One example is the magnetotactic bacterium,[55] in which approximately 2% of the dry mass is iron contained in magnetite (Fe_3O_4) crystals.[56] These bacteria require a low oxygen tension for survival, and their net magnetic moments interact with the geomagnetic field to produce a downward directed motion that carries them into the bottom sediments of their aquatic environment. This fascinating survival mechanism requires that there be opposite polarities of the magnetic moments of these bacteria in the northern and southern hemispheres, and this feature of magnetotactic bacteria has been confirmed experimentally.[55,57,58]

Another example of an intact cell that can be oriented magnetically is the deoxygenated sickled erythrocyte. It has been shown that these cells, in which the deoxygenated hemoglobin is paramagnetic, will align in a 0.35 T field with the long axis of the sickled cell oriented perpendicular to the magnetic flux lines.[59] This equilibrium orientation results from the stacking of the planar haem moieties parallel to the long axis of the sickled erythrocyte, with the net magnetic moment oriented perpendicular to the long axis.

Another type of magnetomechanical interaction is the translation of paramagnetic and ferromagnetic substances in static magnetic field spatial gradients. Denoting the magnetic susceptibility as χ and the volume as V, the force, F(z), experienced in a linear magnetic field gradient, dB/dz, is equal to the product of the net magnetic moment and the gradient:

$$F(z) = \frac{\chi V B}{\mu_o} (dB/dz) \qquad (4)$$

From simple energetic calculations it can be shown that extremely large magnetic fields and gradients must be used to produce a significant translation of individual paramagnetic molecules. A similar conclusion can be drawn for large collections of paramagnetic molecules such as the deoxyhemoglobin contained within a deoxygenated erythrocyte. This theoretical expectation is supported by experimental observations on the magnetic separation of erythrocytes from whole blood following conversion of the diamagnetic hemoglobin to paramagnetic deoxyhemoglobin. In order to achieve an efficient separation of the cells, they must be attracted to a wire mesh that is highly magnetized in a 2 T field to produce a gradient at the surface which exceeds 10^4 T/m.[60,61] Fields and spatial gradients of this magnitude are seldom encountered by man, even in the vicinity of high-field superconducting magnets.

Magnetic field effects on electronic spin states. There are several classes of organic chemical reactions that can be influenced by static magnetic fields in the range of 10-100 mT as a result of effects on the electronic spin states of the reaction intermediates.[15,62,63] One well-studied example of such reactions which involves an important biological process is the photo-induced charge transfer reaction in bacterial photosynthesis.[64-69] This reaction involves a radical pair intermediate state through which electron transfer occurs to the ultimate acceptor molecule, a ubiquinone-iron complex. Under natural conditions the electron transfer occurs within 200 picosec following flash excitation of the bacteriochlorophyll. However, chemical reduction of the acceptor molecules extends the lifetime of the intermediate state to about 10 nanosec. With an extended lifetime, the singlet state of the radical pair intermediate evolves into a triplet state via the hyperfine mechanism. However, in the presence of an external magnetic field greater than approximately 10 mT, the triplet channels are blocked and the resulting yield of triplet product is expected to decrease by two thirds. This predicted blocking of triplet channels by a weak magnetic field has been confirmed experimentally using laser pulse excitation and optical absorption measurements.[67] Although these observations may have implications for naturally occurring biological processes, it should be emphasized that the magnetic field effects studied to date occur only when the photosynthetic system is placed in an abnormal state by chemical reduction of the electron acceptor molecules.

Static Magnetic Fields - Laboratory Studies

Several species of marine animals and various lower life forms possess an inherent sensitivity to static magnetic fields with intensities as low as that of the geomagnetic field, i.e., approximately 50 µT. It has been established experimentally that weak magnetic fields influence direction finding by elasmobranch fish[17-20] and the orientation and swimming direction of magnetotactic bacteria.[55-58] As discussed in the preceding section, the biophysical mechanisms underlying the magnetic field sensitivity of these organisms are well understood. In addition, evidence has been presented that the kinetic movements of mollusks,[70] the waggle dance of bees,[71] and migratory patterns of birds[72-75] are all influenced by weak static fields. The precise mechanism underlying the magnetic field sensitivity of these species has not been determined, although magnetomechanical effects leading to the stimulation of sensory receptors may be involved since small deposits of magnetite have been found in the tooth denticles of mollusks,[76,77] the abdominal region of bees,[78] and the cranium of pigeons.[79,80]

Studies of static magnetic field interactions with higher organisms have produced numerous contradictory findings, and the only effect that is well established at the present time is the induction of electrical potentials in the central circulatory system. Several detailed reviews of the literature on static magnetic field bioeffects have been published by the authors,[4,7,14] in which a number of examples were cited of recent experimental results that contradicted earlier claims of significant magnetic field effects at the cellular and animal levels. Several examples of the disparity between early and recent findings include: (1) the report[81] of cell transformation resulting from exposure to a 0.5 T field at 4 °K was shown to be an artifact resulting from unconventional culture techniques;[82] (2) numerous reports of alterations induced by static magnetic fields in the metabolism, respiration, and growth properties of normal and tumor cells[83-93] have not been successfully replicated;[94-102] (3) genetic and developmental changes in several animal species and lower organisms exposed to magnetic fields[84,103-116] have not been observed in more recent studies;[117-126] (4) adverse effects of static magnetic fields on sensitive target tissues such as the hematologic, immunologic and endocrine systems[85,86,127-149] have not been found in several recent studies;[150-153] (5) several reports of magnetic field effects on physiological regulation and circadian timing[154-161] have not been confirmed in carefully controlled studies with rodents.[14,162-164] One recent example of an effect that could not be replicated in another laboratory is the report that thermoregulation in rodents is influenced by strong magnetic field gradients.[165,166]

During the past decade a significant number of studies have been reported in which the bioeffects of static magnetic fields were examined under well-controlled laboratory conditions, including the use of precise dosimetry, large numbers of experimental subjects, quantitative biochemical and physiological end points, and careful attention to environmental conditions other than the magnetic field that could influence the experimental outcome. Based on this body of literature, the following important biological processes appear not to be influenced by static magnetic fields at levels up to approximately 2 T: (1) cell growth and morphology;[82,94-102] (2) DNA structure and gene expression,[120-123,125,126] (3) reproduction and development (pre- and post-natal),[118,119,124] (4) bioelectric properties of isolated neurons,[37-39] (5) animal behavior,[167] (6) visual response to photic stimulation,[168] (7) cardiovascular dynamics (acute exposures),[29,30] (8) hematological indices,[150-152,162] (9) immune responsiveness,[153] (10) physiological regulation and circadian rhythms.[14,162-164]

Although there is an increasing database which suggests that mammals experience no adverse effects from exposure to fields up to 2 T, additional research is needed in several key areas. These include: (1) studies of cardiovascular performance in mammals exposed chronically to magnetic field levels that induce electrical potentials on the order of 1 mV or larger within the central circulatory system: (2) electroencephalographic measurements of evoked and non-evoked electrical activity in the central nervous system, which has previously been reported to exhibit both excitatory and inhibitory responses to static magnetic fields;[169-172] (3) additional studies are needed to clarify whether adrenergic and cholinergic hormonal responses occur in exposed animals;[146-148] (4) cellular, tissue and animal studies will be required to assess the effects of static magnetic fields at the high intensities of 2 to 10 T that have been proposed for use in NMR in vivo spectroscopy.

TIME-VARYING MAGNETIC FIELDS

Interaction Mechanisms

The primary physical interaction of time-varying magnetic fields with living systems is the induction of electric fields and currents in tissue. In accord with Faraday's law of induction, the relationship between the induced electric field intensity, $\vec{E}$, and the time rate of change of the magnetic flux density is given by the equation:

$$\oint \vec{E} \cdot \vec{d\ell} = - d/dt \iint \vec{B} \cdot \vec{dS} \tag{5}$$

In eqn. (5) the line integral is around a closed curve and $\vec{d\ell}$ is a differential element of length along the curve; $\vec{B}$ is the magnetic flux density and $\vec{dS}$ is a differential surface area element directed normal to the surface enclosed by the curve over which the line integral is taken. For the specific case of a circular loop with radius R intersected by a spatially uniform, time-varying magnetic field orthogonal to the loop, eqn. (5) gives for the magnitude of the average electric field tangent to the loop surface:

$$E = (R/2)\frac{dB}{dt} \tag{6}$$

If the magnetic field is sinusoidal with a frequency υ, then

$$E = \pi \upsilon R B \tag{7}$$

From Ohm's law, the current density, $\vec{J}$, induced in tissue with an average conductivity σ is given by

$$\vec{J} = \sigma \vec{E} \tag{8}$$

The rate of energy dissipation in tissue per unit time, P, is equal to:

$$P = \vec{J} \cdot \vec{E} = \sigma E^2 \tag{9}$$

The metric units of B, E, J and P are Tesla, V/m, A/m^2 and W/m^3, respectively.

Electrical potentials can also be induced magnetically by fields that are static, i.e., not varying in time. One example is the induction of potentials in a moving electrolytic conductor such as blood, which was discussed earlier in this chapter. A magnetically-induced potential can also result from the application of a static field when the area linked by the lines of magnetic flux changes as a function of time. From eqn. (5) the resulting potential ϕ can be estimated as:[29]

$$\phi \approx Bf\Delta S \tag{10}$$

where ΔS is the area change and f is the frequency of motion leading to the change in area and magnetic flux linkage. This type of induced potential results from changes in the area of the chest during breathing, and can be detected in the ECG of animals placed in extremely high fields. The magnitude of ϕ is small, typically being less than 25% of the magnitude of the induced aortic blood flow potential.[29]

Various physical characteristics of time-varying magnetic fields are of importance in assessing their biological effects, including the fundamental field frequency, the maximum and average flux density, the presence of harmonic frequencies, and the waveform and polarity of the signal. Several types of waveforms have been used in biological research with ELF magnetic fields, including sinusoidal, square-wave, and pulsed waveforms. Two characteristics that are of key importance in analyzing the effects of square-wave and pulsed fields are the rise and decay times, which determine the maximum time rate of change of the field and hence the maximum instantaneous current densities induced in tissue.

Time-Varying Magnetic Fields -- Laboratory Studies

Four levels of biological effects from time-varying magnetic fields can be defined on the basis of the electrical currents induced in living tissues: (1) fields that induce current densities above 1 A/m^2 in tissue can be expected to produce rapid, irreversible effects such as cardiac fibrillation; (2) fields inducing current densities above 10 mA/m^2 lead to reversible visual effects (magnetophosphenes and changes in visually evoked potentials) during acute exposures; (3) the chronic application of fields that induce current densities in the range of 10-100 mA/m^2 can produce irreversible alterations in the biochemistry and physiology of cells and organized tissues, an example being the effects of bidirectional pulsed fields used to facilitate bone fracture reunion; (4) fields that induce current densities less than approximately 1-10 mA/m^2, which is the range of endogeneous current densities present in organs such as the brain and heart,[173,174] lead to few (if any) biological effects irrespective of the exposure duration.

<u>Neuromuscular stimulation</u>. In the first class of phenomena described above, direct neuromuscular effects result from large tissue currents induced by a time-varying magnetic field. Several investigators[175-182] have achieved direct neural stimulation using pulsed or sinusoidal magnetic fields that induced tissue current densities in the range of 1-10 A/m^2. In one study involving electromyographic recordings from the human arm,[181] it was found that a pulsed field with dB/dt greater than 10^4 T/sec was required to stimulate the median nerve trunk. The duration of the magnetic stimulus has also been found to be an important parameter in the excitation of nerve and nerve-muscle preparations. Using a 20 kHz sinusoidal field applied in bursts of 0.5 to 50 msec duration, Öberg[178] found that a progressive increase in the magnetic flux density was required to stimulate the frog gastrocnemius neuromuscular preparation when the burst duration was reduced to less than 2-5 msec. A similar rise in threshold stimulus strength has been observed for frog neuromuscular stimulation using pulsed magnetic fields with pulse durations less than approximately 1 msec.[179,182]

The threshold current density required to produce ventricular fibrillation has been studied in several species of laboratory animals in which large currents were induced by sinusoidal voltages applied through contact electrodes.[183-194] From these data it can be estimated that the threshold current density required to produce ventricular fibrillation in the human heart is in the range of 2-10 A/m^2. For sinusoidal voltages, the minimum threshold current densities were observed in the frequency range of 20-200 Hz.[184] In experiments with dog hearts subjected to 60 Hz voltage stimuli it was found that the threshold current required to elicit fibrillation increased by a factor of approximately 140 as the stimulus duration was decreased from 1.6 sec to 16 msec.[189] Dalziel[195] has estimated that the stimulus strength producing cardiac fibrillation varies as the reciprocal square root of the shock duration over the range of exposure times from 8 msec to 5 sec.

The thresholds for several other forms of neuromuscular effects in laboratory animals and man, including the stimulation of seizures, extrasystoles and respiratory tetanus, have been estimated. From electroshock studies in humans it has been estimated that a current density of 30 A/m^2 must be induced for 300 msec to produce convulsive seizures.[196] The threshold current density for stimulation of extrasystoles was found in studies with guinea pig hearts to be 3-5 times lower than the threshold for eliciting ventricular fibrillation.[192,193] However, a prolonged stimulation of extrasystoles was found to ultimately lead to ventricular fibrillation. Based on limited studies with humans, it can be estimated that the threshold stimulus required to produce respiratory tetanus is approximately 10-15 times less than that which produces ventricular fibrillation.[197-199] This estimate suggests that induced current densities in the range of 0.15 - 1.0 A/m^2 could produce tetanic contractions of the muscles involved in breathing.

It is important to note that extremely large values of the magnetic flux density are required to elicit stimulatory effects on the neuromuscular system of animals when sinusoidal waveforms are used. As an example, consider a 60-Hz field that is axially incident on a circular loop of tissue with R = 0.06 m and σ = 0.2 S/m, comparable to the human heart. From eqns. (7) and (8) it can be calculated that the magnetic flux density must be 0.88 T to induce a current density of 2 A/m^2, which is the estimated lower threshold for inducing ventricular fibrillation. The corresponding time rate of change of the magnetic field and the induced electric field intensity are 330 T/sec and 9.95 V/m, respectively. ELF magnetic fields with this magnitude and time variation are seldom, if ever, encountered by man. However, some caution must be taken in assessing the effects of time-varying magnetic fields on potentially sensitive neuromuscular substrates, such as pacemaker cells. In a study with pacemaker neurons from the Aplysia abdominal ganglion, Wachtel[200] demonstrated that an ELF field with a frequency synchronized to the endogenous neuronal firing rate could alter the membrane electrical activity when the induced current density in the extracellular medium exceeded 20 mA/m^2.

Magnetophosphenes and other visual phenomena. One of the most extensively studied effects of time-varying magnetic fields is the induction of a flickering illumination within the visual field known as magnetophosphenes.[201-213] This phenomenon occurs as an immediate response to stimulation by either pulsed or sinusoidal magnetic fields with frequencies less than 100 Hz, and the effect is completely reversible with no apparent influence on visual acuity. The maximum visual sensitivity to sinusoidal magnetic fields has been found at a frequency of 20 Hz in human subjects with normal vision.[210] At this frequency the threshold magnetic field intensity required to elicit phosphenes is approximately 10 mT, as shown in Fig. 3. The corresponding time rate of change of the field is 1.26 T/sec. In studies with pulsed fields having a rise time of 2 msec and a repetition rate of 15 Hz, the threshold values of dB/dt for eliciting phosphenes ranged from 1.3 to 1.9 T/sec in five adult subjects.[213] There was a trend in the data which suggested that the threshold was lower among younger subjects. In related studies it was also observed that the stimulus duration is an important parameter, since pulses of 0.9 msec duration with dB/dt = 12 T/sec did not evoke phosphenes.

Several types of experimental evidence indicate that the magnetic field interaction leading to magnetophosphenes occurs in the retina: (1) magnetophosphenes are produced by time-varying magnetic fields applied in the region of the eye, and not by fields directed toward the visual cortex in the occipital region of the brain;[205] (2) pressure on the eyeball abolishes sensitivity to magnetophosphenes;[205] (3) the threshold magnetic field intensity required to elicit magnetophosphenes in human subjects with defects in color vision was found to have a different dependence on the field frequency than that observed for subjects with normal color vision;[210] (4) in a patient in whom both eyes had been removed as the result of severe glaucoma, phosphenes could not be induced by time-varying magnetic fields, thereby precluding the possibility that magnetophosphenes can be initiated directly in the visual pathways of the brain.[210]

Although experimental evidence has clearly implicated the retina as the site of magnetic field action leading to phosphenes, it is not as yet resolved whether the photoreceptors or the neuronal elements of the retina are the sensitive substrates that respond to the field. In a series of experiments on in vitro frog retinal preparations, extracellular electrical recordings were made from the ganglion cell layer of the retina immediately following termination of exposure to a 20-Hz, 60-mT field.[211] It was found that the average latency time for response of the ganglion cells to a photic stimulus increased by

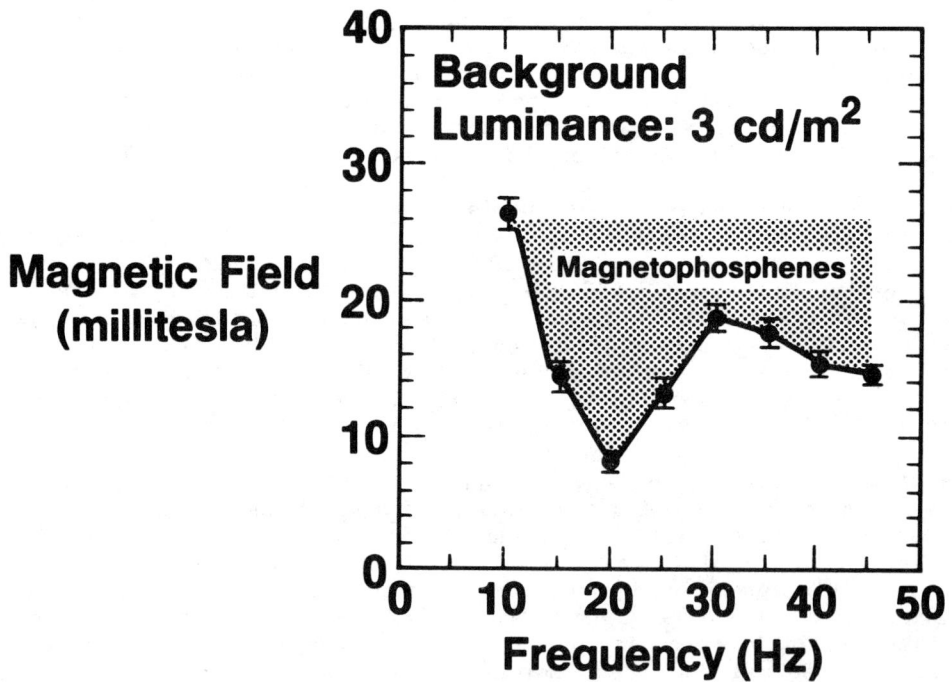

Fig. 3: Threshold values of the magnetic flux density required to elicit magnetophosphenes are plotted as a function of the field frequency. Each data point represents the mean value ± 1 S.E. for 10 volunteers, all of whom were studied with a background white light level of 3 cd/m^2. [Adapted from Fig. 3 of ref. 207.]

5 msec ($p < 0.05$) in the presence of the magnetic field. In addition, the ganglion cells that exhibited electrical activity during photic stimulation ("on" cells) ceased their activity during magnetic field stimulation (i.e., they became "off" cells). The converse behavior of ganglion cells was also observed. These observations indicate that stimulation of the retina by light and by a time-varying magnetic field elicits responses in similar postsynaptic neural pathways.

Several other phenomena related to the sensitivity of the visuosensory system to time-varying magnetic fields have also been studied. In experiments with human subjects it was found that distinct flickering could be elicited in the visual field by sinusoidal magnetic fields in the frequency range 5-60 Hz.[214] The threshold field intensity varied with the field frequency and background light level, but was as low as 5 mT under optimal conditions. Alterations in visually evoked potentials (VEP) have also been reported to occur in sinusoidal ELF magnetic fields at intensity levels that are 5-10 times greater than those which produce magnetophosphenes.[214] The change in VEP is characterized by a reversal of polarity and a decreased amplitude of the three major evoked potentials. These effects were observed within 3 min following onset of the magnetic field exposure, and the VEP returned to normal only after a recovery period of approximately 30-70 min following termination of the exposure. The relationship of these changes in the VEP to the mechanism of magnetophosphene induction is not clear from the evidence that is presently available.

<u>Effects on cellular, tissue and animal systems</u>. A large number of reports have appeared in the literature on the biochemical, physiological and behavioral effects of time-varying magnetic fields in the ELF frequency range.[167,215-284] The information gained in these studies is in many cases difficult to interpret for several reasons: (1) A wide range of field intensities, frequencies, waveforms, and exposure durations have been used. Many of the earlier studies utilized sinusoidal ELF magnetic fields, but recent research has focused increasingly on the effects of pulsed fields with complex waveforms. (2) Few of the findings of positive bioeffects have been verified by independent replication in different laboratories. (3) A number of apparent inconsistencies can be found among the reported behavioral and physiological effects of time-varying magnetic fields. For example, behavioral alterations were observed in a majority of studies with animals exposed to ELF sinusoidal fields that induced maximum current densities of less than 1 mA/m^2 in the cranium.[269-277] In contrast, no effects were noted in several behavioral studies conducted with magnetic fields that induced maximum intracranial current densities of 1 mA/m^2 or larger.[167,222,278-283] Another example of contradictory data are the reports that exposure to a low-intensity ELF magnetic field produced an elevation in serum triglyceride levels in human subjects,[221] but comparable effects were not observed in monkeys.[222]

Although many uncertainties exist in the interpretation of the existing laboratory data on the cellular, tissue and animal effects of time-varying magnetic fields, there is increasing evidence that several biochemical and physiological properties of cells and organized tissues are altered. Briefly summarized, these biological effects include: (1) altered cell growth rate,[229,233,241,245,246,266] (2) decreased rate of cellular respiration,[241-243] (3) altered metabolism of carbohydrates, proteins and nucleic acids,[228,231,236,237,243,248,256,263,264,268] (4) effects on gene expression and genetic regulation of cell functions,[240,251,259] (5) teratological and developmental effects,[219,220,250,261,262] (6) morphological and other nonspecific tissue changes in adult animals, frequently reversible with time following exposure,[216,223,247,249,252,255] (7) endocrine alterations,[217,224,230,232,236,249] (8) altered hormonal responses of cells and tissues, including effects on cell surface receptors,[254,257,260,265] (9) altered immune response to antigens and lectins.[215,225,258]

The results of these studies have been summarized schematically in Fig. 4, in which the observations of bioeffects from exposure to time-varying magnetic fields have been grouped according to estimates of the maximum value of dB/dt and the maximum induced current density in the target tissues that were examined. It is evident that alterations were observed at the cellular and tissue levels in the majority of studies in which the induced current densities exceeded 1 mA/m^2, which is a level typical of the endogenous current densities within living tissues. It should be noted in particular that the investigations in which either square waveforms or pulsed fields that induced tissue current densities greater than 10 mA/m^2 led to findings of positive bioeffects.[240,245,250,251,254,256-263,265,268] The suggestion has been made that these fields may exert electrochemical effects at the cell surface.[254,260] Such effects, in turn, could influence hormone-receptor interactions, adenylate cyclase activity, and the membrane transport and intracellular concentration of calcium ions. These membrane functions have been shown to exert a major influence on cellular metabolism and growth dynamics.

Several investigations using bidirectional pulsed magnetic fields have shown an enhanced synthesis of collagen, decreased intracellular cAMP, and altered synthesis of cell surface glycoproteins in cultures of fibroblasts and bone-forming cells.[256,263,265,268,284] These findings suggest biochemical and biophysical mechanisms through which the stimulation of bone growth may occur in response to pulsed magnetic fields. Beginning in the early 1970's, several clinical reports have indicated that the use of pulsed magnetic fields with repetition frequencies in the ELF range may provide an effective, noninvasive procedure for the treatment of bone nonunions and pseudoarthroses via electrical stimulation.[285-291] Current densities of approximately 20 mA/m^2 can be induced in bone by the pulsed field applicators that are presently used for fracture therapy.[16,292] Although the initial clinical trials yielded success rates up to 85% in achieving bone fracture reunion via magnetic stimulation, a recent report has suggested that prolonged immobilization of a patient wearing the magnetic field applicator may also be an important factor contributing to the success of this procedure.[293]

Time-Varying Magnetic Fields – Cell, Tissue and Animal Studies

- Magnetophosphene and behavioral studies excluded
- Combined electric and magnetic field experiments excluded
- Complete description of field and exposure conditions required
- Quantitative physiological and/or biochemical end points required

dB/dt (T/s)	Findings (+)	Findings (−)
<1	6	8
1→3	3	1
3→20	25	1
>20	9	1

J_{max} (mA/m^2)	Findings (+)	Findings (−)
<1	5	6
1→10	8	2
10→20	10	3
>20	20	0

Positive Effects Reported:
- Altered cell growth rate
- Decreased cellular respiration
- Effects on gene expression
- Developmental effects
- Altered immune response
- Endocrine alterations
- Altered metabolism of carbohydrates, nucleic acids and proteins

Mammalian systems:	42/54
Non-mammalian systems:	12/54
In vivo studies:	32/54
In vitro studies:	22/54
Sinusoidal fields:	39/54
Square-wave fields:	3/54
Pulsed fields:	12/54

Fig. 4. Experimental observations on the bioeffects of time-varying magnetic fields in the ELF frequency range are summarized on the basis of the estimated maximum values of dB/dt and induced current density in the exposed samples. The literature database used in preparing this summary is from refs. 215-268. Criteria employed in the selection of literature are stated at the top, and several of the observed bioeffects are listed on the right side of the figure. A summary is given at the bottom of the general characteristics of the biological systems studied and the magnetic field waveforms that were tested.

RADIOFREQUENCY FIELDS

Interaction Mechanisms

An established mechanism through which RF radiation produces direct cellular and tissue effects is through heating. As discussed in the following section, various nonthermal effects of RF radiation have also been reported. However, controversy still exists in regard to direct biological effects from induced currents and polarization effects (dipole orientation) produced by RF fields with incident power densities sufficiently low that no measurable temperature rise occurs in the exposed tissue.

In the RF frequency range below 100 MHz that is presently used in medical NMR, approximately 90% or more of the absorbed energy results from tissue currents induced by the magnetic component of the field.[294,295] The total energy dissipation is a function of the frequency, RF incident power density, exposure duration, coupling between the RF coil and the specimen, and several properties of the exposed tissue, including conductivity, dielectric constant, specific gravity, size, and orientation relative to the field polarization. Tissue heating is also influenced by the rate of heat loss via thermal conduction and convection mechanisms in the exposed subject.

Under the near-field geometric conditions present in NMR imaging devices, the energy dissipation is best expressed in terms of the specific absorption rate in W/kg, as opposed to the incident power density in W/m^2, which is commonly used for far-field (Fraunhofer) irradiation conditions. The specific absorption rate, SAR, is related to the average induced electric field, $E/\sqrt{2}$, the tissue conductivity, σ, the tissue density, ρ, and the duty cycle, D, of the applied RF field by the equation:

$$\text{SAR} = \frac{\sigma E^2 D}{2\rho} \tag{11}$$

The duty cycle $D = \tau/\delta$, where τ is the pulse duration and δ is the pulse repetition interval. Because the magnetic component of the field is dominant in the low range of RF frequencies used for medical NMR, the induced electric field can be calculated for a circular loop of tissue of radius R using eqn. (7), in which B is now understood to be the magnetic component of the RF field. In addition, the rotating component of the field, B_1, must satisfy the Larmor resonance condition. For a rectangular $\pi/2$ pulse,

$$B_1 = \frac{\pi}{2\gamma\tau} \tag{12}$$

where γ is the gyromagnetic ratio (expressed as an angular frequency in units of Hz/Tesla). Noting that $B = 2B_1$ for conversion from a linear to a rotating field, and using eqns. (7) and (12), the SAR given by eqn. (11) becomes:

$$\text{SAR} = \frac{\pi^4 \sigma \nu^2 R^2}{2\gamma^2 \rho \tau \delta} \tag{13}$$

For proton NMR, the SAR in MKS units of W/kg is given by:

$$SAR = \frac{(6.80 \times 10^{-16})\sigma \upsilon^2 R^2}{\rho \tau \delta} \qquad (14)$$

If the flip angle is π, the SAR is 4 times greater than the value given by eqn. (14). The SAR for an arbitrary flip angle, Θ, can be calculated from eqn. (14) using the multiplicative factor $4\Theta^2/\pi^2$. It is important to note for calculational purposes that the appropriate units of the parameters in eqn. (14) are σ = S/m, υ = Hz, R = m, ρ = kg/m^3 and τ and δ = sec.

The SAR predicted by eqn. (14) is plotted for a human torso model with R = 0.17 m in Fig. 5. The SAR at frequencies from 1 to 100 MHz is presented as a double logarithmic plot with $\tau \cdot \delta = \tau^2/D$ as the abscissa. It is evident that the SAR increases as the pulse repetition interval (δ) decreases and/or the duty cycle (D) increases. At 30 MHz the SAR in the torso model equals the average body basal metabolic rate (in the resting condition) when τ^2/D is approximately 10^{-5} sec^2. The quadratic dependence of the SAR on the loop radius as shown in eqn. (13) has been confirmed experimentally.[296,297]

It should be noted that the SAR given by eqn. (13) represents the peak surface SAR since the attenuation of the RF magnetic field in tissue is neglected. By comparing the results of SAR calculations using this simplified model with the results of a more precise calculation in which attenuation effects were taken into account,[294] Bottomley and Edelstein[298] concluded that eqn. (13) overestimates the true SAR by about 30% at frequencies in the range of 30 - 100 MHz. At lower frequencies a substantially better agreement is achieved.

The average SAR in a three-dimensional element of tissue can be obtained from a volume integration of the surface SAR for simple geometries such as spheres and cylinders with an axial orientation relative to the incident RF field. By this procedure it can be shown[299] that the average SAR in spherical and cylindrical elements of tissue are, respectively, 0.4 and 0.5 times the surface SAR predicted from eqn. (13).

Experimental measurements of SAR have been performed using a number of techniques, including infrared thermography and direct temperature measurements both in living specimens and in phantoms filled with saline or tissue-equivalent materials.[300-307] To determine the SAR associated with the RF fields used in medical NMR, the simplest method is to measure the change in Q (quality factor) of the coil upon introduction of the specimen.[308] For an unloaded coil, $Q_o = 2\pi \upsilon_o L/R_o$, where L and R_o are, respectively, the coil inductance and resistance. The effective resistance, R_s, which the presence of a sample adds to the resistance of the coil is equal to:

$$R_s = 2\pi \upsilon_o L(1/Q_s - 1/Q_o) \qquad (15)$$

In eqn. (15) Q_s is the Q value of the coil with the specimen in place. Using eqn. (15) the fraction of the applied RF power that is dissipated in the specimen can be calculated from the resistance ratio:

$$\frac{R_s}{R_s + R_o} = 1 - Q_s/Q_o \qquad (16)$$

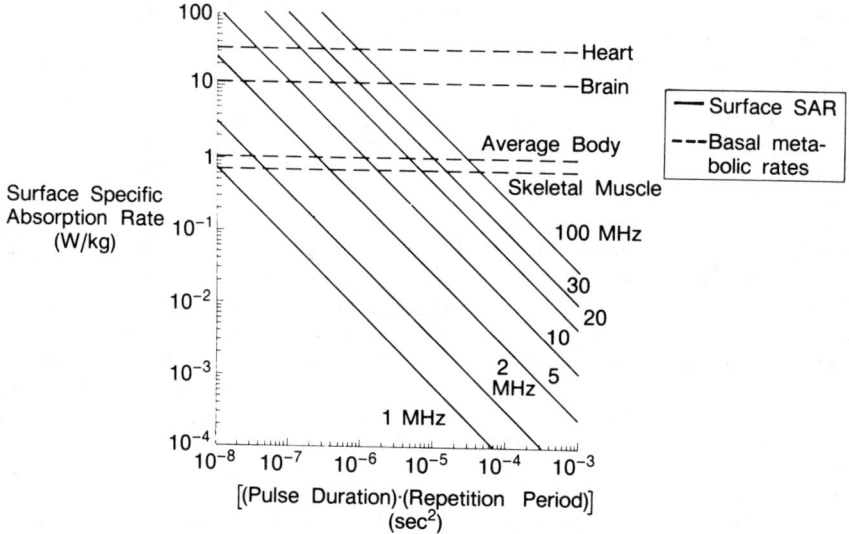

Fig. 5: The peak surface SAR in a human torso model is plotted as a function of the pulse duration (τ) times the pulse repetition interval (δ). Curves calculated from eqn. (14) in the text using conductivity values for muscle tissue are shown for RF field frequencies ranging from 1-100 MHz. Also shown are average basal metabolic rates for the whole body, skeletal muscle, brain and heart. [Adapted from Fig. 3 of ref. 298.]

A calculation of SAR can then be made using eqn. (16) in combination with information on the RF pulse characteristics and the specimen size.

A direct calculation of the expected temperature rise, ΔT, in tissue exposed to RF radiation for a time t (in sec), can be made from the equation:

$$\Delta T = \frac{(SAR) \cdot t}{C} \qquad (17)$$

where C is the heat capacity expressed in J/kg/°C. It should be noted that eqn. (17) does not include terms to account for heat loss via thermal conduction and convection processes. An average value of the soft tissue heat capacity[306] is 0.83 kcal/kg/°C = 3.47 kJ/kg/°C. In the absence of heat loss mechanisms, eqn. (17) predicts that an SAR of 2 W/kg applied for 10 min would lead to a temperature rise of 0.35 °C. Experiments have been performed by one of the authors (T.F.B.) in which fiberoptic probes were used to determine temperature changes in the stomach and subcutaneous tissues during NMR imaging that produced an SAR at the 2 W/kg level.[309] No temperature change was observed in the stomach during a 10 min exposure, but an elevation occurred in the skin temperature as anticipated from the vasodilation response to thermal stress.

At the frequencies used in medical NMR procedures the deposition of RF energy in tissue is expected to be more uniform than that observed at frequencies above 100 MHz, where "hot spots" are theoretically predicted and experimentally observed.[300,307,310,311] Nevertheless, anisotropy and discontinuities in tissue electrical properties can lead to significant nonuniformities in RF heating profiles at frequencies well below 100 MHz.[312] Consideration must also be given to the local RF heating that can occur because of constrictions in the induced current pathways within anatomically thin regions that are not electrically insulated from large current loops, e.g., regions of ischemic tissue. Recent experiments using lucite and wood phantoms constructed to simulate this conditions have confirmed that geometric constraints on current pathways can produce excessive local heating.[297]

RF Fields -- Laboratory Studies

Thermal effects. Tissue heating from exposure to RF radiation produces a series of physiological responses characteristic of stress, with a resultant onset of thermoregulatory mechanisms mediated through the neuroendocrine and cardiovascular systems.[5,313] Thermosensitivity and thermoregulatory responses are associated both with the hypothalamus and with thermal receptors located in the skin and internal regions of the body.[314,315] Afferent signals reflecting temperature change converge in the central nervous system and modify the activity of the major neuroendocrine control systems, thereby triggering the physiological and behavioral responses necessary for the maintenance of homeostasis. These responses have been studied extensively in several animal species, including rodents, dogs and nonhuman primates. In general, laboratory investigations have been conducted with RF radiation at frequencies significantly higher than those used in NMR devices, and with the subjects irradiated under far-field conditions. Nevertheless, tissue heating resulting from NMR imaging procedures can be expected to elicit a similar set of physiological responses.

Neuroendocrine responses to RF heating have been shown to alter the activity and the complex interactions of the hypothalamic, pituitary, adrenal and thyroid systems. At SAR values in excess of 3 W/kg, plasma corticosterone levels are elevated in rats and this endocrine response is dependent upon ACTH secretion by the pituitary.[316,317] Depressed thyroid hormone levels are observed under similar irradiation conditions, and this response has been associated with an inhibition of secretion of thyrotropin (TSH) by the pituitary.[318-321] In both cases, the alteration in hormone levels is reversible upon termination of the exposure.

Exposure of dogs to RF radiation at SAR values in excess of approximately 4 W/kg has revealed a characteristic pattern of thermoregulatory response in which the body temperature initially increases and then stabilizes following the onset of thermoregulatory mechanisms.[313,322-324] The early phase of this response was found to be accompanied by an increase in blood volume due to withdrawal of fluid from the extracellular space into the circulation, and by increases in heart rate and intraventricular blood pressure. These cardiodynamic changes reflect thermoregulatory responses that facilitate the conduction of heat to the body surface. Prolonged exposure of animals to thermalizing levels of RF radiation ultimately led to failure of these thermoregulatory mechanisms.

Several studies with rodents and monkeys have also demonstrated a behavioral component of thermoregulatory responses. It has been shown that rats will turn on a heat lamp less frequently when exposed to RF radiation at an SAR greater than 1 W/kg,[325] and a similar thermoregulatory behavior is exhibited by squirrel monkeys.[326,327] In these monkeys it has been found that altered thermoregulatory behavior commences when the temperature in the preoptic/anterior hypothalamic area increases by as little as 0.2-0.3 $^\circ$C.[328] This brain region is considered to be the control center for normal thermoregulatory processes, and its activity can be modified in response to a small temperature increase under conditions in which the colonic temperature remains constant.[328]

There have been numerous published reports of physiological and behavioral changes occurring as the result of exposure to RF radiation at levels that produce direct thermal effects. Briefly summarized, several of the cellular, tissue and animal responses that have been studied include: (1) alterations in neural and neuromuscular functions;[329-332] (2) increased blood-brain barrier permeability;[333-339] (3) operant behavioral changes;[340-343] (4) cutaneous thermal perception;[344-347] (5) auditory stimulation resulting from a thermoelastic interaction;[348-353] (6) ocular impairment (lens opacification and corneal abnormalities);[354-359] (7) stress-associated effects on the immune system;[5,360-366] (8) hematological alterations;[5,367-371] (9) effects on reproductive organs;[372-374] (10) teratogenic effects;[375-381] (11) effects on cellular morphology, water and electrolyte content, and plasma membrane properties.[382-393]

Although substantial evidence exists for direct thermal injury to cells and tissues exposed to RF radiation at high intensities, it should be noted that there have been many conflicting reports on the threshold field intensities that elicit effects and the relative potency of pulsed versus continuous wave radiation in many systems. Under conditions where the field frequency, waveform, intensity, and exposure duration are similar, the possibility must be considered that inadequate dosimetry may be the origin of divergent findings of positive and negative biological effects. As one example, there were several early reports of chromosomal alterations and genetic changes in cells exposed to RF radiation,[394-397] whereas subsequent research has not led to similar findings.[398-401] Recent studies with NMR fields at frequencies of 15-30 MHz have also shown no evidence for cytogenetic effects in cellular systems.[125,402-404] As emphasized by Michaelson,[405] variations in the exposure system, specimen sizes, and dosimetry procedures used for cellular samples could be the basis of many differing results described in the literature. He further states that several reported genetic effects from exposure to RF radiation at power levels that were presumed not to produce sample heating may, in fact, have been the consequence of direct thermal damage.

<u>Nonthermal effects.</u> Beginning in the 1950's, an increasing body of evidence has been compiled by scientists in the Soviet Union and Eastern European countries that low-intensity RF fields in the microwave band can produce measurable alterations in the nervous, cardiovascular, endocrine, immune, and reproductive systems of mammals.[406-408] Although many of these reports conflict with data obtained by scientists in the United States and Western Europe, the possible existence of nonthermal effects of RF radiation remains an unresolved issue. As described by McRee,[408] U.S. and U.S.S.R. scientists working in collaboration have confirmed the existence of several metabolic and behavioral effects resulting from the chronic exposure of rats to low-intensity microwaves. There are also numerous examples of biological studies conducted by U.S. and Western European scientists in which nonthermal effects of RF radiation were observed, one example being the alteration of rat brain metabolic parameters.[409-411] Reviews of nonthermal RF radiation effects and possible interaction mechanisms have recently been prepared by Taylor[412] and by Postow and Swicord.[413]

An observation on nonthermal effects that has elicited considerable interest among U.S. scientists is the finding that alterations in calcium-ion binding to nerve cell surfaces occurs as the result of exposure to low-intensity RF radiation that is amplitude-modulated at ELF frequencies. In the first publication describing this effect, Bawin et al.[414] reported that the release of preloaded $^{45}Ca^{++}$ was accelerated by exposure of chick brain hemispheres to an amplitude-modulated 147-MHz field. The maximum increase in the release of calcium ions was 10 to 20 percent relative to control samples, and occurred at an ELF modulation frequency of 16 Hz. This finding was subsequently confirmed by Blackman et al.,[415,416] who further observed that the calcium efflux phenomenon was limited to an intensity window for the RF carrier wave that was centered around 0.8 mW/cm^2. Several other carrier frequencies, including 50, 147 and 450 MHz, have also been studied to assess the presence of intensity windows.[417-420] It was found that the intensity window observed with 16-Hz amplitude modulation of the different RF carrier fields shifted in a manner that gave an identical electric field strength within the exposed brain tissue.

Adey et al.[421] have reported that an increased release of preloaded ^{45}Ca^{++} can be produced in the cerebral cortex of an anesthetized cat by exposure to a 450-MHz field with an intensity of 3 mW/cm^2 and amplitude modulation at 16 Hz. In this in vivo study, no attempt was made to determine the presence of windows of sensitivity in either the frequency or intensity domains.

The observations of windowed phenomena described above have led to a number of interesting theoretical concepts concerning possible origins for nonthermal RF radiation effects,[412,413] and they provide a strong impetus for additional biological studies using RF field intensities that do not produce significant tissue heating. However, the implications of these effects for NMR imaging procedures are not clear at the present time. As demonstrated both in the original research on this subject, and in other recent studies,[422,423] ELF amplitude modulation appears to be essential for producing an RF field effect on calcium ion binding to brain tissue. Differences therefore exist in the waveforms that are effective in producing this effect relative to the RF fields used in present NMR imaging devices.

HUMAN HEALTH STUDIES

Static Magnetic Fields

A clinical study of Soviet workers in the magnet production and machine-building industries was reported by Vyalov.[424] The exposure group consisted of 645 workers whose hands were routinely exposed to static fields of 2 to 5 mT, and whose chest and head were in fields of 0.3 to 0.5 mT under normal working conditions. It was estimated that the magnetic field exposure levels were 10 to 50 times larger than the typical values during 10 to 15 percent of the workday. The control group in this study consisted of 138 supervisors in a machine-building plant who were not in contact with magnets. A number of subjective symptoms were reported among the exposed group, including headache, fatigue, dizziness, unclear vision, noise in the ears, and itching and sweating on the palms of the hands. Edema and desquamation on the palms of the hands were also reported. In addition, minor physiological effects including decreased blood pressure and changes in hematological parameters were noted in the exposed group. These studies were qualitative in nature and no statistical analysis was performed on the clinical data. There was also no effort made to assess the possible effects of stressful environmental factors such as high ambient temperature, airborne metallic particles, or the chemical agents used for degreasing and other procedures.

In contrast to the Soviet study, two recent epidemiological surveys in the United States failed to reveal any significant health effects associated with chronic exposure to static magnetic fields.

Marsh et al.[425] conducted a cross-sectional study on the health data of 320 workers in plants using large electrolytic cells for chemical separation processes. The average static field level in the work environment was 7.6 mT and the maximum field was 14.6 mT. The study included a control group of 186 unexposed workers. Among the exposed group, slight decreases were found in the blood leukocyte count and the percent of monocytes, while a small increase occurred in the lymphocyte percentage. However, the mean value of the white cell count for the exposed group remained within the normal range. There was also a slight tendency for elevated systolic and diastolic blood pressures among the black workers in the study. None of the observed changes in blood pressure or hematologic parameters was considered indicative of a significant adverse effect associated with magnetic field exposure.

A recently completed study characterized the prevalence of disease among 792 workers at U.S. National Laboratories who were exposed occupationally to static magnetic fields.[426] The control group consisted of 792 unexposed workers matched for age, race and socioeconomic status. The range of magnetic field exposures was from 0.5 mT for long durations to 2 T for periods of several hours. No significant increase or decrease in the prevalence of 19 categories of disease was observed in the exposed group relative to the controls. Of the 792 exposed subjects, 198 had experienced exposures of 0.3 T or higher for periods of 1 hour or longer. No difference in the prevalence of disease was found between this subgroup and the remainder of the exposed population or the matched controls. No trends were observed in the health data suggestive of a dose-response relationship.

Milham[427] recently reported that workers exposed to large static magnetic fields in the aluminum industry have an elevated leukemia mortality rate. The percentage mortality ratios (PMR) for all forms of leukemia and for acute leukemia among these workers were compared with general population values determined from 438,000 death records of adult males in the state of Washington during the period 1950-1979. The PMR values for all types of leukemia and for acute leukemia were reported to be 189 and 258, respectively, both of which differed significantly from the no-effect level of 100. Because of the large magnetic fields associated with the aluminum reduction process, which have been measured using a magnetic field personal dosimeter and found to be as high as 57 mT during anode changes on prebake cells,[428] Milham suggested that a correlation may exist between exposure to these fields and leukemogenesis.[427] The excess of leukemias observed in Milham's study was confirmed in a subsequent study involving 21,829 workers in 14 aluminum reduction plants.[429] In this second study, an excess incidence of pancreatic, genitourinary and benign tumors was also found among the aluminum workers.

Although these two epidemiological studies have demonstrated an increased cancer risk for persons directly involved in aluminum production, there is at present no clear evidence to indicate the responsible carcinogenic factors within the work environment. The process used for aluminum reduction creates coal tar pitch volatiles, fluoride fumes, sulfur oxides and carbon dioxide. The presence of hydrocarcon particulates, and perhaps other environmental contaminants, must be taken into account in any attempt to relate magnetic field exposure and increased cancer risk among persons working in the aluminum industry.

Time-Varying Magnetic Fields

Several laboratory studies have been conducted with human subjects exposed to sinusoidally time-varying magnetic fields with frequencies in the ELF range.[221,227,253] None of these investigations have revealed adverse clinical or psychological changes in the exposed subjects. Beischer et al.[221] observed an elevation in serum triglycerides at 24 and 48 hours post-exposure, but the subjects were not fasted prior to blood sampling and the change in triglyceride concentration could have resulted from differences in diet or physical activity. In a subsequent study with rhesus monkeys exposed to similar fields, no change in serum triglyceride concentration was observed.[222] The strongest field used in the various laboratory studies with humans was a 5-mT, 50-Hz field to which subjects were exposed for 4 hours by Sander et al.[253] In this investigation no field-associated changes were observed in serum chemistry, blood cell counts, blood gases and lactate concentration, electrocardiogram, pulse rate, skin temperature, circulating hormones (cortisol, insulin, gastrin, thyroxin), and various neuronal measurements including visually evoked potentials recorded in the electroencephalogram.

Recent concern over the possible health effects of time-varying magnetic fields has been raised by several reports of an apparent correlation between cancer incidence and exposure to power-frequency fields. The first publication on this subject appeared in 1979, and reported a correlation between the incidence of leukemia among children living in the Denver, CO, area and exposure to 60-Hz magnetic fields from high-current primary and secondary wiring configurations in the vicinity of their residences.[430] This finding was followed by 12 additional epidemiological studies during the period 1980-1985. Three of these studies involved the analysis of cancer incidence in relation to residential exposure to power-frequency fields.[431-433] In the other nine studies, cancer incidence was analyzed for groups of individuals in various electrical, electronic and telecommunication occupations.[427,434-441] As summarized in Table I, 11 of the 13 epidemiological surveys conducted to date have shown an apparent correlation between the incidence of various forms of cancer and residential and/or occupational exposure to power-frequency fields. In nearly all cases where a positive finding was obtained, the increased risk of cancer among the exposed group of individuals was small, generally less than a factor of two relative to a control group or the general population.

Despite the large number of positive findings that have been reported, it is not possible to conclude at the present time that a definite association exists between the exposure of individuals to ELF electromagnetic fields and their relative risk of contracting leukemia or other forms of cancer. This uncertainty arises from numerous methodological deficiencies in the epidemiological surveys

Table I. Epidemiological studies on the potential relationship of residential and occupational exposure to ELF electric and magnetic fields and cancer

Reference	Subjects	Correlation between increased cancer incidence and residential or occupational exposures
Wertheimer and Leeper, 1979 (Ref. No. 430)	Children (< 19 yr); residential fields [344 cases; 344 controls]	(+)
Fulton et al., 1980 (Ref. No. 431)	Children (< 20 yr); residential fields [119 cases; 240 controls]	(−)
Tomenius et al., 1982 (Ref. No. 432)	Children (< 18 yr); residential fields [716 cases; 716 controls]	(+)
Wertheimer and Leeper, 1982 (Ref. No. 433)	Adults; residential fields [1179 cases; 1179 controls]	(+)
Wiklund et al., 1981 (Ref. No. 434)	Adults; telecommunication workers [Swedish Cancer Registry with 385,000 cases, 1961-1973]	(−)
Milham, 1982 (Ref. No. 427)	Adults; male workers in 11 occupations involving electric and/or magnetic fields [Survey of 438,000 deaths in Washington State men from 1950-1979]	(+)
Wright et al., 1982 (Ref. No. 435)	Adults; male workers in 10 electrical/electronic occupations [Cancer Surveillance Program in Los Angeles County, 1972-1979]	(+)
McDowall, 1983 (Ref. No. 436)	Males aged 15-74; workers in 10 electrical/electronic occupations [Survey of occupational mortality in England and Wales, 1970-1972]	(+)

Table I (cont'd). Epidemiological studies on the potential relationship of residential and occupational exposure to ELF electric and magnetic fields and cancer

Reference	Subjects	Correlation between increased cancer incidence and residential or occupational exposures
Coleman et al., 1983 (Ref. No. 437)	Males aged 15-74; workers in 10 electrical/electronic occupations [South Thames Cancer Registry from 1961-1979]	(+)
Vågarö and Olin, 1983 (Ref. No. 438)	Males and females aged 15-64; workers in electrical/electronic occupations [Swedish Cancer Registry with 385,000 cases from 1961-1973]	(+)
Pearce et al., 1985 (Ref. No. 439)	Adults; male workers in 8 electrical/electronic occupations [546 cases; 2184 controls]	(+)
Milham, 1985 (Ref. No. 440)	Adults; male members of American Radio Relay League in states of Washington and California [1691 male cancer deaths in these two states compared with U.S. age-specific white male death frequencies in 1976]	(+)
Lin et al., 1985 (Ref. No. 441)	Adults; white male workers in 3 electrical/electronic occupations [Brain tumor decedents in state of Maryland from 1969 through 1982]	(+)

conducted to date. Several specific problems are the following: (1) In all of the studies thus far reported, the electric and magnetic field dosimetry was at best qualitative. In studies of residential ELF fields, the neglect of local fields from appliances may have led to incorrect conclusions concerning the peak and average

exposure of individuals to power-frequency fields and the harmonic frequencies that emanate from electrical devices used within the home. (2) The sample populations in many of the epidemiological studies were small, and the reported increases in cancer incidence by a factor of 2 or less might be expected to occur on the basis of chance alone. In these studies, it would have been informative if the authors had presented data on several nonexposed occupational groups in which the sample size was comparable to that of the exposed groups. (3) Control groups were frequently chosen in a nonblind manner involving subjective criteria, and the control population was often not matched with the exposed group on the basis of age, sex, race, socioeconomic class, or urban/rural residential status.
(4) Several of the studies used weak statistical methods such as the calculation of proportionate mortality ratios, which can lead to extremely misleading conclusions for population subgroups in which the overall incidence of disease is low with the exception of one disease class such as cancer (or some specific form of cancer such as leukemia). (5) The existence of confounding factors such as smoking habits and exposure to industrial pollutants of known carcinogenic potential (e.g., aryl hydrocarbons) has been ignored in all of the epidemiological studies that have attempted to relate ELF fields and cancer incidence.

Radiofrequency Fields

There have been several epidemiological studies on military, industrial and foreign service personnel exposed to RF radiation. In a broad study involving Navy personnel who had served during the Korean War,[442] no evidence was obtained for increased illness or mortality rate among a "high-exposure" group (20,109 personnel involved in radar repairs) and a "low-exposure" group (20,781 personnel involved in operating radar equipment). Mortality was assessed from death certificates during the period 1955-1974, and morbidity from (1) "in-service" hospitalization during the period 1950-1959, (2) Veterans Administration hospital admissions during the period 1963-1976, and (3) disability compensation records for 1976. In another case-control study on World War II and Korean War veterans who had worked with radar units, no evidence was found for an elevated incidence of cataracts in the exposed population.[443] These studies of radar workers lacked sufficient dosimetric information to make assignments of exposure levels. However, accidental exposures of Navy personnel to RF power densities exceeding 100 mW/cm^2 have been documented, and some personnel may have been subjected to levels in excess of 10 mW/cm^2 on a routine basis.[444] In a study on adult males occupationally exposed to radar for a period of four years, Robinette et al.[445] also found no evidence for an effect on life span, morbidity or cause of death. A four-year medical surveillance program in the aircraft industry involving 355 employees exposed to radar failed to detect any abnormal change in the general health of these personnel.[446]

One epidemiological study suggested a possible link between microwave exposure and congenital abnormalities. In a case-control study on the incidence of Down's syndrome in Baltimore, MD, it was found that paternal exposure to radar during military service was weakly associated with an increased incidence of this disorder in their offspring.[447] However, further investigation did not confirm the existence of a correlation between radar exposure of fathers and the incidence of Down's syndrome in the offspring.[448]

Effects from controlled RF heating have been studied in the offspring of women treated with diathermy to relieve the pain of uterine contractions during labor. In studies involving 2000 diathermy patients, no adverse short-term or long-term effects on the fetus were observed.[449,450]

The effects of chronic exposure to low-intensity microwaves were studied in 1827 employees who had served in the U.S. embassy in Moscow during the period 1953 to 1976, during which time the embassy was irradiated at RF power densities up to 15 $\mu W/cm^2$. The morbidity and mortality rates among this study group were compared with the rates in a second group of 2561 U.S. employees who had served during the same time period at eight Eastern European embassies or consulates that were not irradiated with microwaves. Based on information gained from personnel records, mail questionnaires and telephone interviews, there were no untoward health effects found among the irradiated study group from the Moscow embassy in comparison with individuals in the unirradiated group.[451,452]

In contrast to reports from the U.S. and Western European countries, epidemiological studies carried out in the Soviet Union and Eastern European countries on workers exposed to RF radiation have led to findings of apparent effects on the nervous and cardiovascular systems.[453-456] The nervous system effects revealed in these studies were characteristic of the neurasthenic syndrome, and included headache, fatigue, irritability, loss of appetite, drowsiness, sweating, memory loss, depression and emotional instability. The cardiovascular effects that were reported among exposed workers included bradycardia and alterations in cardiac conduction properties. The significance of these apparent neural and cardiovascular effects is difficult to assess, especially in view of the fact that a similar symptomatology was generally not observed in U.S. studies on radar workers or in the study on irradiated Moscow embassy personnel.

One aspect of the potential health effects of exposure to RF radiation that has not been satisfactorily addressed in previous studies is the issue of possible carcinogenic risk.[452] In a recent investigation involving 100 rats chronically exposed for 25 months to pulsed 2450-MHz microwaves, a statistically significant increase in primary neoplasms was observed in the exposed group relative to a sham-exposed control group of equal size.[457] Although the investigators concluded that the biological significance of this study is questionable at the present time, it underscores the need for further investigations on the carcinogenic potential of chronic exposure to RF radiation.

NMR Clinical Experience

Because NMR imaging and in vivo spectroscopy are relatively new techniques, the opportunity has not been available for a long-term medical assessment of patients and volunteers subjected to the fields from NMR devices. Based on a six-month follow-up of 181 patients and 70 volunteers ranging in age from 2 to 83, Reid et al.[8] have reported that no unexpected changes in cardiac or neurological functions occurred as the result of imaging with a 0.04 T NMR unit. The cohort of patients included three with epileptic seizures and one with myocardial infarction. A total of 118 patients who received head imaging with the same NMR unit exhibited no visual or central nervous system dysfunctions subsequent to imaging.[458]

PHYSICAL SAFETY FACTORS IN MEDICAL NMR

Metallic Implants

Two types of physical hazard are associated with the interaction of metallic implants and the fields used in NMR imaging devices: (1) forces and torques are exerted on ferromagnetic materials by the static magnetic field, and (2) significant RF heating can occur in materials with a high electrical conductivity. New et al.[459] measured the magnetic forces and torques exerted on 21 hemostatic clips and various other materials such as dental amalgam. Of the 21 clips, 19 of which were aneurysm clips, 16 showed a deflection near the portals of two magnets operating at 0.147 T and 1.44 T, respectively. Five of the 16 magnetic clips exhibited slight deflections of less than $5°$ arc, and 5 others showed marked deflections greater than $45°$ arc. Of the remaining materials tested, only a shunt connector demonstrated significant ferromagnetic properties. The nonmagnetic materials were primarily composed of austenitic stainless steel, which has a high (10 to 20 percent) nickel content that stabilizes the iron in a nonmagnetic form. Clips composed of tantalum or titanium are also non-ferromagnetic.[460] Surgical clips composed of martensitic stainless steels are ferromagnetic and experience significant forces and torques in magnetic fields comparable to those used in NMR devices.[461] Barrafato and Henkelman[462] conducted a systematic study of 54 different types of surgical clips and characterized their magnetic properties based on the rotational torque experienced in a 0.15 T static field, and the force experienced when a 1.5 mT/m field gradient was imposed. These studies confirmed the nonmagnetic character of clips composed of tantalum and various austenitic stainless steel alloys and silver alloys.

A study has been carried out to determine heating effects in surgical clips and hip protheses exposed to rapidly time-varying magnetic fields and to RF fields at intensities greater than used in conventional NMR devices.[463] The maximum temperature rises recorded for copper and steel clips and for individual hip prosthetic devices were less than $1°C$ under these exposure conditions, and it was concluded that no significant heating problem should be encountered during NMR imaging procedures. However, when two hip prostheses were joined together in a saline solution and subjected to the RF field, a temperature increase of several degrees was observed. The authors cautioned against the use of NMR imaging on patients with large implanted prosthetic devices until further research has been performed to assess the extent of possible RF heating problems.

Cardiac Pacemakers

An issue of particular concern is the malfunction of implanted cardiac pacemakers in response to the fields from NMR imaging devices. Because modern pacemakers contain a reed relay switch that can be closed by applying an external magnetic field in order to remotely test the battery strength, it is expected that implanted pacemakers will be influenced by static magnetic fields used for NMR imaging. Based on in vitro tests with demand pacemakers from six major manufacturers, Pavlicek et al.[464] found that fields of 1.7 to 4.7 mT produced closure of the reed switch, thereby resulting in a change from a synchronous to an asynchronous pacing mode. All six of the pacemakers studied were found to experience forces and torques when placed in NMR devices operating at fields up to 0.5 T. Two of the pacemakers experienced a torque that was judged on subjective criteria to be sufficient to cause significant movement within tissue.

A second aspect of pacemaker vulnerability to NMR imaging fields is the electromagnetic interference (EMI) that can result from signals introduced by the time-varying magnetic field or the RF field. Protection against RF fields is provided by a titanium casing and a low-pass input filter that discriminates against high-frequency EMI transmitted through the electrode leads. However, many brands of pacemaker are not protected against EMI in the ELF frequency range. The "unipolar" design of demand pacemakers, in which the cathode lead is implanted in the heart and the pacemaker case serves as the anode, is particularly susceptible to low-frequency EMI. This sensitivity results from the considerable physical separation of the anode and cathode, which thus provides a large antenna for the detection of EMI signals. The "bipolar" pacemaker design is much less sensitive to EMI because both leads are implanted within the heart at a small distance of separation. It has been estimated that among the 350,000 to 500,000 individuals in the United States with implanted pacemakers, approximately 50 percent have models with the unipolar electrode design.[465] It should also be noted that some manufacturers of pacemakers with the unipolar electrode configuration have overcome the problem of low-frequency EMI by incorporating a design feature that automatically decreases the sensitivity of the amplifier circuit when an interference signal is sensed. These specific pacemaker models thereby avoid reversion to an asynchronous mode in response to EMI.[466]

Pavlicek et al.[464] have found that a rapidly-switched gradient field with a time variation of 3 T/sec can induce potentials up to 20 mV in the loop formed by the electrode lead and the case of a unipolar pacemaker. This signal amplitude is sufficiently large to avoid rejection by the pacemaker's EMI discrimination circuitry, and it could therefore be mistakenly recognized as a valid cardiac electrical signal. A total of 26 pacemaker models were examined by Jenkins and Woody[467] for sensitivity to 60-Hz magnetic fields. Twenty of these units were found to revert to an asynchronous mode or to exhibit abnormal pacing characteristics in 60-Hz fields with amplitudes ranging from 0.1 to 0.4 mT. The average threshold field strength for inducing pacemaker malfunction was 0.2 mT, which corresponds to a dB/dt of 0.075 T/sec. This value of dB/dt is significantly less than the time variation of the switched gradient fields used in present NMR devices.

CLINICAL NMR EXPOSURE GUIDELINES

Exposure guidelines for NMR imaging and in vivo spectroscopy issued in the United States,[468] United Kingdom,[469] and the Federal Republic of Germany[470] are summarized in Table II. Recommended limits were given for the static magnetic fields, the time-varying magnetic fields, and the RF fields used in NMR devices. These guidelines are in close agreement on a limit for the static magnetic field of 2 to 2.5 T, but significant differences exist in the recommended exposure limits for time-varying magnetic fields and for

Table II. Exposure guidelines in clinical NMR

Source	B (Tesla)	Time-varying fields	RF fields
National Center for Devices and Radiological Health, DHHS: 1982	2.0	3 Tesla/sec	Specific absorption rate < 0.4 W/kg (whole body) or < 2 W/kg per g of tissue
National Radiation Protection Board, U.K.: 1983	2.5	20 Tesla/sec (r.m.s) for pulses $\geq$ 10 msec; $2t^{-\frac{1}{2}}$ for pulses < 10 msec (t in sec)	Body temperature rise of < 1°C [specific absorption rate < 0.4 W/kg (whole body) or < 4 W/kg per g of tissue]
Federal Health Office, FRG: 1984	2.0	Induced current < 30 mA/m^2 or induced field < 0.3 V/m for pulses $\geq$ 10 msec; induced current < 0.3/t mA/m^2 or induced field < 3/t mV/m for pulses < 10 msec (t in sec)	Specific absorption rate < 1 W/kg (whole body) or < 5 W/kg per kg of tissue (except for the eyes)

RF fields.

A limit of 3 T/sec for the time-varying field was recommended in the U.S./D.H.H.S. guideline[468] based on a review of the known interaction mechanisms and biological effects of time-varying magnetic fields.[4] In contrast, the U.K./N.R.P.B. guideline[469] was set at 20 T/sec (r.m.s.) based on the estimate that a time-varying magnetic field of this magnitude would induce a maximum current density of less than 0.3 A/m^2 (r.m.s.) in any part of the body.[471] This current density was judged to be safe on the basis that it is approximately one order of magnitude less than the threshold for producing cardiac fibrillation. The limit on dB/dt in the U.K./N.R.P.B. guideline is permitted to increase as the reciprocal square root of the pulse duration, i.e., 2/ t in units of T/sec (r.m.s.), for pulses shorter than 10 msec. This specification was based on various measurements of the stimulus strength versus duration relationship for human responses to electric current, as reviewed in an earlier section of this chapter. The F.R.G./F.H.O. guideline for time-varying magnetic fields is not extensively justified on the basis of laboratory data.[470] However, the recommended limits on induced current density and voltage gradient are reasonably consistent with the U.S./D.H.H.S. limit of 3 T/sec, since the maximum current density induced in the human body by a magnetic field with this time rate of change would be approximately 30 mA/m^2. The F.R.G/F.H.O. guideline also permits the induced current density limit to increase as the reciprocal of the pulse duration, i.e. 0.3/t in units of mA/m^2, for pulses less than 10 msec.

The recommended exposure limits for RF fields given in all three sets of guidelines are designed to avoid significant regional or whole-body heating. The maximum whole-body SAR value recommended in the U.S./D.H.H.S. guideline is consistent with recommendations by the American National Standard Institute,[472] whereas the F.R.G./F.H.O. limit is 2.5 times higher. In both sets of NMR exposure guidelines, the recommended limit for absorbed RF power in localized tissue regions is increased by a factor of 5 relative to the whole-body SAR limit. The U.S./D.H.H.S. guideline, however, specifies the local SAR per gram of tissue, whereas the F.R.G./F.H.O. guideline specifies this quantity per kilogram of tissue exclusive of the eyes. The U.K./N.R.P.B. guideline for the whole-body SAR limit is consistent with the U.S./D.H.H.S. recommendation, but the SAR limit per gram of tissue is twice that given in the U.S./D.H.H.S. guideline.

Both the U.K./N.R.P.B. and F.R.G./F.H.O. guidelines discuss the risks of imaging patients with implanted pacemakers, vascular clips, or large prosthetic devices. In addition, the U.K./N.R.P.B. guideline states that it would be prudent to exclude women in the first trimester of pregnancy from NMR imaging procedures.

The one recommendation that relates to staff members operating NMR equipment is the specification in the U.K./N.R.P.B. guideline that the Stanford Linear Accelerator limits on static magnetic field exposure[473] should be applied to these personnel. Under these limits, exposure of the whole body is not to exceed 0.02 T for prolonged periods, and exposure of the arms and hands is limited to 0.2 T. For short periods of less than 15 min duration, these exposure limits are increased to 0.2 T for the whole body and 2 T for the arms and hands.

SUMMARY AND CONCLUSIONS

Based on the review presented in this chapter of interaction mechanisms, laboratory investigations, and human health studies, several summary statements and general conclusions can be drawn regarding biological effects of the static and time-varying magnetic fields and the RF fields used in the present generation of NMR devices:

- Static magnetic fields at levels up to 2 T have not been found to produce adverse behavioral or physiological changes in mammals. Electrical potentials induced within the central circulatory system of laboratory animals placed in fields up to 2 T do not significantly influence cardiac performance during brief exposures. Additional studies are needed to assess the effects of prolonged exposure to fields of this magnitude on the cardiovascular and central nervous systems. Future research should also address the issue of potential effects on cellular, tissue and animal systems resulting from exposure to ultrahigh fields in the range of 2-10 T. Little information exists on the response of biological systems to fields of this magnitude, which have been considered for use in future NMR devices.

- Time-varying magnetic fields that induce tissue current densities less than 10 mA/m^2 have not been demonstrated to produce harmful effects, although some laboratory findings of behavioral and physiological alterations have been reported. A time variation of 1 to 2 T/sec would induce maximum current densities of this magnitude in critical organs such as the heart and brain. Acute visual phenomena that occur in fields with a time rate of change exceeding 1.3 T/sec are completely reversible and produce no harmful long-term effects.

- It is well established that exposure to RF fields can lead to irreversible tissue damage if the regional or whole-body heating exceeds the normal thermoregulatory capacity of the body. Nonthermal effects of low-intensity RF fields have also been reported to occur in the cardiovascular and nervous systems, tissue metabolism, and a variety of other cellular and tissue functions. Windows of sensitivity in the frequency and intensity domains have been observed in studies on the influence of amplitude-modulated RF fields on calcium-ion binding to nerve cell surfaces. The maximum influence on calcium ion binding occurs when the RF field is amplitude modulated in the ELF frequency range, and theoretical calculations indicate that this effect cannot be attributed to a thermal interaction mechanism.[474] Further research is needed to elucidate the physical and chemical processes by which RF fields could exert nonthermal effects on living systems.

- Epidemiological studies on human populations exposed to large static magnetic fields and to RF fields have provided no consistent evidence for adverse health effects. Controversy currently surrounds the issue of elevated cancer risk among individuals exposed residentially and/or occupationally to ELF electric and magnetic fields above the normal ambient levels. A direct correlation between cancer risk and exposure to ELF fields has not been established, and numerous criticisms have been raised of the epidemiological procedures used in the studies reported to date. Among the various methodological deficiences noted in these studies, the failure to account for confounding variables has been the most widely criticized.[475,476] At the present time, there are no direct implications of these epidemiological studies for the safety of patients or operational staff exposed to the time-varying magnetic fields of NMR devices. However, a long-term assessment of the health profiles of these individuals is advisable, and may lend further insight into the issue of potential carcinogenic risk from exposure to electromagnetic fields.

• A serious risk in NMR imaging procedures is associated with the forces and torques exerted by large static magnetic fields and magnetic field gradients on metallic implants such as vascular clips and prosthetic devices. Static magnetic fields greater than 1.5 mT and time-varying fields with dB/dt greater than approximately 75 mT/sec can alter the performance of implanted cardiac pacemakers. These physical interactions of the fields associated with NMR devices constitute a direct health hazard to patients and operational staff with implanted pacemakers, vascular clips, or prostheses.

• Clinical NMR exposure guidelines issued in the U.S., U.K., and F.R.G. impose a reasonable limit of 2 to 2.5 T on the static magnetic field level, and the various RF exposure limits are adequate to protect patients against excessive thermal stress. A 3 T/sec limit recommended in the U.S./D.H.H.S. guideline on the maximum time variation of rapidly-switched gradient fields appears reasonable on the basis of available information from laboratory studies, including several clinical investigations on human subjects. The F.R.G./F.H.O. limits on induced current density and voltage gradient are reasonably consistent with the 3 T/sec limit imposed by the U.S./D.H.H.S. guideline. From available laboratory information on cellular, tissue and animal systems, the 20 T/sec (r.m.s.) limit recommended in the U.S./N.R.P.B. guideline appears to be excessive.

ACKNOWLEDGMENTS

The excellent secretarial assistance of K. Springsteen is gratefully acknowledged. Funding for the authors' research is received from the Office of Energy Research, Health and Environmental Research Division, of the U.S. Department of Energy under Contract No. DE-AC03-76SF00098 with the Lawrence Berkeley Laboratory (T.S.T. and T.F.B.), from the National Institutes of Health (grants HL25840 and HL07367, T.F.B.), from the Electric Power Research Institute (Contract No. RP799-21 and RP2572-5, T.S.T.), and from the IBM Corporation (T.F.B.). We also thank Dr. G. Kambic of the Technicare Corporation (Cleveland, Ohio) for providing technical information on the operating characteristics of commercially available NMR devices, and Dr. M. Roos for several helpful suggestions on the text of this chapter.

REFERENCES

1. Sheppard, A.R., Eisenbud, M.: Biological Effects of Electric and Magnetic Fields of Extremely Low Frequency. New York: New York University Press (1977).
2. Phillips, R.D., Gillis, M.R., Kaune, W.T., Mahlum, D.D., eds.: Proceedings of the Eighteenth Annual Hanford Life Sciences Symposium: Biological Effects of Extremely Low Frequency Electromagnetic Fields. Springfield, VA: NTIS Rep. No. CONF-781016 (1979).
3. Tenforde, T.S., ed.: Magnetic Field Effects on Biological Systems. New York: Plenum Press (1979).
4. Budinger, T.S.: IEEE Trans. Nucl. Sci. 26, 2821 (1979).
5. Michaelson, S.M.: Proc. IEEE 68, 40 (1980).
6. Schwan, H.P., Foster, K.R.: Proc. IEEE 68, 104 (1980).
7. Budinger, T.F.: J. Comp. Assist. Tomogr. 5, 800 (1981).
8. Reid, A., Smith, F.W., Hutchinson, J.M.S.: Br. J. Radiol. 55, 784 (1982).
9. Budinger, T.F., Cullander, C.: Health effects of in vivo magnetic resonance. (In) Clinical Magnetic Resonance Imaging, pp. 303-320. Margulis, A.R., Higgins, C.S., Kaufman, L., Crooks, L.E., eds. San Francisco: Univ. Calif. Printing Dept. (1984).
10. Extremely Low Frequency (ELF) Fields. (WHO Envir. Health Crit. 35). Geneva: World Health Organization (1984).
11. Budinger, T.F., Lauterbur, P.C.: Science 226, 288 (1984).
12. Tenforde, T.S.: Biological effects of ELF magnetic fields. (In) Biological and Human Health Effects of Extremely Low Frequency Electromagnetic Fields, pp. 79-127. Arlington, VA: Am. Inst. Biol. Sci. (1985).
13. Tenforde, T.S.: Mechanisms for biological effects of magnetic fields. (In) Biological Effects and Dosimetry of Non-Ionizing Radiation: Static and ELF Electromagnetic Fields. Grandolfo, M., Michaelson, S.M., Rindi, A., eds. New York: Plenum, in press, 1985.
14. Tenforde, T.S.: Biological effects of stationary magnetic fields. (In) Biological Effects and Dosimetry of Non-Ionizing Radiation: Static and ELF Electromagnetic Fields. Grandolfo, M., Michaelson, S.M., Rindi, A., eds. New York: Plenum, in press, 1985.
15. Frankel, R.B.: Biological effects of static magnetic fields. (In) Handbook of Biological Effects of Electromagnetic Fields. Polk, C., Postow, E., eds. Boca Raton, FL: CRC Press, in press, 1986.
16. Tenforde, T.S.: Interaction of ELF magnetic fields with living matter. (In) Handbook of Biological Effects of Electromagnetic Fields. Polk, C., Postow, E., eds. Boca Raton, FL: CRC press, in press, 1986.
17. Kalmijn, A.J.: The detection of electric fields from inanimate and animate sources other than electric organs. (In) Handbook of Sensory Physiology, pp. 147-200. Autrum, H., Jung, R., Loewenstein, W.R., MacKay, D.M., Teuber, H.L., eds. New York: Springer-Verlag (1974).

18. Kalmijn, A.J.: Experimental evidence of geomagnetic orientation in elasmobranch fishes. (In) Animal Migration, Navigation, and Homing, pp. 347-353. Schmidt-Koenig, K., Keeton, W.T., eds. New York: Springer-Verlag (1978).
19. Kalmijn, A.J.: IEEE Trans. Mag. MAG-17, 1113 (1981).
20. Kalmijn, A.J.: Science 218, 916 (1982).
21. Kolin, A.: Rev. Sci. Instrum. 16, 109 (1945).
22. Kolin, A.: Rev. Sci. Instrum. 23, 235 (1952).
23. Mills, C.J.: Med. Instrum. 11, 136 (1977).
24. Beischer, D.E., Knepton, J.C.: Aerosp. Med. 35, 939 (1964).
25. Togawa, T., Okai, O., Oshima, M.: Med. Biol. Engin. 5, 169 (1967).
26. Beischer, D.E.: Vectorcardiogram and aortic blood flow of squirrel monkeys (Saimiri sciureus) in a strong superconductive electromagnet. (In) Biological Effects of Magnetic Fields, pp. 249-251. Barnothy, M.F., ed. New York: Plenum (1969).
27. Gaffey, C.T., Tenforde, T.S.: Changes in the electrocardiograms of rats and dogs exposed to DC magnetic fields. Lawrence Berkeley Laboratory Report No. 9085. Berkeley, CA: University of California (1979).
28. Gaffey, C.T., Tenforde, T.S., Dean, E.E.: Bioelectromagnetics 1, 209 (1980).
29. Gaffey, C.T., Tenforde, T.S.: Bioelectromagnetics 2, 357 (1981).
30. Tenforde, T.S., Gaffey, C.T., Moyer, B.R., Budinger, T.F.: Bioelectromagnetics 4, 1 (1983).
31. Tenforde, T.S., Gaffey, C.T., Raybourn, M.S.: Influence of stationary magnetic fields on ionic conduction processes in biological systems. (In) Proc. Sixth EMC Symp., pp. 205-210. Dvořák, T., ed. Zurich, Switzerland, Mar. 5-7, 1985.
32. Belousova, L.Y.: Biofizika 10, 365 (1965).
33. Korchevskii, E.M., Marochnik, L.S.: Biofizika 10, 371 (1965).
34. Vardanyan, V.A.: Biofizika 18, 491 (1973).
35. Wikswo, J.P., Barach, J.P.: IEEE Trans. Biomed. Engin. BME-27, 722 (1980).
36. Liboff, R.L.: J. Theor. Biol. 83, 427 (1980).
37. Schwartz, J.-L.: IEEE Trans. Biomed. Engin. BME-25, 467 (1978).
38. Schwartz, J.-L.: IEEE Trans. Biomed. Engin. BME-26, 238 (1979).
39. Gaffey, C.T., Tenforde, T.S.: Radiat. Envir. Biophys. 22, 61 (1983).
40. Maret, G., Schickfus, M.v., Mayer, A., Dransfeld, K.: Phys. Rev. Lett. 35, 397 (1975).
41. Chalazonitis, N., Chagneux, R., Arvanitaki, A.: C.R. Acad. Sci. Paris Ser. D 271, 130 (1970).
42. Hong, F.T., Mauzerall, D., Mauro, A.: Proc. Natl. Acad. Sci. (USA) 68: 1283 (1971).
43. Chagneux, R., Chalazonitis, N.: C.R. Acad. Sci. Paris Ser. D 274, 317 (1972).
44. Chagneux, R., Chagneux, H., Chalazonitis, N.: Biophys. J. 18, 125 (1977).
45. Becker, J.F., Trentacosti, F., Geacintov, N.E.: Photochem. Photobiol. 27, 51 (1978).
46. Hong, F.T.: Biophys. J. 29, 343 (1980).
47. Vilenchik, M.M.: Biofiz. 27, 31 (1982).

48. Arnold, W., Steele, R., Mueller, H.: Proc. Natl. Acad. Sci. (USA) 44, 1 (1958).
49. Geacintov, N.E., VanNostrand, F., Pope, M., Tinkel, J.B.: Biochim. Biophys. Acta 226, 486 (1971).
50. Geacintov, N.E., VanNostrand, F., Becker, J.F., Tinkel, J.B.: Biochim. Biophys. Acta 267, 65 (1972).
51. Becker, J.F., Geacintov, N.E., VanNostrand, F., VanMetter, R.: Biochem. Biophys. Res. Comm. 51, 597 (1973).
52. Breton, J.: Biochem. Biophys. Res. Comm. 59, 1011 (1974).
53. Becker, J.F., Geacintov, N.E., Swenberg, C.E.: Biochim. Biophys. Acta 503, 545 (1978).
54. Neugebauer, D.-Ch., Blaurock, A.E.: FEBS Lett. 78, 31 (1977).
55. Blakemore, R.: Science 190, 377 (1975).
56. Frankel, R.B., Blakemore, E.P., Wolfe, R.S.: Science 203, 1355 (1979).
57. Blakemore, R.P., Frankel, R.B., Kalmijn, A.J.: Nature 286, 384 (1980).
58. Frankel, R.B., Blakemore, R.P., Torres de Araujo, F.F., Esquival, D.M.S.: Science 212, 1269 (1981).
59. Murayama, M.: Nature 206, 420 (1965).
60. Melville, D., Paul, F., Roath, S.: Nature 155, 706 (1975).
61. Paul, F., Roath, S., Melville, D.: Brit. J. Haematol. 38, 273 (1978).
62. Swenberg, C.E.: Theoretical remarks on low magnetic field interactions with biological systems. (In) Magnetic Field Effects on Biological Systems, pp. 89-91. Tenforde, T.S., ed. New York: Plenum (1979).
63. Schulten, K.: Magnetic field effects in chemistry and biology. (In) Festkorperprobleme XXII: Advances in Solid State Physics, pp. 61-83. Aachen, P.G., ed. Munster, Germany: Proc. 46th Ann. Meeting of German Physical Soc., Mar. 29-Apr. 2, 1982.
64. Blankenship, R.E., Schaafsma, T.J., Parson, W.W.: Biochim. Biophys. Acta 461, 297 (1977).
65. Werner, H.-J., Schulten, K., Weller, A.: Biochim. Biophys. Acta 502, 255 (1978).
66. Haberkorn, R., Michel-Beyerle, M.E.: Biophys. J. 26, 489 (1979).
67. Michel-Beyerle, M.E., Scheer, H., Seidlitz, H., Tempus, D., Haberkorn, R.: FEBS Lett. 100, 9 (1979).
68. Hoff, A.J.: Quart. Rev. Biophys. 14, 599 (1981).
69. Ogrodnik, A., Kruger, H.W., Orthuber, H., Haberkorn, R., Michel-Beyerle, M.E., Scheer, H.: Biophys. J. 39, 91 (1982).
70. Ratner, S.C.: Behav. Biol. 17, 573 (1976).
71. Martin, H., Lindauer, M.: J. Comp. Physiol. 122, 145 (1977).
72. Keeton, W.T.: Proc. Natl. Acad. Sci. (USA) 68, 1283 (1971).
73. Wiltschko, W., Wiltschko, R.: Science 176, 62 (1972).
74. Emlen, S.T., Wiltschko, W., Demong, N.J., et al.: Science 193, 505 (1976).
75. Bookman, M.A.: Nature 267, 340 (1977).
76. Lowenstam, H.A.: Geol. Soc. Am. Bull. 73, 435 (1962).
77. Kirschvink, J.L., Lowenstam, H.A.: Earth Planet. Sci. Lett. 44, 193 (1979).
78. Gould, J.L., Kirschvink, J.L., Deffeyes, K.A.: Science 201,

1026 (1978).
79. Walcott, C., Gould, J.L., Kirschvink, J.L.: Science 205, 1027 (1979).
80. Presti, D., Pettigrew, J.D.: Nature 285, 99 (1980).
81. Malinin, G.I., Gregory, W.D., Morelli, L., et al.: Science 194, 844 (1976).
82. Frazier, M.E., Andrews, T.K., Thompson, B.B.: In vitro evaluation of static magnetic fields. (In) Biological Effects of Extremely Low Frequency Electromagnetic Fields, pp. 417-435. Phillips, R.D., Gillis, M.F., Kaune, W.T., Mahlum, D.D., eds. Springfield, VA: NTIS Rep. No. CONF-781016 (1979).
83. Mulay, I.L., Mulay, L.N.: Nature 190, 1019 (1961).
84. Mulay, I.L., Mulay, L.N.: Effects on Drosophila melanogaster and S-37 tumor cells; postulates for magnetic field interactions. (In) Biological Effects of Magnetic Fields, Vol. 1, pp. 146-169. Barnothy, M.F., ed. New York: Plenum (1964).
85. Reno, V.R., Nutini, L.B.: Nature 198, 204 (1963).
86. Reno, V.R., Nutini, L.G.: Tissue respiration. (In) Biological Effects of Magnetic Fields, Vol. 1, pp. 211-217. Barnothy, M.F., ed. New York: Plenum (1964).
87. Pereira, M.R., Nutini, L.G., Fardon, J.C., Cook, E.S.: Proc. Soc. Exp. Biol. Med. 124, 573 (1967).
88. Cook, E.A., Fardon, J.C., Nutini, L.G.: Effects of magnetic fields on cellular respiration. (In) Biological Effects of Magnetic Fields, Vol. 2, pp. 67-78. Barnothy, M.F., ed. New York: Plenum (1969).
89. D'Souza, L., Reno, V.R., Nutini, L.G., Cook. E.S.: The effect of a magnetic field on DNA synthesis by ascites Sarcoma 37 cells. (In) Biological Effects of Magnetic Fields, Vol. 2, pp. 53-59. Barnothy, M.F., ed. New York: Plenum (1969).
90. Gerencer, V.F., Barnothy, M.F., Barnothy, J.M.: Nature 196, 539 (1962).
91. Butler, B.C., Dean, W.W.: Am. J. Med. Electron. 3, 125 (1964).
92. Barnothy, J.M.: Rejection of transplanted tumors in mice. (In) Biological Effects of Magnetic Fields, Vol. 1, pp. 100-108. New York: Plenum (1964).
93. Gross, L.: Lifespan increase of tumor-bearing mice through pretreatment. (In) Biological Effects of Magnetic Fields, Vol. 1, pp. 132-139. New York: Plenum (1964).
94. Montgomery, D.J., Smith, A.E.: Biomed. Sci. Instrum. 1, 123 (1963).
95. Halpern, N.H., Green, A.E.: Nature 202, 717 (1964).
96. Hall, E.J., Bedford, J.S., Leask, M.J.M.: Nature 203, 1086 (1964).
97. Greene, A.E., Halpern, M.H.: Aerosp. Med. 37, 251 (1966).
98. Rockwell, S.: Int. J. Radiat. Biol. 31, 153 (1966).
99. Iwasaki, T., Ohara, H., Matsumoto, S., Matsudaira, H.: J. Radiat. Res. 19, 287 (1978).
100. Nath, R., Schulz, R.J., Bongiorni, P.: Int. J. Radiat. Biol. 38, 285 (1980).
101. Eiselein, B.S., Boutell, H.M., Biggs, M.W.: Aerosp. Med. 32, 383 (1961).
102. Chandra, S., Stefani, S.: Effect of constant and alternating

magnetic fields on tumor cells in vitro and in vivo. (In) Biological Effects of Extremely Low Frequency Electromagnetic Fields, pp. 436-446. Phillips, R.D., Gillis, M.F., Kaune, W.T., Mahlum, D.D., eds. Springfield, VA: NTIS Rep. No. CONF-781016 (1979).
103. Levengood, W.C.: Nature 209, 1009 (1966).
104. Levengood, W.C.: Biophys. J. 7, 297 (1967).
105. Tegenkamp, T.R.: Mutagenic effects of magnetic fields on Drosophila melanogaster. (In) Biological Effects of Magnetic Fields, Vol. 2, pp. 189-206. Barnothy, M.F., ed. New York: Plenum (1969).
106. Perakis, N.: Acta Anat. 4, 225 (1947).
107. Neurath, P.W.: Nature 219, 1358 (1968).
108. Amer, N.M.: The Effects of Homogeneous Magnetic Fields, Ambient Gas Composition and Temperature on Development of Tribolium confusum. Lawrence Radiation Laboratory Rep. No. UCRL-16854. Berkeley, CA: University of California (1965).
109. Levengood, W.C.: J. Embryol. Exp. Morphol. 21, 23 (1969).
110. Ueno, S., Harada, K., Shiokawa, K.: IEEE Trans. Mag. MAG-20, 1663 (1984).
111. Lee, P.H., Weis, J.J.: Biol. Bull. 159, 681 (1980).
112. Joshi, M.Y., Khan, M.Z., Damle, P.S.: Differentiation 10, 39 (1978).
113. Brewer, H.B.: Biophys. J. 28, 305 (1979).
114. Strand, J.A., Abernathy, C.S., Skalski, J.R., Genoway, R.G.: Bioelectromagnetics 4, 295 (1983).
115. Barnothy, J.M.: Development of young mice. (In) Biological Effects of Magnetic Fields, Vol. 1, pp. 93-99. Barnothy, M.F., ed. New York: Plenum (1964).
116. Nakagawa, M.: Jap. J. Hyg. 34, 488 (1979).
117. Mild, K.H., Sandström, M., Løvtrup, S.: Bioelectromagnetics 2, 199 (1981).
118. Sikov, M.R., Mahlum, D.D., Montgomery, L.D., Decker, J.R.: Development of mice after intrauterine exposure to direct-current magnetic fields. (In) Biological Effects of Extremely Low Frequency Electromagnetic Fields, pp. 462-473. Phillips, R.D. Gillis, M.F., Kaune, W.T., Mahlum, D.D., eds. Springfield, VA: NTIS Rep. No. CONF-781016 (1979).
119. Kelman, B.J., Mahlum, D.D., Decker, J.R.: Effects of exposure to magnetic fields on the pregnant rat. Presented at the 4th Ann. Meeting of the Bioelectromagnetics Soc., Los Angeles, June 28-July 2, 1982.
120. Kale, P.G., Baum, J.W.: Envir. Mutagen. 1, 371 (1979).
121. Mittler, S.: Mutat. Res. 13, 287 (1971).
122. Diebolt, J.R.: Mutat. Res. 57, 169 (1978).
123. Baum, J.W., Schairer, L.A., Lindahl, K.L.: Tests in the plant Tradescantia for mutagenic effects of strong magnetic fields. (In) Magnetic Field Effects on Biological Systems, pp. 22-24. Tenforde, T.S., ed. New York: Plenum (1979).
124. Mahlum, D.D., Sikov, M.R., Decker, J.R.: Dominant lethal studies in mice exposed to direct-current magnetic fields. (In) Biological effects of Extremely Low Frequency Electromagnetic Fields, pp. 474-484. Phillips, R.D., Gillis, M.F., Kaune, W.T.,

Mahlum, D.D., eds. Springfield, VA: NTIS Rep. No. CONF-781016 (1979).
125. Wolff, S., Crooks, L.E., Brown, P., et al.: Radiol. 136, 707 (1980).
126. Roots, R.J., Kraft, G.H., Farinato, R.S., Tenforde, T.S.: Electrophoretic and electrooptical studies on the conformation and susceptibility to psoralen crosslinking of magnetically oriented DNA. Lawrence Berkeley Laboratory Rep. No. 13601. Berkeley, CA: University of California (1982).
127. Barnothy, J.M., Barnothy, M.F., Boszormenyi-Nagy, I.: Nature 177, 577 (1956).
128. Barnothy, M.F., Sümegi, I.: Effects of the magnetic field on internal organs and the endocrine system of mice. (In) Biological Effects of Magnetic Fields, Vol. 2, pp. 103-126. Barnothy, M.F., ed. New York: Plenum (1969).
129. Barnothy, M.F., Sümegi, I.: Nature 221, 270 (1969).
130. Nakagawa, M., Muroya, H., Matsuda, Y., Tsukamoto, H.: J. Transport. Med. 34, 376 (1980).
131. Tvildiani, D.D., Kurashvili, R.B., Chlaidzye, T.I., et al.: Soobsh. Akad. Nauk Gruz. SSR 110, 413 (1983).
132. Demetskiy, A.M., Surganova, S.F., Popova, L.I., Gavilovich, P.F.: Zdravookhr. Belorus. 12, 3 (1979).
133. Rusyayev, V.F.: Prob. Gematol. Pereliv. Krovi 2, 19 (1979).
134. Markuze, I.I., Ambartsumyan, R.G., Chibrikin, V.M., Piruzyan, L.A.: Izv. Akad. Nauk SSSR (Ser. Biol.) 2, 281 (1973).
135. Tvildiani, D.D., Chlaidze, T.I., Dolidze, N.V., et al.: Soobsh. Akad. Nauk Gruz. SSR 101, 169 (1981).
136. Hanneman, G.D.: Changes in sodium and potassium content of urine from mice subjected to intense magnetic fields. (In) Biological Effects of Magnetic Fields, Vol. 2, pp. 127-135. Barnothy, M.F., ed. New York: Plenum (1969).
137. Rabinovich, E.Z., Taran, Y.P., Usacheva, M.D., et al.: Biofiz. 28, 693 (1983).
138. Galaktionova, G.V., Strzhizhovskiy, A.G.: Kosm. Biol. Med. 7, 49 (1973).
139. Strzhizhorskiy, A.D., Galaktionova, G.V., Cheremnykh, P.A.: Tsitol. 2, 205 (1980).
140. Bucking, J., Herbst, M., Piontek, P.: Radiat. Envir. Biophys. 11, 79 (1974).
141. Wordsworth, O.J.: Radiat. Res. 57, 442 (1974).
142. Strzhizhovskiy, A.K., Mastryukova, V.M.: Izv. Akad. Nauk SSR (Ser. Biol) 3, 437 (1983).
143. Kholodov, Y.A., Shishlo, M.A.: Electromagnetic Fields in Physiology. Moscow: Nauka (1980).
144. Kandil, A., Elashmawy, H.: J. Drug. Res. 12, 127 (1981).
145. Pautrizel, R., Priore, A., Berlureau, F., Pautrizel, A.N.: Comp. Rend. Acad. Sci. (Ser. D) 268, 1889 (1962).
146. Friedman, H., Carey, R.J.: Physiol. Behav. 9, 171 (1972).
147. Klimovskaya, L.D., Maslova, A.F.: Kosm. Biol. Aviakosm. Med. 15, 74 (1981).
148. Klimovskaya, L.D., Maslova, A.F.: Izv. Akad. Nauk SSR (Ser. Biol.) 4, 606 (1983).
149. Hayek, A., Guardian, C., Guardian, J., Obarski, G.: Biochem.

Biophys. Res. Comm. 122, 191 (1984).
150. Nahas, G.G., Boccalon, H., Berryer, P., Wagner, B.: Aviat. Space Envir. Med. 46, 1161 (1975).
151. Viktora, L., Fiala, J., Petz, R.: Physiol. Bohemoslov. 25, 359 (1976).
152. Battocletti, J.H., Salles-Cunha, S., Halbach, R.E., et al.: Med. Phys. 8, 115 (1981).
153. Tenforde, T.S., Shifrine, M.: Bioelectromagnetics 5, 443 (1984).
154. Brown, F.A., Jr., Skow, K.M.: J. Interdiscipl. Cycle Res. 9, 137 (1978).
155. Kavaliers, M., Ossenkopp, J.-P., Hirst, M.: Physiol. Behav. 32, 261 (1984).
156. Bliss, V.L., Heppner, F.H.: Nature 261, 411 (1976).
157. Semm, P., Schneider, T., Vollrath, L.: Nature 288, 607 (1980).
158. Semm, P., Schneider, T., Vollrath, L., Wiltschko, W.: Magnetic sensitive pineal cells in pigeons. (In) Avian Navigation, pp. 329-337. Papi, F., Wallraff, H.G., eds. New York: Springer-Verlag (1982).
159. Semm, P.: Comp. Biochem. Physiol. 76A, 683 (1983).
160. Welker, H.A., Semm, P., Willig, R.P., et al.: Exp. Brain Res. 50, 426 (1983).
161. Raybourn, M.S.: Science 220, 715 (1983).
162. Tenforde, T.S., Levy, L., Veklerov, E.: Monitoring of circadian waveforms in rodents exposed to high-intensity static magnetic fields. Presented at the 23rd Hanford Life Sci. Symp., Richland, WA, Oct. 2-4, 1984.
163. Tenforde, T.S., Levy, L., Dols, C.G., Banchero, P.G.: Measurements of circadian temperature variations in mice exposed to a 1.5 Tesla stationary magnetic field. Presented at the 4th Ann. Meeting of the Bioelectromagnetics Soc., Los Angeles, June 28-July 2, 1982.
164. Tenforde, T.S., Levy, L.: Circadian regulation of body temperature in mice subjected to continuous or intermittent exposures to a 1.5-Tesla stationary magnetic field. Presented at the 6th Ann. Meeting of the Bioelectromagnetics Soc., Atlanta, July 15-19, 1984.
165. Sperber, D., Oldenbourg, R., Dransfeld, K.: Naturwiss. 71, 100 (1984).
166. Tenforde, T.S., Levy, L.: Thermoregulation in rodents exposed to homogeneous (7.55 Tesla) and gradient (60 Tesla/meter) DC magnetic fields. Presented at 7th Ann. Meeting of the Bioelectromagnetics Soc., San Francisco, June 16-20, 1985.
167. Davis, H.P., Mizumori, S.J.Y., Allen, H., et al.: Bioelectromagnetics 5, 147 (1984).
168. Gaffey, C.T., Tenforde, T.S.: Electroretinograms of cats and monkeys exposed to large stationary magnetic fields. Presented at the 6th Ann. Meeting of the Bioelectromagnetics Soc., Atlanta, July 15-19, 1984.
169. Beischer, D.E., Knepton, J.C., Jr.: The electroencephalogram of the squirrel monkey (Saimiri sciureus) in a very high magnetic field. Naval Aerosp. Med. Inst. Rep., NASA Order No. R-39, Pensacola, FL (1966).

170. Kholodov, Y.A.: Effects on the central nervous system. (In) Biological Effects of Magnetic Fields, Vol. 1, pp. 196-200. Barnothy, M.F., eds. New York: Plenum (1964).
171. Kholodov, Y.A.: The Effect of Electromagnetic and Magnetic Fields on the Central Nervous System. NASA Rep. TT F-465. Springfield, VA: Clearinghouse for Fed. and Tech. Inform. (1966).
172. Kholodov, Y.A., Alexandrovskaya, M.M., Lukjanova, S.N., Udarova, N.S.: Investigations of the reactions of mammalian brain to static magnetic fields. (In) Biological Effects of Magnetic Fields, Vol. 2, pp. 215-225. Barnothy, M.F., ed. New York: Plenum (1969).
173. Bernhardt, J.: Radiat. Envir. Biophys. $\underline{16}$, 309 (1979).
174. Bernhardt, J.H.: On the rating of human exposition to electric and magnetic fields with frequencies below 100 kHz. (In) Protection against Microwave and Radiofrequency Radiations, Electric and Magnetic Fields. Notes from ISPRA Course, November 14-18, 1983.
175. Kolin, A., Brill, N.Q., Bromberg, P.J.: Proc. Soc. Exp. Biol. Med. (N.Y.) $\underline{102}$, 251 (1959).
176. Irwin, D.D., Rush, S., Evering, R., et al.: IEEE Trans. Mag. $\underline{MAG-6}$, 321 (1970).
177. Maass, J.A., Asa, M.M.: IEEE Trans. Mag. MAG-6, 322 (1970).
178. Öberg, P.Å.: Med. Biol. Engin. $\underline{11}$, 55 (1973).
179. Ueno, S., Matsumoto, S., Harada, K., Oomura, Y.: IEEE Trans. Mag. $\underline{MAG-14}$, 958 (1978).
180. Ueno, S., Lövsund, P., Öberg, P.Å.: On the effect of alternating magnetic fields on action potential in lobster giant axon. Presented at 5th Nordic Meeting on Med. Biol. Engin., Linköping, Sweden, June 10-13, 1981.
181. Polson, M.J.R., Barker, A.T., Freeston, I.L.: Med. Biol. Engin. Comput. $\underline{20}$, 243 (1982).
182. Ueno, S., Harada, K., Ji, C., Oomura, Y.: IEEE Trans. Mag. $\underline{MAG-20}$, 1660 (1984).
183. Osypka, P.: Elektromed. $\underline{8}$, 153 and 193 (1963).
184. Geddes, L.A., Baker, L.E., Moore, A.G., Coulter, T.W.: Med. Biol. Engin. $\underline{7}$, 289 (1969).
185. Watson, A.B., Wright, J.S., Loughman, J.: Med. J. Aust. $\underline{1}$, 1179 (1973).
186. Irnich, W., Silny, J., deBakker, J.M.T.: Biomed. Technik $\underline{19}$, 62 (1974).
187. Jacobsen, J., Buntenkötter, S., Reinhard, H.J., et al.: Deut. Tierärzt. Wochenschr. $\underline{81}$, 214 (1974).
188. Roy, O.Z., Scott, J.R., Park, G.C.: IEEE Trans. Biomed. Engin. $\underline{23}$, 45 (1976).
189. Roy, O.Z., Park, G.C., Scott, J.R.: IEEE Trans. Biomed. Engin. $\underline{24}$, 430 (1977).
190. Kugelberg, J.: Scan. J. Thorac. Cardiovasc. Surg. $\underline{10}$, 237 (1976).
191. Schwan, H.P.: Ann. N.Y. Acad. Sci. $\underline{303}$, 198 (1977).
192. Antoni, H.: Funkt. Biol. Med. $\underline{1}$, 39 (1982).
193. Weirich, J., Hohnloser, S., Antoni, H.: Pflügers Arch. Suppl. $\underline{392}$, 3 (1982).

194. Weirich, J.: Cardiol. 70, 19 (1983).
195. Dalziel, C.F.: Trans. AIEE 79, 667 (1960).
196. Fink, M. Convulsive Therapy: Theory and Practice. New York: Raven Press (1979).
197. Dalziel, C.F.: IRE Trans. Med. Electron. PGME-5, 44 (1956).
198. Lee, W.R.: Proc. IRE 113, 144 (1966).
199. Tenforde, T.S.: Physical properties of high-voltage ELF electromagnetic fields and their interaction with living systems. Proc. Workshop on Electric Energy Systems Research, Washington, D.C., April 24-26, 1985.
200. Wachtel, H.: Firing-pattern changes and transmembrane currents produced by extremely low frequency fields in pacemaker neurons. (In) Biological Effects of Extremely Low Frequency Electromagnetic Fields, pp. 132-146. Phillips, R.D., Gillis, M.F., Kaune, W.T., Mahlum, D.D., eds. Springfield, VA: NTIS Rep. No. CONF-781016 (1979).
201. d'Arsonval, M.A.: C.R. Soc. Biol. (Paris) 3 (100 Ser.), 450 (1896).
202. Thompson, S.P.: Proc. Roy. Soc. Lond. (Ser. B) 82, 396 (1909-1910).
203. Dunlap, K.: Science 33, 68 (1911).
204. Magnusson, C.E., Stevens, H.C.: Am. J. Physiol. 29, 124 (1911-1912).
205. Barlow, H.B., Kohn, H.I., Walsh, E.G.: Am. J. Physiol. 148, 372 (1947).
206. Seidel, D., Knoll, M., Eichmeier, J.: Pflüg. Arch. 229, 11 (1968).
207. Lövsund, P., Öberg, P.Å., Nilsson, S.E.G.: Acta Ophth. 57, 812 (1979).
208. Lövsund, P., Öberg, P.Å., Nilsson, S.E.G.: Radio Science 14(6S), 125 (1979).
209. Lövsund, P., Öberg, P.Å., Nilsson, S.E.G.: Med. Biol. Engin. Comp. 18, 758 (1980).
210. Lövsund, P., Öberg, P.Å., Nilsson, S.E.G., Reuter, T.: Med. Biol. Engin. Comp. 18, 326 (1980).
211. Lövsund,, P., Nilsson, S.E.G., Öberg P.Å.: Med. Biol. Engin. Comp. 19, 679 (1981).
212. Lövsund, P., Öberg, P.Å., Nilsson, S.E.G.: Radio Science 17(5S), 35S (1982).
213. Budinger, T.F., Cullander, C., Bordow, R.: Switched magnetic field thresholds for the induction of magnetophosphenes. Presented at 3rd Ann. Meeting of Soc. Mag. Res. Med., New York, Aug. 13-17, 1984.
214. Silny, J.: Changes in VEP caused by strong magnetic fields. (In) Evoked Potentials II: The Second International Evoked Potentials Symposium, pp. 272-279. Nodar, R.H., Barber, C., eds. Boston: Butterworth (1984).
215. Odintsov, Y.N.: Tr. Tomskogo. Vaktsyn. Syvorotok 16, 234 (1965).
216. Druz, V.A., Madiyevskii, Yu.M.: Biofiz. 11, 631 (1966).
217. Riesen, W.H., Aranyi, C., Kyle, J.L., Valentino, A.R., Miller, D.A.: A pilot study of the interaction of extremely low frequency electromagnetic fields with brain organelles. (In)

Compilation of Navy-Sponsored ELF Biomedical and Ecological Research Reports, Vol. 1, Tech. Memo. No. 3 (IITRI Proj. E6185). Bethesda, Naval Med. Res. Develop. Command (1971).
218. Tarakhovsky, M.L., Sambroskaya, E.P., Medvedev, B.M., et al.: Fiziol. Zh. Kiev. Akad. Nauk Ukr. (RSR) 17, 452 (1971).
219. Krueger, W.F., Bradley, J.W., Giarola, A.J., Daruvalla, S.R.: ISA Trans. BM 72335, 183 (1972).
220. Ossenkopp, K.-P., Koltek, W.T., Persinger, M.A.: Develop. Psychobiol. 5, 275 (1972).
221. Beischer, D.E., Grissett, J.D., Mitchell, R.R.: Exposure of man to magnetic fields alternating at extremely low frequency. Rep. No. NAMRL-1180. Pensacola: Naval Aerosp. Med. Res. Lab. (1973).
222. deLorge, J.: A psychobiological study of rhesus monkeys exposed to extremely low-frequency low-intensity magnetic fields. Rep. No. NAMRL 1203 (NTIS No. AD/A000078). Pensacola: Naval Aerosp. Med. Res. Lab. (1974).
223. Toroptsev, I.V., Garganeyev, G.P., Gorshenina, T.I., Teplyakova, N.L.: Pathologoanatomic characteristics of changes in experimental animals under the influence of magnetic fields. (In) Influence of Magnetic Fields on Biological Objects, pp. 95-104. Kholodov, Yu.A., ed. Springfield, VA: NTIS Rep. No. JPRS 63038 (1974).
224. Udintsev, N.A., Moroz, V.V.: Byull. Eksp. Biol. Med. 77, 51 (1974).
225. Mizushima, Y., Akaoka, I., Nishida, Y.: Experientia 21, 1411 (1975).
226. Beischer, D.E., Brehl, R.J.: Search for effects of 45 Hz magnetic fields on liver triglycerides in mice. Rep. No. NAMRL-1197. Pensacola: Naval Aerosp. Res. Lab. (1975).
227. Mantell, B.: Untersuchungen über die Wirkung eines magnetischen Wechselfeldes 50 Hz auf den Menschen (Investigations into the effects on man of an alternating magnetic field at 50 Hz). Ph.D. diss., University of Freiburg, Germany (1975).
228. Udintsev, N.A., Kanskaia, N.V., Shchepetil'nifova, A.I., et al.: Byull. Eksp. Biol. Med. 81, 670 (1976).
229. Batkin, S., Tabrah, F.L.: Res. Comm. Chem. Pathol. Pharmacol. 16, 351 (1977).
230. Sakharova, S.A., Ryzhov, A.I., Udintsev, N.A.: Dokl. Vyssh. Shkoly. Biol. Nauki 9, 35 (1977).
231. Kartashev, A.G., Kalyuzhin, V.A., Migalkin, I.V.: Kosm. Biol. Aviakosm. Med. 12, 76 (1978).
232. Kolesova, N.I., Voloshina, E.I., Udintsev, N.A.: Patol. Fiziol. Eksp. 6, 71 (1978).
233. Tabrah, F.L., Guernsey, D.L., Chou, S.-C., Batkin, S.: T.-I.-T. J. Life Sci. 8, 73 (1978).
234. Persinger, M.A., Lafreniere, G.F., Carrey, N.J.: Int. J. Biometeor. 22, 67 (1978).
235. Persinger, M.A., Coderre, D.J.: Int. J. Biometeor. 22, 123 (1978).
236. Udintsev, N.A., Serebrov, V.Yu., Tsyrov, G.I.: Byull. Eksp. Biol. Med. 86, 544 (1978).
237. Udintsev, N.A., Khlynin, S.M.: Ukr. Biol. Zh. 50, 714 (1979).
238. Kronenberg, S.S., Tenforde, T.S.: Cell growth in a

low-intensity, 60-Hz magnetic field. Lawrence Berkeley Laboratory Rep. No. 10056. Berkeley, CA: University of California (1979).
239. Chandra, S., Stefani, S.: Effects of constant and alternating magnetic fields on tumor cells in vitro and in vivo. (In) Biological Effects of Extremely Low Frequency Electromagnetic Fields, pp. 436-446. Phillips, R.D., Gillis, M.F., Kaune, W.T., Mahlum, D.D., eds. Springfield, VA: NTIS Rep. No. CONF-781016 (1979).
240. Chiabrera, A., Hinsenkamp, M., Pilla, A.A., et al.: J. Histochem. Cytochem. 27, 375 (1979).
241. Goodman, E.M., Greenebaum, B., Marron, M.T.: Radiat. Res. 78, 485 (1979).
242. Greenebaum, B., Goodman, E.M., Marron, M.T.: Radio Sci. 14(6S), 103 (1979).
243. Kolodub, F.A., Chernysheva, O.N.: Ukr. Biokhim. Zh. (Kiev) 3, 299 (1980).
244. Fam, W.Z.: IEEE Trans. Mag. MAG-17, 1510 (1981).
245. Aarholt, E., Flinn, E.A., Smith, C.W.: Phys. Med. Biol. 26, 613 (1981).
246. Ramon, C., Ayaz, M., Streeter, D.D., Jr.: Bioelectromagnetics 2, 285 (1981).
247. Toroptsev, I.V., Soldatova, L.P.: Arkh. Patol. (Moscow) 43, 33 (1981).
248. Kolodub, F.A., Chernysheva, O.N., Evtushenko, G.I.: Kardiol. 21, 82 (1981).
249. Sakharova, S.A., Ryzhov, A.I., Udintsev, N.A.: Kosm. Biol. Aviakosm. Med. 15, 52 (1981).
250. Delgado, J.M.R., Leal, J., Monteagudo, J.L., Garcia-Garcia, M.G.: J. Anat. 134, 533 (1982).
251. Aarholt, E., Flinn, E.A., Smith, C.W.: Phys. Biol. Med. 27, 606 (1982).
252. Soldatova, L.P., Arkh. Anat. Gistol. Embriol. 83, 12 (1982).
253. Sander, R., Brinkmann, J., Kuhne, B.: Laboratory studies on animals and human beings exposed to 50 Hz electric and magnetic fields. Paper 36-01 presented at Int. Cong. Large High Voltage Elect. Syst., Paris, Sept. 1-9, 1982.
254. Lubin, R.A., Cain, C.D., Chen, M.C.-Y., et al.: Proc. Natl. Acad. Sci. (USA) 79, 4180 (1982).
255. Shober, A., Yank, M., Fischer, G.: Zbl. Bakt. Hyg. B176, 305 (1982).
256. Norton, L.A.: Clin. Orthop. Rel. Res. 167, 280 (1982).
257. Dixey, R., Rein, G.: Nature 296, 253 (1982).
258. Conti, P., Gigante, G.E., Cifone, M.G., et al.: FEBS Lett. 162, 156 (1983).
259. Goodman, R., Bassett, C.A.L., Henderson, A.S.: Science 220, 1283 (1983).
260. Jolley, W.B., Hinshaw, D.B., Knierim, K., Hinshaw, D.B.: Bioelectromagnetics 4, 103 (1983).
261. Ramirez, E., Monteagudo, J.L., Garcia-Gracia, M., Delgado, J.M.R.: Bioelectromagnetics 4, 315 (1983).
262. Ubeda, A., Leal, J., Trillo, M.A., et al.: J. Anat. 137, 513 (1983).

263. Archer, C.W., Ratcliffe, N.A.: J. Exp. Zool. 225, 243 (1983).
264. Liboff, A.R., Williams, T., Jr., Strong, D.M., Wistar, R., Jr.: Science 223, 818 (1984).
265. Cain, C.S., Luben, R.A., Adey, W.R.: Pulsed electromagnetic field effects on PTH stimulated cAMP accumulation and bone resorption in mouse calvariae. Presented at 23rd Ann. Hanford Life Sci. Symp., Richland, WA, Oct. 2-4, 1984.
266. Winters, W.D., Phillips, J.L.: Enhancement of human tumor cell growth by electromagnetic and magnetic fields. Presented at 6th Ann. Bioelectromagnetics Soc. Meeting, Atlanta, GA, July 15-19, 1984.
267. Winters, W.D., Phillips, J.L.: Monoclonal antibody detection of tumor antigens in human colon cancer cells following electromagnetic field exposures. Presented at 6th Ann. Bioelectromagnetics Soc. Meeting, Atlanta, GA, July 15-19, 1984.
268. Murray, J.C., Farndale, R.W.: Biochim. Biophys. Acta 838, 98 (1985).
269. Friedman, H., Becker, R.O., Bachman, C.H.: Nature 213, 949 (1967).
270. Persinger, M.A.: Develop. Psychobiol. 2, 168 (1969).
271. Persinger, M.A., Foster, W.S.: Arch. Met. Geoph. Biokl. (Ser. B) 18, 363 (1970).
272. Persinger, M.A., Pear J.J.: Develop. Psychobiol. 5, 269 (1972).
273. Persinger, M.A., Ossenkopp, K.-P., Glavin, G.B.: Int. J. Biometeor. 16, 155 (1972).
274. Medvedev, M.A., Urazaev, A.M., Kulakov, I.U.A.: Zh. Vyssh. Nerv. Deiat. 26, 1131 (1976).
275. Smith, R.F., Justesen, D.R.: Radio Science 12(6S), 279 (1977).
276. Brown, F.A. Jr., Scow, K.M.: J. Interdiscipl. Cycle Res. 9, 137 (1978).
277. Delgado, J.M.R., Monteagudo, J.L., Ramiriz, E.: Non-invasive magnetic stimulation of the monkey cerebellum. Presented at the 5th Ann. Meeting of the Bioelectromagnetics Soc., Boulder, CO, June 12-16, 1983.
278. deLorge, J.: Operant behavior of rhesus monkeys in the presence of low-frequency low-intensity magnetic and electric fields: experiment 1. Rep. No. NAMRL-1155 (NTIS No. AD754058). Pensacola: Naval Aerosp. Med. Lab. (1972).
279. deLorge, J.: Operant behavior of rhesus monkeys in the presence of low-frequency low-intensity magnetic and electric fields: experiment 2. Rep. No. NAMRL 1179 (NTIS No. AD764532). Pensacola: Naval Aerosp. Med. Res. Lab. (1973).
280. deLorge, J.: Operant behavior of rhesus monkeys in the presence of low-frequency low-intensity magnetic and electric fields: experiment 3. Rep. No. NAMRL 1196 (NTIS No. AD774106). Pensacola: Naval Aerosp. Med. Res. Lab. (1973).
281. deLorge, J.: Effects of magnetic fields on behavior in nonhuman primates. (In) Magnetic Field Effects on Biological Systems, pp. 37-38. Tenforde, T.S., ed. New York: Plenum (1979).
282. deLorge, J.: Behavioral studies of monkeys in electric and magnetic fields at ELF frequencies. (In) Biological Effects and Dosimetry of Non-ionizing Radiation: Static and ELF Electromagnetic Fields. Grandolfo, M., Michaelson, S.M., Rindi,

A., eds. New York: Plenum, in press, 1985.
283. Tucker, R.D., Schmitt, O.H.: IEEE Trans. Biomed. Engin. BME-25, 509 (1978).
284. Fitton-Jackson, S., Bassett, C.A.L.: The response of skeletal tissues to pulsed magnetic fields. (In) Tissue Culture in Medical Research (II), pp. 21-28. Richards, R.J., Rajan, K.T., eds. New York: Pergamon (1980).
285. Bassett, C.A.L.: Pulsing electromagnetic fields: a new approach to surgical problems. (In) Metabolic Surgery, pp. 255-306. Buchwald, H., Varco, R.L., eds. New York: Grune and Stratton (1978).
286. Bassett, C.A.L., Pawluk, R.J., Pilla, A.A.: Ann. N.Y. Acad. Sci. 238, 242 (1974).
287. Bassett, C.A.L., Pilla, A.A., Pawluk, R.J.: Clin. Orthop. 124, 128 (1977).
288. Watson, J., Downes, E.M.: Japan J. Appl. Phys. 17, 215 (1978).
289. Bassett, C.A.L., Mitchell, S.N., Gaston, S.R.: J. Am. Med. Assoc. 247, 623 (1982).
290. Bigliani, L.U., Rosenwasser, M.P., Caulo, N., et al.: J. Bone Joint Surg. 65, 480 (1983).
291. Barker, A.T., Lunt, M.J.: Clin. Phys. Physiol. Meas. 4, 1 (1983).
292. Lunt, M.J.: Med. Biol. Engin. Comput. 20, 501 (1982).
293. Barker, A.T., Dixon, R.A., Sharrard, W.J.W., Sutcliffe, M.L.: Lancet 1 (8384), 994 (1984).
294. Bottomley, P.A., Andrew, E.R.: Phys. Med. Biol. 23, 630 (1978).
295. Hoult, D.I., Lauterbur, P.C.: J. Mag. Res. 34, 425 (1979).
296. Bottomley, P.A.: RF power deposition in NMR imaging. Presented at 3rd Ann. Meeting of Soc. Mag. Res. Med., New York, Aug. 13-17, 1984.
297. Budinger, T.F., Pavlicek, W., Faul, D.D., Guy, A.W.: RF heating at 1.5 Tesla and above in proton NMR imaging. Presented at 4th Ann. Meeting of Soc. Mag. Res. Med., London, Aug. 19-23, 1985.
298. Bottomley, P.A., Edelstein, W.A.: Med. Phys. 8, 510 (1981).
299. Bottomley, P.A., Redington, R.W., Edelstein, W.A., Schenck, J.F.: Mag. Res. Med., in press, 1985.
300. Guy, A.W.: IEEE Trans. Microwave Theory Tech. MTT-19, 205 (1971).
301. Chou, C.K., Guy, A.W.: Microwave and RF dosimetry. (In) The Physical Basis of Electromagnetic Interactions with Biological Systems, pp. 214-216. Taylor, L.S., Cheung, A.Y., eds. Rockville, MD: HEW Publ. (FDA) 78-8055 (1978).
302. Cetas, T.C.: Thermometry in strong electromagnetic fields. (In) The Physical Basis of Electromagnetic Interactions with Biological Systems, pp. 261-281. Taylor, L.S., Cheung, A.Y., eds. Rockville, MD: HEW Publ. (FDA) 78-8055 (1978).
303. Deficis, A., Priou, A.: Non-perturbing microprobes for measurements in electromagnetic fields. (In) The Physical Basis of Electromagnetic Interactions with Biological Systems, pp. 283-293. Taylor, L.S., Cheung, A.Y., eds. Rockville, MD: HEW Publ. (FDA) 78-8055 (1978).
304. Cain, C.A., Chen, M.M., Lam, K.L., Mullin, J.: The viscometric thermometer. (In) The Physical Basis of Electromagnetic

Interactions with Biological Systems, pp. 295-308. Taylor, L.S., Cheung, A.Y., eds. Rockville, MD: HEW Publ. (FDA) 78-8055 (1978).
305. Olsen, R.G., Hammer, W.C.: Thermographic comparison of temperature probes used in microwave dosimetry studies. Presented at Symp. on Electromagnetic Fields in Biological Systems, Ottawa, Canada, June 27-30, 1978.
306. Durney, C.H., Johnson, C.C., Barber, P.W., et al.: Radiofrequency Radiation Handbook, 2nd ed., Rep. No. SAM-TR-768-22. Salt Lake City, UT: University of Utah Elec. Engin. Dept. (1978).
307. Wilkening, G.M., Barnes, F.S., Bowman, R.R., et al.: Radiofrequency Electromagnetic Fields: Properties, Quantities and Units, Biophysical Interaction, and Measurements. Washington, D.C.: National Council on Radiation Protection and Measurements Rep. No. 67 (1981).
308. Hoult, D.I.: Medical imaging by NMR. (In) Magnetic Resonance in Biology, Vol. 1, pp. 70-109. Cohen, J.S., ed. New York: Wiley (1980).
309. Pavlicek, W., Budinger, T.F., Kramer, D., et al.: unpublished data from studies on RF heating in human subjects during NMR proton imaging at Cleveland Clinic, 1984.
310. Kritikos, H.N., Schwan, H.P.: IEEE Trans. Biomed. Engin. $\underline{\text{BME-19}}$, 53 (1972).
311. Kritikos, H.N., Schwan, H.P.: IEEE Trans. Biomed. Engin. $\underline{\text{BME-22}}$, 457 (1975).
312. Gandhi, O.P., DeFord, J.F., Kanai, H.: IEEE Trans. Biomed. Engin. $\underline{\text{BME-31}}$, 644 (1984).
313. Michaelson, S.M.: Biological effects and health hazards of RF and MW energy: fundamentals and overall phenomenology. (In) Biological Effects and Dosimetry of Nonionizing Radiation, pp. 337-357. Grandolfo, M., Michaelson, S.M., Rindi, A., eds. New York: Plenum (1983).
314. Hammel, H.T., Hardy, J.D., Fusco, M.M.: Am. J. Physiol. $\underline{198}$, 481 (1960).
315. Brengelmann, G.: Temperature regulation. (In) Physiology and Biophysics, Vol. III (20th ed.), pp. 105-135. Ruch, T.C., Patton, H.D., eds. Philadelphia: Saunders (1974).
316. Lotz, W.G., Michaelson, S.M.: J. Appl. Physiol. Resp. Envir. Exercise Physiol. $\underline{44}$, 438 (1978).
317. Lotz, W.G., Michaelson, S.M.: J. Appl. Physiol. Resp. Envir. Exercise Physiol. $\underline{47}$, 1284 (1979).
318. Parker, L.N.: Am. J. Physiol. $\underline{224}$, 1388 (1973).
319. Vetter, R.J.: Proc. Natl. Electron. Conf. $\underline{30}$, 237 (1975).
320. Lu, S.-T., Lebda, N., Pettit, S., et al.: Radio Sci. $\underline{12(6S)}$, 147 (1977).
321. Lu, S.-T., Lotz, W.G., Michaelson, S.M.: Proc. IEEE $\underline{68}$, 73 (1980).
322. Lu, S.-T., Bogardus, R., Cohen, J., et al.: Thermogenetic and cardiodynamic regulation in dogs cranially exposed to 2450-MHz (CW) microwaves. (In) IEEE S-MIT Int. Symp. Dig. Tech. Papers, pp. 102-103. Gaylord, T.K., ed. (1974).
323. Kinnen, E., Bogardus, R., Lu, S.-T., Michaelson, S.: Proc.

Natl. Electron. Conf. 30, 233 (1975).
324. Michaelson, S.M.: Neurosci. Res. Prog. Bull. 15, 98 (1977).
325. Stern, S., Margolin, L., Weiss, B., et al.: Science 206, 1198 (1979).
326. Adair, E.R.: J. Appl. Physiol. 42, 559 (1977).
327. Adair, E.R., Adams, B.W.: Bioelectromagnetics 1, 1 (1980).
328. Adair, E.R., Adams, B.W., Akel, G.M.: Bioelectromagnetics 5, 3 (1984).
329. McRee, D.I., Wachtel, H.: Radiat. Res. 82, 536 (1980).
330. Modak, A.T., Stavinoha, W.B., Deam, A.P.: Bioelectromagnetics 2, 89 (1981).
331. Hjeresen, D.L., Guy, A.W., Petracca, F.M., Diaz, J.: Bioelectromagnetics 4, 341 (1983).
332. Yee, K.C., Chou, C.K., Guy, A.W.: Bioelectromagnetics 5, 263 (1984).
333. Frey, A.H., Feld, S.R., Frey, B.: Ann. N.Y. Acad. Sci. 247, 433 (1975).
334. Oscar, K.J., Hawkins, T.D.: Brain Res. 126, 281 (1977).
335. Merritt, J.H., Chamness, A.F., Allen, S.J.: Radiat. Envir. Biophys. 15, 367 (1978).
336. Preston, E., Vavasour, E.J., Assenheim, H.M.: Brain Res. 174, 109 (1979).
337. Justeson, D.R.: Proc. IEEE 68, 60 (1980).
338. Ward, T.R., Elder, J.A., Long, M.D., Svendsgaard, D.: Bioelectromagnetics 3, 371 (1982).
339. Goldman, H., Lin, J.C., Murphy, S., Lin, M.F.: Bioelectromagnetics 5, 323 (1984).
340. deLorge, J.O., Ezell, C.S.: Bioelectromagnetics 1, 183 (1980).
341. Lebovitz, R.M.: Bioelectromagnetics 2, 169 (1981).
342. Thomas, J.R., Schrot, J., Banvard, R.A.: Bioelectromagnetics 3, 227 (1982).
343. deLorge, J.O.: Bioelectromagnetics 5, 233 (1984).
344. Cook, H.F.: J. Physiol. 118, 1 (1952).
345. Hendler, E., Hardy, J.D., Murgatroyd, D.: Skin heating and temperature sensation produced by infrared and microwave irradiation. (In) Temperature Measurement and Control in Science and Industry, pp. 221-230. Hardy, J.D., ed. New York: Reinhold (1963).
346. Hendler, E.: Cutaneous receptor response to microwave radiation. (In) Thermal Problems in Aerospace Medicine, pp. 149-161. Hardy, J.D., ed. Surrey: Unwin Ltd. (1968).
347. Justeson, D.R., Adair, E.R., Stevens, J.C., Bruce-Wolfe, V.: Bioelectromagnetics 3, 117 (1982).
348. Frey, A.H.: Aerosp. Med. 32, 1140 (1961).
349. Sharp, J.C., Grove, H.M., Gandhi, O.P.: IEEE Trans. Microwave Theory Tech. 22, 583 (1974).
350. Foster, K.R., Finch, E.D.: Science 185, 256 (1974).
351. Guy, A.W., Chou, C.K., Lin, J.C., Christensen, D.: Ann. N.Y. Acad. Sci. 247, 194 (1975).
352. Lin, J.C.: Microwave Auditory Effects and Applications. Springfield, IL: C.C. Thomas (1978).
353. Lin, J.C.: Proc. IEEE 68, 67 (1980).
354. Birenbaum, L., Kaplan, I.T., Metlay, W., et al.: J. Microwave

Power 4, 232 (1969).
355. Guy, A.W., Lin, J.C., Kramer, P.O., Emery, A.F.: IEEE Trans. Microwave Theory Tech. MIT-23, 492 (1975).
356. Appleton, B., Hirsch, S.E., Brown, P.V.K.: Ann. N.Y. Acad. Sci. 247, 125 (1975).
357. Kramer, P., Harris, C., Emery, A.F., Guy, A.W.: J. Microwave Power 11, 135 (1976).
358. Cleary, S.F.: Proc. IEEE 68, 49 (1980).
359. Kues, H.A., Hirst, L.W., Lutty, G.A., et al.: Bioelectromagnetics 6, 177 (1985).
360. Liburdy, R.P.: Radiat. Res. 77, 34 (1979).
361. Liburdy, R.P.: Radiat. Res. 83, 66 (1980).
362. Smialowicz, R.J., Rogers, R.R., Garner, R.J., et al.: Bioelectromagnetics 4, 371 (1983).
363. Yang, H.K., Cain, C.A., Lockwood, J., Tompkins, W.A.F.: Bioelectromagnetics 4, 123 (1983).
364. Rao, G.R., Cain, C.A., Lockwood, J., Tompkins, W.A.F.: Bioelectromagnetics 4, 141 (1983).
365. Rao, G.R., Cain, C.A., Tompkins, W.A.F.: Bioelectromagnetics 5, 377 (1984).
366. Rao, G.R., Cain, C.A., Tompkins, W.A.F.: Bioelectromagnetics 6, 41 (1985).
367. Michaelson, S.M., Thomson, R.A.F., Tamami, M.Y.El., et al.: Aerosp. Med. 35, 824 (1964).
368. Michaelson, S.M., Thomson, R.A.F., Howland, J.W.: Biologic Effects of Microwave Exposure, p. 138. Rome, N.Y.: Griffiss Air Force Base Rep. No. ASTIA AD824-242 (1967).
369. Baranski, S.: Aerosp. Med. 42, 1196 (1971).
370. Czerski, P.: Ann. N.Y. Acad. Sci. 247, 232 (1975).
371. Roberts, N.J. Jr.: Radiofrequency and microwave effects on immunological and hematopoietic systems. (In) Biological Effects and Dosimetry of Nonionizing Radiation, pp. 429-459. Grandolfo, M., Michaelson, S.M., Rindi, A., eds. New York: Plenum (1983).
372. Imig, C.J., Thomson, J.D., Hines, H.M.: Proc. Soc. Exp. Biol. 69, 382 (1948).
373. Gorodetskaya, S.F.: Fiziol. Zh. 9, 394 (1963).
374. Ely, T.S., Goldman, D., Hearon, J.Z., et al.: IEEE Trans. Biomed. Engin. BME-11, 123 (1964).
375. Brent, R.L., Franklin, J.B., Wallace, J.P.: Teratol. 4, 48A (1971).
376. Rugh, R., Ginns, E.I., Ho, H.S., Leach, W.M.: Radiat. Res. 62, 225 (1975).
377. Rugh, R.: J. Microwave Power 11, 127 (1976).
378. Chernovetz, M.E., Justesen, D.R., Oke, A.F.: Radio Sci. 12(6S), 191 (1977).
379. Berman, E., Kinn, J.B., Carter, H.B.: Health Phys. 35, 791 (1978).
380. O'Connor, M.E.: Proc. IEEE 68, 56 (1980).
381. Lary, J.M., Conover, D.L., Johnson, P.H., Burg, J.R.: Bioelectromagnetics 4, 249 (1983).
382. Allis, J.W., Sinha, B.L.: Bioelectromagnetics 2, 13 (1981).

383. Mikolajczyk, H.: Bioelectromagnetics 2, 51 (1981).
384. Stensaas, L.J., Partlow, L.M., Bush, L.G., et al.: Bioelectromagnetics 2, 141 (1981).
385. Furmaniak, A.: Bioelectromagnetics 4, 55 (1983).
386. Sultan, M.F., Cain, C.A., Tompkins, W.A.F.: Bioelectromagnetics 4, 115 (1983).
387. Sultan, M.F., Cain, C.A., Tompkins, W.A.F.: Bioelectromagnetics 4, 157 (1983).
388. Dardalhon, M., More, C., Averbeck, D., Berteaud, A.J.: Bioelectromagnetics 5, 247 (1984).
389. Liburdy, R.P., Penn, A.: Bioelectromagnetics 5, 283 (1984).
390. Barsoum, Y.H., Pickard, W.F.: Bioelectromagnetics 3, 193 (1982).
391. Barsoum, Y.H., Pickard, W.F.: Bioelectromagnetics 3, 393 (1982).
392. Gokhale, A.V., Brunkard, K.M., Pickard, W.F.: Bioelectromagnetics 5, 357 (1984).
393. Shnyrov, V.L., Zhadan, G.G., Akoev, I.G.: Bioelectromagnetics 5, 411 (1984).
394. Janes, D.E., Leach, W.M., Mills, W.A., et al.: Nonioniz. Radiat. 1, 125 (1969).
395. Heller, J.H.: Cellular effects of microwave radiation. (In) Biological Effects and Health Implications of Microwave Radiation, pp. 116-121. Cleary, S.F., ed. Bethesda: U.S.H.E.W./P.H.S. (BRH/DBE) Rep. No. 70-2 (1970).
396. Chen, K.M., Samuel, A., Hoopingavner, R.: Envir. Lett. 6, 37 (1974).
397. Yao, K.T.S.: Genetics 83, 584 (1976).
398. Averbeck, D., Dardalhon, M., Berteaud, A.J.: J. Microwave Power 11, 143 (1976).
399. Baranski, S., Debiec, H., Kwarecki, K., Mezykowski, T.: J. Microwave Power 11, 146 (1976).
400. Huang, A.T., Engle, M.E., Elder, J.A., et al.: Radio Sci. 12(6S), 173 (1977).
401. Correlli, J.C., Gutmann, R.J., Kohazi, S., Levy, J.: J. Microwave Power 12(6S), 141 (1977).
402. Geard, C.R., Osmak, R.S., Hall, E.J., et al.: Radiol. 152, 199 (1984).
403. Thomas, A., Morris, P.G.: Brit. J. Radiol. 54, 615 (1981).
404. Cooke, P., Morris, P.G.: Brit. J. Radiol. 54, 622 (1981).
405. Michaelson, S.M.: Mutagenic and developmental effects of microwave radiofrequency (MW/RF) energies. (In) Biological Effects and Dosimetry of Nonionizing Radiation, pp. 461-484. Grandolfo, M., Michaelson, S.M., Rindi, A., eds. New York: Plenum (1983).
406. Gordon, Z.V., ed.: Biological Effects of Radiofrequency Electromagnetic Fields. JPRS Rep. No. 63321 (1974).
407. Minin, B.A.: Microwaves and Human Safety. JPRS Rep. No. 65506-1 (1975).
408. McRee, D.I.: Proc. IEEE 68, 84 (1980).
409. Sanders, A.P., Schaefer, D.J., Joines, W.T.: Bioelectromagnetics 1, 171 (1980).
410. Sanders, A.P., Joines, W.T.: Bioelectromagnetics 5, 63 (1980).

411. Sanders, A.P., Joines, W.T., Allis, J.W.: Bioelectromagnetics 6, 89 (1985).
412. Taylor, L.S.: Bioelectromagnetics 2, 259 (1981).
413. Postow, E., Swicord, M.L.: Modulated field and "window" effects. (In) Handbook of Biological Effects of Electromagnetic Fields. Polk, C., Postow, E., eds. Boca Raton, FL: CRC Press, in press, 1986.
414. Bawin, S.M., Kaczmarek, L.K., Adey, W.R.: Ann. N.Y. Acad. Sci. 247, 74 (1975).
415. Blackman, C.F., Elder, J.A., Weil, C.M., et al.: Radio Sci. 14(6S), 93 (1979).
416. Blackman, C.F., Benane, S.G., Elder, J.A., et al.: Bioelectromagnetics 1, 35 (1980).
417. Blackman, C.F., Benane, S.G., Joines, W.T., et al.: Bioelectromagnetics 1, 227 (1980).
418. Joines, W.T., Blackman, C.F.: Bioelectromagnetics 1, 271 (1980).
419. Joines, W.T., Blackman, C.F.: Bioelectromagnetics 2, 411 (1981).
420. Weil, C.M., Spiegel, R.J., Joines, W.T.: Bioelectromagnetics 5, 293 (1984).
421. Adey, W.R., Bawin, S.M., Lawrence, A.F.: Bioelectromagnetics 3, 295 (1982).
422. Shelton, W.W., Merritt, J.H.: Bioelectromagnetics 2, 161 (1981).
423. Merritt, J.H., Shelton, W.W., Chamness, A.F.: Bioelectromagnetics 3, 475 (1982).
424. Vyalov, A.M.: Clinco-hygienic and experimental data on the effects of magnetic fields under industrial conditions. (In) Influence of Magnetic Fields on Biological Objects, pp. 163-174. Kholodov, Yu.A., ed. Springfield, VA: NTIS Rep. No. JPRS 63038 (1974).
425. Marsh, J.L., Armstrong, T.J., Jacobson, A.P., Smith, R.G.: Am. Indust. Hyg. Assoc. J. 43, 387 (1982).
426. Budinger, T.F., Bristol, K.S., Yen, C.K., Wong, P.: Biological effects of static magnetic fields. Presented at 3rd Ann. Meeting Soc. Mag. Res. Med., New York, Aug. 4-6, 1984.
427. Milham, S.: New Eng. J. Med. 307, 249 (1982).
428. Tenforde, T.S.: Magnetic field applications in modern technology and medicine. Proc. Symp. Biological Effects of Static and Extremely-Low-Frequency Magnetic Fields. Neuherberg, West Germany, May 13-15, 1985.
429. Rockette, H.E., Arena, V.C.: J. Occup. Med. 25, 549 (1983).
430. Wertheimer, N., Leeper, E.: Am. J. Epidemiol. 109, 273 (1979).
431. Fulton, J.P., Cobb, S., Preble, L.: Am. J. Epidemiol. 111, 392 (1980).
432. Tomenius, L., Helström, L., Enander, B.: Electrical constructions and 50 Hz magnetic field at the dwellings of tumour cases (0-18 years of age) in the county of Stockholm. Presented at the Int. Symp. Occup. Health and Safety in Mining and Tunnelling, Prague, June 21-25, 1982.
433. Wertheimer, N., Leeper, E.: Int. J. Epidemiol. 11, 345 (1982).
434. Wiklund, K., Einhorn, J., Eklund, G.: Int. J. Epidemiol. 10,

373 (1981).
435. Wright, W.E., Peters, J.M., Mack, T.M.: Lancet 2(8308), 1160 (1982).
436. McDowall, M.E.: Lancet 1(8318), 246 (1983).
437. Coleman, M., Bell, J., Skeet, R.: Lancet 1(8332), 982 (1983).
438. Vågerö, D., Olin, R.: Brit. J. Ind. Med. 40, 188 (1983).
439. Pearce, N.E., Sheppard, R.A., Howard, J.K., et al.: Lancet 1(8432), 811 (1985).
440. Milham, S.: Lancet 1(8432), 812 (1985).
441. Lin, R.S., Dischinger, P.C., Conde, J., Farrell, K.P.: J. Occup. Med. 27, 413 (1985).
442. Occupational Exposure to Microwave Radiation (Radar). Final rep. for Contract No. EDA 223-76-6003 to Food and Drug. Admin., Natl. Acad. Sci., Natl. Res. Council (1978).
443. Cleary, S.F., Pasternack, B.S., Beebe, G.W.: Arch. Envir. Health 11, 179 (1965).
444. Glaser, Z.R., Heimer, G.M.: IEEE Trans. Microwave Theory MIT-19, 232 (1971).
445. Robinette, C.D., Silverman, C., Jablon, S.: Am. J. Epidemiol. 112, 39 (1980).
446. Barron, C.I., Baraff, A.A.: J. Am. Med. Assoc. 168, 1194 (1958).
447. Sigler, A.T., Lilienfeld, A.M., Cohen, B.H., et al.: Bull. Johns Hopkins Hosp. 117, 374 (1965).
448. Cohen, B.H., Lilienfeld, A.M., Kramer, S., et al.: Parental factors in Down's Syndrome -- results of the second Baltimore case-control study. (In) Population Cytogenetics, Studies in Humans, pp. 301-352. Hook, E.B., Porter, I.H., eds. New York: Academic Press (1977).
449. Daels, J.: Obstet. Gyn. 42, 76 (1973).
450. Daels, J.: J. Microwave Power 11, 166 (1976).
451. Lilienfeld, A.M., Tonascia, J., Tonascia, S., et al.: Foreign Service Health Status Study -- Evaluation of Health Status of Foreign Service and Other Employees from Selected Eastern European Posts. Final rep. for Contract No. 6025-619073, U.S. State Dept. Springfield, VA: NTIS Rep. No. PB-288163 (1978).
452. Silverman, C.: Proc. IEEE 68, 78 (1980).
453. Gordon, Z.V.: Biological Effect of Microwaves in Occupational Hygiene. NASA Transl. No. TTF-663 (1970).
454. Petrov, I.R., ed.: Influence of Microwave Radiation on the Organism of Man and Animals. NASA Transl. No. TTF-708 (1972).
455. Sadchikova, M.N.: Clinical manifestations of reactions to microwaves: irradiation in various occupational groups. (In) Biologic Effects and Health Hazards of Microwave Radiation, pp. 261-267. Czerski, P., Ostrowski, K., Silverman, C., et al., eds. Warsaw: Polish Med. Publ. (1974).
456. Baranski, S., Czerski, P.: Biological Effects of Microwaves. Stroudsburg, PA: Dowden, Hutchinson, Ross (1976).
457. Kunz, L.L., Johnson, R.B., Thompson, D., et al.: Effects of Long-Term Low-Level Radiofrequency Radiation Exposure on Rats. Vol. 8: Evaluation of Longevity, Cause of Death, and Histopathological Findings. Brooks A.F.B., TX: U.S.A.F. School of Med. Rep. No. USAFSAM-TR-85-11 (1985).

458. Smith, F.W.: Lancet 1(8278), 974 (1982).
459. New, P.F.J., Rosen, B.R., Brady, T.J., et al.: Radiol. 147, 139 (1983).
460. Zimmermann, B.H., Paul, D.D.: Diag. Imag. Clin. Med. 53, 53 (1984).
461. Dujovny, M., Kossovsky, N., Kossovsky, R, et al.: Am. Coll. Surg., Surg. Forum XXXIV, 525 (1983).
462. Barrafato, D., Helkelman, M.: Canad. J. Surg. 27, 509 (1984).
463. Davis, P.L., Crooks, L., Arakawa, M., et al.: Am. J. Roentgenol. 137, 857 (1981).
464. Pavlicek, W., Geisinger, M., Castle, L., et al.: Radiol. 147, 149 (1983).
465. Griffin, J.C.: The effects of ELF electric and magnetic fields on artificial cardiac pacemakers. (In) Assessments and Viewpoints on the Biological and Human Health Effects of Extremely Low Frequency (ELF) Electromagnetic Fields, pp. 173-183. Washington, D.C.: Am. Inst. Biol. Sci. (1985).
466. Butrous, G.S., Male, J.C., Webber, R.S., et al.: Pacing and Clin. Electrophysiol. 6, 1282 (1983).
467. Jenkins, B.M., Woody, J.A.: IEEE Int. Symp. on Electromag. Comp. EMC-S 78, 273 (1978).
468. Guidelines for Evaluating Electromagnetic Exposure Risk for Trials of Clinical NMR Systems. F.D.A./D.H.H.S. letter from J.C. Villforth, Director, BRH. Feb. 12, 1982.
469. Natl. Radiol. Protection Board ad hoc Adv. Group on NMR Clinical Imaging: Br. J. Radiol. 56, 974 (1983).
470. Bernhardt, J.H., Kossel, F.: Clin. Phys. Physiol. Meas. 6, 65 (1985).
471. Saunders, R.D., Orr, J.S.: Biologic effects of NMR. (In) Nuclear Magnetic Resonance (NMR) Imaging, pp. 383-396. Partain, C.L., James, A.E., Rollo, F.D., Price, R.R., eds. Philadelphia: Saunders (1983).
472. American National Standards Institute: Safety Levels with Respect to Human Exposure to Radiofrequency Electromagnetic Fields, 300 kHz to 100 GHz. New York: IEEE Rep., ANSI Comm. C.95.1 (1982).
473. Panofsky, W.K.H.: Limits on Human Exposure in Static Magnetic Fields. Palo Alto, CA: Guidance letter to Stanford Linear Accelerator staff, May 6, 1970.
474. Tenforde, T.S.: J. Theor. Biol. 83, 517 (1980).
475. Bonnell, J.A.: Lancet 1(8334), 1168 (1983).
476. Seager, J.: Lancet 1(8537), 1095 (1985).

APPENDIX A

ELECTRICITY AND MAGNETISM FOR NMR - A REVIEW OF BASIC CONCEPTS

Kenneth E. Ekstrand, and Robert L. Dixon
Department of Radiology, Bowman Gray School of Medicine
Winston-Salem, North Carolina 27103

ABSTRACT

We present a review of classical electricity and magnetism with emphasis on its application to the nuclear magnetic resonance phenomenon. Starting from the fundamental laws of electromagnetism, Maxwell's equations, we explore electrostatics and magnetostatics paying particular attention to the behavior of a magnetic dipole in a uniform magnetic field. We then discuss the passive circuit elements (capacitors, inductors, and resistors) and the resonant LRC circuit in the detection of oscillating electromagnetic signals. We then consider the effects of electric and magnetic fields on material media, concluding with an examination of the detection of time-varying changes in the magnetization of a material body.

INTRODUCTION

Nuclear magnetic resonance (NMR) is an inherently quantum mechanical phenomenon; yet many of its effects can be understood in terms of classical physics. For this reason a thorough understanding of classical electromagnetism is important to the study of NMR. This paper begins with a review of the fundamental laws of electromagnetism followed by a discussion of the applications of these laws to situations which are relevant to NMR.

Classical electromagnetism owes its origin to the work of many individuals, but it was Faraday who first emphasized the action of the "field of force" surrounding an electrically charged body or current-carrying wire. Maxwell's further development of the field concept culminated in the four equations which now bear his name. It is thus appropriate to begin our review of electricity and magnetism with an examination of these equations.

MAXWELL'S EQUATIONS AND ELECTROMAGNETIC RADIATION

Since electric and magnetic fields are vectorial in nature, the differential equations which describe them utilize the vector differential operators divergence and curl. In a region of space that is empty aside from the presence of a charge density ρ (coulombs/meter^3) and a current density $\vec{J}$ (amps/meter^2) these equations are in the SI system of units,

$$\text{div}\,\vec{E} = \nabla \cdot \vec{E} = \rho/\epsilon_0 \tag{1}$$

$$\text{div}\,\vec{B} = \nabla \cdot \vec{B} = 0 \tag{2}$$

$$\text{curl } \vec{E} = \nabla \times \vec{E} = -\partial \vec{B}/\partial t \qquad (3)$$

$$\text{curl } \vec{B} = \nabla \times \vec{B} = \mu_0 \vec{J} + \mu_0 \epsilon_0 \partial \vec{E}/\partial t \qquad (4)$$

where $\vec{E}$ is the electric field strength (in volts/meter) and $\vec{B}$ is the magnetic induction (in tesla). The constant ϵ_0 is called the permittivity of free space and μ_0 is the permeability of free space. These equations provide a complete description of the behavior of the fields in terms of their sources. One additional principle is necessary to describe the influence of the fields on charges and currents. This is the Lorentz force law shown in Eq. (5),

$$\vec{F} = q(\vec{E} + \vec{v} \times \vec{B}) \qquad (5)$$

where $\vec{F}$ is the force on a charge q moving with velocity $\vec{v}$.

One remarkable consequence of Maxwell's equations is the inference of the existence of electromagnetic radiation. In a region of space in which there are no charges or currents Eqs. (1 to 4) become symmetrical with respect to $\vec{E}$ and $\vec{B}$. In addition, Eqs. (3) and (4), which couple spatial derivatives with time derivatives, can be transformed to describe $\vec{E}$ and $\vec{B}$ as waves propagating with the velocity $C = 1/\sqrt{\epsilon_0 \mu_0}$ (the velocity of light). At NMR frequencies the wavelength of electromagnetic radiation is large compared with the distance from the pickup coil to the source of signal and therefore considerations of wave behavior of the signal are not relevant. This is not true in the case of electron spin resonance.

ELECTROSTATICS AND MAGNETOSTATICS

If we restrict our attention to the electrostatic case in which the fields are static or slowly varying, the time derivatives in Maxwell's equations can be neglected and we find that $\vec{E}$ and $\vec{B}$ are no longer coupled to each other. Electric fields are determined solely by the distribution of charges and the magnetic induction arises from currents. In this case Eq. (3) simplifies to

$$\nabla \times \vec{E} = 0 \qquad (6)$$

An important consequence which can be derived from Eq. (6) is that the electric field is the gradient of a scalar potential function[1], V(r), whose units are volts. That is

$$\vec{E} = -\nabla V \qquad (7)$$

The minus sign is used for consistency with the expression for the potential energy of a charged particle being acted upon by an electric force. The work done in moving charge q from point r_1 to point r_2 is

$$W = \int_{r_1}^{r_2} \vec{F} \cdot d\vec{r} = q \int_{r_1}^{r_2} \vec{E} \cdot d\vec{r}$$
$$= q(V(r_1) - V(r_2))$$

In the case of magnetostatics Eq. (4) becomes

$$\nabla \times \vec{B} = \mu_0 \vec{J} \tag{8}$$

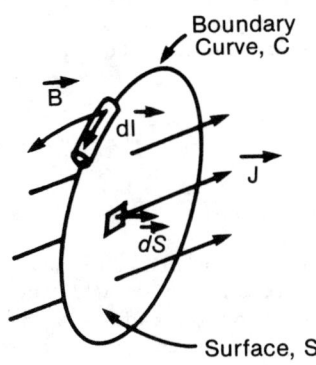

Figure 1. Illustration of Stokes' theorem applied to Eq. (8).

An equivalent integral form can be obtained by integrating the quantities on both sides of Eq. (8) over a surface through which the current flows, as indicated in Fig. 1. We can then apply Stokes' theorem[1], which states that the integral of the curl of a vector field over a surface is equal to the line integral of the same vector field over the boundary of the surface. The result is that Eq. (8) becomes

$$\oint_C \vec{B} \cdot d\vec{l} = \mu_0 \int_S \vec{J} \cdot d\vec{S} = \mu_0 I \tag{9}$$

where I is the total current flowing through the surface. Equation (9) is frequently referred to as Ampere's circuital law. We can use it to determine the value of the magnetic induction from a long straight wire carrying a steady current I. If we choose a cylindrical coordinate system with the wire as the axis, then $\vec{B}$ only has an angular (ϕ) component. Integrating B_ϕ over the circumference of a circle of radius r we have

$$B_\phi \cdot 2\pi r = \mu_0 I$$

or

$$B_\phi = \frac{\mu_0 I}{2\pi r}$$

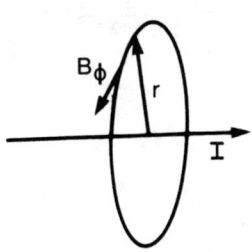

Figure 2. Ampere's law for a long straight wire.

Equation (9) is useful only in situations with a high degree of spatial symmetry. For a general arrangement of current carrying wires, $\vec{B}$ can be calculated by integrating the value from individual current elements using the equation

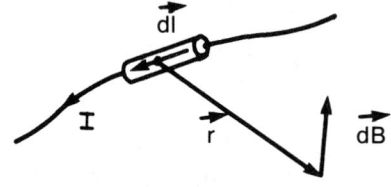

$$d\vec{B} = \frac{\mu_0}{4\pi} I \frac{d\vec{\ell} \times \vec{r}}{|r|^3} \qquad (10)$$

Equation (10), the Biot-Savart law, is occasionally called Ampere's law. It can be shown to be equivalent to Eq. (8).[2]

Figure 3. Illustration of the Biot-Savart law.

THE MAGNETIC MOMENT OF A CURRENT LOOP

The Biot-Savart law can be used to calculate the magnetic induction from a loop of current. For simplicity we will consider only the field on the axis of a circular loop of radius a carrying a current I as shown in Fig. 4. Since the vector $\vec{r}$ is always orthogonal to $d\vec{\ell}$ we have, from equation (10),

$$|dB| = \frac{\mu_0 I}{4\pi r^2} d\ell$$

When the integration is carried out the components of $\vec{B}$ perpendicular to the axis will vanish. The axial component of $d\vec{B}$ is

$$dB_z = \frac{\mu_0 I}{4\pi r^2} \cos\phi \, d\ell$$

$$= \frac{\mu_0 I}{4\pi r^3} a \, d\ell$$

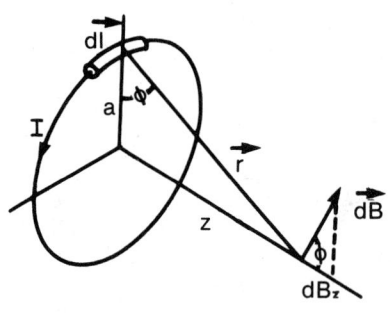

Figure 4. Calculation of $\vec{B}$ on the axis of a current loop

Integrating over the circumference of the loop we have

$$B_z = \frac{\mu_0 I a^2}{2 r^3} = \frac{\mu_0 I \cdot A}{2\pi r^3} \qquad (11)$$

where A is the area enclosed by the loop. The product I·A is called the magnetic moment of the current loop. Off the axis, in the case where the diameter of the loop is small compared with r, the equation for the magnetic induction takes the form [2]

$$\vec{B} = \frac{\mu_0}{4\pi}\left(\frac{3\vec{r}(\vec{r}\cdot\vec{m})}{r^5} - \frac{\vec{m}}{r^3}\right) \quad (12)$$

where $\vec{m}$ is the magnetic moment vector with a magnitude I·A and a direction perpendicular to the loop. Equation (12) is identical in algebraic form to that for the electric field from an electric dipole, i.e., a positive and negative charge separated by a short distance, and thus $\vec{m}$ is often called the magnetic dipole moment. A more general definition of the magnetic moment of any current distribution $\vec{J}(r)$ is[2]

$$\vec{m} = \frac{1}{2}\int \vec{r} \times \vec{J}(\vec{r})\, dv \quad (13)$$

Of particular significance to the magnetic resonance phenomenon is the calculation of the torque on a magnetic moment from an external uniform magnetic field. From the Lorentz force law [Eq. (5)] identifying $q\vec{v}$ with $Id\vec{\ell}$ we find that the force on the current element due to a magnetic induction $\vec{B}$ is

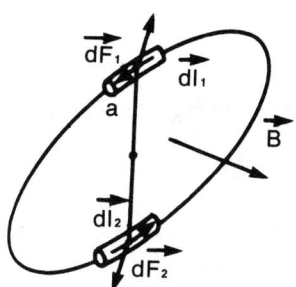

$$d\vec{F} = I\,d\vec{\ell} \times \vec{B}$$

Figure 5. Forces on a current loop in a $\vec{B}$ field.

It is clear that the net force on a rigid current loop will be zero since every force element due to a current element $Id\ell_1$ will be balanced by an oppositely directed force element from the diagonally opposite current element $Id\ell_2$ (Fig. 5).

An incremental element of torque (force x lever arm) on the current loop, taking its origin at the center of the loop of radius a, is

$$d\vec{T} = \vec{a} \times d\vec{F} = I\vec{a} \times (d\vec{\ell} \times \vec{B})$$

The total torque is therefore

$$\vec{T} = I\oint \vec{a} \times (d\vec{\ell} \times \vec{B}) \quad (14)$$

where the integral is evaluated over the entire loop. To simplify this integral we make use of an identity for the triple vector product[1]

$$\vec{a} \times (\vec{b} \times \vec{c}) = (\vec{a} \cdot \vec{c})\vec{b} - (\vec{b} \cdot \vec{a})\vec{c} \qquad (15)$$

Thus Eq. (14) becomes

$$\vec{T} = I \oint (\vec{a} \cdot \vec{B}) d\vec{\ell} - I \oint \vec{B}(\vec{a} \cdot d\vec{\ell}) \qquad (16)$$

Since $\vec{a}$ is always perpendicular to $d\vec{\ell}$, the second integral vanishes. To evaluate the first integral we adopt a coordinate system in which the current loop lies in the x-y plane, $\vec{B}$ having an arbitrary direction.

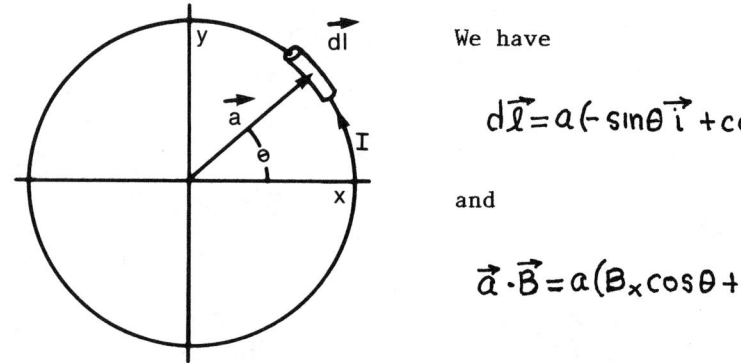

We have

$$d\vec{\ell} = a(-\sin\theta \vec{i} + \cos\theta \vec{j})d\theta$$

and

$$\vec{a} \cdot \vec{B} = a(B_x \cos\theta + B_y \sin\theta)$$

Figure 6. Coordinate system for evaluating Eq. (16).

where $\vec{i}$ and $\vec{j}$ are unit vectors in the x and y directions. In this coordinate system Eq. (16) is

$$\vec{T} = Ia^2 \int_0^{2\pi} (B_x \cos\theta + B_y \sin\theta)(-\sin\theta \vec{i} + \cos\theta \vec{j}) d\theta .$$

The integral is readily evaluated to yield

$$\vec{T} = \pi a^2 I (-B_y \vec{i} + B_x \vec{j}) = I \cdot A \vec{k} \times \vec{B}$$

where A is the area enclosed by the loop and $\vec{k}$ is a unit vector perpendicular to the loop. In view of our previous definition of the magnetic moment we have

$$\vec{T} = \vec{m} \times \vec{B} \qquad (17)$$

Equation (17) can be shown to be valid for an arbitrary distribution of current using Eq. (13) for the definition of $\vec{m}$.[2]

When the magnetic moment is aligned with the external field there is no net torque since the cross product is zero.

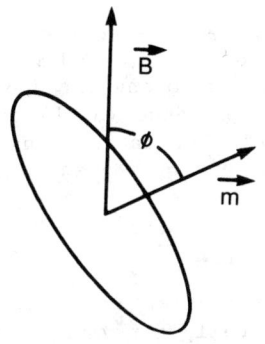

If the loop is rotated from the equilibrium position through an angle ϕ, work must be expended and the magnitude is given by

$$W = \int_0^\phi T d\phi' = \int_0^\phi mB \sin\phi' d\phi'$$

$$= mB \cos\phi$$

Figure 7. Rotation of magnetic moment from its equilibrium position

Thus a magnetic moment making an angle ϕ with an external magnetic field is said to have a potential energy U given by

$$U = -\vec{m}\cdot\vec{B} \qquad (18)$$

In classical electromagnetic theory, a continuous distribution of energy levels from -mB to +mB is possible. Magnetic resonance however, is a quantum mechanical phenomenon and therefore the potential energy is restricted to discrete levels. Equation (18) does remain valid in the quantum mechanical description of NMR.[3]

CAPACITANCE, INDUCTANCE, AND TUNED CIRCUITS

We will now shift our emphasis to the study of electrical devices used in the observation of NMR. The simplest type of capacitor, a device for storing charge, consists of a pair of parallel conducting plates. If a quantity of charge q is removed from one plate and added to the other, the excess positive and negative charges will distribute themselves uniformly over the inside surfaces of the plates. Neglecting edge effects, the electric field between the plates will be constant and equal to $q/\varepsilon_0 A$ where A is the area of the plate. If a charge Δq is moved a distance d from plate to plate the work done is expressed by

$$W(\Delta q) = \int_0^d \Delta q \vec{E}\cdot d\vec{r} = \Delta q \frac{qd}{\varepsilon_0 A}$$

and a change of this magnitude occurs in the potential energy. In terms of the electrostatic potential V (the potential energy divided by the charge) we have

$$V = \frac{g d}{\varepsilon_0 A} = g/C$$

where the constant of proportionality between the charge and the potential is called the capacitance, C, and is expressed in farads. The concept of capacitance can be generalized to any arrangement of two conducting surfaces. Since work must be done in charging a capacitor, energy is stored by the field. By integrating the effect of incremental charges, we find the energy stored to be

$$W = \int_0^g V \, dg' = \frac{1}{2} g^2/C = \frac{1}{2} C V^2$$

A device for storing energy in a magnetic field is the inductor. A solenoid (a long cylindrical coil) carrying a constant current produces a uniform (neglecting end effects) magnetic field. The magnetic induction within the solenoid is

$$B = \mu_0 \frac{N}{\ell} I \tag{19}$$

where I is the current in the wire, N is the number of loops in the coil and ℓ is its length. This result can be obtained by integrating the individual contributions to the field for each turn of wire, using Eq. (11), or more simply by applying Ampere's circuital law [Eq. (9)] over the length of the solenoid.

The effect of an inductor in an electric circuit can be understood in terms of Faraday's law of induction, Eq. (3). If the magnetic field in a region of space varies with time then an electric field is induced in that region.

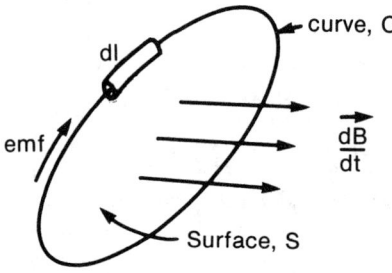

If we transform Eq. (3) into its equivalent integral form using Stokes' theorem, we find that

$$\text{emf} = \oint_c \vec{E} \cdot d\vec{\ell}$$
$$= -\frac{\partial}{\partial t} \int_s \vec{B} \cdot d\vec{s}$$
$$= -\frac{\partial \Phi}{\partial t} \tag{20}$$

Figure 8. Illustrating the integral form of Faraday's law.

where Φ is the flux of magnetic induction through the surface. The line integral of the electric field is called the electromotive force or emf. The units of the emf are volts, although it is not a potential in the sense of Eq. (7), since the potential applies only to the case of static charges. The work done on a charge q is

$$W = \int_q \vec{E} \cdot d\vec{r}$$

whether the integral is an induced emf or a potential difference.

If A is the cross-sectional area for a single loop of a solenoid, $\Phi = B \cdot A$, hence

$$emf = -A \frac{\partial B}{\partial t}$$

For N loops of the solenoid we have

$$emf = -NA \frac{\partial B}{\partial t}$$

Using Eq. (19) for the value of B we have

$$emf = -\mu_0 \frac{N^2}{\ell} A \frac{dI}{dt} = -L \frac{dI}{dt}$$

where L is called the inductance of the coil. As with capacitance, inductance can be generalized to any form of current-carrying circuit element.

If an element of charge, dq, tranverses a circuit with inductance L, the work done on it is

$$dW = -emf \, dq = L \frac{dI}{dt} dq$$

and the work done per unit time is

$$\frac{dW}{dt} = LI \frac{dI}{dt}$$

Integrating this equation from an initial condition of zero current to a final value of I we find that the energy stored in the magnetic field of an inductor is

$$W = \frac{1}{2} L I^2$$

A third type of electrical circuit element, one which dissipates energy rather than storing it, is a resistor. The voltage across an ideal resistor is proportional to the current and the constant of proportionality is the resistance, R, in units of ohms, i.e., the voltage-to-current relationship is V=IR. The energy lost by a charge element dq traversing a voltage V is Vdq. Thus the rate at which a resistor dissipates energy is

$$\frac{dW}{dt} = V \frac{dq}{dt} = VI = RI^2$$

If we combine the three circuit elements discussed above with an external source of electrical energy, an external emf, we have a driven LRC circuit.

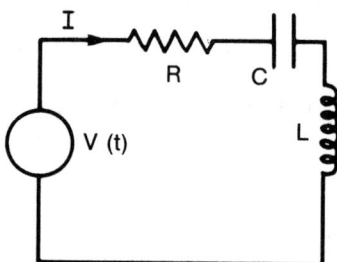

The simplest circuit is that in which all the elements are connected in series such that the current through each device is the same. The equation governing the flow of current through the circuit is

$$V(t) = L\frac{dI}{dt} + RI + q/C \qquad (21)$$

Figure 9. The series LRC circuit

Equation (21) follows from equating the rate of energy supplied by the driving emf which is V(t)I with the rate of change of stored energy and the rate of energy dissipation by the resistor.

If V(t) varies sinusoidally it is easiest to solve Eq. (21) by representing V(t) by $V_o e^{i\omega t}$, realizing that the real part of the solution represents the observed situation. Since I = dq/dt we can rewrite Eq. (21) as

$$V_o e^{i\omega t} = L\frac{d^2q}{dt^2} + R\frac{dq}{dt} + q/C \qquad (22)$$

The solution will be of the form $q = Ae^{i(\omega t - \alpha)}$. Substituting this representation for q into Eq. (22) and solving the resulting algebraic equation we find

$$q = \frac{CV_o e^{i(\omega t - \alpha)}}{\sqrt{(1 - LC\omega^2)^2 + \omega^2 R^2 C^2}}$$

$$\alpha = \tan^{-1}\frac{\omega RC}{1 - LC\omega^2}$$

Since I = dq/dt the current is

$$I = \frac{i\omega CV_o e^{i(\omega t - \alpha)}}{\sqrt{(1 - LC\omega^2)^2 + \omega^2 R^2 C^2}}$$

The true current is the real part of this expression.

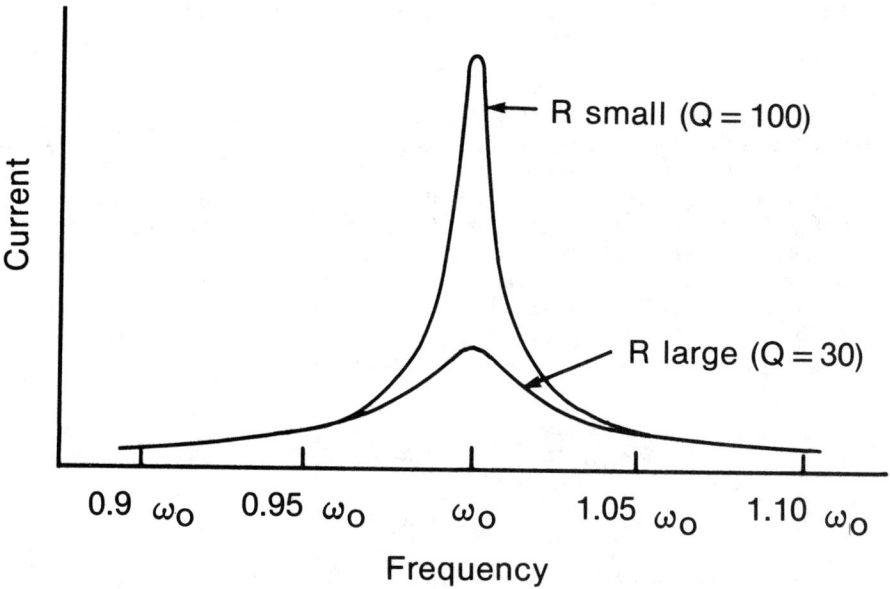

Figure 10. Plot of the amplitude of current for varying excitation frequency.

Figure 10 shows plots of the amplitude of I versus angular frequency w for different values of resistance R. We see that in any case, |I| is a maximum when the angular frequency satisfies the resonance condition

$$\omega = \frac{1}{\sqrt{LC}} = \omega_o$$

The efficiency of the tuned circuit, that is, one whose resonance frequency matches the excitation frequency, is usually denoted by the symbol Q and has the value

$$Q = \omega_o L / R = \frac{1}{R}\sqrt{\frac{L}{C}}$$

Q is the ratio of the stored energy to the energy dissipated in one cycle when the resonance condition is satisfied. In addition, Q is related to the width of the resonance according to the equation

$$\frac{\Delta\omega}{\omega_o} = \sqrt{3}/Q$$

where $\Delta\omega$ is the width of the resonance curve at half-height. Circuits which have a narrow resonance have a large value of Q and little energy dissipation.

The driving emf, V(t), in NMR is usually produced within the pickup coil by a rotating magnetization in the material within the coil. In addition, the coil is the principal source of resistance within the circuit. Thus V(t), R, and L are all produced in a single physical element and the signal that is accessible to the observer is that which appears across the capacitor. At resonance, the amplitude of the voltage at the capacitor is

$$V_{cap} = \frac{V_o}{\omega_o RC} = QV_o$$

A high Q circuit results in a greater detected signal.

ELECTRIC AND MAGNETIC FIELDS IN MEDIA

In our discussion of inductance and capacitance we have assumed empty space between the plates of the capacitor and within the coil of the inductor. If material media are inserted in these places the electric and magnetic fields are altered due to the presence of induced electric dipoles and currents. In the case of an electric field impressed on a nonconducting (dielectric) medium, induced molecular dipoles will tend to align with the field. Although these charges are bound within the dielectric, there will be a net charge on the surfaces of the material which will decrease the electric field within it.

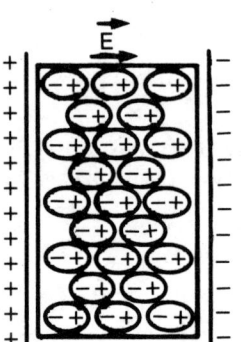

In discussions of electromagnetism in media a second electric field quantity, the electric displacement $\vec{D}$ is frequently introduced. The displacement, whose units are coulombs/meter^2 is independent of the polarization of the medium. Its value depends solely on charges which are external to the medium.

Figure 11. Induced dipoles in material within a capacitor

An analogous situation occurs with material in a magnetic field. When an electron orbits an atom a current loop is created, and when placed in a magnetic field a torque is impressed on the orbit in accordance with Eq. (17). This torque causes the orbit to precess about an axis defined by the applied field. The current created by this precessing motion creates a magnetic field whose direction opposes the applied field. Thus ordinary materials are diamagnetic, that is, the magnetic induction within the material is decreased with respect to the value for empty space. As in the case of electric displacement, a second magnetic field quantity, called the magnetic field strength, $\vec{H}$, is introduced. It is defined by the relation

$$\vec{H} = \vec{B}/\mu = \frac{\vec{B}}{(1+\chi)\mu_0}$$

where μ is the permeability of the material and χ is the magnetic susceptibility. The units of $\vec{H}$ are ampere/meter. $\vec{H}$ is dependent solely on external currents, not on currents or magnetic moments within the substance. In ordinary diamagnetic materials $\chi < 0$.

There are, however, certain materials in which $\chi > 0$. These are called paramagnetic materials (for ferromagnetic materials χ is not defined since the relationship between $\vec{H}$ and $\vec{B}$ is neither linear nor single valued). Paramagnetism is caused by the presence of unpaired electron spins within the molecules of the substance. As can be seen from Eq. (18), the energy for a magnetic moment in a magnetic field is lowest when the moment is aligned with the field. There will be a statistical tendency for individual magnetic moments in paramagnetic substances to maintain this alignment. The result will be an increase in the magnetic induction within the material compared with that in empty space. In paramagnetic substances the contribution to $\vec{B}$ from the aligned moments overwhelms the diamagnetic contribution from the electron orbits and $\chi > 0$.

The magnetization $\vec{M}$ of a material is the net magnetic moment per unit volume. The relationship between $\vec{M}$ and the two magnetic field quantities is

$$\vec{B} = \mu_0(\vec{H} + \vec{M})$$

Therefore $\vec{B}$ in a medium is made up of contributions from an external applied field $\vec{H}$ plus an internal magnetization $\vec{M}$. In tissue, $B \cong \mu_0 H$, that is, $\vec{M}$ is very small and the two field quantities are used interchangeably by many authors. (In the cgs system of units B and H have the same numerical value.)

In certain substances there is a small contribution to $\vec{M}$ from nuclear moments. When the nuclear magnetization is displaced from equilibrium a sinusoidally varying component to $\vec{M}$ occurs. The detection of this signal is the essence of the NMR experiment.

EMF INDUCED IN A COIL DUE TO A PRECESSING MAGNETIZATION (B/I RULE)

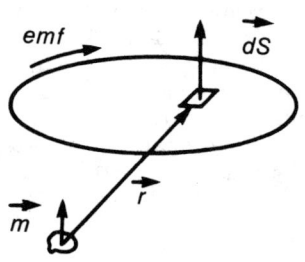

Figure 12. Time varying magnetic moment near a coil.

We will derive an expression for the emf produced in a receiver coil due to such a time varying magnetization. First we will derive a theorem concerning the emf due to a magnetic moment in the vicinity of a coil.[4] This will be done in some detail since justifications for this theorum are difficult to find in the literature.

We first consider the magnetic flux from $\vec{m}(t)$ through a surface enclosed by this coil (Fig. 12). Using Faraday's law of induction [Eq. (20)] and Eq. (12) we have

$$emf = -\frac{\partial}{\partial t}\int_S \frac{\mu_o}{4\pi}\left(\frac{3\vec{r}\,(\vec{r}\cdot\vec{m})}{r^5} - \frac{\vec{m}}{r^3}\right)\cdot d\vec{S}$$

This equation can be transformed into

$$emf = \frac{\partial}{\partial t}\int_S \frac{\mu_o}{4\pi}\nabla\times\left(\frac{\vec{r}\times\vec{m}}{r^3}\right)\cdot d\vec{S} \tag{23}$$

This can be seen as follows

$$\nabla\times\left(\frac{\vec{r}\times\vec{m}}{r^3}\right) = \frac{1}{r^3}\nabla\times(\vec{r}\times\vec{m}) + \nabla\left(\frac{1}{r^3}\right)\times(\vec{r}\times\vec{m})$$

but $\nabla\left(\frac{1}{r^3}\right) = -3\vec{r}/r^5$ and $\nabla\times(\vec{r}\times\vec{m}) = -2\vec{m}$ thus

$$\nabla\times\left(\frac{\vec{r}\times\vec{m}}{r^3}\right) = -\frac{2\vec{m}}{r^3} - \frac{3}{r^5}\vec{r}\times(\vec{r}\times\vec{m})$$

Using Eq. (15) for the triple vector product we have

$$\nabla\times\left(\frac{\vec{r}\times\vec{m}}{r^3}\right) = -\frac{3\vec{r}\,(\vec{r}\cdot\vec{m})}{r^5} + \frac{\vec{m}}{r^3}$$

Applying Stokes' theorem to Eq. (23) we have

$$emf = \frac{\partial}{\partial t}\oint \frac{\mu_o}{4\pi}\left(\frac{\vec{r}\times\vec{m}}{r^3}\right)\cdot d\vec{\ell}$$

Then using the vector identity $(\vec{a} \times \vec{b}) \cdot \vec{c} = -(\vec{a} \times \vec{c}) \cdot \vec{b}$ we have

$$emf = -\frac{\partial}{\partial t}\left(\oint \frac{\mu_o}{4\pi} \frac{\vec{r} \times d\vec{\ell}}{r^3}\right) \cdot \vec{m}$$

The line integral in this equation can be recognized, from the Biot-Savart law [Eq. (10)], as the magnetic induction at $\vec{m}$ from a unit current flowing in the loop. This is called the field-to-current ratio, B/I.[5] Thus we have the theorem

$$emf = -\frac{\partial}{\partial t}\left[(\vec{B}/I) \cdot \vec{m}\right]$$

The emf from the entire sample is found by replacing $\vec{m}$ by $\vec{M}dv$, where M is the magnetization, and integrating over the volume of the sample. Recognizing that B/I is time independent (it depends only on the coil geometry) the electromotive force is

$$emf = \int \vec{B}/I \cdot \frac{d\vec{M}}{dt} dv$$

To illustrate the use of this equation we consider the example of a body of volume V with magnetization $\vec{M}$ placed in a solenoidal coil with n turns per unit length wrapped along the X-axis. From Eq. (19), $B/I = \mu_o n$. If $\vec{M}$ is precessing about the Z-axis then $M_x = M_o \sin(\omega t)$ and therefore

$$emf = V\mu_o n \omega M_o \cos(\omega t).$$

With this result we conclude our review of classical electromagnetism. We hope it has helped the reader in establishing a foundation for the further study of nuclear magnetic resonance both in terms of the phenomenon itself and the instrumentation used to observe it.

REFERENCES

1. Hildebrand FR. *Advanced Calculus for Applications*, 2nd ed. Prentice Hall (1976).

2. Jackson JD. *Classical Electrodynamics*, 2nd ed. Wiley (1975).

3. Dixon RL and Ekstrand KE. Med Phys 9; 807-818 (1982).

4. Hoult DI and Richards RE. J Magn Reson 24; 71-85 (1976).

5. King KF and Moran PR. Med Phys 11; 1-14 (1984).

APPENDIX B

Glossary of NMR Terms

Prepared under the auspices of:

Subcommittee on NMR Nomenclature and Phantom Development
Leon Axel, Ph.D., M.D., Chairman

Committee on NMR Imaging Technology and Equipment
Alexander R. Margulis, M.D., Chairman

Commission on Nuclear Magnetic Resonance
Thomas F. Meaney, M.D., Chairman

American College of Radiology
1891 Preston White Drive
Reston, Virginia 22091

1983

INTRODUCTION

This glossary of conventional NMR-related terms, along with the accompanying table of basic quantities in electricity and magnetism, are offered by the American College of Radiology for the use of physicians, medical physicists, and manufacturers. For physicians and physicists, being familiar with this glossary will aid in reading scientific papers and manufacturers' product descriptions; it is also hoped that potential authors will use the suggested definitions and conventions as standards in writing papers of their own. For manufacturers, the glossary provides a standard set of terms and symbol and display conventions to use in product descriptions and display design. Although technically accurate, no effort has been made to formalize the definitions. Only those concepts most directly related to medical NMR have been included. Important related areas, such as digital data processing, have been purposely omitted. In order to simplify the notation, the use of subscripts and Greek letters has been minimized (it may be clearer to use some symbols in subscripted forms when writing equations).

This Glossary has been produced under the auspices of the American College of Radiology's Subcommittee on NMR Nomenclature and Phantom Development under the chairmanship of Leon Axel, Ph.D., M.D.

Commission on NMR

Thomas F. Meaney, M.D., Chairman
Stanley Baum, M.D.
Thomas F. Budinger, M.D.
Richard H. Greenspan, M.D.
A. Everette James, Jr., M.Sc., J.D., M.D.
Alexander R. Margulis, M.D.
Juan M. Taveras, M.D.
James E. Youker, M.D.

Committee on NMR Imaging Technology and Equipment

Alexander R. Margulis, M.D., Chairman
Leon Axel, Ph.D., M.D.
Morry Blumenfeld, Ph.D.
Lawrence E. Crooks, Ph.D.
Waldo S. Hinshaw, Ph.D.
Leon Kaufman, Ph.D.
James A. Nelson, M.D.

Subcommittee on NMR Nomenclature and Phantom Development

Leon Axel, Ph.D., M.D., Chairman
Lawrence E. Crooks, Ph.D.
Andre Luiten, Ph.D.
Manfred Pfeiler, Ph.D.
John F. Schenck, M.D., Ph.D.
Stephen R. Thomas, Ph.D.

GLOSSARY OF NMR TERMS

Acquisition time-see Image acquisition time.

ADC-see Analog to digital converter.

Adiabatic fast passage (AFP)-technique of producing rotation of the macroscopic magnetization vector by sweeping the frequency of an irradiating RF wave (or the strength of the magnetic field) through resonance (the Larmor frequency) in a time short compared to the relaxation times. Particularly used for inversion of the spins. A continuous wave NMR technique.

Adiabatic rapid passage-see Adiabatic fast passage.

AFP-see Adiabatic fast passage.

Analog to digital converter (ADC)-part of the interface that converts ordinary (analog) voltages, such as the detected NMR signal, into digital number form, that can be read by the computer.

Angular frequency(ω)-frequency of oscillation or rotation (measured, e.g., in radians/second) commonly designated by the Greek letter ω: $\omega = 2\pi f$, where f is frequency (e.g., in hertz (Hz)).

Angular momentum-a vector quantity given by the vector product of the momentum of a particle and its position vector. In the absences of external forces, the angular mementum remains constant, with the result that any rotating body tends to maintain the same axis of rotation. When a torque is applied to a rotating body, the resulting change in angular momentum results in precession. Atomic nuclei possess an intrinsic angular momentum referred to as spin, measured in multiples of Planck's constant.

Antenna-device to send or receive electromagnetic radiation. Electromagnetic radiation per se is not relevant to NMR, as it is the magnetic vector alone that couples the spins and the coils, and the term coil should be used instead.

Array processor-optional component of computer system specially designed to speed up numerical calculations like those needed in NMR imaging.

Artifacts-false features in the image produced by the imaging process.

B_o-a conventional symbol for the constant magnetic (induction) field in an NMR system. (Although historically used, H_o (units of magnetic field strength, ampere/meter) should be distinguished from the more appropriate B_o (units of magnetic induction, tesla).)

B_1-a conventional symbol for the radiofrequency magnetic induction field used in an NMR system (another symbol historically used is H_1). It is useful to consider it as composed of two oppositely rotating vectors, usually in a plane transverse to B_o. At the Larmor frequency, the vector rotating in the same direction as the precessing spins will interact strongly with the spins.

Bloch equations-phenomenological "classical" equations of motion for the macroscopic magnetization vector. They include the effects of precession about the magnetic field (static and RF) and the T1 and T2 relaxation times.

Boltzmann distribution-if a system of particles which are able to exchange energy in collisions is in thermal equilibrium, then the relative number of particles, N_1 and N_2, in two particular energy states with corresponding energies, E_1 and E_2, is given by

$$\frac{N_1}{N_2} = \exp[-(E_1-E_2)/kT]$$

where k is Boltzmann's constant and T is absolute temperature. For example, in NMR of protons at room temperature in a magnetic field of 0.25 tesla, the difference in numbers of spins aligned with the magnetic field and against the field is about one part in a million; the small excess of nuclei in the lower energy state is the basis of the net magnetization and the resonance phenomenon.

Carr-Purcell (CP) sequence-sequence of a 90° RF pulse followed by repeated 180° RF pulses to produce a train of spin echoes; useful for measuring T2.

Carr-Purcell-Meiboom-Gill (CPMG) sequence-modification of Carr-Purcell RF pulse sequence with 90° phase shift in the rotating frame of reference between the 90° pulse and the subsequent 180° pulses to reduce accumulating effects of imperfections in the 180° pulses. Suppression of effects of pulse error accumulation can alternatively be achieved by alternating phases of the 180° pulses by 180°.

Chemical shift (δ)-the change in the Larmor frequency of a given nucleus when bound in different sites in a molecule, due to the magnetic shielding effects of the electron orbitals. Chemical shifts make possible the differentiation of different molecular compounds and different sites within the molecules in high-resolution NMR spectra. The amount of the shift is proportional to magnetic field strength and is usually specified in parts per million (ppm) of the resonance frequency relative to a standard.

Coherence-maintenance of a constant phase relationship between rotating or oscillating waves or objects. Loss of phase coherence of the spins results in a decrease in the transverse magnetization and hence a decrease in the NMR signal.

Coil-single or multiple loops of wire (or other electrical conductor, such as tubing, etc.) designed either to produce a magnetic field from current flowing through the wire, or to detect a changing magnetic field by voltage induced in the wire.

Computer-as used for NMR, can be divided into central processing unit (DPU), consisting of instruction interpretation and arithmetic unit plus fast access memory, and perpheral devices such as bulk data storage and input and output devices (including, via the interface, the spectrometer). Under software control, the computer controls the RF pulses and gradients necessary to acquire data, and processes the data to produce spectra or images. (Note that devices such as the spectrometer may themselves incorporate small computers.)

Continuous wave NMR (CW)-a technique for studying NMR by continuously applying RF radiation to the sample and slowly sweeping either the RF frequency or the magnetic field through the resonance values; now largely superceded by pulse NMR techniques.

Contrast-contrast can be defined as the relatvie difference of the signal intensities in two adjacent regions. In a general sense, we can consider image contrast, where the strength of the image intensity in adjacent regions of the image is compared, or object contrast, where the relative values of a parameter affecting the image (such as spin density or relaxation time) in corresponding adjacent regions of the object are compared. If the two intensitites are J_1 and J_2, a useful quantitative definition of contrast is $(J_1-J_2)/(J_1+J_2)$. Relating image contrast to object contrast is more difficult in NMR imaging than in conventional radiography, as there are more object parameters affecting the image and their relative contributions are very dependent on the particular imaging technique used. As in other kinds of imaging, image contrast in NMR will also depend on region size, as reflected through the modulation transfer function (MTF) characteristics.

CP-see Carr-Purcell.

CPMG-see Carr-Purcell-Meiboom-Gill.

CPU-see Computer.

Crossed-coil-coil pair arranged with their magnetic fields at right angles to each other in such a way as to minimize their mutual electromagnetic interaction.

Cryomagnet-see Superconducting magnet.

Cryostat-an apparatus for maintaining a constant low temperature (as by means of liquid helium). Requires vacuum chambers to help with thermal isolation.

CW-see Continuous wave.

DAC-see Digital to analog converter.

Data system-see Computer.

dB/dt-the rate of change of the magnetic field (induction) with time. Because changing magnetic fields can induce electrical fields, this is one area of potential concern for safety limits.

Demodulator-another term for detector, by analogy to broadcast radio receivers.

Dectector-portion of the receiver that demodulates the RF NMR signal and converts it to a lower frequency signal. Most detectors now used are phase sensitive (e.g. quadrature demodulator/detector), and will also give phase information about the RF signal.

Diamagnetic-a substance that will slightly decrease a magnetic field when placed within it (its magnetization is oppositely directed to the magnetic field, i.e., with a small negative magnetic susceptibility).

Diffusion-the process by which molecules or other particles intermingle and migrate due to their random thermal motion. NMR provides a sensitive technique for measuring diffusion of some substances.

Digital to analog converter (DAC)-part of the interface that converts digital numbers from the computer into analog (ordinary) voltages or currents.

Echo-see Spin echo.

Echo planar imaging-a technique of planar imaging in which a complete planar image is obtained from one selective excitation pulse. The FID is observed while periodically switching the y-gradient field in the presence of a static x-gradient field. The Fourier transform of the resulting spin echo train can be used to produce an image of the excited plane.

Eddy currents-electric currents induced in a conductor by a changing magnetic field or by motion of the conductor through a magnetic field. One of the sources of concern about potential hazard to subjects in very high magnetic fields or rapidly varying gradient or main magnetic fields. Can be a practical problem in the cryostat of superconducting magnets.

Excitation-putting energy into the spin system; if a net transverse magnetization is produced, an NMR signal can be observed.

f-see Frequency.

Faraday shield-electrical conductor interposed between transmitter and/or receiver coil and patient to block out electric fields.

Fast Fourier transform (FFT)-an efficient computational method of performing a Fourier transform.

Ferromagnetic-a substance, such as iron, that has a large positive magnetic susceptibility.

FFT-see Fast Fourier transform.

FID-see Free induction decay.

Field gradient-see Gradient magnetic field.

Field lock-a feedback control used to maintain the static magnetic field at a constant strength, usually by monitoring the resonance frequency of a reference sample or line in the spectrum.

Filling factor-a measure of the geometrical relationship of the RF coil and the body. It affects the efficiency of irradiating the body and detecting NMR signals, thereby affecting the signal-to-noise ratio and, ultimately, image quality. Achieving a high filling factor requires fitting the coil closely to the body, thus potentially decreasing patient comfort.

Filtered back projection-mathematical technique used in reconstruciton from projections to create images from a set of multiple projection profiles. It essentially involves "correcting" the projection profiles by convolving them with a suitable mathematical filter and then back projecting the filtered projections into image space. Widely used in conventional computer tomography (CT).

Flip angle-amount of rotation of the macroscopic magnetization vector produced by an RF pulse, with respect to the direction of the static magnetic field.

Fourier transform (FT)-a mathematical procedure to separate out the frequency components of a signal from its amplitudes as a function of time, or vice versa. The Fourier transform is used to generate the spectrum from the FID in pulse NMR techniques and is essential to most imaging techniques.

Fourier transform imaging-NMR imaging techniques in which at lease one dimension is phase encoded by applying variable gradient pulses along that dimension before "reading out" the NMR signal with a gradient magnetic field perpendicular to the variable gradient. The Fourier transform is then used to reconstruct an image from the set of encoded NMR signals. An imaging technique of this type is spin warp imaging.

Free induction decay (FID)-if transverse magnetization of the spins is prduced, e.g., by a $90°$ pulse, a transient NMR signal will result that will decay toward zero with a characteristic time constant T2 (or T2*); this decaying signal is the FID. In practice, the first part of the FID is not observable due to residual effects of the powerful exciting RF pulse on the electronics of the receiver.

Free induction signal (FIS)-see Free induction decay.

Frequency (F)-the number of repetitions of a periodic process per unit time. For electromagnetic radiation, such as radio waves, the old unit, cycles per second (CPS), has been replaced by the SI unit, hertz, abbreviated Hz. It is related to angular frequency, ω, by $f = \omega/2\pi$.

FT-see Fourier tranform.

G-see Gauss.

G_x, G_y, G_z-conventional symbols for gradient magnetic field. Used with subscripts to denote spatial direction component of gradient, i.e., direction along which the field changes.

Gauss (G)-a unit of magnetic flux density in the older (CGS) system. The Earth's magnetic field is approximately one half gauss to one gauss, depending on location. The cureently preferred (SI) unit is the tesla (T) (1 T = 10,000 G).

Golay coil-term commonly used for a particular kind of gradient coil, commonly used to create gradient magnetic fields, perpendicular to the main magnetic field.

Gradient-the amount and direction of the rate of changes in space of some quantity, such as magnetic field strength.

Gradient coils-current carrying coils designed to produce a desired gradient magnetic field (so that the magnetic field will be stronger in some locations than others). Proper design of the size and configuration of the coils is necessary to produce a controlled and uniform gradient.

Gradient magnetic field-a magnetic field which changes in strength in a certain given direction. Such fields are used in NMR imaging with selective excitation to select a region for imaging and also to encode the location of NMR signals received from the object being imaged. Measured (e.g.) in teslas per meter.

Gradient pulse—briefly applied gradient magnetic field.

Gyromagnetic ratio (γ)—the ratio of the magnetic moment to the angular momentum of a particle. This is a constant for a given nucleus.

H_o—conventional symbol historically used for the constant magnetic field in an NMR system; it is physically more correct to use B_o. A magnet provides a field strength, H; however, at a point in an object, the spins experience the magnetic induction, B.

H_1—conventional symbol historically used for the radiofrequency magnetic field in an NMR system; it is physically more correct to use B_1. It is useful to consider it as composed of two oppositely rotating vectors. At the Larmor frequency, the vector rotating in the same direction as the precessing spins will interact strongly with the spins.

Hardware—electrical and mechanical components of computer.

Helmholtz coil—pair of current carrying coils used to create uniform magnetic field in the space between them.

Hertz (Hz)—the standard (SI) unit of frequency; equal to the old unit cycles per second.

Homogeneity—uniformity. In NMR, the homogeneity of the static magnetic field is an important criterion of the quality of the magnet. Homogeneity requirements for NMR imaging are generally lower than the homogeneity requirements for NMR spectroscopy, but for most imaging techniques must be maintained over a larger region.

Hz—see Hertz.

I—see Nuclear spin number.

Image acquisition time—time required to carry out an NMR imaging procedure comprising only the data acquisiton time. The additional image reconstruction time will also be important to determine how quickly the image can be viewed. In comparing sequential plane imaging and volume imaging techniques, the equivalent image acquisition time per slice must be considered, as well as the actual image aquisition time.

Inductance—measure of the magnetic coupling between two current carrying loops (mutual) (reflecting their spatial relationship) or of a loop (such as a coil) with itself (self). One of the principal determinants of the resonance frequency of an RF circuit.

Inhomogeneity—degree of lack of homogeneity, for example the fractional deviation of the local magnetic field from the average value of the field.

Interface-set of devices that enables the interaction of the computer and the spectrometer. Particularly, this includes an analog to digital converter (ADC), which turns the analog voltages, such as the output of the RF receiver, into numbers that can be read by the computer. It also includes a digital to analog converter (DAC), which does the reverse, enabling the computer to produce control voltages.

Interpulse time-times between successive RF pulses used in pulse sequences. Particularly important are the inversion time (TI) in inversion recovery, and the time between a $90°$ pulse and the subsequent $180°$ pulse to produce a spin echo, which will be approximately one half the spin echo time (TE). The time between repetitions of pulse sequences is the repetition time (TR).

Inversion-a nonequilibrium state in which the macroscopic magnetization vector is oriented opposite to the magnetic field; usually produced by adiabatic fast passage or $180°$ RF pulses.

Inversion-recovery (IR)-pulse NMR technique which can be incorporated into NMR imaging, wherein the nuclear magnetization is inverted at a time on the order of T1 before the regular imaging pulse-gradient sequences. The resulting partial relaxation of the spins in the different structures being imaged can be used to produce an image that depends strongly on T1. This may bring out differences in the appearance of structures with different T1 relaxation times. Note that this does <u>not</u> directly produce an image of T1. T1 in a given region can be calculated from the change in the NMR signal from the region due to the inversion pulse compared to the signal with no inversion pulse or an inversion pulse with a different inversion time (T1).

Inversion time (TI)-time between inversion and subsequent $90°$ pulse to elicit NMR signal in inversion-recovery.

Inversion transfer-see <u>Saturation transfer</u>.

k-Boltzmann's constant: appears in Boltzmann distribution.

kHz-see <u>Kilohertz</u>.

Kilohertz (kHz)-unit of frequency; equal to one thousand hertz.

Larmor equation-states that the frequency of precession of the nuclear magnetic moment is proportional to the magnetic field.

$$\omega_o = -\gamma B_o \text{ (radians per second)}$$

$$\text{or } f_o = -\gamma B_o/2\pi \text{ (hertz)}$$

where ω_o or f_o is the frequency, γ is the gyromagnetic ratio, and B_o is the magnetic induction field. The negative sign indicates the direction of the rotation.

Larmor frequency (ω_o or f_o)-the frequency at which magnetic resonance can be excited; given by the Larmor equation. By varying the magnetic field across the body with a gradient magnetic field, the corresponding variation of the Larmor frequency can be used to encode position. For protons (hydrogen nuclei), the Larmor frequency is 42.58 MH_z/tesla.

Lattice-by analogy to NMR in solids, the magnetic and thermal environment with which nuclei exchange energy in longitudinal relaxation.

Line imaging-see Sequential line imaging.

Line scanning-see Sequential line imaging.

Line width-width of line in spectrum; related to the reciprocal of the transverse relaxation time (T2* in practical systems). Measured in units of frequency, generally at the half-maximum points.

LMR-see Localized magnetic resonance.

Localized magnetic resonance (LMR)-a particular technique for obtaining NMR spectra, for example, of phosphorus, from a limited region by creating a sensitive volume with inhomoogeneous applied gradient magnetic fields, which may be enhanced with the use of surface coils.

Longitudinal magnetization (M_z)-component of the macroscopic magnetization vector along the static magnetic field. Following excitation by RF pulse, M_z will approach its equilibrium value M_o, with a characteristic time constant T1.

Longitudinal relaxation-return of longitudinal magnetization to its equilibrium value after excitation; requires exchange of energy between the nuclear spins and the lattice.

Longitudinal relaxation time-see T1.

Lorentzian line-usual shape of the lines in an NMR spectrum, characterized by a central peak with long tails; proportional to $1/[(1/T2)^2+(f-f_o)^2]$, where f is frequency and f_o is the frequency of the peak (i.e., central resonance frequency).

M-conventional symbol for macroscopic magnetization vector.

M_{xy}-see Transverse magnetization.

M_z-see Longitudinal magnetization.

M_o-equilibrium value of the magnetization; directed along the direction of the static magnetic field. Proportional to spin density, N.

Macroscopic magnetic moment-see <u>Macroscopic magnetization vector</u>.

Macroscopic magnetization vector-net magnetic moment per unit volume (a vector quantity) of a sample in a given region, considered as the integrated effect of all the individual microscopic nuclear magnetic moments. Most NMR experiments actually deal with this.

Magnetic dipole-north and south magnetic poles separated by a finite distance. An electric current loop, including the effective current of a spinning nucleon or nucleus, can create an equivalent magnetic dipole.

Magnetic field (H)-the region surrounding a magnet (or current carrying conductor) is endowed with certain properties. One is that a small magnet in such a region experiences a torque that tends to align it in a given direction. Magnetic field is a vector quantity; the direction of the field is defined as the direction that the north pole of the small magnet points when in equilibrium. A magnetic field produces a magnetizing force on a body within it. Although the dangers of large magnetic fields are largely hopothetical, this is an area of potential concern for safety limits.

Formally, the forces experienced by moving charged particles, current carrying wires, and small magnets in the vicinity of a magnet are due to magnetic induction (B), which includes the effect of magnetization, while the magnetic field (H) is defined so as not to inlcude magnetization. However, both B and H are often loosely used to denote magnetic fields.

Magnetic field gradient-see <u>Gradient magnetic field</u>.

Magnetic induction (B)-also called magnetic flux density. The net magnetic effect from an externally applied magnetic field and the resulting magnetization. B is proportional to H(B= H), with the SI unit being the tesla.

Magnetic moment-a measure of the net magnetic properties of an object or particle. A nucleus with an intrinsic spin will have an associated magnetic dipole moment, so that it will interact with a magnetic field (as if it were a tiny bar magnet).

Magnetic resonance-see <u>Nuclear magnetic resonance</u> (NMR). Another magnetic resonance phenomenon is electron spin resonance (ESR).

Magnetic susceptibility ( )-measure of the ability of a substance to become magnetized.

Magnetization (see also <u>Macroscopic magnetization vector</u>)-the magnetic polarization of a material produced by a magnetic field (magnetic moment per unit volume).

Magnetogyric ratio-see Gyromagnetic ratio.

Maxwell coil-a particular kind of gradient coil, commonly used to create gradient magnetic fields along the direction of the main magnetic field.

Megahertz (MHz)-unit of frequency, equal to one million hertz.

Meiboom-Gill sequence-see Carr-Purcell-Meiboom-Gill sequence.

MHz-see Megahertz.

Multiple line-scan imaging (MLSI)-variation of sequential line imaging techniques that can be used if selective excitation methods that do not affect adjacent lines are employed. Adjacent lines are imaged while waiting for relaxation of the first line toward equilibrium, which may result in decreased imaging time. A different type of MLSI uses simultaneous excitation of two or more lines with different phase encoding followed by suitable decoding.

Multiple plane imaging-variation of sequential plane imaging techniques that can be used with selective excitation techniques that do not affect adjacent planes. Adjacent planes are imaged while waiting for relaxation of the first plane toward equilibrium, resulting in decreased imaging time.

Multiple sensitive point-sequential line imaging technique utilizing two orthogonal oscillating magnetic field gradients, an SFP pulse sequence, and signal averaging to isolate the NMR spectrometer sensitivity to a desired line in the body.

N (H)-see Spin density.

NMR-see Nuclear magnetic resonance.

NMR imaging (see also Zeugmatography)-creation of images of objects such as the body by use of the nuclear magnetic resonance phenomenon. The immediate practical application involves imaging the distribution of hydrogen nuclei (protons) in the body. The image brightness in a given region is usually dependent jointly on the spin density and the relaxation times, with their relative importance determined by the particular imaging technique employed. Image brightness is also affected by motion such as blood flow.

NMR signal-electromagnetic signal in the radiofrequency range produced by the precession of the transverse magnetization of the spins. The rotation of the transverse magnetization induces a voltage in a coil, which is amplified and demodulated by the receiver; the signal may refer only to this induced voltage.

Nuclear magnetic resonance (NMR)-the absorption or emission of electromagnetic energy by nuclei in a static magnetic field, after excitation by a suitable RF magnetic field. The peak resonance frequency is proportional to the magnetic field, and is given by the Larmor equation. Only nuclei with a non-zero spin exhibit NMR.

Nuclear signal-see NMR signal.

Nuclear spin (see also Spin)-an intrinsic property of certain nuclei that gives them an associated characteristic angular momentum and magnetic moment.

Nuclear spin quantum number (I)-property of all nuclei related to the largest measurable component of the nuclear angular momentum. Non-zero values of nuclear angular momentum are quantized (fixed) as integral or half-integral multiples of (h/2), where h is Planck's constant. The number of possible energy states for a given nucleus in a fixed magnetic field is equal to 2I+1.

Nucleon-generic term for a neutron or proton.

Nutation-a displacement of the axis of a spinning body away from the simple coneshaped figure which would be traced by the axis during precession. In the rotating frame of reference, the nutation caused by an RF pulse appears as a simple precession, although the motion is more complex in the stationary frame of reference.

Orientation-a suggested standard orientation for the presentation of NMR images is: 1) transverse: patient's right on the left side of the image, anterior or ventral on top, 2) coronal: patient's right to left side of image, superior or head to the top, 3) sagittal: patient's head to the top, anterior to the left side of image. R, L, S and A should be shown on the screen, as appropriate. In displaying sagittal images, it is helpful to indicate whether a slice is to the left or right of the midline.

Paramagnetic-a substance with a small but positive magnetic susceptibility (magnetizability). The addition of a small amount of paramagnetic substance may greatly reduce the relaxation times of water. Typical paramagnetic substances usually possess an unpaired electron and include atoms or ions of transition elements, rare earth elements, some metals, and some molecules including molecular oxygen and free radicals. Paramagnetic substances are considered promising for use as contrast agents in NMR imaging.

Partial saturation (PS)-excitation technique applying repeated RF pulses in times on the order of or shorter than T1. In NMR imaging systems, although it results in decreased signal amplitude, there is the possibility of generating images with increased contrast between regions with different relaxation times. It does <u>not</u> directly produce images of Tl. The change in NMR signal from a region resulting from a change in the interpulse time, TR, can be used to calculate Tl for the region. Although partial saturation is also commonly referred to as saturation recovery, that term should properly be reserved for the particular case of partial saturation in which recovery after each excitation effectively takes place from true saturation.

Permanent magnet-a magnet whose magnetic field originates from permanently magnetized material.

Permeability (μ)-tendency of a substance to concentrate magnetic field, $\mu = B/H$.

Phantom-an artificial object of known dimensions and properties used to test aspects of an imaging machine.

Phase-in a periodic function (such as rotational or sinusoidal motion), the position relative to a particular part of the cycle.

Phase sensitive detector-see <u>Demodulator</u>.

Pixel-acronym for a picture element; the smallest discrete part of a digital image display.

Planar spin imaging-one particular technique of planar imaging that creates an NMR image of a plane from one excitation sequence by selectively exciting a grid of points within the plane and then applying a gradient magnetic field so that each point has a different Larmor frequency. Fourier transformation of the FID can then be used to separate the signals from each selected point and create the image.

Planar imaging-imaging technique in which image of a plane is built up from signals received from the whole plane. See also <u>Sequential plane imaging</u>.

Point imaging-see <u>Sequential point imaging</u>.

Point scanning-see <u>Sequential point imaging</u>.

Precession-comparatively slow gyration of the axis of a spinning body so as to trace out a cone; caused by the application of a torque tending to change the direction of the rotation axis, and continuously directed at right angles to the plane of the torque. The magnetic moment of a nucleus with spin will experience such a torque when inclined at an angle to the magnetic field, resulting in precession at the Larmor frequency. A familiar example is the effect of gravity on the motion of a spinning top or gyroscope.

Precessional frequency-see <u>Larmor frequency</u>.

Probe-the portion of an NMR spectrometer comprising the sample container and the RF coils, with some associated electronics. The RF coils may consist of separate receiver and transmitter coils in a crossed-coil configuration, or, alternatively, a single coil to perform both functions.

Program-see Software.

Progressive saturation-see Saturation recovery.

Projection profile-spectrum of NMR signal whose frequency components are broadened by a gradient magnetic field. In the simplest case (negligible line width, no relaxation effects, and no effects of prior gradients), it corresponds to a one-dimensional projection of the spin density along the direction of the gradient; in this form it is used in reconstruction from projections imaging.

PS-see Partial saturation.

Pulse, 90° ($\pi/2$ **pulse**)-RF pulse designed to rotate the macroscopic magnetization vector 90° in space as referred to the rotating frame of reference, usually about an axis at right angles to the main magnetic field. If the spins are initally aligned with the magnetic field, this pulse will produce transverse magnetization and an FID.

Pulse, 180° (π **pulse**)-RF pulse designed to rotate the macroscopic magnetization vector 180° in space as referred to the rotating frame of reference, usually about an axis at right angles to the main magnetic field. If the spins are initially aligned with the magnetic field, this pulse will produce inversion.

Pulse, RF-see RF pulse.

Pulse length (width)-time duration of a pulse. For an RF pulse near the Larmor frequency, the longer the pulse length, the greater the angle of rotation of the macroscopic magnetization vector will be (greater than 180° can bring it back toward its original orientation).

Pulse NMR-NMR techniques that use RF pulses and Fourier transformation of the NMR signal; have largely replaced the older continuous wave techniques.

Pulse programmer-part of the spectrometer or interface that controls the timing, duration, and amplitude of the pulses (RF or gradient).

Pulse sequences-set of RF (and/or gradient) magnetic field pulses and time spacings between these pulses; used in conjunction with gradient magnetic fiels and NMR signal reception to produce NMR images. See also Interpulse times.

Pulsed gradients-see Gradient pulse.

Q-see Quality factor.

Quadrature detector-a phase sensitive detector or demodulator that detects the components of the signal in phase with a reference oscillator and 90° out of phase with the reference oscillator.

Quality factor (Q)-applies to any electrical circuit component; most often the coil Q is limiting. Inversely related to the fraction of the energy in an oscillating system lost in one oscillation cycle. Q is inversely related to the range of frequency over which the system will exhibit resonance. It affects the signal-to-noise ratio, because the detected signal increased proportionally to Q while the noise is proportional to the square root of Q. The Q of a coil will depend on whether it is unloaded (no patient) or loaded (patient).

Quenching-loss of superconductivity of the current carrying coil that may occur unexpectedly in a superconducting magnet. As the magnet becomes resistive, heat will be released that can result in rapid evaporation of liquid helium in the cryostat. This may present a hazard if not properly planned for.

Radian-dimensionless unit of angular measure; $360° = 2$ radians.

Radiofrequency (RF)-wave frequency intermediate between auditory and infra red. The RF used in NMR studies is commonly in the megahertz (MHz) range. The principal effect of RF magnetic fields on the body is power deposition in the form of heating, mainly at the surface; this is a principal area of concern for safety limits.

Readout delay-see TE.

Receiver-portion of the NMR apparatus that detects and amplifies RF signals picked up by the receiving coil. Includes a preamplifer, amplifier, and demodulator.

Receiver coil-coil of the RF receiver; "picks up" the NMR signal.

Reconstruction from projections imaging-NMR imaging technique in which a set of projection profiles of the body is obtained by observing NMR signals in the presence of a suitable corresponding set of gradient magnetic fields. Images can then be reconstructed using techniques analogous to those used in conventional computed tomography (CT), such as filtered back projection. It can be used for volume imaging or, with plane selection techniques, for sequential plane imaging.

Refocusing-see Spin echo.

Relaxation rates-reciprocals of the relaxation times.

Relaxation times-after excitation, the spins will tend to return to their equilibrium distribution, in which there is no transverse magnetization and the longitudinal magnetization is at its maximum value and oriented in the direction of the static magnetic field. It is observed that in the absence of applied RF, the transverse magnetization decays toward zero with a characteristic time constant T2, and the longitudinal magnetization returns toward the equilibrium value M_o with a characteristic time constant T1.

Repeated FID-a form of NMR imaging in which repeated 90° pulses are applied. Results in partial saturation if interpulse times are of the order of or less than T1. Strictly speaking, applies only if NMR signal is detected as an FID.

Repetition time-see TR.

Rephasing gradient-gradient magnetic field applied for a brief period after a selective excitation pulse, in the opposite direction to the gradient used for the selective excitation. The result of the gradient reversal is a rephasing of the spins (which will have gotten out of phase with each other along the direction of the selection gradient), forming an echo by "time reversal," and improving the sensitivity of imaging after the selective excitation process.

Resistive magnet-a magnet whose magnetic field originates from current flowing through an ordinary (nonsuperconducting) conductor.

Resolution, spatial-although generally referring to the ability of the imaging process to distinguish adjacent structures in the object (an important measure of image quality), the specific criterion of resolution to be used depends on the type of test used (e.g. bar pattern or contrasting detail phantom). As the ability to separate or detect objects depends on their contrast, and the differen NMR parameters of objects will affect image contrast differently for different imaging techniques, care must be taken in comparing the results of resolution phantom tests of different machines and no single simple measure of resolution can be specified.

Resonance-a large amplitude vibration in a mechanical or electrical system caused by a relatively small periodic stimulus with a frequency at or close to a natural frequency of the system; in NMR apparatus, resonance can refer to the NMR itself or the tuning of the RF circuitry.

Resonant frequency-frequency at which resonance phenomenon occurs; given by the Larmor equation for NMR; determined by inductance and capacitance for RF circuits.

RF-see Radiofrequency.

RF coil-used for transmitting RF pulses and/or receiving NMR signals. Most commonly used in saddle coil or solenoid configurations for NMR imaging.

RF pulse-brief burst of RF magnetic field delivered to object by RF transmitter. For RF frequency near the Larmor frequency, it will result in rotation of the macroscopic magnetization vector in the rotating frame of reference (or a more complicated nutational motion in the stationary frame of reference). The amount of rotation will depend on the strength and duration of the RF pulse; commonly used examples are $90°$ ($\pi/2$) and $180°$ (π) pulses.

Rotating frame of reference-a frame of reference (with corresponding coordinate systems) that is rotating about the axis of the static magnetic field B_o (with respect to a stationary ("laboratory") frame of reference) at a frequency equal to that of the applied RF magnetic field, B_1. Although B_1 is a rotating vector, it appears stationary in the rotating frame, leading to simpler mathematical formulations.

Rotating frame zeugmatography-technique of NMR imaging that uses a gradient of the RF excitation field (to give a corresponding variation of the flip angle along the gradient as a means of encoding the spatial location of spins in the direction of the RF field gradient) in conjunction with a static gradient magnetic field (to give spatial encoding in an orthogonal direction). It can be considered to be a form of Fourier transform imaging.

Saddle coil-RF coil configuration design commonly used when the static magnetic field is coaxial with the axis of the coil along the long axis of the body (e.g. superconducting magnets and most resistive magnet) as opposed to solenoid or surface coil.

Saturation-a nonequilibrium state in NMR, in which equal numbers of spins are aligned against and with the magnetic field, so that there is no net magnetization. Can be produced by repeatedly supplying RF pulses at the Larmor frequency with interpulse times short compared to T1.

Saturation recovery (SR)-particular type of partial saturation pulse sequence in which the preceding pulses leave the spins in a state of saturation, so that recovery at the time of the next pulse has taken place form an initial condition of no magnetization.

Saturation transfer (or Inversion transfer)-nuclei can retain their magnetic orientation through a chemical reaction. Thus, if RF radiation is supplied to the spins at a frequency corresponding to the chemical shift of the nuclei in one chemical state so as to produce saturation or inversion, and chemical reactions transform the nuclei into another chemical state with a different chemical shift in a time short compared to the relaxation time, the NMR spectrum may show the effects of the saturation or inversion on the corresponding, unirradiated, line in the spectrum. This technique can be used to study reaction kinetics of suitable molecules.

SE-see Spin echo.

Selective excitation-controlling the frequency spectrum of an irradiating RF pulse (via tailoring) while imposing a gradient magnetic field on spins, such that only a desired region will have a suitable resonant frequency to be excited. Originally used to excite all but a desired region; now more commonly used to select only a desired region, such as a plane, for excitation.

Selective irradiation-see Selective excitation.

Sensitive plane-technique of selecting a plane for sequential plane imaging by using an oscillating gradient magnetic field and filtering out the corresponding time dependent part of the NMR signal. The gradient used is at right angles to the desire plane and the magnitude of the oscillating gradient magnetic field is equal to zero only in the desired plane.

Sensitive point-technique of selecting out a point for sequential point imaging by applying three orthogonal oscillating gradient magnetic fields such that the local magnetic field is time dependent everywhere except at the desired point, and then filtering out the corresponding time dependent portion of the NMR signal.

Sensitive volume-region of the object from which NMR signal will preferentially be acquired because of strong magnetic field inhomogeneity elsewhere. Effect can be enhanced by use of a shaped RF field that is strongest in the sensitive region.

Sequence time-see TR.

Sequential line imaging (Line scanning, Line imaging)-NMR imaging techniques in which the image is built up from successive lines through the object. In various schemes, the lines are isloated by oscillating gradient magnetic fields or selective excitation, and then the NMR signals from the selected line are encoded for position by detecting the FID or spin echo in the presence of a gradient magnetic field along the line; the Fourier transform of the detected signal then yields the distribution of emitted NMR signal along the line.

Sequential plane imaging (Plane imaging)-NMR imaging technique in which the image of an object is built up from successive planes in the object. In various schemes, the planes are selected by oscillating gradient magnetic fields or selective excitation.

Sequential point imaging (Point scanning)-NMR imaging techniques in which the image is built from successive point positions in the object. In various schemes, the points are isolated by oscillating gradient magnetic fields (sensitive point) or shaped magnetic fields.

SFP-see Steady state free precession.

Shim coils-coils carrying a relatively small current that are used to provide auxiliary magnetic fields in order to compensate for inhomogeneities in the main magnetic field of an NMR system.

Shimming-correction of inhomogeneity of the magnetic field produced by the main magnet of an NMR system due to imperfections in the magnet or to the presence of external ferromagnetic objects. May involve changing the configuration of the magnet or the addition of shim coils or small pieces of steel.

SI (International System of Units)-the preferred international standard system of physical units and measures.

Signal-to-noise ratio (SNR or S/N)-used to describe the relative contributions to a detected signal of the true signal and random superimposed signals ("noise"). One common method to improve (increase) the SNR is to average several measurements of the signal on the expectation that random contributions will tend to cancel out. The SNR can also be improved by sampling larger volumes (with a corresponding loss of spatial resolution) or, within limits, by increasing the strength of the magnetic field used. S/N will depend on the electrical properties of the sample or patient being studied.

Simultaneous volume imaging-see Volume imaging.

Skin depth-time dependent electromagnetic fields are significantly attenuated by conducting media (including the human body); the skin depth gives a measure of the average depth of penetration of the RF field. It may be a limiting factor in NMR imaging at very high frequencies (high magnetic fields). The skin depth also affects the Q of the coils.

S/N-see Signal-to-noise ratio.

SNR-see Signal-to-noise ratio.

Software-the set of instructions, or programs, that controls the activities of the computer. Programs may be written in machine language (sequences of numbers directly interpretable by the computer), assembly language, or higher level languages such as Fortran of Basic. The software includes overall supervising "executive" programs, data acquisition programs, data processing programs (including image reconstruction), and display programs.

Solenoid coil-a coil of wire wound in the form of a long cylinder.

When a current is passed through the coil, the magnetic field within the coil is relatively uniform. Solenoid RF coils are commonly used when the static magnetic field is perpendicular to the long axis of the body.

Spectrometer-the portions of the NMR apparatus that actually produce the NMR phenomenon and acquire the signals, including the magnet, the probe, the RF circuitry, etc. The spectrometer is controlled by the computer via the interface under the direction of the software.

Spectrum-an array of the frequency components of the NMR signal according to frequency. Nuclei with different resonant frequencies will show up as peaks at different corresponding frequencies in the spectrum, or "lines."

Spin-the intrinsic angular momentum of an elementary particle, or system of particles such as a nucleus, that is also responsible for the magnetic moment; or, a particle or nucleus possessing such a spin. The spins of nuclei have characteristic fixed values. Pairs of neutrons and protons align to cancel out their spins, so that nuclei with an odd number of neutrons and/or protons will have a net nonzero rotational component characterized by an integer of half integer quantum "nuclear spin number" (I).

Spin density (N)-the density of resonating spins in a given region; one of the principal determinants of the strength of the MNR signal from the region. The SI units would be moles/m^3. For water, there are about 1.1×10^5 moles of hydrogen per m^3, or .11 moles of hydrogen/cm^3. True spin density is not imaged directly, but must be calculated from signals received with different interpulse times.

Spin echo-reappearance of an NMR signal after the FID has died away, as a result of the effective reversal of the dephasing of the spins ("refocusing") by such techniques as reversal of a gradient magnetic field (often referred to as a form of "time reversal"), or by specific RF pulse sequences such as the Carr-Purcell sequence (applied in a time shorter than or on the order of T2). Multiple spin echoes or a series of spin echoes at different times can be used to determine T2 without contamination by effects of the inhomogeneity of the magnetic field.

Spin-echo imaging-any of many NMR imaging techniques in which the spin echo NMR signal rather than the FID is used. Can be used to create images that depend strongly on T2. Note that spin echoes do not directly produce an image of T2.

Spin-lattice relaxation time-see T1.

Spin number, nuclear-see Nuclear spin number.

Spin-Spin relaxation time-see T2.

Spin tagging-nuclei will retain their magnetic orientation for a time on the order of T1 even in the presence of motion. Thus, if the nuclei in a given region have their spin orientation changed, the altered spins will serve as a "tag" to trace the motion of any fluid that may have been in the tagged region for a time on the order of T1.

Spin warp imaging-a form of Fourier transform imaging in which phase encoding gradient pulses are applied for a constant duration but with varying amplitude. This is distinct from the original FT imaging methods in which phase encoding is performed by applying gradient pulses of constant amplitude but varying duration. The spin warp method, as other Fourier imaging techniques, is relatively tolerant of nonuniformities (inhomogeneities) in the static or gradient magnetic fields.

SR-see Saturation recovery.

SSFP-see Steady state free precession.

Steady state free precesion (SFP or SSFP)-method of NMR excitation in which strings of RF pulses are applied rapidly and repeatedly with interpulse intervals short compared to both T1 and T2. Alternating the phases of the RF pulses by $180°$ can be useful in obtaining maximal signal strength.

Superconducting magnet-a magnet whose magnetic field originates from current flowing through a superconductor. Such a magnet must be enclosed in a cryostat.

Superconductor-a substance whose electrical resistance essentially disappears at temperatures near absolute zero. A commonly used superconductor in NMR imaging system magnets in niobium-titanium, embedded in a copper matrix to help protect the superconductor from quenching.

Surface coil NMR-a simple flat RF receiver coil placed over a region of interest will have an effective selectivity for a volume approximately subtended by the coil circumference and one radius deep from the coil center. Such a coil can be used for simple localization of sites for measurement of chemical shift spectra, especially of phosphorus, and blood flow studies. Some additional spatial selectivity can be achieved with gradient magnetic fields.

Susceptibility-see Magnetic susceptibility.

T-see Tesla.

T1 ("T-one")-spin-lattice or longitudinal relaxation time; the characteristic time constant for spins to tend to align themselves with the external magnetic field. Starting from zero magnetization in the z direction, the x magnetization will grow 63% of its final maximum value in a time T1.

T2 ("T-two")-spin-spin or transverse relaxation time; the characteristic time constant for loss of phase coherence among spins oriented at an angle to the static magnetic field, due to interactions between the spins, with resulting loss of transverse magnetization and NMR signal. Starting from a non zero value of the magnetization in the xy plane, the xy magnetization will decay so that it loses 63% of its initial value in a time T2.

T2* ("T-two-star")-the characteristic time constant for loss of phase coherence among spins oriented at an angle to the static magnetic field due to a combination of magnetic field inhomogeneities, B, and spin-spin transverse relaxation with resultant more rapid loss in transverse magnetization and NMR signal. NMR signal can still be recovered as a spin echo in times less than or on theorder of T2. $1/T2^* = 1/T2 + \Delta\omega/2; \Delta\omega = \gamma \Delta B$.

Tailored excitation-see Selective excitation.

Tailored pulse-shaped pulse whose magnitude is varied with time in predetermined manner. Affects the frequency componenets of an RF pulse in a manner determined by the Fourier transform of the pulse.

TE-echo time. Time between middle of $90°$ pulse and middle of spin echo production. For multiple echoes, use TE1, TE2....

Tesla (T)-the preferred (SI) unit of magnetic flux density. One tesla is equal to 10,000 gauss, the older (CGS) unit.

Thermal equilibrium-a state in which all parts of a system are at the same effective temperature, in particular where the relative alignment of the spins with the magnetic field is determined solely by the thermal energy of the system (in which case the relative numbers of spins with different alignments will be given by the Boltzmann distribution).

TI-inversion time. Time after middle of inverting RF pulse to middle of $90°$ pulse to detect amount of longitudinal magnetization.

Time reversal-technique of producing a spin echo by subjecting excited spins to a gradient magnetic field, and then reversing the direction of the gradient field. All methods of spin echo production can be viewed as effective time reversal.

Torque-the effectiveness of a force in setting a body into rotation. It is a vector quantity given by the vector product of the force and the position vector where the force is applied; for a rotating body, the torque is the product of the moment of inertia and the resulting angular acceleration.

TR-repetition time. The period of time between the beginning of a pulse sequence and the beginning of the succeeding (essentially identical) pulse sequence.

Transmitter—portion of the NMR apparatus that produces RF current and delivers it to the transmitting coil.

Transmitter coil—coil of the RF transmitter.

Transverse magnetization (M_{xy})—component of the macroscopic magnetization vector at right angles to the static magnetic field (B_o). Precession of the transverse magnetization at the Larmor frequency is responsible for the detectable NMR signal. In the absence of externally applied RF energy, the transverse magnetization will decay to zero with a characteristic time constant of T2 or T2*.

Transverse relaxation time—see T2.

Two-dimensional Fourier transform imaging (2DFT)—a form of sequential plane imaging using Fourier transform imaging.

Tuning—process of adjusting the resonant frequency, e.g., of the RF circuit, to a desired value, e.g., the Larmor frequency. More generally, the process of adjusting the components of the spectrometer for optimal NMR signal strength.

Tunnel—opening into NMR imaging machine to place patient into imaging region.

Vector—a quantity having both magnitude and direction, frequently represented by an arrow whose length is proportional to the magnitude and with an arrowhead at one end to indicate the direction.

Volume imaging—imaging techniques in which NMR signals are gathered from the whole object volume to be imaged at once, with appropriate encoding pulse/gradient sequences to encode positions of the spins. Many sequential plane imaging techniques can be generalized to volume imaging, at least in principle. Advantages include potential improvement in signal-to-noise ratio by including signal from the whole volume at once; disadvantages include a bigger computational task for image reconstruction and longer image acquisition times (although the entire volume can be imaged from the one set of data). Also called simultaneous volume imaging.

Voxel—volume element; the element of 3-D space corresponding to a pixel, for a given slice thickness.

x—dimension in the stationary (laboratory) frame of reference in the plane orthogonal (at right angles) to the direction of the static magnetic field (B_o), z, and orthogonal to y, the other dimension in this plane.

x^1-dimension in the rotating frame of reference in the plane at right angles to the direction of the static magnetic field (B_o), z; defined to be in the direction of the magnetic vector of the RF field (B_1).

y-dimension in the stationary (laboratory) frame of reference in the plane orthogonal to the direction of the static magnetic field (B_o and H_o), z, and orthogonal to x, the other dimension in this plane.

y^1-dimension in the rotating frame of reference in the plane orthogonal (at right angles) to the direction of the static magnetic field (B_o and H_o), z, and orthogonal to the other dimension in this plane, x^1.

z-dimension in the direction of the static magnetic field (B_o and H_o), in both the stationary and rotating frames of reference.

Zeugmatography-term for NMR imaging coined from Greek roots suggesting the role of the gradient magnetic field in joining the RF magnetic field to a desired local spatial region through nuclear magnetic resonance.

2DFT-see Two-dimensional Fourier transform.

γ-see Gyromagnetic ratio.

δ -see Chemical shift.

μ -see Permeability.

ς -often used to denote different time delays between RF pulses. See Interpulse times.

χ-see Magnetic susceptibility.

ω-see Angular frequency.

ω_0-see Larmor frequency.

INDEX

A

Abdomen, imaging of, 300, 350
Acceptance testing, 414, 437, 449, 451–457
Adiabatic fast passage (AFP), 566
Adrenal gland, imaging of, 357
Analog to digital converter (ADC), 166, 183–185, 191, 566
Angular momentum, 3, 566
Artifacts, 75, 150, 167, 287, 332, 347, 456, 566
ATP (Adenosine Tri Phosphate), 249

B

Bandwidth, 144, 145, 217, 218
Biological effects, 493–523
Biological tissues, relaxation times in, 20, 57, 67
Biot-Savart Law, 114, 133, 552
B/I ratio, 563
Bladder, imaging of, 360
Bloch equations, 14 16, 201, 567
Blood flow, 326–338, 343, 351
Boltzmann distribution, 13, 567
Bone, imaging of, 374
Bowel, imaging of, 296, 361
Brain, imaging of, 229, 232–240
Breast, imaging of, 367–371, 377

C

Carbon-13, 250, 256, 295
Cardiac gating, 333, 340
Cardiac, imaging of, 339–349
Carr-Purcell (CP) sequence, 23, 65, 567
Carr-Purcell-Meiboom-Gill (CPMG) sequence, 23, 65, 567
Chemical shift
    definition of, 251, 567
    imaging, 253, 281–288
    methods of, 282–286
Chest, imaging of, 364–367
Computed Tomography (CT), 25
Computer interface, 197–198
Computer requirements/architecture, 188–189, 199, 200
Contrast, tissue, 68, 416, 440, 442, 568
    agents, 289–325, 295, 416
Contrast-to-noise, 220–226
Crossed ellipse coil, 157
Cross-relaxation, magnetic, 209, 210
Cryostat, 105–107, 568

D

Demodulator, 569
Deuteration, 210
Diamagnetic, 292, 561, 569
Diffusion, 66, 208–209, 569
Digital to analog converter (DAC), 569
Direct memory access (DMA), 185

E

Echo planar imaging, 79, 285, 569
Economic factors, 289, 403, 447, 476–492
Eddy currents, 569
Eigen states, 201–203
Equilibrium magnetization, 74, 81
Exchange model, relaxation times, 57, 210

F

Faraday shield, 149, 406, 570
Fast Fourier transform (FFT), 570
Ferromagnetic, 292, 396, 415, 561
Fetus, imaging of, 376, 378
Field gradients, 24, 113–115, 570
Field lock, 252, 570
Filling factor, 146–149, 217, 570
Filtered back projection, 25, 570
Filtering, low pass, 156, 168, 174
Flip angle, 150, 163, 443, 570
Flow, imaging of, 326–338
Fluorine-19, 269–276
    nuclear sensitivity and properties of, 269
    imaging with, 272–275, 287, 295

Fluorodeoxyglucose (FDG), 270–272
Fourier transform (FT), 12, 73, 75, 570
Free induction decay (FID), 17, 62, 143, 571
Free radicals, 298
Fringe field, 89–91, 393, 396

G

Gallbladder, imaging of, 352
Gating, cardiac, 333, 340
Gd-DTPA, 306, 309, 416
Golay coil, 121, 571
Gradient coils, 111–141, 134, 571
    axial, 115–118
    transverse, 118–124
Gradient pulse, 123, 124, 139, 327, 572
Gyromagnetic ratio (γ), 2, 251, 572

H

Hamiltonian, 4, 33, 113, 201–202
    dipolar, 206
Head, imaging of, 229, 232
Helmholtz coil, 572
Homogeneity,
    static field, 112–113, 437, 572
    RF field, 148, 150–157

I

Image acquisition time, 220, 572
Image methods,
    choice of, 232
    classification and description of, 71–80
    comparison of, 112
    contrast to noise considerations in, 220–226, 440–441
    echo-planar methods in, 79, 285
    for fluid flow, 326–338
    general principles of, 24–25, 71
    image distortion in 124–127, 433–437
    multiplanar two dimensional methods in, 78–79
    power absorption in, 525
    projection reconstruction methods in, 74–75, 122, 125
    resolution in, 419–420
    sensitive line methods in, 73
    sensitive point methods in, 72, 282
    signal to noise considerations in, 192, 217–228, 439–440
    slice selection in, 30, 73–74
    three dimensional scanning method in, 77–78
    two dimensional Fourier transform (2DFT) methods in, 75–77, 78–79, 127, 132, 218, 588
Imaging time, effects of relaxation times, 68–69
Impedance matching, 159–161
Inductance, 148–149, 557, 572
Inversion recovery, 20, 26, 224, 573

K

Kidney imaging of, 290, 302, 351, 356

L

Larmor frequency (ω_0) definition of, 3–4, 251, 574
Liver, imaging of, 352, 353, 380
Lorentzian line, 54, 574
Losses,
    coil, 146, 149–151
    dielectric, 146–147
    magnetic, 146
    patient, 146–147
Lymph nodes, imaging of, 358

M

Macroscopic magnetization vector (M), 3, 561, 575
Magnetic dipole, 5, 40, 145, 396, 553, 575
Magnetic field, 396, 575
    biologic effects of, 395, 493–509
    effect on equipment, 91, 399–401
    radio frequency B_1, 142, 145–157, 162
Magnetic induction (**B**), 549–557, 561, 575

Magnetic susceptibility, 561, 575
Magnetization (see Macroscopic magnetization vector)
Main magnet, 85–110, 391–398, 446–477
    access, 88–89
    manufacture of, 100–109
    safety precautions for, 394
    static homogeneity of, 87, 91–99, 252, 394
    temporal stability of, 88
Maxwell coil, 117, 133, 576
Maxwell pair gradient coil spacing, 118
Maxwell's equations for electromagnetic field, 549
Multiple line-scan imaging (MLSI), 576
Multiple plane imaging, 181, 576
Multiple sensitive point, 576

N

Nitroxide spin labels, 298
Noise, 72, 80, 145, 159–160
Nuclear magnetic resonance (see also Imaging methods), 577
    biomagnetic effects of, 395, 493–528
    field gradient coils in, 111–141
    main magnet in, 85–110
    oscillator for, 166–167
    pulse controller in, 187
    radio-frequency coil design for, 142–163
    radio-frequency field-biomagnetic effects in, 395
    receiver system for, 173–179
    time-dependent field-biomagnetic effects in, 395, 518–522
Nuclear spin quantum number, 32–36, 113, 577
Nutation, 9, 10, 577

P

Pacemakers, effect of magnetic field on, 91, 342, 395, 524
Pancreas, imaging of, 296, 355
Paramagnetic elements, 415, 561, 577
    contrast agents, 291
    effect on relaxation, 15, 211, 293, 417

Partial saturation (PS), 81, 577
Pelvis, imaging of, 358
Perfluorocarbon compounds (PFCs), 272–275
Permanent magnet, 108, 578
Permeability, 396, 403, 550, 561, 578
Phantoms, 414–444, 457
Phase, 75, 330, 578
Phase encoding, 76
Phase sensitive detector, 20, 177
Phosphocreatine, 256
Phosphorus-31, 249–250
    imaging of, 253, 287
Pixel, 25, 218, 419, 578
Power absorption, in NMR imaging, 395, 510–516
Power considerations, for main magnet, 107–108, 389
Precession, 4, 142, 145, 578
Pre-market approval, 448
Projection profile, 24, 122, 579
Prostate, imaging of, 358
Pulse programmer, 187, 579
Pulse sequences, 59–70, 132, 193, 220–224, 579
    definitions, 25–30
    effect on clinical image, 232, 350
Purchase contracts, writing of, 450, 457
Purchasing specifications, 445, 461

Q

Quadrature detection, 580
    reception/excitation, 149–150, 157
Quality assurance, 414, 443
    image quality, 453
Quality factor (Q), 143, 144, 147, 559–560, 580
Quenching, 104–105, 580

R

Radio-frequency amplifier, 160–161
Radio-frequency coil, design, 147–158, 253
Radio-frequency modulation,
    amplitude, 169
    phase, 168–170

Radio-frequency penetration, 150
Radio-frequency shielding, 405–406
Receiver, 158, 580
Receiver coil, 142–143, 560, 580
    spectrometer interface, 159–161
Reciprocity, principle of, 145
Refocusing, 331
Relaxation times, 442, 581
    exchange model in, 210
    in normal and malignant human tissue, 68
    paramagnetic impurity effect on, 211, 415–417
    spin-lattice relaxation, 14, 51, 60, 205–206, 208, 210
    value for water of, 56
        frequency dependence of, 55, 208, 211–213, 224–226
        in the rotating frame $T_{1\rho}$, 61
    spin-spin, 16, 49, 61, 206, 208, 209
Repeated FID, 26, 581
Rephasing gradient, 30, 581
Resistive magnet, 107–108, 391, 581
    coil design, 92–99
Resolution, spatial, 77, 80, 87, 112, 182, 193, 419, 581
Resonance, 8, 143, 559, 581
Resonators,
    bird cage, 156–157
    slotted tube, 154–155
Rotating frame of reference, 7, 8, 582
Rotating frame chemical shift imaging, 283

S

Saddle coil, 121, 582
Safety, 394, 523–526
    precautions, 89–91, 395
    recommendations, 395
Sample volume, 145–149
Sampling process, 182–183, 196
Saturation, 582
Saturation recovery (SR), 62–63, 81, 582
Selective excitation, 30, 73, 285, 328, 583
Selective pulses, 79
Sensitive plane, 72, 122, 583
Sensitive point, 282, 583
Sensitive volume, 583

Shielding
    RF, 149, 254, 405–406
    magnetic, 402–405
Shim coils, 97–99, 389, 584
Shimming, 112, 252 584
SI (International System of Units), 549, 584
Signal averaging, 218
Signal-to-noise ratio (SNR or S/N), 12, 72, 80, 143, 144–147, 150, 160, 162–163, 218–221, 439, 584
Sinc function, 74, 84
Site planning, 387–413
Skin depth, 12, 584
Slice geometry, 425–432
Solenoid coil, 148, 151–152, 556, 584
Spatial resolution, (see Resolution, spatial)
Specifications, system, 389
Spectrometer, 166–179, 252, 585
Spectroscopy, 250
Spectrum, 585
Spin, 2, 32, 250
Spin density (N), 223, 585
Spin echo, 21–24, 220–222, 585
Spin-echo imaging, 27–29, 220–222, 350, 585
Spin labels, 298
Spin-lattice relaxation time (see T_1)
Spin-spin relaxation time (see T_2)
Spin warp imaging, 75, 84, 586
Spine, imaging of, 229, 240–245, 381–385
Steady state free precession (SFP or SSFP), 63, 586
Stray capacitance (electric field), 146, 148–149
Superconducting magnet, 100–107, 390, 586
Superconductor, 102–103, 586
Surface coil, 161–163, 254, 282, 586

T

T_1 ("T-one"), 14, 20, 51, 60, 81, 203, 205–208, 210, 213, 293, 442, 586
T_2 ("T-two"), 16, 49, 54, 61, 82, 203, 205–209, 293, 442, 587
T_{2^*} ("T-two-star"), 19, 61, 587
Tailored pulses, 30, 587

TE, definition of, 28, 64, 221, 587
Thermal equilibrium, 45, 587
Thermal imaging, 273
TI, definition of, 26, 62, 221, 587
Tissue contrast, 220–227
Torque, 2, 553, 554, 587
TR, definition of, 26, 62, 221, 587
Transition probabilities, 205
Transmitter, 158, 167–173, 588
    isolation of, 171–172
Transmitter coils, 142–143, 588
    design of, 150
Transverse field gradients, 96–97
Transverse magnetization, 150, 202, 203, 205, 208, 588
Tumor discrimination,
    relaxation times and, 68

Tuning, 158–162, 588
Two-dimensional Fourier transform
    imaging (2DFT), 127, 132, 218, 588

U

Uterus, imaging of, 359

V

Voxel, 147, 162, 217, 588

Z

Zeugmatography, 181, 589

SUFFOLK UNIVERSITY
MILDRED F. SAWYER LIBRARY
8 ASHBURTON PLACE
BOSTON, MA 02108